COUNSELING PEOPLE OF AFRICAN ANCESTRY

This volume advances a uniquely Africentric, sociocultural understanding of health maintenance and risk reduction in African cultural heritage populations. It unites a diverse group of leading African and Africanist scholars in an exploration of common cultural values in African heritage communities and their practical applications in contemporary counseling. The chapters highlight the prominent health issues faced in Africanist settings today and use real-world experiences to illustrate core lessons for effective community action. The approach spans complex cultural milieus, from diversity counseling to conflict resolution. Each chapter includes field-based experiential exercises, discussion boxes, research boxes, and case studies, which serve as valuable resources in both coursework and casework. *Counseling People of African Ancestry* is an essential primer for community health workers, counselors, researchers, and educators seeking a better understanding of African cultural heritage settings to promote health, well-being, and development.

Elias Mpofu is professor and head of discipline of rehabilitation counseling at the University of Sydney, Australia. Formerly a professor of rehabilitation services at the Pennsylvania State University, he has also held professorial appointments at the University of Botswana and the University of Zimbabwe. He was awarded three national research awards, in rehabilitation in 2007, by the American Rehabilitation Counseling Association (ARCA), U.S. National Council on Rehabilitation Education (NCRE), and U.S. National Institute on Disability and Rehabilitation Research (NIDRR). Also, his research and education expertise recognitions include an awarded honorary doctoral degree in education by the University of Pretoria, South Africa (2010), and the rehabilitation educator of the year award by the U.S. NCRE (2010). He is also on several awarded research grants by the U.S. National Institutes of Health investigating the interface of faith and health in several African communities. Mpofu has more than twenty years of research and health education experience in sub-Saharan Africa and has published more than eighty research articles in peer-refereed journals, fifty book chapters, and eight books in the last sixteen years. He is the lead co-editor of *Rehabilitation and Health Assessment: Applying ICF Guidelines* (2010) and *Assessment in Rehabilitation and Health* (2010).

COUNSELING PEOPLE OF AFRICAN ANCESTRY

Edited by

Elias Mpofu
University of Sydney

CAMBRIDGE
UNIVERSITY PRESS

CAMBRIDGE
UNIVERSITY PRESS

Shaftesbury Road, Cambridge CB2 8EA, United Kingdom

One Liberty Plaza, 20th Floor, New York, NY 10006, USA

477 Williamstown Road, Port Melbourne, NY 3207, Australia

314–321, 3rd Floor, Plot 3, Splendor Forum, Jasola District Centre, New Delhi – 110025, India

103 Penang Road, #05–06/07, Visioncrest Commercial, Singapore 238467

Cambridge University Press is part of Cambridge University Press & Assessment, a department of the University of Cambridge.

We share the University's mission to contribute to society through the pursuit of education, learning and research at the highest international levels of excellence.

www.cambridge.org
Information on this title: www.cambridge.org/9780521887229

First published 2011

A catalogue record for this publication is available from the British Library

Library of Congress Cataloging-in-Publication data
Counseling people of African ancestry / [edited by] Elias Mpofu.
p. ; cm.
Includes bibliographical references and index.
ISBN 978-0-521-88722-9 (hardback : alk. paper)
1. Psychiatry, Transcultural. 2. Cross-cultural counseling. 3. Africans – Psychology.
I. Mpofu, Elias. II. Title.
[DNLM: 1. African Continental Ancestry Group – psychology. 2. Counseling – methods.
3. Cultural Competency. 4. Health Promotion – methods. 5. Medicine, African Traditional – psychology. WA 300.1]
RC455.4.E8C68 2011
616.89008996073–dc22 2011001812

ISBN 978-0-521-88722-9 Hardback

This book is dedicated to all people contributing to the health and well-being of African heritage communities around the globe.

Contents

Contributors . . . . . . *page* ix
About the Editor xi
Editorial Board xii
Foreword xiii
Fred J. van Staden
Preface xv
Elias Mpofu
Acknowledgments xix

PART 1. FOUNDATIONS OF COUNSELING IN AFRICAN SETTINGS
Section Editor – Lisa Lopez Levers

1. **Indigenous Healing Practices in Sub-Saharan Africa 3**
Elias Mpofu, Karl Peltzer, and Olaniyi Bojuwoye

2. **The Role of the Oral Tradition in Counseling People of African Ancestry 22**
Jacobus G. Maree and Cecilia M. du Toit

3. **Assessment for Counseling Intervention 41**
Lynne Radomsky, Sofoh Hassane, Michelle Hoy-Watkins, and Chiwoza Bandawe

4. **Research on Counseling in African Settings 57**
Lisa Lopez Levers, Michelle May, and Gwen Vogel

5. **Deconstructing Counseling Psychology for the African Context 75**
Anbanithi Muthukrishna and David Lackland Sam

6. **Racial Oppression, Colonization, and Identity: Toward an Empowerment Model for People of African Heritage 93**
Alex L. Pieterse, Dennis Howitt, and Anthony V. Naidoo

PART 2. CONTEXTS OF COUNSELING
Section Editor – Terri Bakker

7. **School Counseling 111**
Elias Mpofu, Jacobus G. Maree, Joseph M. Kasayira, and Carol Noela Van der Westhuizen

8. **Counseling Students at Tertiary Institutions 126**
Ilse Ruane, Joseph M. Kasayira, and Elizabeth N. Shino

9. **Family Therapy within the African Context** 142
Vinitha Jithoo and Terri Bakker

10. **Pastoral Care and Counseling** 155
Daniël Johannes Louw

11. **African Refugees: Challenges and Prospects of Resettlement Programs** 166
Clemente Abrokwaa, Mary Shilalukey Ngoma, Edward Shizha, and Elias Mpofu

12. **Counseling Orphans and Vulnerable Children in Africa** 180
Gertie Pretorius, Brandon Morgan, Magen Mhaka-Mutepfa, Mary Shilalukey Ngoma, and Thokozile Mayekiso

13. **Diversity Counseling with African Americans** 193
Debra A. Harley and Kim L. Stansbury

14. **Resolving Conflict in Africa: In Search of Sustainable Peace** 209
Joleen Steyn-Kotze and Gerrie Swart

PART 3. COUNSELING APPLICATIONS
Section Editor – Elias Mpofu

15. **Counseling for Trauma** 229
David J. A. Edwards and Linda Eskell Blokland

16. **HIV and AIDS Counseling** 249
Lisa Lopez Levers, Elias Mpofu, Ronél Ferreira, and Joseph M. Kasayira

17. **Substance Use Disorder Counseling** 265
Monika M. L. dos Santos, Solomon T. Rataemane, Elias Mpofu, and Andreas Plüddemann

18. **Career Counseling People of African Ancestry** 281
Mark Watson, Mary McMahon, Nhlanhla Mkhize, Robert D. Schweitzer, and Elias Mpofu

19. **Counseling People with Disabilities** 294
Elias Mpofu, Grace Ukasoanya, Anniah Mupawose, Debra A. Harley, John Charema, and Kayi Ntinda

PART 4. THE FUTURE OF COUNSELING IN AFRICAN HERITAGE SETTINGS

20. **Counseling in African Cultural Heritage Settings: The Challenges and Opportunities** 313
Elias Mpofu, Terri Bakker, and Lisa Lopez Levers

Counseling People of African Ancestry Multiple Choice Answers 317
Index 319

Contributors

Clemente Abrokwaa, PhD
The Pennsylvania State University, USA

Terri Bakker, PhD
University of Pretoria, South Africa

Chiwoza Bandawe, PhD
University of Cape Town, South Africa

Linda Eskell Blokland, PhD
University of Pretoria, South Africa

Olaniyi Bojuwoye, PhD
University of the Western Cape, South Africa

Monika M. L. dos Santos, PhD
Vista Clinic and University of South Africa

Cecilia M. du Toit, PhD
University of Pretoria, South Africa

David J. A. Edwards, PhD
Rhodes University, South Africa

Ronél Ferreira, PhD
University of Pretoria, South Africa

Debra A. Harley, PhD
University of Kentucky, USA

Sofoh Hassane, PhD
United Arab Emirates University, UAE

Dennis Howitt, PhD
Loughborough University, UK

Vinitha Jithoo, PhD
University of Witswatesrand, South Africa

Joseph M. Kasayira, MSc
University of Malawi, Malawi

Lisa Lopez Levers, PhD
Duquesne University, USA

Daniël Johannes Louw, PhD
University of Stellenbosch, South Africa

Jacobus G. Maree, PhD, D.Ed, D.Phil
University of Pretoria, South Africa

Michelle May, PhD
University of South Africa, South Africa

Thokozile Mayekiso, PhD
Nelson Mandela Metropolitan University, South Africa

Mary McMahon, PhD
University of Queensland, Australia

Magen Mhaka-Mutepfa, M.Ed
University of Zimbabwe, Zimbabwe

Nhlanhla Mkhize, PhD
University of Kwazulu Natal, South Africa

Brandon Morgan, MA
University of Johannesburg, South Africa

Elias Mpofu, PhD, D.Ed
The University of Sydney, Australia

Anniah Mupawose, MA
University of Witswatersrand, South Africa

Anbanithi Muthukrishna, PhD
University of Kwazulu Natal, South Africa

Anthony V. Naidoo, PhD
University of Stellenbosch, South Africa

Mary Shilalukey Ngoma, MD
University of Zambia, Zambia

Kayi Ntinda, MSW
University of Botswana, Botswana

Karl Peltzer, PhD
Human Sciences Research Council, South Africa

Alex L. Pieterse, PhD
University of Albany, USA

Andreas Plüddemann, PhD
Medical Research Council of South Africa, South Africa

Gertie Pretorius, PhD
University of Johannesburg, South Africa

Lynne Radomsky, PhD
University of the Western Cape, South Africa

Solomon T. Rataemane, MD
University of the Lmpopopo, South Africa

Ilse Ruane, PhD
University of Pretoria, South Africa

David Lackland Sam, PhD
University of Bergen, Norway

Robert D. Schweitzer, PhD
Queensland University of Technology, Australia

Elizabeth N. Shino, PhD
University of Namibia, Namibia

Edward Shizha, PhD
Wilfrid Laurier University, Canada

Kim L. Stansbury, PhD
Eastern Washington University, USA

Joleen Steyn-Kotze, PhD
Nelson Mandela Metropolitan University, South Africa

Gerrie Swart, PhD
University of Stellenbosch, South Africa

Grace Ukasoanya, PhD
University of Manitoba, Canada

Carol Noela Van der Westhuizen, PhD
University of Pretoria, South Africa

Gwen Vogel, PhD
University of Denver, USA

Mark Watson, PhD
Nelson Mandela Metropolitan University, South Africa

Michelle Hoy-Watkins, PhD
University of Chicago, USA

About the Editor

Elias Mpofu, PhD, D.Ed, CRC is professor and head of discipline of rehabilitation counseling at the University of Sydney, Australia. A native of Zimbabwe, Professor Mpofu has achieved professorial appointments at seven universities across the globe in the past decade, including The Pennsylvania State University, University of Botswana, and the University of Zimbabwe. He is the Editor of the *Journal of Psychology in Africa* and the *Australian Journal of Rehabilitation Counselling*. Professor Mpofu has more than twenty years of research and education experience in sub-Saharan Africa. Professor Mpofu has published more than eighty research articles in peer-refereed journals, thirty book chapters, and six books in the last sixteen years. Professor Mpofu has chaired several plenary sessions and invited symposium on international health at conferences of the International Congress of Psychology. He is the international representative of the National Council on Rehabilitation Education (NCRE: USA) and Secretary of the Australian Society of Rehabilitation Counsellors (ASORC). Professor Mpofu's primary teaching assignment at The University of Sydney is counseling theories and techniques.

Editorial Board

Foreword

Africa is embracing itself.

This volume of multifaceted counseling approaches, problems, contexts, and practices is saying just that – Africa is embracing itself.

Proudly and eloquently, it presents the case of existing practices of nurturance and support grounded in belief systems founded among people of African ancestry. Also, it shows the affinity that exists among these practices, whether indigenous or exogenous in origin.

By pulling the complex strands of the twenty contributions from all over Africa and elsewhere into a coherent unified framework, the editor, Professor Elias Mpofu, has reconfirmed his stature as an eminent African scholar in the fullest sense of the word, one with foresight, energy, tenacity, and a passion for his profession. With his vision of compiling a volume on present counseling practices for people of African ancestry, he afforded us the opportunity to look inward, to discover that there really is a "best practice" for counseling conditions, specifically for people of African ancestry. With this work, he and the other contributors laid the foundations for Africans, wherever we may find ourselves in the world, to look at each other, across borders and nations, and to discover that we have much in common, sharing counseling challenges and practices.

The rich mosaic of Africanist voices contained in this publication aimed at the subject specialist yield connectivities, inform each other, and help us to understand how the human condition, in its multicultural African expressions, can be strengthened. Most tellingly, they also speak with a common voice, attesting to the existence of a holistic, systemic indigenous counseling psychology in African contexts – a psychology that promotes optimal functioning through acknowledging diversity along with communality, a psychology that pays homage to African spirituality and recognizes African historical, cultural, and sociopolitical dimensions of being.

My reading of the text evoked the following thought:

There is a certain
Being-of-Africa-in-the-world.
It contains the earliest
of all human presences
of survival,
of transformation.

It is in Africa where our human eyes were opened,
Forging the first glimmers
of greater understanding,
of greater awareness
of our being-human-in-the-world.

It is this most ancient legacy of all,
that continues guiding Africa
to embrace itself,
to heal itself
to celebrate its well being.

Finally, in the words of the Zulu people from South Africa, the restorative nature of our counseling practices continues to take us by the hand, guiding us to the following state of being:

> *Nathi sesidabuka nge njabulo*
> (We also originate with joy)
> *Sithi abese kunjalo kakhulu, khehla*
> (We say, Lo! It is well so, Old One)
> *Kakhulu kakhulo!*
> (Very well so!)

Congratulations to the forty-eight authors who contributed to this text. It embodies a major step forward in our arsenal of systematic knowledge on counseling customs and challenges among people of African ancestry. It marks a significant shift in, and focus on, interrogating, engaging, and strengthening our approaches to health promotion.

It is my hope that this volume will lead to a succession of publications over years to come. The unfolding of our knowledge of continued and changing challenges, in counseling people of African ancestry, should be never-ending.

Fred J. van Staden, Ph.D.
Department of Psychology,
University of South Africa
August 2009

Preface

The book addresses critical information needs for counselors working with Africans, people of African ancestry, or with an African cultural heritage. People of "African ancestry" are individuals whose cultural heritage is rooted in Africa. By implication, an African ancestry identity goes beyond race, skin color, or geographic location to include anyone who proclaims an African selfhood. In this book, the term "counseling people of African ancestry" refers to a way of working with people whose identities are embedded in an African cultural heritage. Having grown up in an African village, and lived in the United States and several other countries, I have observed significant, broad similarities in my cultural assumptions with those of African Americans and other people with an African cultural heritage across the globe. It appeared to me there was some continuity in the underlying cultural values in people of an African cultural heritage that sustained across time and contexts, and that needed to be addressed in the context of help seeking and giving to people of that cultural heritage. This book was written, in part, in response to that perceived need.

Contributors to the book are leading African and Africanist scholars from the African continent, Australia, the European Union, Middle East, and North America and provide the rich perspectives on help seeking, giving, and health from their diverse African cultural heritages. Members of the book's editorial board are renowned Africanist scholars and contributed invaluable insights that shaped the scope of the book.

GOALS OF THE BOOK

The book has three main aims. First, the book seeks to advance an Afrocentric sociocultural understanding of functioning, disability and health, and culturally grounded approaches to health maintenance, protection, and risk reduction in African cultural heritage populations. This book is a timely publication in view of the severe health service limitations with diverse people of African ancestry and the apparent lack of documented, culturally responsive counseling treatments with them. Negative health disparities, involving people of African ancestry, have been reported both in the developed and developing countries (Haviland, Morales, Dial, & Pincus, 2005; Hwang & Mpofu, 2009; Smedley, Stith, & Nelson, 2003). Yet, little usable information on culturally sensitive treatments, with a rich African cultural core, is available to counselors and other health service providers (Harley, 2005; Mpofu, 2005).

Second, the book seeks to provide a resource for students and professionals with an interest in promoting health and well-being in people of an African cultural heritage in their diversity. It seeks to achieve this goal by underscoring the broad underlying themes important to understanding influences on health concepts and participation by people of African ancestry. In this regard, the book adds to the growing body of scholarship on resources to promote health and well-being in people of African ancestry in the various life domains and contexts.

Finally, an aim of this book is to highlight health protection and promotion practices salient to African cultural settings. Also, the book provides suggestions useful to the growth and development in the provision of culturally responsive health services in African contexts.

FOR WHOM THE BOOK IS INTENDED

The book is intended for use by senior undergraduate and graduate students of African and African American studies, psychology, education, public health, anthropology, and related disciplines. Health service providers in the private and public sectors, and international aid agencies will find the book an invaluable resource for counselor preparation for their health promotion and development work with people of African ancestry. The chapters of the book are extensively referenced, and students and health service professionals seeking a deeper understanding of specific themes will find the reference list helpful. Instructors and other trainers on health giving to people of African ancestry will find the teaching-learning support exercises provided useful to their efforts to engage their students in meaningful learning.

THE BOOK'S APPROACH

The book is in four parts. The first part (Chapters 1–6) illuminates the cultural foundations important for understanding contemporary counseling issues in African cultural heritage settings. Specific issues considered in this section include help seeking and giving in tradition-led African settings (Chapter 1), the significance of oral traditions to the ownership and enactment of health and well-being by people of African ancestry (Chapter 2), and influences of colonial heritages on the theory and practice of counseling practice in Africanist settings (Chapters 5 and 6). Also, the first part of the book explores the research evidence for counseling practice in African settings and the importance for provision of consumer responsive counseling interventions in those settings (Chapters 3 and 4).

This articulation of the foundations of counseling practice in Africanist settings sets the stage for comprehending the subsequent sections of the book, *Contexts of Counseling* and *Counseling Applications*. Whereas the first part of the book introduces the reader to the foundations and cultural context of counseling people of African descent; the second part (Chapters 7–14) discusses some of the contexts in which counseling services are provided: families (Chapter 9), communities (Chapters 11 and 12), faith-based organizations (Chapter 10), and educational institutions (Chapters 7 and 8). The discussion covers the type of institutions where counselors work, the primary focus area of the counseling process within each of the settings, and typical service models. African heritage contexts are complex in their cultural diversity. This second part of the book addresses counseling services for complex cultural milieus such as diversity counseling (Chapter 13) and conflict resolution (Chapter 14).

The third part of the book comprises five chapters (Chapters 15–19) on counseling applications. The focus of these chapters is on counseling approaches for specific health conditions, statuses, and populations. The section surveys counseling applications with a selection of conditions or statuses for which there are significant counseling needs in many Africanist contexts including counseling approaches for people with trauma (Chapter 15), HIV and AIDS (Chapter 16), career development (Chapter 18), and people with disabilities (Chapter 19). The book concludes with an epilogue that reflects on the core themes covered in this volume, and prospects for the advancement of counseling in Africanist settings.

The contributing authors were required to follow a common framework for the chapter contents so that each chapter covered similar issues spanning importance and definition of terms, historical aspects, current practices, and issues for research scholarship. A common chapter outline for the book chapter was intended to enable readers to have a greater appreciation of the similarities and differences in the development and status of counseling practice across themes. To the extent possible, each chapter addresses perspectives from a variety of counseling traditions, including indigenous and modern counseling theory. Also, each chapter addresses unique health service delivery practices that may influence counseling in reference to the chapter topic. Pertinent legislation or international conventions are cited as necessary to highlight national, regional, or international importance to the counseling issues being discussed.

INSTRUCTIONAL FEATURES

Each chapter includes several types of instructional features to help the reader process the key concepts presented: self-check exercises, field-based experiential exercises, discussion boxes, research boxes, and case studies. *Discussion boxes* describe a current hot issue, dilemma, or controversy pertinent to the chapter content. At the end of this description, there are some questions intended to encourage readers to demonstrate an understanding of the nature of the issue presented and to propose how it may be resolved. The discussion boxes are intended to enhance learning in readers by encouraging an appreciation of the fact that experts may disagree or hold diverse views regarding counseling issues, thus challenging readers to acquire and hold their own views based on the best evidence available. Briefly, the *research boxes* describe significant research on a counseling issue, and thereby highlight the importance of specific counseling features. The description of the research is followed by questions intended to encourage readers to demonstrate an understanding of the importance of the research and, if presenting a research controversy, to propose how the controversy may be resolved.

Self-check exercises provide readers opportunities to assess their understanding of the chapter content. *Field-based experiential exercises and case studies* assist readers to test their application of the key concepts and practices from the chapter readings.

Elias Mpofu
August 05, 2009

REFERENCES

Harley, D. A. (2005b). African Americans and indigenous counseling. In D. A. Harley & J. M. Dillard (Eds.), *Contemporary mental health issues among African Americans* (pp. 293–306). Alexandria, VA: American Counseling Association.

Haviland, M. G., Morales, L. S., Dial, T. H., & Pincus, H. A. (2005). Race/ethnicity socioeconomic status, and satisfaction with health care. *American Journal of Medical Quality*, *20*, 195–203.

Hwang, K., & Mpofu, E. (2009). Health care quality measures. In E. Mpofu & T. Oakland (Eds.), *Rehabilitation and health assessment: Applying ICF guidelines* (pp. 141–61). New York: Springer.

Mpofu, E. (2005). Selective interventions in counseling African Americans with disabilities. In D. A. Harley & J. M. Dillard (Eds.), *Contemporary mental health issues among African Americans* (pp. 237–53). Alexandria, VA: American Counseling Association.

Smedley, B. D., Stith, A. Y., & Nelson, A. R. (2003). *Unequal treatments: Confronting racial and ethnic disparities in health care*. Washington, DC: National Academies Press.

Acknowledgments

I would like to express my gratitude to Eric Schwartz, Simina Calin, and Jeanie Lee, at Cambridge University Press, for their support in the development of this book project, and also to the more than forty authors who contributed to the writing of the chapters comprising this volume. Additionally, my special thanks goes to Drs. Terri Bakker and Lisa Lopez Levers for their great assistance with supporting many of the authors with manuscript development and reviewing their contributed manuscripts. Also, I thank Dr. Beverly Vandiver and Jacobus G. Maree for networking with several key authors who contributed chapters to this volume.

PART 1
FOUNDATIONS OF COUNSELING IN AFRICAN SETTINGS

Section Editor
Lisa Lopez Levers

1 Indigenous Healing Practices in Sub-Saharan Africa

Elias Mpofu, Karl Peltzer, and Olaniyi Bojuwoye

OVERVIEW. Healers seek to help patients understand the sociocultural basis of their health conditions, and how they can recognize, activate, or utilize resources and/or support systems necessary to alleviate their suffering. Treatment modalities include relaxation techniques, use of herbs, psychocultural education, dream interpretation, storytelling, use of proverbs, cleansing, libation, music, and ceremonies. In this chapter, we consider the importance of indigenous healing systems, history of research into traditional health care in Africa, national and international influences on African indigenous healing systems, current practices, legal and professional issues, and issues for research on African indigenous healing systems.

LEARNING OBJECTIVES

By the end of the chapter, the reader should be able to:

1. Define indigenous healing.
2. Outline traditionalist African core beliefs about health and well-being.
3. Discuss the major approaches and techniques to healing by indigenous healers and their rationale.
4. Differentiate among consultation procedures with African indigenous healers.
5. Evaluate prospective areas of research that would advance knowledge of African indigenous healing systems.

INTRODUCTION

Through the ages, human societies have developed systems for responding to health problems and for improving the quality of life. As evidence, every region of the world has a form of traditional or indigenous healing system, either formal or nonformal (Gielen, Fish, & Draguns, 2004; Harley, 2006). The World Health Organization (WHO, 1978, 2001) defined traditional healing as knowledge and practices, whether explicable or not, used in the diagnosis, prevention, and elimination of physical, mental, and social imbalance and relying exclusively on practical experiences and observations handed down from generation to generation, mostly verbally, but also, to some limited extent, in writing. Indigenous healing systems are those locally developed, recognized, and used by most of the inhabitants of a historical community, which they believe to incorporate their health concepts and needs (Levers, 2006a; Mpofu, 2006). Thus, the development of systems to maintain well-being or respond to ill health is tied to the historical, social, and environmental conditions in which they occur.

IMPORTANCE, DEFINITION, AND SCOPE OF KEY TERMS AND CONCEPTS

There currently is increasing recognition of the value to health care of traditional or indigenous healing systems (Marks, 2006; Moodley & West, 2005; WHO, 2001). In fact, the vast majority of the world's population uses indigenous healing systems for their health care (Mpofu, 2006; UNESCO, 1994; WHO, 2001). For the purpose of the discussion in this chapter, the terms "indigenous health care" or "traditional healing" are used interchangeably to refer to systems of health care rooted in the sociocultural contexts of the communities.

Africans have developed systems of responding to disease or ill health that are grounded in local culture (Conserveafrica, 2006; Levers, 2006a). The health care systems evolved from the beliefs, attitudes, customs, methods, and established practices for improving human conditions or elevating the quality of human life. As a result of recent advances in the fields of environmental sciences, immunology, medical botany, and pharmacognosy, health care policy designers have come to appreciate the effectiveness of African traditional health care (Conserveafrica, 2006).

We recognize the diversity and complexity of people of African cultural heritage in their help-seeking preferences. For example, Africans with Western education may prefer mostly modern biomedical health care rather than indigenous, traditional health care systems (Levers, 2006b; Mpofu & Harley, 2002), although a significant minority of them would also consult the indigenous health care system. Tradition-directed Africans or those who subscribe to a predominantly metaphysical explanation for well-being are likely to use the indigenous healing services that we discuss in this chapter.

Indigenous healing incorporates techniques with the potential role of facilitating increased level of well-being in one or more of the levels of body, mind, emotions, and spirit (Atherton, 2007). These techniques include traditional intervention strategies for promotion of health, prevention of ill health, and treatment of ill health. Intervention strategies by healers are intended to produce changes (especially in behavior patterns) in the affected, their primary and associational groups (e.g., family), as well as in the community in general.

An important consideration in discussion about African indigenous healing is the role of provider(s) of the services (in this regard the traditional healers) and the recipient(s) of the treatment (i.e., the patients or clients). The scope of practice for the African indigenous healer is not just the sick person(s) but also the sick person's primary and associational groups and the community in general (Edwards & Edwards, 2009). Second, indigenous healing intervention is also defined by the presumed purposes and methods of intervention. For example, in Africa, the act of healing is typically a religious act. Thus, when a traditionalist African patient takes a herbal infusion, he or she perceives healing from the belief in the spiritual or ancestral power to make the medicine work to treat the debilitating health condition. The spiritual significance is perceived important, perhaps more than the bioactive properties of the remedy. Many patients with a belief in the power of (ancestral) spirits to divine the causes of illness and problems find an anamnestic investigation in the Western sense uncalled for (Kleinmann 1980). Thus, African indigenous healing practices are informed by prevalent cultural theories of diseases or ill health, available sociocultural resources, perceived needs and problems, as well as traditional coping strategies.

HISTORY OF RESEARCH IN TRADITIONAL HEALTH CARE IN AFRICA

Much of what is known to African indigenous healers about their practices is passed on by oral history or folklore. This orally transmitted knowledge about healing is usually known only to initiated traditional healers and is taught to others by the healers themselves or spiritual agents (e.g., by ancestral spirits: Peltzer, 1992). Therefore, researching and documenting traditional healing methods used by native Africans may be difficult (Krauss 1990; Peltzer 1987, 1992). Historically, most formal research on African indigenous healing has been conducted by Europeans and North Americans (e.g., Bascom 1969; Edgerton, 1980; Gelfand, 1964; Green, 1994; Janzen, 1978; Levers, 2006a; McMillen, 2004; Peltzer, 1987; Prince, 1966; Warren, 1974; Zempléni, 1969). A growing cohort of African scientists are engaged in research on indigenous healing (e.g., Anumonye, 1973; Chavunduka, 1978; Kayombo, Mbwambo, & Massila, 2005; Makanjuola, 1987; Mpofu, 2003; Ngubane, 1977; Ovuga, Boardman, & Oluka, 1999; Twumasi, 1975, 1984). African traditional healers as researchers are sparsely represented in the literature (e.g., Mume, 1977). Research on indigenous healing systems has centered on types of conditions for which healing is sought and on concepts of well-being and disease.

Research on Types of Conditions for Which Treatment Is Sought

Most of the research literature on traditional healing in Africa is on mental disorders (Corin & Bibeau, 1980). In reality, in an African traditional healing context, healers consider spiritual or mental and physical disorders to be comorbid, necessitating the use of interventions believed to heal the body, mind, and soul. Most traditional healing methods are geared toward ameliorating psychosomatic, psychosocial, or family collective problems (Good & Kimani, 1980; Peltzer, 1987; Sabuni, 2007).

Indigenous healers typically treat a variety of mental, physical, and spiritual disorders (Peltzer, 1987). For example, they treat mental health conditions including hysteria, anxiety, and functional psychotic disorders. They also treat psychosomatic disorders or conditions or psychological conditions believed to manifest as physical conditions. Indigenous healers also treat numerous physical conditions (see Discussion Box 1.1).

However, very few studies have examined outcomes for patients in the long-term care of traditional healers (Assen, 1991; Peltzer, 1987).

Case Study 1.1: Patient with Psychosomatic Illness

A Nigerian patient, Mr. Mogaji, complained of a number of bodily ailments, especially when he stayed in the house of some of his relatives. He believes these relatives are against him and are trying to bewitch him. Therefore, he stopped going to visit and stay at their house. His therapist assured him in various ways and encouraged him go to the very house to greet one of the women whom he believed caused his illness. At first, the patient refused, even though he would not have to stay there, but he eventually went. On return, he was very happy because he not only managed to greet the woman but also to stay there overnight without developing his usual bodily symptoms.

Questions

1. Explain the therapeutic effects on Mr. Mogaji of greeting the woman he believed caused him illness from a traditionalist, spiritual perspective. How would the symptom relief be explained from a secular, Western perspective?

Discussion Box 1.1: Types of Conditions and Problems in Consultation with Traditional Health Practitioners

Two-hundred and twenty-seven patients exiting a traditional health practitioner's practice (n = 17) were interviewed on their reasons for consultation. The practice settings were two purposefully chosen urban sites in KwaZulu-Natal, South Africa (Peltzer & Mngqundaniso, 2008)

The table reports the type of conditions for which consultation was sought.

	N	%
Bad luck, reverse bad luck	47	21.2
Acute conditions (diarrhea, fever, flu, headaches, cough, other)	41	18.5
Generalized pain (stomach, muscle, or other nonspecific pain)	30	13.5
Chronic pain in joints/arthritis (joints, back, neck)	27	12.2
Psychosocial problem (marital, mental, ancestors' problems; spirit illness)	27	12.2
Magic poisoning	25	11.3
Problems with breathing	21	9.5
Communicable disease: HIV	18	8.1
Infertility	16	7.2
Children's problems	13	5.9
Weakness of the body, dizziness	12	5.4
Communicable disease: STI (other than HIV)	11	5.0
Other	8	3.6
High blood pressure/hypertension	4	1.8
Diabetes or related complications	4	1.8
Epilepsy	3	1.4
Cancer	3	1.4
Depression or anxiety	3	1.4
Stroke/sudden paralysis of one side of body	2	0.9
Problems with mouth, teeth, or swallowing	2	0.9
Sexual dysfunction	2	0.9

Questions

1. Characterize the conditions or problem areas for which consultation was sought by the patients in terms of body, mind, and soul aspects.
2. Explain from the perspective of African traditional medicine emphasis or priority ordering of consultation needs.

African indigenous healers appear relatively more successful in treating mental health conditions compared to physical conditions (Last & Chavunduka, 1986; Mpofu & Harley, 2006). Their effectiveness with physical conditions is limited in part by the fact that they typically do not use laboratories to study the disease-causing agents and their treatment. Treatment interventions by traditional healers use mostly episodic consultation, with no documentation to trace treatment effects over time.

Well-being and Disease Concepts

An allied line of research involvement has been on typologies of traditional healers and theories or concepts of illness (Chavunduka, 1978; Janzen, 1978; Makanjuola, 1987; Mshana et al., 2006; Warren, 1974). For example, research has documented that healers believe "spiritual" processes cause illnesses and guide treatment interventions. They believe in the use of spiritual power of ancestral spirits or gods to name the patient's problem and to divine the appropriate healing regimen.

An area of study that has received considerable research attention is the process of divination in the diagnosis of illness (Bascom, 1969; Chavunduka, 1987; Peltzer 1981, 1982, 1987; Prince 1966; Reynolds-Whyte, 1991). For example, Chavunduka (1978) described the case of a woman with a seizure disorder from a family with healing traditions. A traditional healer in a trance or possession by a spirit diagnosed two competing ancestral spirits wanting to possess the woman. One of spirits was believed to be a departed maternal grandfather courting her to become a witch, and the other the paternal grandfather resisting the overtures. The healer divined that the battle between the two spirits to possess the patient caused epileptic fits in her.

In traditional medicine, the diagnostic process of naming the affliction and determining its causation often involves elaborate procedures in which a diagnostician-diviner,

Research Box 1.1: Tradition-led Treatment Approaches

Mzimkulu, K. G., & Simbayi, L. C. (2006). Perspectives and practices of Xhosa speaking African traditional healers when managing psychosis. *International Journal of Disability, Development and Education, 53,* 417–32.

Objective: The study investigated symptoms defining psychosis from the perspective of four indigenous healers in the Xhosa (South Africa) tradition. The healers were affiliated with a psychiatric treatment center at a South African hospital.

Method: Qualitative interviews were conducted in Xhosa and the data used to construct themes from their practice in treating psychosis, inclusive of diagnosis, etiology, and treatment.

Results: Symptoms of psychosis identified by the Xhosa healers were similar to those in the *Diagnostic and Statistical Manual of Mental Disorders*, Fourth Edition (*DSM-IV-TR*). The healers explained psychosis in their patients as resulting from spiritual influences, witchcraft, and genetic predisposition. Treatment approaches emphasized purgatives, cleansing rituals, and spirit evocation through singing.

Conclusion: The Xhosa indigenous healers were complex in their understanding of psychosis and treatment methods.

Questions

1. Explain the fact that Xhosa traditional healers were consistent with *DSM-IV-TR* in their identification of symptoms of psychosis and divergent in their attribution of etiology and treatment.
2. How may treatment approaches preferred by the traditional healers be aligned to their theory of etiology?
3. What patient safety issues would be relevant from the use of purgatives and cleansing rituals to treat psychosis?
4. What additional information would you need about the study to understand better diagnosis, etiology, and treatment of psychosis by the Xhosa healers? How would that additional information enhance your understanding of treatment approaches for psychosis in the Xhosa tradition?

Case Study 1.2: Ancestral Spirits Counter Claims

Mrs. Majako has two types of ancestral spirits: two Vadzimu (ancestral spirits; sg. Mudzimu) and one Shave (stranger spirit). During the course of the pretraining illness, Mrs. Majako became initially possessed by the Mudzimu of her grandfather, one month later by the Mudzimu of her grandmother, and finally by a Shave. Usually Vadzimu are spirits of deceased parents or grandparents, especially the grandfather. The Mudzimu is believed to cause and cure illnesses as well as solve problems. In addition, the Mudzimu protects the individual and the family from evil influences (cf. Gelfand 1964). The Shave is a stranger spirit that causes minor illnesses and brings luck in work and love (Gelfand 1964). Mrs. Majako's Shave assists the Vadzimu in healing and is a good dancer and singer. Majako-Mudzimu/grandfather knows herbal ailments, especially for infertility, abdominal complaints, and evil spirits; and Majako-Mudzimu/grandmother is specialized in "diagnosis" through Kufemba, that is, smelling the patient. This is done on Tuesdays, Thursdays, and Saturdays, especially for people with witchcraft and family problems.

At the beginning of the ceremony, the musicians start playing and Mrs. Majako gets involved in dancing. As the sound increases, her head starts shaking rhythmically, and slowly she begins to smell the patient from his feet to abdomen, up and down, until she becomes possessed by her own and later by the patient's spirits. Her spirit "Majako-Mudzimu" starts speaking: "I have lived at your home. There I often went together with chief S. to the same church … Your father uses bad medicine …" Later on she becomes possessed by witchcraft spirits (Varoyi; sg. Muroyi) that stem from the patient's relatives. After a long divining process, the mother-in-law of the patient is identified as a witch who, supported by the patient's father's second wife, "killed" the patient's mother and is now also after the patient's life.

Questions

1. Describe the full constellation of people presumed to be involved in the client's problems.
2. Explain any disease or illness concepts related to the client's presenting problem.

patient, and kinspeople participate. Although designed to lead to the choice of appropriate remedial action, the naming process itself has significant therapeutic aspects (Jilek, 1993). In the naming process, the patient's feelings and experiences are restructured into a culturally validated image system. The patient is provided with a language in which ineffable psychic states can be expressed and chaotic experiences reorganized, thereby becoming

Discussion Box 1.2: The Art of Divination

To analyze the principles of the naming process, a traditional healer (Malongo) was invited to divine or name fifty-eight nursing students in Malawi. Malongo explained that he spiritually identifies himself with his client, his family, his house, his place of work, etcetera. His "spirit actually goes" to the focus of the problem and "collects the information" needed for the naming of the client's problems. In the nursing college, each student had the opportunity to see Malongo for twenty minutes, and was asked to write a report on the consultation, stating the contents of the divination, whether it was correct or not, and his or her general impression on the encounter. It was found that only 35% of the students accepted the healer's explanatory model (e.g., "I was very anxious, because they can tell you all about your problems."), whereas 30% were ambivalent (e.g., "Many things he said were surprisingly true, and I doubt whether to believe in it or not.") and 35% discrepant (e.g., "His diagnosis procedure was based on guesswork."). Evaluation of the divinations found that 56% were reported as wrong and 44% were correct. Generally, the more precise the healer was, the more often he was incorrect (e.g., in the number of siblings of the student), and the more general he was, the more he was correct (e.g., "Your boyfriend loves you ..." or "If you work hard you are going to pass your exams ...") (Peltzer, 1987).

Questions

1. Comment on the conceptual equivalence of traditional healers' spiritual identification with the client and his surroundings with the Western concept of empathy in psychotherapy.
2. Discuss the influences of the perceived validity of the naming or divinatory process by the (a) healers and their clients, (b) researchers; and (c) practitioners of Western medicine.

intelligible and manageable (Levi-Strauss, 1963). The divinatory process can be conducted in the form of instrumental divination or medium divination. In the case of instrumental divination, the healer employs a material vehicle (or instrument) from which he or she draws conclusions according to a series of mantic configurations based on spiritual power (Sow, 1980: e.g., a bottle filled with herbs and water). In medium divination, all techniques of so-called possessions are included, aiming ultimately at plumbing the deeper psychic layers of the healer for treatment effects (Sow, 1980).

NATIONAL AND INTERNATIONAL INFLUENCES

African indigenous healing systems at present have wider recognition and dissemination than before (Last & Chavunduka, 1986; Marks, 2006). For example, in 1964, the Organization of African Unity (OAU) set up the Scientific and Technical Research Commission (STRC) to spearhead research into indigenous healing. Subsequently, in 1968, the STRC hosted an international symposium in Dakar, Senegal to study the use and development of medicinal plants in Africa. The outcome of the symposium led to seventeen research centers being set up all over Africa to stimulate research on the proof of efficacy of African medicinal plants. The African Advisory Committee for Health Research and Development (AACHRD, 2000) recommended the revitalization of research on traditional medicine, particularly for common problems such as HIV/AIDS, tuberculosis, malaria, and childhood illnesses. At a Summit Meeting in Abuja, Nigeria, in 2001, the Organization of African Unity (OAU) Heads of State declared that research on traditional medicine should be made a priority. Later in the same year at a Summit Meeting in Lusaka, Zambia, the OAU declared the period 2001–2010 as the decade for African Traditional Medicine.

Countries that are reported to be conducting research on evaluation of herbal preparations for the management of HIV/AIDS include Benin, Burkina Faso, DRC, Ghana, Côte d'Ivoire, Kenya, Mali, Nigeria, South Africa, Tanzania, Togo, Uganda, and Zimbabwe. Jayasuriya and Jayasuriya (2002) reported that several African countries have statutory responsibility to undertake research relating to medicinal plants including the National Pharmaceutical Bureau of Burundi, the Central Laboratory at Mototo in Guinea, the National Institute for Medical Research of Tanzania, the Institute of Medicinal Research and Medicinal Plants of Cameroon, and the National Institute for Research on Traditional Pharmacopoeia and Traditional Medicine of Mali.

The Eastern and Southern African Regional Initiative on Traditional Medicine and AIDS convened a regional consultation in May 2003, which produced a series of proposed standards around three main themes related to traditional medicine and HIV and AIDS: the systematic evaluation of traditional medicines; spiritual aspects of healing: HIV prevention and care; processing and packaging of traditional remedies; protection of indigenous knowledge; and intellectual property rights related to traditional medicine. (Homsy et al., 2004). Bodies such as the Traditional and Modern Health Practitioners Together Against AIDS (Uganda), the Association for the Promotion of Traditional Medicine (Senegal), the Zimbabwe National Traditional Health Practitioner Association (Zimbabwe), and the Global Initiative for Traditional Systems of Health are

Discussion Box 1.3: The Case of Mrs. Mhlauzi

Mrs. Mhlauzi (age seventy-nine), a peasant farmer, had apparent senile dementia. She had a history of going on unplanned trips considerably away from home for the past eight years. On occasion, she would return from these escapades with bodily bruises, suggesting falls she could not explain. She would claim to have visited the great tribal ancestral shrine to pay homage, and would also claim to be visiting the state president. Her children and grandchildren and neighbors alike observed that she appeared to be overly forgetful and to have undergone some personality change. For example, family members reported that she appeared to have become more secretive and untrusting of those around her. She also publicly accused her son-in-law from the same village of stealing her livestock, and arbitration by fellow villagers was not helpful in resolving the matter. In the past two months, she left the village without informing anyone of her destination and has not returned since. A missing person's report was filed with the local police.

Family members consulted a traditional healer to divine just where she might be and the cause of her apparent mental illness. The traditional healer divined that she had lost her mental functions from a malevolent spirit that possessed her, and that was unhappy with her care. Consequently, the malevolent spirit had driven her away from home; and she would not return unless some rituals to chastise and expel the offending goblin were carried out. The healer further explained that several divorced mothers in the extended family were so because of the spell of the same malevolent spirit. The healer also observed that members of the family with high-paying professional jobs would not prosper from the influence of the malevolent spirit that would impoverish everyone. For a fee, the healer would treat the malevolent spirit and restore well-being to the whole family.

Questions

1. Consult any source on senile dementia. What symptoms from the case description are consistent with senile dementia?
2. Explain the traditional healer's diagnosis from a traditionalist African perspective.
3. What health beliefs in the family would support the healer's diagnosis and proposed treatment?
4. What evidence, if any, would falsify the healers' proposed etiology for the mental illness in Mrs. Mhlauzi?

making major inroads in fostering promotion of traditional medicine (Chavunduka, 1986; Romero-Daza, 2002).

CURRENT PRACTICES

African indigenous healing is deeply rooted in the physical, emotional, and spiritual aspects of being and is inextricably linked to religion or belief systems (Edwards & Edwards, 2009). It seeks to provide health, sanity, spiritual solace, and other valued family or community collective virtues (including a return to traditional family values). In this section, we consider the fundamental causation of disease and illness from a traditionalist African perspective. We follow this up by discussing the treatment techniques mostly used by indigenous healers and their patients. We briefly consider the treatment of HIV/AIDS by traditional healers in the sub-Saharan subregion to illustrate the practical application of some of the health care concepts we consider in this chapter.

The Fundamental Etiology of Health Conditions

Most tradition-directed African clients believe that the problem or illness originates from outside themselves in the environment, including the actions of malevolent people, spirits, or acts of witchcraft (Sabuni, 2007) and that divination will reveal the true cause of their lack of well-being. Regardless of the fact that an environmental pathogen is recognized to cause an illness in a person, healers and their patients believe that the illness is explained by the fact that the pathogen would not have infected the particular individual had not a spirit enabled it to result in the health condition. Similarly, victims of occupational accidents are believed to sustain injury because a spirit set the stage for the accident to happen. The spirit can be a malevolent one cast by others of ill will or a benevolent one demanding recognition for the many good things it does for the living family.

Since the fundamental causation of wellness or ill health is explained in metaphysical terms, healers and their patients prefer directive treatments or those using mostly external oriented techniques (e.g., ritual cleaning, enactment, sacrifices). However, internally oriented therapies such as scarification or making bodily incisions, aroma therapy, vomiting, and purging are also used, but mostly in their perceived function to keep evil spirits, witches, and bad luck at bay.

Emphasis on Holistic Treatment

A prominent quality of African traditional healing is its holistic nature. A holistic model of health care has several advantages, among which is the recognition that (1) an illness does manifest across various levels of the community and (2) physical problems can also cause psychological or spiritual problems (Levers, 2006b; Marks, 2006). As previously observed, health-related beliefs held by traditionalist Africans encompass the family or community collective as a major resource for well-being (Jahoda, 1961; Mpofu, 2003; Simwaka, Peltzer, & Banda, 2007; Teuton, Bentall, & Dowrick, 2007). Problems and illness are not individualized but interpreted within the social system, kinship, traditional, and cultural norms (Schmidbauer, 1969; Staugard, 1986). To be effective in his or her practice, the healer must have a comprehensive knowledge of his or her culture, tradition, and the environment in general. His or her task is to convey cultural ideals on the basis of mythological structures to the clients (Schmidbauer, 1969).

Treatments

Healers tend to achieve their treatment effects through a secondary process. Healing by secondary process is directed primarily to the reactions to the illness by significant others rather than to the primary symptoms by the patient (Prince, 1974). The patient is abrogated of any responsibility for the illness and is a neutral observer of a social healing process (Chavunduka, 1978). The healer achieves secondary process treatment effects in part by validating the implicit theories held by the patient and significant others about the illness and appropriate treatment by his or her active therapeutic procedures (Mpofu, 2003).

Treatment methods used by healers can be classified as follows: (1) physical activity with management of interpersonal relationships; (2) use of expectation; (3) use of symbolism and enactment; (4) use of naming; (5) dream interpretation; and (6) cleansing, libation, and scarification. We briefly consider each of these treatments next.

Use of Physical Activity with Orchestration of Interpersonal Relationships

Traditional healers consider treatments that provide vigorous activities or interpersonal interactions more effective than those that fail to actively engage the body and generate interpersonal synergy (Butler, 1998). These physical activities often involve groups of others who support the client and healer in the treatment efforts. Significant others (e.g., family and friends) also actively participate to reinforce treatment effects. Typical group healing ceremonies involve vigorous physical exercises, such as dancing, clapping of hands, and singing. These physical activities help energize the patient and significant others in their adherence to intervention for wellness.

Bodily movement therapies are often used in the context of cultural–spiritual rituals. For example, during dance ceremonies accompanied by possession trance, the bar is lowered on everyday conduct of behavior so that the patient can express his or her repressed affects and behavior pattern. Flexible regression to earlier behavioral–emotional developmental stages or the sudden discharge or catharsis of strong affects is systematically encouraged by the healer through verbal exhortations. These exhortations include naming to the patient significant ancestors believed to be prime mediators of the power of healing and asking them to help the patient achieve rapid healing.

Healers use the group as a behavioral change agent (Parrott, 1999). Group activities make possible social networking for the reconstruction of people's physical, social, and spiritual environments. In group activities, such as African traditional healing ceremonies, the dynamics of human relationships move from competition to collaboration (Comaroff, 1980). For example, family members and patients strengthen their emotional bonds from the group therapy, creating a more supportive environment to sustain healing after the intensive group therapy.

Use of Expectation

Healers use expectation to win and motivate patients to engage in treatment. Expectation is a treatment effect from the belief by the patient that a therapist's procedures will successfully treat a condition for which consultation is being sought. Healers achieve significant expectation effects through donning of impressive regalia during consultation (Lesolang-Pitje, 2000). The regalia typically include garments from animal products such as skins, body parts, or droppings. It could also include garments and head gear made from brightly colored clothing (pure white or blood red) bedecked with charm objects. Dressing with at least the skin from a major cat (e.g., leopard, lion) or bird (eagle) adds to a high expectation. Clients hold the belief that the healer or his or her agents must have killed a major cat, which itself is a powerful accomplishment. Moreover, the attire also points to the healer's association with spiritual beings or supernatural endowment.

A traditional healer with multilingualism (implying ability to call to the treatment effort spirits from many cultures) and gender accessibility (i.e., ability to call to possession either a male or female spirit) also conjures high expectation effects in clients. Healers with ease of use of dramatic flair, gesture, or oratory ability in making their observations will likely have desired expectation effects in their clients. Minimally, healers should have expert socioemotional skills to engage patients to reap expectation benefits. Their clairvoyant abilities add to the expectation by clients that they would provide the kind of services clients need to achieve health (Katz & Wexler, 1989).

Use of Symbolism and Enactment

Healers use herbal extracts to convey symbolic messages. For example, Makanjuola (1987) identified nine symbolic associations that healers and their clients believe to be potent in treating a variety of health conditions. These include: (1) meaning of the name of the remedy, (2) sound of the name of the remedy, (3) form or appearance of the remedy, (4) physical qualities, (5) behavior of the remedy (e.g., leaves that "go to sleep"), (6) referent part of the remedy (e.g., strong skull or head of an animal believed to fortify from migraine headache), (7) symbolic holism (e.g., pepper or salt, believed to be anti-spell agents, is sprinkled on a surface or object with a spell), and (8) color symbolism (e.g., a castaway black hen carries an offending malevolent spirit cast out of a person). Healers also use ritual enactment to represent and cast away an unwanted spiritual influence (Mpofu, 2006b). With ritual enactment, a patient with a named health-compromising spiritual influence works with a healer to name and symbolically cast the malevolent spirit away in the wilds or to inhabit a domesticated animal (e.g., goat, fowl). With the patient believing the malevolent spirit cast away or banished to the wilds or into an animal, he or she may experience significant relief of symptoms or cure.

Use of Naming

Healers use verbal techniques to help patients directly experience certain emotions or states of consciousness believed to be therapeutic. For instance, in their use of naming (as previously discussed), healers use verbal techniques to provide a rich label to a health condition to explain both its *etiology* and necessary treatment. Typically, as part of the divination, the healer will name a variety of different problems and watch the patient's reaction to each specific precision. The precisions can be differentiated according to symptomatic precision (e.g., "Your body is not good...you have pain in your shoulder"), situational precision (e.g., "When you are surrounded by people you get pain in your shoulders."), or temporal precision (e.g., "When you wake up in the mornings you have pain in your shoulder") (Peltzer, 1995, p. 106). Once the illness is put into a cultural frame, definite expectations are aroused in the patient and his or her family. The healer follows up by identifying the patient with others who have been cured of similar conditions and thereby adding to patient expectation and his or her own credibility.

Patients expect healers to name their problems to provide a scaffold for the healing process. Through naming, the healer provides the patient with a language in which unexpressed states can be directly expressed. Through naming, negative events are explained and personifications are provided, and the patient is initiated to enter the treatment process. In the naming process, ancestors of the patient and healer become part of the healing intervention in the world of the living. Patients may experience a reduction in symptoms after a naming procedure (Pfeiffer, 1974). Therefore, the act of naming can be considered as therapeutic (Torrey, 1986).

Naming is different from the diagnostic process. According to Western medicine, the patient is first examined physically and psychologically before a diagnosis is made. However, the traditional healer does not usually undertake an investigation on the patient before diagnosis, since it is assumed that the healer's spirits already know the cause of the problem or illness. This, however, does not mean that the healer diagnoses without any examination, but the diagnostic process is basically identical with the naming process wherein physical examination and questions are made to appear as if they play only a subordinate role. Only questions before the naming of problems can be considered as anamnestic questions, and if such questions are asked, they seem to have low anamnestic relevance. An exception to this rule is the situation of a patient who is possessed when entering the healing interaction. Consider the case of an interaction between the healer and a twelve-year-old girl who is diagnosed as a witch (Peltzer, 1987):

HEALER: "What is your name?"
PATIENT'S(SPIRIT): "I have told you this already."
HEALER: "I said, what is your name?"
PATIENT'S(SPIRIT): "I was not given any name."
HEALER: "What about the name of your mother?"
PATIENT'S(SPIRIT): "Tiyega is my mother."
HEALER: "What is your mission and what do you want 'in' the girl?"
PATIENT'S(SPIRIT): "We have been asked to kill a person."
HEALER: "I see; that is what you want ..."
PATIENT'SWITCHSPIRIT: "We want to kill."
HEALER: "Whom did you kill?"
PATIENT'SWITCHSPIRIT: "Many." ...

In this case the status of being a witch will be ascribed after a line of diagnostic questioning culturally consistent with identifying a witch.

Dream Interpretation

It is common to consult a healer when the dreaming is excessive or the dreams are unclear, complicated, or frightening. Tradition-directed Africans believe that dreams have a special influence on most waking activities and that dreams cause illness and misfortunes at work or in personal relationships. To them, dreams that appear to have high vision or trance qualities are communicating a reality that cannot be ignored. For example, a dream in the form of a visual image of an ancestor is perceived by both healers and clients to be a revealed spiritual or absolute truth about that particular ancestor's present involvement in the life events of the client. The following example illustrates interpretations of a bad dream by two healers (Peltzer, 1985):

Description of a Dream

Client: I dreamt about a snake chasing me, and I had to climb a tree for safety, and it followed me onto the tree.

Discussion Box 1.4: Healer Naming Practices

The traditional healer with a traditional patient (Peltzer, 2005, p. 107)

TRADITIONAL HEALER (TH): When you write, you sometimes feel as though there is darkness in your eyes – especially when you are writing.
PATIENT (PT): Yes
TH: Also when you are reading you have tears coming from your eyes – does that happen?
PT: Yes.
TH: And when you sit somewhere you find that you start perspiring – sweating too much, is it true?
[The following is summarized] Sometimes you feel very cold …
Sometimes after you have eaten, you suddenly feel hungry …
Your leg feels sometimes as though it is paralyzed …
PT: Yes.
TH: You sometimes feel as though you are alone – although there may be people chatting to you, you still do not talk; you remain silent. Am I lying?
PT: No.
TH: Vyanusi [spiritually caused acute confusional state] is in the background but foremost is vimbuza [spirit disorder: conversion or dissociation disorder or depressive neurosis]; it is not witchcraft. Your uncle used to look for medicine for you – ages ago – he used to help a lot of people. Am I lying?
PT: No.
TH: Sometimes when you wake up in the morning you feel pain in your arms when you stretch them. Am I lying?
PT: No.
TH: Sometimes when you wake up you feel as though you want to fall when you stand up. Then you say that you want to remain standing or seated for a long time before you walk – there is some witchcraft involved – jealousy – that money – they feel you have a lot of money and your fellow villagers feel they want to fix you. At work there is little cooperation – that is where it all starts from. But then when you have the money, you do not know how to spend it wisely. Something goes wrong inside your head. You cannot hold your capital. You have a big vimbuza problem, that is why you sometimes feel dizzy… Anything else – any complaints?
PT: No, none.

Reprinted with permission from *Journal of Psychology in Africa*, *15*(1), 105–108.

Questions

1. Discuss the diagnostic process in contrast to the naming process.
2. Discuss the healer–patient relationship effects apparent from this interview.

I jumped down and it stopped chasing me. After that a bee stung me and I cried.

Interpretations

1. **Healer Bwanali**: The dream symbolizes people (witches) who are responsible for your diseases.
2. **Healer Kumpolota**: At first, the dream is bad because he is chased by a snake, then it becomes good because he can escape from the snake. However, the bee shows that the danger is still there and it is therefore a dream with a bad omen.

Another example is that of a patient who dreamt that his mother and father, who had both died some time back, were speaking to him. They wanted *nsima* (staple food) made from white maize flour, with meat and vegetables. The healer interpreted the dream saying that he (the patient) should hold an ancestral feast. The patient prepared food, invited people from the village, and after the feasting, the spirits were pacified. Had the feast not taken place, both the healer and the patient believed the spirits would have come back to torment the patient, making him fall ill again (Peltzer, 1985). The patient has therapeutic dependency on the perceived spiritual authority of the healer in dream interpretation. Individual motivations are suspended for culturally prevalent interpretations of good or bad dreams (Peltzer, 1985).

Healers and their clients may hold common symbolic meanings for the contents of dreams from their cultural socialization (Crapanzano, 1975; Peltzer, 1987). For example the Chewa of Malawi believe that dreaming of a "snake" means bad luck or plotting enemies. However, other symbolism is culturally mixed in meaning. For example, in Malawi, dreaming of "giving birth to a child" symbolized good luck in one cultural community and witchcraft or danger in another (Peltzer, 1987). The healer dream interpreter selects certain dream symbols that are perceived to be significant in terms of shared fantasies with the client. It would seem that dream symbols formulate conflicts that are influenced by spiritual activities involving the ancestors and other aliens.

Cleansing, Libation, and Scarification

Cleansing measures include herbal emetics and laxatives administered with copious amounts of fluid, sweat baths, steam baths, and fumigation with incense or smoke. These procedures are intended by the healer, and understood by the patient, as purifying and cleansing measures to get rid of "polluting" or otherwise pathogenic substances (Jilek, 1993). Healers may also give patients culturally validated symbolism, such as amulets, charms, talismans, or medicine bundles, which have been blessed or otherwise "worked on" by the healer to help psychologically sustain the cleansing effects in the patients. Patients may experience a higher sense of well-being after the cleansing from the belief that the cleaning washed away the cause of their ailment. Patients may also receive special magico-religious formulas. Such objects and formulas are universally assumed to protect the bearer from illness and evil influence, affording him or her tranquillity and peace of mind (Jilek, 1993).

Healers may use sacrificial rites as part of the cleansing process. Sacrificial rites are performed to appease and recompense supernatural or ancestral powers, and to urge their withdrawal of a punishing illness or to supplicate their intervention on behalf of the patients. Rituals of sacrifice are often associated with confession of having broken divine or ancestral rules (taboos) or with public admission of transgressions against community members, followed by a promise of appropriate rectification (Jilek, 1993). The sacrificial ritual often ends with a communal meal in which the healer, patient, and kinspeople partake of the sacrificed animal's meat in a symbolic act sealing conciliation with supernatural beings or ancestors (Prince, 1974).

Scarification or the making of body incisions to administer herbal treatments directly into the bloodstream is widely practiced by traditional healers in Africa. The medicines typically include burned up residues of herbs believed to prevent disease, cure the cause, or protect against disease-causing malevolent spiritual influences.

Cleansing, Aromatherapy, or Fumigation

Because the cause of ill health in tradition-directed Africans is attributable mostly to angry ancestral spirits, or witchcraft, treatment emphasis is on freeing the patient of the evil spirits causing the ill health. A typical treatment strategy, in this connection, is cleansing treatment performed to remove whatever is causing the ill health either from the inside or outside of the body of the patient and from the environment (living and nonliving) of the patient.

Mzimkulu's (2000) study of the treatment of psychotic patients by some Xhosa traditional healers in South Africa revealed a five-stage process of traditional cleansing treatment. The first stage involves administering to the patient herbal fumes or fragrances through inhalation. The healer intends for the aromatherapy to relax the patient, create treatment expectation effects, and encourage treatment adherence. The second stage of treatment is the cleansing of the inside of the head of the patient to remove evil spirits from that part of the body. The general belief is that the head (or the mind) influences the health of the body. Healers typically administer a liquid herbal mixture to the patient's face, some of which is allowed to get into the eyes and the nostrils with the belief that the herbal treatment would aggravate the malevolent spirits inhabiting the head (or mind) enough to cause the spirits to want to leave the patient. The third stage involves removing evil spirits from inside the body of the patient by administering a purgative to induce diarrhea, vomiting, and sweating. Finally, the outside of the body is cleansed by subjecting the patient to steaming or a bath with herbal mixtures.

Tradition-directed Africans believe that causes of ill health inhabit the physical environment, and total treatment must rid the physical habitat of threats to well-being. Healers typically use fumigation with herbal medicines to treat habitats suspected to cause illness in persons. For example, they may burn herbs in houses or sprinkle liquid herbal mixtures on the walls and floors of the house or habitat. Family members and the patient may also be fumigated or sprinkled.

An animal sacrifice may cap the elaborate treatment regimen. The consumption of the meat from the animal sacrifice is accompanied by a ceremony involving music, singing, and dancing in which family members, together with the patient and the healer, participate. The consumption of the meat from the animal sacrifice often is accompanied with the pouring or sprinkling of the specially brewed local beer on the ground in a symbolic gesture inviting the rest of the elements of the cosmos (especially ancestral spirits and deities) to partake in the activities of the ritual ceremony. The healers and their patients believe that invited ancestral spirits or deities would use their influence to promote good family and communal relationships as well as harmony between living beings and all elements of the cosmos.

HIV/AIDS Treatment

A smaller proportion of traditional healers engage in HIV/AIDS treatment. For example, only 6 percent of a sample of traditional healers in KwaZulu-Natal self-identified to treat HIV/AIDS. However, a larger proportion of healers treat opportunistic infections from HIV/AIDS that they ascribe to witchcraft, breaking of taboos, or the influence of bad or aggrieved spirits. For example, among 618 HIV-infected patients before initiation of antiretroviral therapy in three public hospitals in KwaZulu-Natal, South Africa, 29.6 percent had been taking herbal remedies. Herbal therapies were the most expensive, costing on average 128 Rand per month (1 US$ = 7.60 Rand) (Peltzer, Friend-du Preez, Ramlagan, & Fomundam, 2008).

Discussion Box 1.5: Patient Adherence

The Mlothwas consulted a traditional healer to treat what appeared to be a psychosomatic illness in Nozipho, their twenty-two-year-old daughter. The condition was persistent, and exceeded family expertise in herbal treatments. The traditional healer repeatedly administered an herbal mix that caused Nozipho hot flushes, heart palpitations, bowel movements, and excruciating abdominal pain. Nosipho let her parents and siblings know of the pain the medication caused her. The traditional healer was insistent that the medicine caused Nozipho pain because it was working to eliminate disease in her that was the source of her ill health, and that if she was well, she would not experience any pain from the medication. The family believed the traditional healer. However, after Nozipho continued to complain of pain from taking the herbal mix, her eldest brother Ntolwana volunteered to take the herbal mix to see if it would cause him no pain since he was not a patient. Ntolwana fell ill from taking the medication, and was relieved only from vomiting the medicine. He advised Nozipho not to take the herbal mix any more and to seek alternative treatment. The traditional healer protested that his medicine worked and that Ntolwana had dishonored him by taking his medicine without his personal prescription. He refused payment for his services.

Questions

1. Explain the fact that Nozipho continued to take a potentially poisonous herbal mix despite the negative side effects.
2. What benefits and risks do patients carry from their perception that the traditional healer's authority in herbal treatments is final?
3. How may questions about the potentially life-threatening herbal treatment be best addressed while maintaining harmony between the traditional healer and Nozipho's family?
4. What are the implications of payment refusal by a traditional healer for the well-being of the patient and family?

The evidence about the effectiveness of traditional healers in treating HIV/AIDS is inconclusive (Levers, 2006b; Peltzer & Mngqundaniso, 2008). For example, in the mid-1990s there were claims that the *mchape* concoction by a cult leader would cure AIDS, and at present *chambe* and *malawix* are on the market as AIDS cures in Malawi (Simwaka, Peltzer, & Banda, 2007). Liu (2007) systematically assessed the beneficial and harmful effects of herbal medicines in people with HIV infection and AIDS and reported that some herbal medicines seemed to be effective in symptom improvement, although with no significant effects on antiviral or immunity enhancement.

Consultation Procedures

The patient may consult the traditional healer as an individual, although family consultation is often preferred. As previously observed, African indigenous theories on wellness consider the health of individuals to be spiritually tied to that of the family collective. For instance, the healer and patients believe that social tensions and stress in the patient and within the family or community cause certain problems of living or illnesses. They also believe that family or cultural consensus about the cause of illness and the appropriate healing process would resolve the difficulties experienced. Deeply rooted motives and problems of the family or kinship are projected onto the healer (spirit) and through transference can then be acted out. Consequently, the family is integrated into the help-seeking and treatment process.

The help-seeking behavior of African clients certainly suggests confidence in the traditional healers. It is also informed by cultural attitudes toward ill health, especially in terms of acceptance and utilization of help as well as acceptance of the cultural theories of ill health and cure.

Healer–Patient Treatment Dynamics

African indigenous healers use mostly directive approaches to treatment. They stage the entire treatment session and pace it to the perceived needs of the patient. Patients are likely to perceive a healer who is prescriptive and directive as more competent than one who is less directive. The patient is motivated by the perceived charisma and spiritual powers of the healer. These characteristics serve as emotional arousals, triggering hope and willingness to participate actively in the healing process. The patient considers the healer as a responsible and authoritative father figure administering therapeutic functions (Pfeiffer, 1991). As a result, the patient typically adheres to the prescribed treatment regimen or other corrective measures, much more so than if a family member had given him or her health advice.

Patient adherence to treatment is reinforced by the client's belief in the healer as a supernatural authority (Sow, 1980). In fact, the world of the dead or ancestors is seen as authoritative in all human matters, so that health predictions and statements made by the healer's ancestral spirits are seen as divine revelations. The healer, as a medium between the authority of the ancestors and the living, reemphasizes and depicts ideal social norms and values. He or she mediates between cultural ideals and human or individual failure, and is able to create hope in the people concerned (Pfeiffer, 1974). Healers are perceived by their clients as custodians of their cultural knowledge and histories.

Consultation Procedures with Traditional Healers

Consultation is believed by both healer and patient to have the oversight of the ancestral spirits, who add to the vision of the healer in selecting the appropriate treatment and enable the patient's responsiveness to treatment. The consultation settings of African traditional healing methods can be distinguished mainly according to time coordinates of the healer–patient interaction: (1) episodic outpatient, (2) continuous outpatient, and (3) inpatient setting (Kleinman, 1980). We consider each of these in turn.

The episodic outpatient setting

In the episodic outpatient setting, patients consult on an "as-needed" basis at the healer's home. The healer typically uses a part of his or her house as a practice clinic. A less common form of an episodic outpatient setting is a healer's home visits, since normally the patient should be taken to the healer. For example, a healer may perform a "kufemba" (smell the illness out) (Shona, Zimbabwe/Mozambique) ceremony during home visits accompanied only by musicians who influence the spiritual sphere of the consultation (Peltzer, 1989). Home visits also take place if the patient is unable to come to the healer. With home visits, the treatment is often preventive but also curative for particular members of the family or the whole family. For example, a healer was called by a collective client (e.g., family, village, business enterprise) to perform group divination and treatment of the institution (Peltzer, 1987). In this instance, the family-owned hotel of a patient had almost burnt down the previous year and the performed ritual was to protect the family from future misfortune (Peltzer, 1996a). The particular consultation methods used were as follows:

1. Day 1. The walls of the family house and the domestic animals were sprinkled with holy water in the belief that specific ancestors would protect the house from evil influences.
2. Day 2. The healer and family addressed the family's ancestors, requesting them to fulfill specific wellness wishes. This could include sacrificing an animal (e.g., goat, ox) and ritual preparation and eating of sacrificed animals by the participants in the ceremony symbolizing the ancestors (Peltzer, 1996a). After these episodic interventions, the collective patients' misfortunes were expected to resolve promptly.

A rare form of outpatient treatment is the identification of witchcraft among a whole community, village, or a school class. In this case, a witch finder cleanses whole villages and communities of witches and wizards. For example, Peltzer (1987) described a village cleansing ceremony by healer Bwanali in Malawi for the purpose of detecting the witch(es) whom the villagers believed to cause frequent child deaths. In the process, all village inhabitants are summoned and asked to surrender their witchcraft instruments on the understanding that if they did not, then great misfortunes would befall them and their families soon after.

There are variations in the specific rituals that accompany the village cleansing process. In some instances, villagers will pass by the healer, and those who lose consciousness and collapse in line or as they pass the healer are presumed to be witches spiritually weighed by their evil medicines. In actual fact, some villagers may lose consciousness from exhaustion, anxiety, or actual conviction of guilt due to some wrongs done, or something that should have been done, even if in an unrelated situation. In other instances, villagers may be asked to drink an herbal concoction mixed by the healer, and those who fall sick from the drink are presumed to be witches. It is likely that some of the villagers may fall sick from being allergic to the chemical properties of the herbal mix or the lack of hygienic preparation of the concoction. In some cases, villagers allied to the traditional healer could fix the witch-hunting ceremony to identify someone with whom they have prior disagreements or whom they want evicted from the village for some personal reason. Nonetheless, the healer typically provides villagers with preventive medicine to protect them from witchcraft or assuming their erstwhile witchcraft practices.

The continuous outpatient consultation

This mode of consultation is typically for treatment of possession cults. The belief is that symptoms in a patient are caused by a potentially good spirit, and the benevolent spirit wishes to be recognized. The spirit can be expressed in possession or possession trance of the patient. An initiation in a possession cult under the continuous supervision of the healer is required (Peltzer, 1996b). Traditional healers, with renown in spirit mediation, tend to provide this form of consultation. Examples of traditional healer groups with this expertise include the "Zar" in Ethiopia (Taha, Ahmed, & Mohamed, 1989), "Rab" in Senegal (Zempléni, 1969), and "Vimbuza" in northern Malawi (Peltzer, 1987). The Orisa cults in Nigeria have a similar function (Prince, 1974). Often healers who are members of these spirit mediation cults perform dances accompanied by drumming, clapping hands, and songs leading to a kinetic trance.

Sacrificial rituals are prevalent with traditional healers who provide continuous outpatient consultation (Machleidt & Peltzer, 1991; Prince, 1966;Zempléni, 1977). An example of a sacrifial ceremony in Malawi includes the following stages: (1) symbolic or token sacrifice; (2) calling the spirits and spirit possession; (3) preparations and songs; (4) the killing of the sacrifice; (5) preparation, fumigation, and eating of the sacrifice; and (6) protection rites (Peltzer, 1987). The expression of strong affects during sacrificial or possession rites is common, and patients may experience total psychic and physical exhaustion for which close supervision by the healer is required (Machleidt & Peltzer, 1991).

Traditional healers in the spirit mediation cult profession may, as part of the socialization process of their trainees (who are patients presumed to be possessed by yet unrecognized benevolent spirits), model advanced techniques in spiritual mediation. For example, the healer may speak to several spiritual agents to access one that would be most divining of the patient's problems. In the case of a daughter in-law with a psychosomatic illness believed to be influenced by departed members of the extended family, the indigenous healer could demonstrate the following sequence of possession by spiritual agents relevant to the patient's case: (1) healer intercedes with unknown (nonfamily) spirit to name the cause of the illness; and (2) the healer intercedes with the family-of-origin spirit (e.g., that of a departed mother or grandmother) to check on any grievances (which could include not paying regular homage to the spirit through family get-togethers). The patient could be possessed during the treatment by a spirit wanting to assert itself, demand recognition, or suggest a treatment regimen. Continuous healer supervision is needed for this mode of consultation as part of the socialization process into ritual possession, to ensure that support for the patient is readily available in times of recurring symptoms, and to assist the patient to explore or express deeper emotions that may occur with spiritual possession (Peltzer, 1995).

The inpatient setting

Inpatient treatment can take place in the family house of the healer or in a specifically erected house in the village or community of the healer. The inpatient treatment in the house of the healer is usually possible only for one to three patients, often including relatives. According to observations of the second author in Ghana, Nigeria, and Zimbabwe (Peltzer, 1992) such a treatment setting can be used specifically for mentally ill patients. Occasionally, a traditional healer can treat five to ten inpatients in his or her family house (Peltzer, 1992).

Mentally ill patients with aggression or severe hallucinations may be physically restrained outside the healer's house during the daytime hours. However, the patients are able to communicate freely with their environment (e.g., with pedestrians passing by) (Peltzer, 1992). Inpatient treatment in healing centers or villages is also available for patients presenting with acute symptoms of a physical or psychosomatic illness. For example, the healer Patriensa of the Ashanti region in Ghana owned a large cocoa plantation including a primary school and other infrastructure for her inpatient clients (Appiah-Kubi, 1981).

The organization of treatment centers in such healing communities involves a chief healer in his or her instrumental and emotional expressive healing function, healer assistants (or trainees), patients, and relatives. The environment is typically a village milieu that offers, on the one hand, real-life situations with activities like fetching water, washing, or cooking and, on the other hand, a modified milieu due to the healing activities taking place. The treatment goal is a progressive resocialization of the patient into culturally adapted forms of community life, including spiritual solidarity with the ancestors. A relative cares for the patient in the healing center to facilitate the assessment and treatment of the familial context of the psychosocial disorder (Peltzer, 1987).

LEGAL AND PROFESSIONAL ISSUES

As noted previously, traditional healers are recognized medical practitioners in many jurisdictions across Africa (Inggs, 2007; Jayasuriya & Jayasuriya, 2002; Lazarus et al., 2006). For example, Jayasuriya and Jayasuriya (2002) reported statutory definitions of traditional medicine and traditional health care practitioner in the 1994 Public Health Code of Burkina Faso and the 1997 Public Health Code of Guinea. These definitions derive from the WHO definition as previously cited. The Guinean Code also has definitions for traditional therapists, traditional midwives, herbalists, and medico-druggists.

Traditional health care practitioners, in preparation for professional practice, are taught by village elders, herbalists, or diviners. Lesolang-Pitje (2000) and Rudnick (2000) observed that the training to become a traditional healer is a long, complex, and highly demanding process. Although the training of traditional healers is mainly via apprenticeship and informal, it nevertheless covers both theoretical and practical aspects. Rudnick also notes further that training is paced in accordance with the individual's needs and talents.

There are current efforts to organize training of traditional health workers through formal instruction. For instance, the Medical School of the University of Kwazulu-Natal recently conducted a series of training workshops for traditional healers in efforts to improve their role in health care delivery and as a prelude to integration of traditional health care systems into the mainstream system. WHO has sponsored seminars and workshops to train traditional birth attendants and midwives in many African countries. Provincial governments in South Africa have set up directorates to help the public access registered traditional healers (Packree, 2007).

The marketing of traditional medicines is also being formally regulated in some African countries. For example, in Mali, one of the statutory responsibilities of the Office of Pharmacy is to promote the research and manufacture of medicines, particularly drugs based on medicinal plants. The National Pharmaceutical Office of Benin is required to oversee the export of medicinal plants; the Universal Medicimen and Herbalist Council of Lesotho is in charge of licensing traditional healers including herbalists, while in Morocco there is a statutory prohibition on the simultaneous practice of the profession of physician, dental surgeon, and midwife, on the one hand, and that of herbalist, on the other (Jayasuriya & Jayasuriya, 2002).

Ethical practices among traditional healers vary widely. For example, most treatments by healers are in the public domain and involve other patients or unrelated people seeking help from the same healer. For example, others witnessing the treatment may be asked to facilitate ritual ceremonies through song and dance. Some healers may seek to enhance their credibility by telling patients of their successful treatment of similar conditions in well known people in the community. Some traditional healers have committed sexual offenses on their patients after convincing the patients that the sexual molestation was part of the treatment. However, there are many traditional healers who practice with distinction and the highest ethical standards.

ISSUES FOR RESEARCH AND OTHER FORMS OF SCHOLARSHIP

Conducting research on various aspects of African traditional healing can help find out "modern truth in ancient wisdom" (Atherton, 2007). The question of the efficacy of African traditional healing methods remains a significant issue for research. For example, few studies have examined the mechanisms of action by which indigenous healing achieves its effects (Bibeau, 1979; Peltzer 1987, 1992; Prince, 1966). For example, the psychic treatment effects of herbal remedies have not been studied much, although a number of healers use plants with active psychotropic components (Makanjuola & Jaiyeola 1987). Although these efforts have greatly enhanced the development of research in medicinal plants and in biochemical medicine, research into the efficacy of the specific healing techniques employed by the healers received very little attention (Sabuni, 2007). Research to understand better the religious framework of African healing, especially with regard to the moral, emotional, and spiritual aspects of healing and the consideration of beliefs, attitudes, environmental influences and natural remedies in the treatment of ill health, is also needed. It seems important not only to study both the repertoire of herbal remedies (Harjula, 1980; Iwu, 1986), but also to investigate in-depth culture-specific treatment methods (Peltzer & Machleidt, 1992; Twumasi, 1984).

Research can also provide a better understanding of some implicit theories of causation of ill health or recovery held by African indigenous healers that parallel those by Western theoreticians (Mpofu, 2003). Drawing the parallels potentially could lead to better collaboration between African indigenous health care systems and Western systems to the benefit of the patients or clients.

Traditional healers may be called to provide expert testimony in court proceedings where witchcraft is alleged in some jurisdictions such as Zimbabwe. The types of evidence from metaphysical explanations may conflict with the transparent and verifiable evidence scrutiny required by modern law or science.

Research should determine the authenticity of alternative ways of knowing where the dignity and integrity of individuals is likely to be compromised from claims or allegations of witchcraft or other forms of supernatural possession.

SUMMARY AND CONCLUSIONS

The health care needs of a majority of tradition-directed Africans are provided by indigenous healers. They use a variety of physical, psychological, and spiritual resources to treat debilitating health conditions. Indigenous healers are often the first choice for health care needs, although most Africans would also consult the modern biomedical health system for some types of illness or those not responsive to healing by traditional healers. National and regional governments on the African continent recognize the traditional healers as partners in health service provision. There is growing support for the work of indigenous healers through legislation and policy, the professionalization of indigenous healing, and research funding.

Research on indigenous healing has thus far focused mostly on concepts of illness and disease and also conditions for which indigenous healing appears to be efficacious. Research into the effectiveness of specific treatments for known health conditions is evolving. A minority of traditional healers are engaged in research into the indigenous treatments they provide.

Indigenous healers use both inpatient and outpatient consultation with clients of patients. Mainly, the consultations are episodic or on an as-needed basis. Inpatient consultations are typical with people with chronic illness or disease. Village treatment centers are less prevalent than those in which healers consult and treat at their homes or the homesteads of clients.

Treatment approaches used by traditional healers encompass family therapy, group therapy, biofeedback techniques, herbal therapy, scarification, music therapy, and spiritual interventions. These treatments are provided within a family or community collective milieu. Family is defined broadly to include the living and also departed ancestors. Healers have the highest respect of their clients or patients, and are perceived to intercede in health issues with the ancestors.

Case Study 1.3: Woman "Flew" in Basket on Witchcraft Mission (Retrieved from NewZimbabwe.com)

A Harare (Zimbabwe) magistrate called in witchcraft experts after a woman from a rural village about 120 km outside the city was found naked outside her brother-in-law's house in a suburb of the city. She claimed she flew there in a winnowing basket with two others on a mission to kill him.

The woman was seen by passers-by outside the house wearing "red headgear" and "some black strings around the waist" just after 6 a.m. on a Sunday morning. Dozens of people soon gathered, some throwing stones at her until the brother-in-law she was on a mission to kill rescued her from the mob.

The woman admitted to a charge of public indecency because of nudity, and prosecutors recommended that the woman be given a noncustodial sentence. Prosecutors said the woman will now be a state witness in a future prosecution of her father-in-law and aunt, whom she claims "flew her" to Harare on the mission to kill her brother-in-law. She also claimed the trio "took off" from a cemetery in a neighboring village in the dead of the night, but once they got to the suburb in Harare on their mission to kill, she balked when asked to carry out the killing. Her father-in-law and aunt then flew off, leaving her stranded at the property.

Refusing to take chances, a Harare magistrate assigned the trial said the woman should be remanded in custody just in case she "flies back" to her village. He also tasked the prison service to ensure that she did not escape or fly back to her village. Experts from the Zimbabwe Traditional Healers Association (ZINATHA) were expected in court to provide guidance on the bizarre case. The practice of witchcraft is illegal in Zimbabwe after witchcraft laws were changed in 2006. Under the colonial-era laws that existed before then, it was a crime to accuse anyone of practicing witchcraft. Under the Zimbabwe Criminal Law (Codification and Reform) Act of 2004, anyone accusing another individual of witchcraft must show proof of the allegations and judicial officers can rely on expert evidence to determine whether or not a practice constitutes witchcraft.

The woman's father-in law and aunt are expected to appear in court to answer to charges of practicing witchcraft.

Questions

1. What alternative explanations are possible for the woman's behavior?
2. What evidence would traditional healer experts likely draw on in this case? How credible and trustworthy would the evidence be to:
   - Other traditional healers?
   - The lay public?
   - The accused?
   - The judicial system?
   - Human rights advocates?
3. Should modern African courts be involved in trying witchcraft cases? Support your answer with reasons.
4. What alternative services should be available to people believing to be engaged in witchcraft or to have been bewitched?

REFERENCES

Africa Advisory Committee for Health Research and Development, AACHRD, (2000). Enhancing research into traditional medicine in the Africa region. A working paper prepared for the 21st Session of the African Advisory Committee for Health Research and Development AACHRD, Port Louis, Mauritius, April 22–25, 2000.

Anumonye, A. (1973). *Nigerian traditional healers and management of psychiatric illness*. Lagos: University of Lagos.

Appiah-Kubi, K. (1981). *Man cures, God heals: Religion and medical practice among the Akans of Ghana*. New York: Friendship Press.

Assen, G. P. M. (1991). Social consequences of psychosis for psychotic patients in Western Province, Kenya, after treatment. In S. O. Okpaku (Ed.), *Mental health in Africa and the Americas today* (pp. 33–52). Nashville, TN: Chrisolith Books.

Atherton, K. (2007). *Holistic healing*. Pindari Herb Farm. Retrieved October 27, 2010 from http://pindariherbfarm.com/healing/holiheal.htm

Bascom, W. (1969). *If a divination: Communication between gods and men in West Africa*. Bloomington: Indiana University Press.

Bibeau, G. (1979). *De la maladie à la guérison: Essai d'analyse systémique de la medicine des Angbandi du Zaire*. Doctoral dissertation, Laval University.

Butler, K, (1998). Beyond the rational. *NETWORKER – Family Therapy*, *24*(1), 24–37.

Chavunduka, G. L. (1978). *Traditional healers and the Shona patient*. Gwelo, Zimbabwe: Mambo Press.

Comaroff, J. (1980). Healing and the cultural order. The case of Baralong Boo Ratshidi of Southern Africa. *American Ethnologist*, 7, 637–57.

Conserveafrica (2006). Overview of medicinal plants and traditional medicine in Africa. Retrieved October 27, 2010 from http://www.conserveafrica.org.uk/medical_plants.pdf/

Corin, E., & Bibeau, G. (1980). Psychiatric perspectives in Africa. Part II: The traditional viewpoint. *Transcultural Psychiatric Research Review*, *17*, 205–33.

Crapanzano, V. (1975). Saints, Jnun, and dreams: An essay in Moroccan ethnopsychology. *Psychiatry*, *38*, 145–59.

Edgerton, R. O. (1980). Traditional treatment for mental illness in Africa. *Culture, Medicine & Psychiatry*, *4*, 167–90.

Edwards, S., & Edwards, D. (2009). Jung's breath-body and African spiritual healing. *Journal of Psychology in Africa*, *20*, 561–64.

Gelfand, M. (1964). *Witchdoctor: Traditional medicine man of Rhodesia*. London: Harvill.

Gielen, U. P., Fish, J. M., & Draguns, J. G. (Eds). (2004). *Handbook of culture, therapy, and healing*. Mahwah, NJ: Lawrence Erlbaum & Associates.

Good, C. M., & Kimani, V. V. (1980). Urban traditional medicine: A Nairobi case-study. *East African Medical Journal*, *57*, 301–16.

Green, E. (1994). *AIDS and STIs in Africa: Bridging the gap between traditional healers and modern medicine*. Boulder, CO: Westview Press.

Harjula, R. (1980). *Mirau and his practice: A study of the ethnomedicinal repertoire of a Tanzanian herbalist*. London: Tri-med.

Harley, D. A. (2006). Indigenous healing practices among rural elderly African Americans. *International Journal of Disability, Development and Education*, *53*, 433–52.

Homsy, J., King, R., Tenywa, J., Kyeyune, P., Opio, A., & Balaba, D. (2004). Defining minimum standards of practice for incorporating African traditional medicine into HIV/AIDS prevention, care, and support: A regional initiative in Eastern and Southern Africa. *The Journal of Alternative and Complementary Medicine*, *10*(5), 905–10.

Inggs, M. (2007). Plant strippers threaten traditional healing. *Sunday Tribune*, Sunday September 9, 2007, Durban, South Africa: The Independent Newspapers Limited, p. 2.

Iwu, M. M. (1986). *African ethnomedicine*. Enugu: Snaap Press.

Jahoda, G. (1961). Traditional healers and other institutions concerned with mental illness in Ghana. *International Journal of Social Psychiatry*, *7*, 245–68.

Janzen, J. (1978). *The quest for therapy in Lower Zaire*. Berkeley: University of California Press.

Jayasuriya, D. C., & Jayasuriya, S. (2002). Legislation and regulation of traditional systems of medicine – systems, practitioners and herbal products. In R. R. Chaudhury & U. M. Rafei (Eds.), *Traditional medicine in Asia* (pp. 195–208). New Delhi: World Health Organization.

Jilek, W. G. (1993). Traditional medicine relevant to psychiatry. In N. Sartorius, G. Girolamo, G. Andrews, & G. A. German (Eds.), *Treatment of mental disorders* (pp. 341–90). Washington, DC: American Psychiatric Press.

Katz, R., & Wexler, A. (1989). Healing and transformations: Lessons from indigenous people (Botswana). In K. Peltzer & P. O. Ebigbo (Eds.), *Clinical psychology in Africa* (pp. 19–46). Frankfurt/Maim: IKO Verlag.

Kayombo, E. J., Mbwambo, Z. H., & Massila, M. (2005). Role of traditional healers in psychosocial support in caring for the orphans: A case of Dar-es Salaam City, Tanzania. *Journal of Ethnobiology and Ethnomedicine*, *1*:3 doi:10.1186/1746-4269–1.

Kleinman, A. (1980). *Patients and healers in the context of culture*. Berkeley: University of California Press.

Krauss, G. (1990). *Kefu Elak: Traditionelle Medizin in Oku (Kamerun)*. Gőttingen: Edition Re.

Last, M., & Chavunduka, G. L. (1986). *The professionalization of African medicine*. Manchester, UK: Manchester University Press.

Lazarus, S., Bojuwoye, O., Chireshe, R., Myambo, K., Akotia, C., Mogaji, A., & Tchombe, T. (2006). Community psychology in Africa: Views from across the continent. *Journal of Psychology in Africa*, *16*(2), 147–60.

Lesolang-Pitje, N. (2000). Initiation into traditional healing: A personal experience. In S. N. Madu, P. K. Baguma, & A. Pritz (Eds.), *Psychotherapy and African reality* (pp. 120–35). Sovenga: University of the North Press.

Levers, L. L. (2006a). Traditional healing as indigenous knowledge: Its relevance to HIV/AIDS in Southern AFRICA and implications for counselors. *Journal of Psychology in Africa.*, *16*, 87–100.

Levers, L. L. (2006b). Samples of indigenous healing: The path of good medicine. *International Journal of Disability, Development and Education*, *53*, 479–88.

Levi-Strauss, C. (1963). *Structural anthropology*. New York: Basic Books.

Liu, J. (2007). The use of herbal medicines in early drug development for the treatment of HIV infections and AIDS. *Expert Opinion on Investigative Drugs*, *16*(9), 1355–64.

Machleidt, W., & Peltzer, K. (1991). The Chilopa ceremony: A sacrificial ritual for mentally (spiritually) ill patients in a traditional healing centre in Malawi. *Psychiatria Danubina: An International Multidisciplinary Journal*, *3*, 205–27.

Makanjuola, R. O. A. (1987). Yoruba traditional healers in psychiatry: I. Healers' concepts of the nature and aetiology of mental disorders. *African Journal of Medicine & Medical Sciences*, *16*, 53–9.

Makanjuola, R. O. A., & Jaiyeola, A. A. (1987). Yoruba traditional healers in Psychiatry: II Management of psychiatric disorders. *African Journal of Medicine & Medical Sciences*, *16*, 61–73.

Marks, L. (2006). Global health crisis: Can indigenous healing practices offer a valuable resource. *International Journal of Disability, Development and Education*, *53*, 453–70.

McMillen, H. (2004). The adapting healer: Pioneering through shifting epidemiological and sociocultural landscapes. *Social Science & Medicine*, *59*, 889–902.

Moodley, R., & West, W. (Eds.). (2005). *Integrating traditional healing practices into counseling and psychotherapy*. Thousand Oaks, CA: SAGE Publications.

Mpofu, E. (2003). Conduct disorder in children: Presentation, treatment options and cultural efficacy in an African setting. *International Journal of Disability, Community and Rehabilitation, 2*(1). Retrieved November 18, 2010 from http://www.ijdcr.ca/Vol.02_01_CAN/articles/mpofu.shtml

Mpofu, E. (2006). Majority world health care traditions intersect indigenous and complementary and alternative medicine. *International Journal of Disability, Development and Education*, *53*, 375–80.

Mshana, G., Plummer, M. L., Wamoyi, J., Zachayo, S., Ross, D. A., & Wight, D. (2006) 'She was bewitched and caught an illness similar to AIDS': AIDS and sexually transmitted infection causation beliefs in rural northern Tanzania. *Culture, Health & Sexuality*, *8*(1), 45–58.

Mune, J. O. (1977). How I acquired the knowledge of traditional medicine. In P. Singer (Ed.), *Traditional healing: new science or new colonialism?* (pp. 54–9). New York: Conch.

Mzimkulu, K. G. (2000). *An investigation of perspectives and practices of African traditional healers when managing psychosis.* Master of Psychology degree thesis, University of the Western Cape, Bellville, South Africa.

Mzimkulu, K. G., & Simbayi, L. C. (2006). Perspectives and practices of Xhosa-speaking African traditional healers when managing psychosis. *International Journal of Disability, Development and Education*, *53*, 417–32.

Ngubane, H. (1977). *Body and mind in Zulu medicine.* London: Academic Press.

Ovuga, E., Boardman, J., & Oluka, E. G. A. (1999). Traditional healers and mental illness in Uganda. *Psychiatric Bulletin*, *23*, 276–9.

Packree, S. (2007). Traditional healing directorate set up. *Daily News*, Thursday August 30, 2007, Durban, South Africa: The Independent Newspaper Limited, p. 5.

Parrott, C. (1999). Towards an integration of science, art and morality: The role of values in psychology. *Counselling Psychology Quarterly*, *12*, 5–24.

Peltzer, K. (1981/82). Die Arbeit der Nana Afua Saah, einer traditionellen Heilerin aus Kumasi. *Ethnomedizin*, *7*, 47–89.

Peltzer, K. (1985). Traditionelle Traumtherapie in Malawi (Traditional dream therapy in Malawi). *Schreibheft: Zeitschrift für Literatur*, *25*, 763–95.

Peltzer, K. (1987). *Traditional healing and psychosocial health care in Malawi.* Heidelberg: Asanger.

Peltzer, K. (1989). The description and analysis of healing interactions of some traditional healers in Zimbabwe. *Sociologus: A Journal for Empirical Ethno-sociology and Ethno-psychology*, *39*, 113–22.

Peltzer, K. (1992). *Traditionelle Heilkunde bei Ashanti und Shona* (Traditional healing in Ashanti and Shona). Bremen: Informationszentrum Afrika.

Peltzer, K. (1995). *Psychology and health in African cultures: Examples of ethnopsychotherapeutic practice.* Frankfurt/Maim: IKO Verlag.

Peltzer, K. (1996a). Arbeit und Organisation von traditionellen Heilkundigen in Lesotho (Work and organisation of traditional healers in Lesotho). *Kölner Beiträge zur Ethnopsychologie und Transkulturellen Psychologie*, *2*, 67–92.

Peltzer, K. (1996b). Psychotherapy and culture in Africa. *World Health*, *49*, 18–19.

Peltzer, K. (2005). African socialisation: The application of cross-cultural methodology. *Journal of Psychology in Africa*, *15*(1), 105–8.

Peltzer, K., Friend-du Preez, N., Ramlagan, S., & Fomundam, H. (2008) Use of Traditional, Complementary and Alternative Medicine (TCAM) for HIV patients prior to initiating antiretroviral therapy in KwaZulu-Natal, South Africa. *BMC Public Health*, 8(1), 255; DOI:10.1186/1471-2458-8-255.

Peltzer, K., & Machleidt, W. (1992). A traditional (African) approach towards the therapy of schizophrenia and its comparison with western models. *The International Journal for Therapeutic and Supportive Organisations*, *13*, 203–17.

Peltzer, K., & Mngqundaniso, N. (2008) Patients consulting traditional health practitioners in the context of HIV/AIDS in urban areas in KwaZulu-Natal, South Africa. *African Journal of Traditional, Complementary and Alternative Medicine*, *5*(4), 370–9.

Pfeiffer, W. M. (1974). "Primitive" und moderne Psychotherapie. *Hippokrates*, *45*, 415–32.

Pfeiffer, W. M. (1991). Wodurch wird ein Gespräch therapeutisch? Zur kulturellen Bedingtheit psychotherapeutischer Methoden. *Psychotherapie, Psychosomatik, Medizinische Psychologie*, *41*, 93–154.

Prince, R. H. (1966). *Ifa: Yoruba divination and sacrifice.* Ibadan: University Press.

Prince, R. H. (1974). Indigenous Yoruba psychiatry. In A. Kiev (Ed.), *Magic, faith and healing* (pp. 155–92). New York: Free Press.

Reynolds-Whyte, S. R. (1991). Knowledge and power in Nyole divination. In P. M. Peek (Ed.), *African divination systems: Ways of knowing* (pp. 153–72). Bloomington: Indiana University Press.

Romero-Daza, N. (2002). Traditional medicine in Africa. *The ANNALS of the American Academy of Political and Social Science*, *583*, 173–6.

Rudnick, H. (2000). *Traditional healing in South Africa. Johannesburg, South Africa:* Rank Afrikaans University Press.

Sabuni, L. P. (2007). Dilemma with the local perception of causes of illnesses in Central Africa: Muted concept but prevalent in everyday life. *Qualitative Health Research*, *17*(9), 1280–91.

Schmidbauer, W. (1969) Schamanismus und Psychotherapie. *Psychologische Rundschau*, *20*, 29–47.

Simwaka, A., Peltzer, K., & Banda, D. (2007) Indigenous healing in Malawi. *Journal of Psychology in Africa*, *17*(1/2), 155–62.

Sow, I. (1980). *Anthropological structures of madness in Africa.* New York: International Universities Press.

Staugard, F. (1986). *Traditional healthcare in Botswana.* In M. Last & G. Chavunduka (Eds.), *The professionalization of African medicine* (pp.51–86). Manchester, UK: Manchester University Press.

Taha, E. B., Ahmed, A. H. A., & Mohamed, F. O. (1989) A study of the therapeutics of Zar. In K. Peltzer, & P. O. Ebigbo (Eds.), *Clinical psychology in Africa* (pp. 451–61). Frankfurt/Maim: IKO Verlag.

Teuton, J., Bentall, R., & Dowrick, C. (2007) Conceptualizing psychosis in Uganda: The perspective of indigenous and religious healers. *Transcultural Psychiatry*, *44*(1), 79–114.

Torrey, E. F. (1986). *Witchdoctors and psychiatrists: The common roots of psychotherapy and its future.* Northvale, NJ: Emerson Hall Publishers.

Twumasi, P. A. (1975). *Medical systems in Ghana.* Accra: Ghana Publishing Co.

Twumasi, P. A. (1984) *Professionalization of traditional medicine in Zambia.* Lusaka: Institute for African Studies.

UNESCO (1994). *Traditional knowledge into the twenty-first century, nature & resources*, Vol. 30, no. 2. Paris: UNESCO.

Warren, D. M. (1974). *Disease, medicine, and religion among the Techiman Bono of Ghana.* Doctoral dissertation, Indiana University.

World Health Organization (WHO). (1978). *The promotion and development of traditional medicine.* Technical reports services, 666. Geneva: Authors.

World Health Organization (WHO). (2001). Legal status of traditional medicines and complementary/alternative medicine: A world review. Retrieved November 12, 2010 from http://whqlibdoc.who.int/hq/2001/WHO_EDM-TRM-2001.2.pdf

Zempléni, A. (1969). *L'interprétation et la thérapie traditionelle du désordre mental chez les Wolof et les Lébou (Sénegal).* Doctoral dissertation, Paris University.

Zempléni, A. (1977) From symptom to sacrifice: the story of Khady Fall. In V. Crapanzano & V. Garrison (Eds.), *Case studies in spirit possession* (pp. 87–139). New York: John Wiley & Sons.

SELF-CHECK EXERCISES

1. Define indigenous healing. How does context inform the notion of indigenous healing?
2. Outline the core beliefs about health and well-being that influence African indigenous healing practices.
3. Consider any three major approaches to healing used by African indigenous healers.What is the rationale of each of these methods? Speculate on how they likely achieve their therapeutic effects.
4. Distinguish between consultation procedures used by African traditional healers and their patients.
5. What is the evidence for the efficacy of indigenous healing practices?

FIELD-BASED EXPERIENTIAL EXERCISES

1. Interview a traditional healer to determine his or her area of expertise and perceptions of effective treatments for the conditions he or she treats. How are his or her treatments explained by his or her theory of well-being or disease?
2. Interview a patient of a traditional healer to find out (a) how he or she was referred to the traditional healer; (b) presenting health condition and personal story about the etiology of the condition; (c) perceived efficacy of the treatment from the consulting traditional healer; (d) sources of healer credibility that influence treatment participation; and (e) history of prior healer consultations and projected outcomes from the current consultation.
3. Consult three different divinatory agents with the same problem (e.g., relationship problem) and compare their responses.
4. Find two examples of dreams with a traditional dream interpretation and discuss culturally different concepts of dream interpretations.
5. Observe a traditional healer in practice to discover the process of naming or diagnosis, especially with regard to how the healer gathers information using a divination instrument, divination songs, physical examination, and observation for the identification/clarification of presenting problem and how he or she arrives at the conclusion with regard to intervention strategies to address the problem.

MULTIPLE-CHOICE QUESTIONS

1. Diagnosis is an essential treatment procedure for the gathering of information about a patient's health conditions and for arriving at a conclusion as to appropriate interventions based on the information gathered. In the diagnosis of a patient's health conditions, all except which of the following is not a process employed by traditional healers?
   a. Dream interpretation
   b. Divination
   c. Physical examination of patient
   d. Interview
   e. Administration of herbal mixtures
2. Which one of the following is not a treatment method, or intervention strategy, employed by traditional health care practitioners?
   a. Physical activity with management of interpersonal relationships
   b. Use of expectation
   c. Use of symbolism and enactment
   d. Dream interpretation, proverbs, and story telling
   e. Herbal infusion with the aid of a syringe and needle
3. Cleansing treatment typifies the holistic nature of African traditional health care delivery because it:
   a. Involves the whole person including body, mind, emotions, and spirit
   b. Takes place in the healer's residence
   c. Involves the cleaning of the head, stomach, and the outer body of the patient
   d. Involves interactions with the family
   e. Involves interaction with the environment
4. The regalia worn by traditional healers is related to the use of expectation as treatment strategy. Which of the following is NOT an attribute of the traditional healer's regalia contributing to the patient's expectation regarding the capability of the healer?
   a. Indicates the healer is no ordinary person but with elevated status in the society
   b. Indicates the presence of spiritual beings
   c. Indicates supernatural powers
   d. Identified with unusual brightly colored garment
   e. Evidence of great accomplishment that must be respected
5. Research and practice in traditional health care must be guided by ethical considerations including all EXCEPT which of the following requirements?
   a. Traditional health care practice should conform to the traditional customary laws and ethics.
   b. Healers should respect the principle of obtaining individual and collective consent in accordance with established procedures.
   c. Treatment should be conducted in a mutually understood and agreed on language.
   d. Research and professional practice in traditional health care must avoid the contentious issue of intellectual property rights.
   e. Healers must respect confidentiality of information including proper agreement on the boundaries of use of information.
6. Salient features that should be captured by legislations guiding professional practice in traditional health care should be all BUT which of the following?
   a. Traditional health care must have criteria for identifying practitioners.

b. Roles of consultation, diagnosis, and care procedures making use of traditional and nontraditional methods should be specified.
c. Training of the practitioners in an informal context should be supplemented with that in structured, formal settings.
d. Traditional medicine has no efficacy for the treatment of mental illness.
e. Healer perspectives of disease and treatment in accordance with the traditions of their practice must be respected.

Answers to the multiple-choice questions are provided at the back of the book

2 The Role of the Oral Tradition in Counseling People of African Ancestry

Jacobus G. Maree and Cecilia M. du Toit

OVERVIEW. In this chapter, we consider the role of the oral tradition in counseling people of African ancestry. We first analyze the meaning and significance of aspects of the oral tradition and some of its constituent genres, such as myth, legend, and fable, in an African context. Second, we contemplate the potential place of the oral tradition in actual counseling with clients of African ancestry. More particularly, we reconsider the role that the oral tradition can play in the healing process of people of African ancestry, who may have lost the sense of connectedness to a past that provided support in a variety of cultural contexts and traditional structures. We conclude by investigating two folktales and their role in a counseling session.

LEARNING OBJECTIVES

By the end of the chapter, the reader should be able to:

1. Discuss some of the different forms the oral tradition in an African context may assume.
2. Explain the role of the oral tradition in counseling clients of African ancestry.
3. Analyze the meaning and significance of the oral tradition and some of its constituent genres, such as myth, legend, and fable, in an African context.
4. Critique the unwarranted emphasis on a positivist approach to counseling in an African context.
5. Express an understanding of the importance to utilize the oral tradition in the counseling of people of African ancestry.
6. Discuss the interventive use of folklore (diagnosis, well-being, and development) in counseling.

INTRODUCTION

Archbishop Desmond Tutu has the following to say regarding the way in which (telling stories of) the past shapes the present and future of both individuals and countries: "The past, it has been said, is another country. The way its stories are told and the way they are heard change as the years go by. The spotlight gyrates, exposing old lies and illuminating new truths. As a fuller picture emerges, a new piece of the jigsaw puzzle of our past settles into place" (Tutu, 1999a, p. 4). The oral traditions, as an integral element of Africa's (past, present, and future) story, present a vast but hitherto largely untapped counseling resource for people of African ancestry, as we attempt to explicate in this chapter.

Even today, in both urban and rural Kwa-Zulu Natal province, South Africa, havoc caused by floods following in the wake of the tropical storms that regularly hit the Indian Ocean coastline leads to the retelling of an ancient legend. When homes in low-lying areas and settlements on the riverbanks are swept away by the torrents of swollen rivers, Zulu elders and younger compatriots alike trace in the sky the path the Great Snake has once again taken in its search for a new pool of water to make its lair. In such times, the destitution of the victims in the aftermath of a natural disaster is likened to the helplessness of humans who fall prey to the inexorable actions of the Great Snake. Since ancient times, in all parts of the world, calamitous forces of nature have been considered "acts of God" and a form of divine retribution for a variety of human transgressions. Throughout the millennia, notions of prosperity or adversity were linked to the relationship an individual, or in ancient and Biblical times, a whole nation, has with God. In most African countries today, notions of health and well-being are inextricably linked to a person's relations with the other, whether the divine or with members of the family or clan (Watson, McMahon, Mkhize, Schweitzer, & Mpofu, 2009). In traditional African communities, adversity and suffering are viewed by most people as the result of the disregard of God (*Utixho*) and the ancestors. Without restitution, the influence of negative forces will continue unabated, resulting not only in illness, but also in death.

As stated earlier, this chapter considers the role that the oral tradition can play in the healing process of people of African ancestry, who may have lost the sense of connectedness to a past that provided succour in a variety of cultural contexts and traditional structures. Here, the term *oral tradition* includes the full range of the oral tradition, viz. *folklore*, *orality*, *orature*, *storytelling*, *folktales*, *fairy tales*, *myths*, and *fables*.

A key element lost in the African Diaspora is the notion of *Ubuntu* (Watson et al., 2009), which, *inter alia*, refers to a common humanity, an interconnectedness that used to provide relief and a meaningful engagement in communal life and supported the ethical–moral self. This, then, is what forms part of a counselor's commitment to a client, and it is this aspect that plays a central role in the African oral tradition. (In this chapter, the word *counselor* is used interchangeably with the word *psychologist*.) Further, our perspective on the way in which the concept *counseling* can best be defined, maybe summed up by Savickas' (2007a) definition of counseling as a focus on "the daily life adjustment issues faced by reasonably well-adjusted people, particularly as they cope with career transition and personal development" (p. 183). He advocates establishing a cross-national professional identity for the field, encouraging indigenous models, methods, and materials and promoting international collaboration (Savickas, 2007a; see also Leong & Ponterotto, 2003; Skovholt, Hansen, Goh, Romano, & Thomas 2005).

Counseling Questions

In the context of the current chapter, some typical counseling questions may be:

- Is the oral tradition still "valid" and used in the twenty-first century, especially in urban environments?
- Can the oral tradition be utilized to identify the person's personality traits internally and externally?
  - If so, how can this be done?
- How can the oral tradition be used to illustrate persons' patterns of addressing internal and external challenges?
- How can exploitation of the oral tradition (including storytelling) be used to facilitate sustained well-being in clients of African ancestry?
- What outcomes of clients' stories can be activated to construct more positive futures?

BACKGROUND

For thousands of years before the advent of writing systems, indigenous knowledge and tribal customs were kept alive through an oral tradition that was passed on from generation to generation. Living with a particular group of people endowed an individual with common terminology, ethnic-specific skills, and traditions that helped the tribe survive in a unique environment. The shared understanding acquired by such a band of people throughout the ages was carried best by a distinctive oral tradition that preserved and perpetuated the spiritual, ethical, cultural, and moral wisdom of the community. While the oral tradition served preindustrial communities by giving emotional support, its delights were also spontaneously experienced by all members of a society who participated in the recounting and communal listening experiences of a cache of narratives.

The central role as chroniclers of a society was performed by poets and storytellers. While entertaining or instructing their audiences in private consultation or public performance, the shamans, medicine men, and sangomas were also, in Jungian terms, the curators of traditions. The public voice of the folklorist served the collective conscience, because the tales that were recounted symbolically depicted the unconscious processes of the psyche (Jung, 1959). Jung indicated that in fictional narratives, characters with strong archetypal features would subconsciously resonate with a large audience. He had the following to say about the essence of tribal lore: "Tribal lore is always sacred and dangerous ... They contain a revealed knowledge that was originally hidden, and they set forth the secrets of the soul in glorious images" (Jung, 1959, p. 5).

Jung distinguished between archetypes, and what he called "archetypal ideas" (1959, p. 5). The term *archetype*, according to Jung, applies indirectly to collective representations because it designates "only those psychic contents which have not yet been submitted to conscious elaboration." He, however, pointed out that while "on the higher levels of esoteric teaching" (Jung, 1959, p. 5), archetypes appear in forms that clearly reveal the critical and evaluating influence of conscious elaboration, manifestations of archetypes as encountered in visions, dreams, and myths are more immediate and naïve.

While archetypes can be found in nearly all forms of literature, archetypal motifs predominate in the oral tradition. The succour of myth and the oral tradition, however, can be superseded in a modern urban setting, and consequently a negation of their value can cause people of African ancestry to feel they have lost the very traditions that had shaped their psyche throughout the ages.

However, where proponents of the oral tradition are still practicing their ancient profession today, as is the case with Gcina Mhlope, the highly acclaimed itinerant storyteller in South Africa, the effects are as immediate and mesmerizing as they have been throughout the ages:

> One of my favourite stories is about the woman who went down to the bottom of the sea to look for stories to bring back for the human world. I have told this tale to audiences in different countries all over the world, and so many times I have had the response: "You know, that story has made me realise that to find the answers I am looking for in my life, I need to look deep inside myself. I must search the depths of the ocean that is my own heart and soul." (Mhlope, 2003)

Based on earlier research, we use a number of working assumptions to guide this chapter (Ebersöhn & Eloff, 2006; Maree, 2005; Maree & Ebersöhn, 2002, 2006, 2008; Maree & Molepo, 2006). First, clients have a natural preference to be happy – and to tell their stories. Second, clients have access to a wide array of internal and external resources (or, if you will, stories), which could be pulled together to facilitate counseling. Whereas challenges that may have an impact on the achievement of happiness occur in clients

Discussion Box 2.1: Antiquity's Most Ancient Riddle

Once upon a time a most fearful creature, a Sphinx, sat at the gates of a Grecian city and asked a passers-by a riddle. If they failed to answer correctly, as all people did, the Sphinx killed and ate them on the spot. One day a brave stranger wished to enter the city and the Sphinx barred his way. "You will first answer the following question," the Sphinx said, baring his sharp teeth. "What monster has four legs in the morning, two legs in the afternoon, and three legs at night?" The young man, Oedipus was his name, thought deeply for a moment while watching the Sphinx rub his paws hungrily. "Ah," said Oedipus. "Man, of course. In the morning of his life he is a baby, crawling on all fours. When he grows older, he walks on two legs. As an old man he needs a crutch to help him walk." The Sphinx was so angry that he unfolded his wings and flew away, never to plague the city again, and Oedipus was taken into the city in triumph, to become king.

and their environments, storytelling, and the (re-)writing of their life stories can be successfully implemented by counselors to mediate an understanding of individual and collective strengths and assist clients to negotiate these challenges to facilitate healing and well-being (happiness) by building on existing strengths and dealing with weaknesses and barriers. Further, storytelling can be used to enhance counseling opportunities for clients via networking and collaboration skills; it can help clients negotiate major life transitions (e.g., dealing with loss) and assist practitioners to administer (viable, affordable) counseling to all clients by linking life stories and life choices.

In attempting to facilitate the development of clients, we attempt to effect personal agency by viewing clients as active agents in their personal development.

DEFINING THE ORAL TRADITION

One of the "uses of enchantment," as pointed out by Bettelheim (1976, p. 4) in his seminal work, is the value of literature – and specifically the genres myth, legend, folk, and fairy tale – in finding the "deeper meaning" in life, in the transcending of the "narrow confines of a self-cenetred existence." He goes on to say that the belief that the acquisition of "meaning" thus attained is

> necessary if a person is to be satisfied with himself and with what he is doing. In order not to be at the mercy of the vagaries of life, one must develop one's inner resources, so that one's emotions, imagination, and intellect mutually support and enrich one another. Our positive feelings give us the strength to develop our rationality: only hope for the future can sustain us in the adversities we unavoidably encounter. (Bettelheim, 1976, p. 4)

Bettelheim, together with his precursors Freud and Jung, wrote in the Euro-American tradition, and the question here arises to what extent the aesthetics of storytelling, myth, and legend shape the production of narrative in African contexts. This chapter asks what role the oral tradition can play in the lives of Africans today, and whether bespoke oral tradition can speak to the realities of contemporary, urban Africa and to people of African ancestry in the Diaspora. To do so, the chapter attempts to investigate the value of continuing traditional elements in a modern, largely urban, de-Africanized setting. It is easy to argue that the traditional African oral tradition, if not entirely lost in modernity, has been almost unrecognizably transformed through globalization, technocratization, and urbanization, thereby losing its power to provide a means through which people can attain some understanding of aspects that affect their lives.

RATIONALE FOR THE STUDY OF ORAL TRADITION

Even though the contents of folktales differ from context to context and from culture to culture, our research confirms the findings of others that, by and large, a number of universal themes emerges from any analysis of folktales, irrespective of context or culture. For the purpose of this chapter, the folktale, as a genre of the oral tradition, is selected and not one of the other, also distinctly event-cenetred categories such as the panegyric (praise poetry or eulogies delivered by court poets or *imbongi*), elegiac poetry, topical and political songs, or other more consciously literary genres such as rhymes, prose narratives, proverbs, riddles, and oratory. There are various reasons for selecting the folktale, with the limitations set by a single chapter being the most obvious. A more justifiable reason is that the folktale is the most visceral, least cerebral of the oral tradition's genres, and therefore, for want of a better word, perhaps more intuitive and ideally suited to our purpose. A subcategory of the folktale, namely the *memorate*, which Hollis, Pershing, and Young (1993) describe as a derivative of legend that is based on personal experience, more happily features in therapy as an individual attempts to communicate artfully to a therapist a specific experience or notion.

Aspects of the oral tradition have traditionally been used as an educational aid for successfully teaching children skills or basic knowledge (such as numbers, naming, or alphabet rhymes). Even older children could learn correct spelling or the number of days in the month through simple rhymes. The oral tradition could instil good behavior in adolescents and have a potentially significant impact on the socialization process and the values or belief systems that ensue and permeate throughout adulthood. It therefore needs to be taken into account that most people – and

Discussion Box 2.2: Two Brothers

Once there were two brothers. Kasanko was the older brother. He was a good man and a hard worker; and he was well liked by all. The younger brother, Zanzele, was his mother's favorite; and he was spoiled by the ladies in the kraal because he was a beautiful, fat, and shiny baby, who became a strong young man with broad shoulders. Kasanko loved his younger brother and always kept an eye on him. When Zanzele needed a spear, Kasanko made him one. When Zanzele needed a hut, Kasanko built him one. When Zanzele needed a pot, Kasanko fetched clay from the river bank and made pots for him. When Kasanko took a wife, Zanzele married two sisters. When Kasanko fathered three children, Zanzele did not. For this reason, Zanzele became angry and hated his brother. One day, when Kasanko was sitting alone by the river, Zanzele hit him over the head with a stone and pushed his body into the water. When the people started looking for Kasanko, Zanzele led the search party. When the women wailed at the funeral, Zanzele cried louder than they. One night Zanzele couldn't sleep. He went outside the hut because he became thirsty. When he lifted the cool water, he saw Kasanko looking up at him from inside the pot. He threw the pot down and screamed loudly. His wives came outside and asked him what was wrong. Zanzele said the pot burnt his hands and he had to throw it down and break it. The next night, Zanzele tried to sleep, but the walls of the hut came closer and closer and he screamed that they were going to crush him. His wives woke and asked him what was wrong. Zanzele said the hut was getting too small for all of them and he was going to sleep next to the fire from now on. One day Zanzele was hunting with the men and he threw his spear at an antelope. The spear flew through the air toward the animal; then it turned around and came straight back to Zanzele. Zanzele fell to the ground and the spear went past his head. He lay trembling and the men stood silent around him because they saw the strange path of the spear. They shook their heads and said: "Ay, bad things are happening to Zanzele. Perhaps, he is not well. If only his brother, Kasanko, were here to look after him." Then, Zanzele started shouting and pointed at the sky: "The eye! Look at the eye!" The men looked up at the sky but could only see the sun. "Look, look! Kasanko is looking after me. Look at his eye. His eye, his eye is watching me." The men whispered that Zanzele was mad. "No! No! Stop looking at me, Kasanko," he shouted. "Please help me, friends. Hide me from the eye of my brother." The men tried to carry Zanzele back to the kraal, but Zanzele escaped from their hands and ran to the river. As he ran he covered his head and shouted: "Ay, the stone hurts! Stop hitting me!" The men ran after him and saw him jump into the river. As the water closed over Zanzele, they could still hear him scream.

Questions

1. Discuss the symbol of the "eye" in the story.
2. Guilt and self-recognition are two central themes in the story. Discuss the extent to which this story can serve a modern client.
3. What are the parallels and differences between the story of the two brothers and the biblical Cain and Abel?
4. What reasons does the story offer to explain the differences in the character of the two brothers?

in this case, especially people of African ancestry – have been exposed to the oral tradition (e.g., folktales) from an early and impressionable age.

In the course of a previous study on the oral tradition (Malimabe-Ramagoshi, Maree, Molepo, & Alexander, 2007), we confirmed the supposition that the majority of oral tradition constituents are meant to have a moral message. After investigating some well-known folktales in South Africa, for instance, we found that the hero in folktales is often flawed; for example, the rabbit (called Hasie in the tale of the rabbit and the tortoise) is portrayed as the clever one because he knows how to lie, steal, cheat, and "get away with murder." This delightfully devious character is also universally found in the figure of the Trickster. The folktales exemplified most types of unacceptable behavior warned against by parents and elders, and written about in the popular press. Even though folktales are allegedly passed from one generation to the next with the primary aim of teaching children good behavior and the cultural/traditional way of doing things in society, we did not encounter many instances of good behavior. In fact, the research indicated that very few folktales, of the ones that we read, dealt with *Ubuntu/Botho* or the positive and exemplary behavior that is meant to take place in society.

A PERSPECTIVE ON THE LITERATURE OF FOLKLORE

Like all other cultures, Africa has both a written and an unwritten tradition. Whereas the written literature can be studied and neatly categorized, just as Western literary works are, even from ancient times, Africa's unwritten tradition remains something of an enigma; although, it is now regularly and studiously recorded by scholars and anthologized in compendiums. The main reason why the literature of the oral tradition remains tantalizingly fluid and ambiguous is that it is, by its very definition, dependent on a performer who designs and adapts a narrative for a very specific audience of listeners every time the tale is told. Oral literature's primary aspect is the fact that it requires a live transmission to an alert audience for its continued existence, making a textual study of the oral tradition something of an anomaly. The oral tradition in Africa, however, is not unique in this respect. Literacy has never been a universal attainment, not only in Africa, but also in Europe. Until the mid-nineteenth century, the majority of poor, even middle-class, Europeans had been illiterate or semi-literate. Until this time, narratives, like knowledge, were orally transmitted in all peasant and lower classes, either communally, or from parent to child. Up to well after the Renaissance, fairy and folk tales had existed only in an oral form, until collectors like Charles Perrault in France and the Grimm brothers in Germany started to record the folk literature of their people by preserving them in print. Until fixed in print, like butterflies pinned to an exhibition board, these tales had a flexible structure and variants, depending on both teller and audience. After the nineteenth century, fairy tales were Bowdlerized in compilations so that they were deemed "suitable" to be read to children. In these sanitized and moralizing – and inevitably rather anemic – versions of traditional fairy and folk tales, the sexual elements were the first to be eliminated, followed by descriptions of violent punishments, cannibalistic practices, and overly gruesome or brutal descriptions. The Mother Goose collections of Victorian England increased the didacticism to an even greater extent, giving rise to a self-conscious, rather than a visceral, interpretation of seminal tales such as Little Red Riding Hood, who is rescued from the wolf's stomach, together with a shaken but undigested grandmother.

The literary forms performed by a storyteller for a very particular audience were thus committed to paper as text and became inflexible documents that fail to give life to tone, gesture, the dramatic use of rhythm, distinctive facial expressions, the passionate voice, or the pregnant pause. In a study of this nature, then, it is the outline of folktales that can be examined, in full knowledge that they can only come to life when recreated by a teller, in the company of a listener. Although the African folktale is contextually different from the European, it is in seminal aspects entirely similar, opening it to Jungian analysis, focused on those archetypes that can serve therapy well. In this regard, Dasen (1993), the Swiss cross-cultural psychologist, voices the concern that

> [restrictive] indigenous psychologies, while relevant in each particular cultural context, will be just as parochial, and ethnocentric, as Western psychology is at the moment. The mere multiplication of independently developed streams of psychology is not the answer, because we need to study universal aspects of behaviour as well as culturally relative ones. People from around the world are not only different from each other in interesting ways, they are also similar, or the same, in important ways. (pp. 152–153)

As early as the nineteenth century, researchers such as the renowned Wilhelm Bleek (Lewis-Williams, 2002), noted the parallelism between African and European tales. Toward the end of the nineteenth century, an early compiler, Chatelain (cited in Finnegan, 1970), took this further by confirming the notion of the similarities between African myths, thereby making a case for the universality of folkloric elements: "Myths, characters and incidents known elsewhere also occur in African narratives … African [oral tradition] is thus a 'branch of the universal tree'" (Chatelain, 1894, quoted in Finnegan, 1970, p. 29). For instance, in the preamble, the Great Snake is a Zulu figure and is variously called *inhlwathi*, or *inkosi yamakhosi omkhulu*, which means Great Lord of Lords, or Lord of the Sky. SeSotho-speaking people attribute flood damage to the monstrous river snake *khanyapa*, and tribes in Tonga call their Great River God *Nyaminyami*. In the Congo, *kabwe* is cruel river python, as is the *mpumina* who, like Ancient Greece's Medusa, or the Medieval Europe's basilisk, causes immediate death when sighted.

There are compelling reasons for considering the implications of myth across a variety of healing modalities. However, before focusing on the utilization of folklore in counseling, we need to define a number of concepts that are central to the current chapter.

Fairy Tales

Although this chapter does not deal with fairy tales, chiefly because in their narrowest sense, fairies (and gnomes, leprechauns, trolls, ogres, nymphs, and other woodland beings) are essentially European creatures, it is useful to distinguish the fairy tale from myth, fable, and legend. Fairy tales were the earliest written texts for Western children, but they, too, were originally composed for a general audience before passing – in simplified form – into the domain of children's literature. The earliest form of fairy tale had been told and enjoyed around the European fireside by old and young alike since time immemorial. It is important to distinguish between the tales about magical folk, told in family circles, which contained traditional characters and archetypes and the artistic, consciously created fairy tale. The traditional fairy tale was never composed by a professional writer. In the seventeenth century, however, Charles Perrault documented existing fairy tales and created a norm for the future, namely the fairy tales as genre. Others followed, with the Brothers Grimm publishing more than 200 tales in the nineteenth century, thereby creating a fairy tale market in Europe. Other authors, such as Hans Christian Anderson, further developed this publishing tradition (and cashed in on its success) and recreated the fairy tale as a work of art. Although Freud and Jung both often referred to the plots of the artistic fairy tale, these mostly imaginative tales are often moralizing, self-conscious, and coy (see Example 2) and devoid of the startling, visceral power of the traditional folktale (see Example 1). Early folktales were the precursors of literary fairy tales. Magical agents of change in folktales (e.g., good fairies, angelic godmothers, talking birds) took care of princes and princesses, orphans, and foundlings – hence the term "fairy tales." Sanchez (2006) maintains that fairy tales were not universal or timeless; rather, they reflected the status quo of a given culture at a specific time (when they were told) and place (where they were told).

Myths

Myths are stories, usually of ancient origin, that seek to explain natural phenomena such as thunder, life, death, and seasonal change. Myths also ponder the origin of the world and the creation of man, and they do so in simple language and universal metaphor. The forces of nature are described in terms of the relations between humans and natural forces (e.g., the myth of the Great Sky Snake, Zeus, or Thor hurling his thunderbolts at recalcitrant humans; the San's role in the procurement of fire; or the flight of shooting stars.) Myths, above all, provide accounts of the epic struggles between the powers of the inner world and the hostile or immovable conditions of the outer world.

Legends

Legends are stories that have some basis in historical truth. They usually feature a larger-than-life hero who embodies qualities idealized in a particular culture, but who is also vulnerable and fallible. Legends often include magical elements, for instance, in the medieval tales about the Holy Grail, King Arthur's wizard Merlin, and the Knights of the Round Table. In South Africa, although legends of Shaka Zulu or other powerful chieftains are richly populated with sangomas, cannibals, and fanciful birds, they remain focused on the impressive character of the protagonist, who is usually a highly idealized individual.

Fables

Fables are one of the most widespread and enduring forms of literary endeavor since their earliest forms are found in Ancient Egypt and in the Rig Vedas of India. They are a didactic literary mode consisting of short stories that illustrate a moral truth or an acceptable mode of behavior. In many fables, animals portray human virtues or failings to make identification possible. Western culture's most famous early fables were purportedly written – or collected – by the ancient Greek freed slave, Aesop. During the seventeenth century, Jean de la Fontaine compiled a European compendium of fables. South African animal fables are similar in character to the fables of European folklore, but with distinctly African animals such as elands, hyenas, ostriches, meerkats, dassies, leopards, and porcupines, in addition to universally common animals such as rabbits, foxes (or their South African counterpart, the jackal), and a variety of birds. Animal tales of the San, for instance, are peopled not only by creatures of the African veld such as the praying mantis and eland, but also by mythical creatures and cosmic figures.

Folklore

An overview of the literature reveals that there seems to be little agreement on the meaning or definition of the term folklore, apart from the view that it appears to be an umbrella term for a number of loosely related concepts. Ben-Amos (1971), in his seminal article on the topic, asserts that folklore (in its cultural context), is "a definite realistic, artistic, and communicative process" (p. 10). The typical opening and closing formulas of tales and songs denote the actions that occur in-between as a different and "distinct category of narration" (p. 10), which should not be confused with reality. Further, folklore can be found in any communicative medium, viz. musical, visual, kinetic, and dramatic, and is limited to the small group social context. Jung argued furthermore that folklore may pertain to subconscious psychological patterns, instincts, or archetypes, often including fantastic components (e.g., magic, ethereal beings, and the personification of inanimate objects).

Folktales

There are numerous schools of thought that influence the classification of folktales and each advances its own set of requirements. Scheub (in Jordan, 2004) classifies folktales in Southern Africa into three distinct genres: *iintsomi*, which refer to the fictitious, mythological, and fantastic; *amabali*, the legendary; and lastly, *imilando*, which group together historical or time-honored accounts. The first two classes reflect the more conventional categorization into myth and legend, while the *imilando* represents the chronicling aspect of folktales. A constructivist approach more firmly distinguishes between myths, legends, and fables. Lynch-Brown and Tomlinson (1993) define folktales as traditional narratives that stem from the lives and imaginations of persons or groups. According to Carney (2006), folktales originated in an attempt to explain the temporal and the spiritual world. The telling of stories appears to be a universal cultural phenomenon, and folktales do not differ noticeably from culture to culture. Comparative studies have consistently revealed striking similarities in the themes and narrative techniques that characterize folktales, as amply illustrated by Freud and Jung and their many acolytes. Just as in the case of fairy tales, folktales form part of a centuries-old tradition, which make them ideal vehicles for the confirmation, or challenging, of the status quo of the storyteller's society.

Types of folktales

Carney (2006) distinguishes between the following categories of folktales:

- *Cumulative tales*, the simplest types of folktales, have no central plot and events are linked in a logical way in patterns of intonation and repetition.
- *Talking beast stories*, in which animals (and other creatures) talk like human beings. These stories mostly

contain lessons that imply that courage, independence, and resourcefulness are rewarded.
- *Amusing tales* are intended to entertain listeners.
- *Realistic stories* contain little exaggeration and no magic is involved.
- *Religious tales* can be didactic, moralistic, or humorous.
- In *romances*, enchantments and unachievable tasks separate lovers, while magic may reunite them.
- Tales in which magic predominates are considered *fairy tales*.

Windling (1995) asserts that folktales do not shy away from topics that are considered taboo, arguing that they rather address the same truths, realities, and problems that have been in existence for thousands of years.

The use of folktales to communicate complex dilemmas

In contemporary African society, folktales are often used to address complex problems (e.g., child abuse and HIV/AIDS). In Swaziland, for example, "protectors" are sent into rural areas to work with children. These professionals, dubbed *mahlombe lekhukalela* ("a shoulder to cry on") by the children, use folktales to convey simple messages instead of the jargon of psychology and sociology (UN Integrated Regional Networks, 2002). A story entitled "How the children of Chakijane put an end to brother Snake's abuse" is about a deceitful visitor (a snake) from the city that convinces Chakijane (a rock rabbit) that it is acceptable for him to sleep with his 12-year-old daughter. Humorous at times, the story, however, has a tragic ending: The snake is beheaded, the father is banished, and the girl dies. After the story has been recited, protectors are chosen from local communities and they proceed to tell the story to others.

BRIEF LITERATURE OVERVIEW OF THE STATUS OF COUNSELING IN THE TWENTY-FIRST CENTURY

To appreciate the many challenges facing the counseling profession in the twenty-first century, we must first trace some of the major developments in the field over the past twenty years. Since we believe that the prevailing political, social, and economic culture in which any practice evolves has a great impact on the advancement of epistemology (theory) and practice, our discussion is embedded in and framed by examples from real-life experiences.

Epistemological Changes

Some epistemological changes have occurred in the field of counseling during the past twenty years. Because counseling theories have generally been accepted in South Africa, with much of their application focused on white South Africans only (Stead & Watson, 2006), few psychometric tests have been designed specifically for South Africa's diverse population. In addition, counseling in South Africa traditionally has an objective (positivist) orientation, which virtually excludes use of the oral tradition. To help rectify this state of affairs, people like Watson and Fouche (2007) call for a profession that is assertive in its advocacy, that will become more integrated, and that will address diversity as well as theoretical and research issues.

A rapidly changing global situation and the shift in values following innovation in communication technology necessitate a changed approach to counseling, requiring counselors to adjust their theory and practice to accommodate a changing and changed context. The modified discipline needs to reflect more innovative counseling methods, techniques, and structures to ensure effective counseling (Amundson, Niles, & Harris-Bowlsbey, 2004; Maree, Bester, Lubbe, & Beck, 2001). This requires a reframing of counseling structures, including collaboration with the client, to help clients seize opportunities that come their way, as a joint socio-moral practice and a meaning-making process (Mkhize, 2004).

The quest is for an approach that "enables rather than fits" (Savickas, 1993, p. 211), and this clearly implies exploitation of the oral tradition in counseling, especially with clients of African ancestry.

On a macro level, scholars are calling for a creative rather than a reactive approach to the current technological society and for international networking to meet the needs of marginalized groups such as the unemployed, disabled, contract workers and other disenfranchised people. The scope of counseling should be broadened to include the full spectrum of diversity in South Africa (e.g., irrespective of class, gender, religion, creed, and race), with the emphasis on actively engaging people in constructing meanings for planning the future (Amundson, 2003; Watson & Stead, 2002). In attempting to facilitate development, psychologists should view clients as active agents in their own personal development: Counseling should therefore continue to address the needs and diversity of individual persons. Furthermore, in a diverse context, it is especially crucial to acquire a sound knowledge of indigenous knowledge systems, if a counselor is to stand any chance of "getting through" to clients. Counselors are allowed the freedom to implement existing as well as new approaches and methods to lead their clients to active participation in the process of counseling.

The consensus view is that the adoption of a combined qualitative–quantitative approach to counseling needs to be addressed as a minimum requirement for the positive development of counseling in South Africa (Leach, Akhurst, & Basson, 2003). In fact, counseling in South Africa has begun to adapt and to develop its own indigenous practices, whereas most counseling interventions elsewhere are informed by a Western world view that focuses on individual as opposed to group needs (Nicholas, Naidoo, & Pretorius, 2006).

The development of an indigenous, African-oriented counseling practice is advocated by Abdi (1975, p. 230). According to Straker (1988, p. 6), the "Western notion

Discussion Box 2.3: Illustrating Epistomological Pluralism

Case Study (Mpofu, 2003): Diagnosis and intervention that were conceptualized and developed in the Western world are more well known and likely to be implemented globally than those conceptualized and developed in non-Western countries. A case study is presented in which a creative mix of the two approaches is demonstrated.

Background Information: Lebo (pseudonym), an eight-year-old boy in Grade Three, from a low-socioeconomic, Shona cultural background, lived with his father an stepmother in a small southeastern Zimbawean town. Although working in the city, the parents maintained a rural home. The school referred Lebo on account of his severely disruptive behavior. Contact was first made through a "contact person," viz. Lebo's niece, who invited the parents, on behalf of the counselor, to join him for "exchange of ideas" (oral tradition being an essential feature of (traditional) Africa.

Assessment Findings: Lebo had not mastered even the most basic letter and number recognition. A history of disruptive behavior at home also became clear.

Family's Implicit Theory about the Disorder: The father opined that the boy's troubled behavior was caused by the protesting spirit of Lebo's biological mother, since the extended family to which Lebo belonged had failed to perform the required spiritual rituals to bring her back to the family.

Clinical Impressions and Treatment Recommendations: Early Onset Conduct Disorder was diagnosed and a multifaceted treatment strategy was tailored to suit Lebo's needs.

Spiritual Intervention: The family was requested to perform the required spiritual rituals to bring Lebo's late mother back to the family.

Special Educational Placement: Placement in a unit for children with special needs was recommended.

Family Support: Monthly consultations (*kupana mazano*, or sharing of ideas) with the counselor on Lebo's behavioral adjustment to enhance parenting skills were proposed. As the Shona proverb says: "Mazano marairamwa," or "One learns plans best by sharing it with others."

Results: After three months, improvement was noted for impulse control, abusive behavior, and truancy.

Discussion: Success in identifying and treating conduct disorder in children from a traditional Shona background might be facilitated by an approach that incorporates elements of both a traditional and a modern nature.

Questions

1. In which core ways might the traditional and modern approaches to behavioral problems (e.g., conduct disorder) be applied in a non-Western environment to complement each other?
2. How typical is the type of approach to behavioral problems in your own country?
3. Elaborate on your views with regard to the need to develop a theory base in psychology that is specifically relevant for clients of African ancestry.

of a talking cure is alien to many Black people in South Africa." Malott (2008) believes that not only the Western versus non-Western paradigm should be addressed but also the challenge of cultural differences across Western countries. He supports Levers' (1997) call for "psychological pluralism" to include indigenous practices in the counseling curriculum. Indigenization could "enable scholars to accept both traditional and imported psychological perspectives" (Sinha, as cited in Stead & Watson, 2006, p. 188).

NEED FOR THE ESTABLISHMENT OF ETHNOPSYCHOLOGY IN COUNSELING

Hickson, Biesheuvel, Turton, and Buhrmann (in Tlali, 1999, p. 36) argue that it has become imperative to establish ethnopsychology (or indigenous psychology) in a South African context on account of the following reasons:

- Frequent communication breakdowns occur between client and counselor.
- Counselors often make negative judgments on their clients.
- Counselors often inadvertently harm their clients instead of helping them.
- Both counselor and client experience the counseling process as frustrating and anxiety provoking.
- Counselors set inappropriate therapy and process goals.

The aforementioned makes it clear that meaningful participation and meaning-making in the counseling relationship are aims that should be optimized to facilitate helpful assessment of personality characteristics. Quantitative measurement, observation of behavior, and a qualitative analysis of test results should be combined to enable psychologists to enter the phenomenological world of the testee.

Case Study 2.1: Tebogo

In 2003, Tebogo, an extremely bright young man, the second of two children from a village in deep Sekhukhuneland, an impoverished region in the Limpopo Province of South Africa, was offered a bursary to study at the University of Pretoria. A few months after arriving in the city, however, Tebogo began to present with feelings of sadness and anger and he was subsequently referred to a counselor (inter alia on account of his inadequate academic achievement). During the first session, Tebogo was reluctant to talk; instead, he simply responded tersely to all questions. The counselor then requested Tebogo's permission to involve two more students from an adjacent region. Furthermore, he decided to consult the students in a forest-like park, a few kilometers from the university where the three were staying at the time. He began the session by asking a number of narrative questions, based on the model proposed by Savickas (2007a). Initially, Tebogo would listen to the others' responses first and only then offer his own responses in a soft, sad tone. Then, in reply to the following question: "What are your earliest recollections from your childhood?" he remarked: "I remember the day I took my (older) brother's clothes and wore them. When I went outside, however, people laughed at me: 'You look so funny, you make us laugh.' At first, I just ignored them, because I was proud of my attire. However, after a while I became self-conscious and realized that I had made a fool of myself." From then on, he began to open up and shared his desire to be home with the counselor and the other two students. Prompted by the counselor, Tebogo eventually divulged the story of the tsetse fly and the elephant, a story that his mother told him when he was still very young. After a lengthy discussion that took place in the course of a few more sessions, he was able to remark: "I have realized that I can tackle many obstacles and problems in my life and my studies."

Tebogo qualified in 2007 and he has subsequently returned to his home region, where he applies his trade and spends much time motivating adolescents.

Questions

1. What are the similarities between Tebogo's story and that of the refugees in Schwartz and Melzak's story (see Research Box 2.1)?
2. In which ways can the strategy employed in the case under discussion be employed in similar contexts?

DEVELOPING AND USING APPROPRIATE ASSESSMENT INSTRUMENTS TO FACILITATE COUNSELING

Research on the identification of appropriate assessment instruments in a diverse context is in its infancy and needs to be broadened considerably. A case in point concerns the use of early anecdotes. In clinical cases, we have found that, in educationally marginalized clients, early anecdotes could be a potentially powerful technique to facilitate engagement and expression of the self in this narrative mode. Despite the fact that very little research has been done, in this regard in an African context, and the fact that very few counselors feel comfortable with this technique, it could be used to tap into prior experience to reveal core life themes culminating in a confident mode of self-expression. It lends itself exceptionally well to help clients take up agency to "write" or "rewrite" their life stories. When clients are particularly uncommunicative or overly protective of their stories during the early stages of therapy, the recounting of a *memorate* (Hollis et al., 1993, p. xi) will go a long way toward unveiling the layers of life themes and fostering the client's confidence. The telling of a well-loved folktale is also an ideal ice-breaker in an early session.

Possible Value of a Narrative Approach in Counseling

In tandem with the introduction of a narrative framework that combines facets of a quantitative approach with life construction, postmodern approaches have become essential in South Africa (Amundson, 2006; Niles & Harris-Bowlsbey, 2002). Such a framework could be used to build and promote counseling in traditional South African society where the focus is on the group, storytelling, and *Ubuntu*, thus empowering counselors to assist individuals to achieve self-actualization and make social contributions through work (Savickas, 2007b). This approach is useful for clients other than upper- and middle-class individuals who have access to state-of-the-art counseling and a wide array of counseling opportunities (Winslade, 2007).

Chen (2001) indicates that individual psychology theorists (e.g., Adler), person-centered theorists (e.g., Rogers), and existential philosophy (e.g., Frankl) all contributed, directly or indirectly, to the growing notion of meaning-making in counseling psychology. The needs of the client come first, with the sole view of empowering him/her to make his/her own decisions about the future. A narrative approach is adopted, by which the client creates his/her own life story, with a view to creating an ideal story as close as possible to the ideal. This narrative comprises a consultative process of counseling with all clients, irrespective of race, gender, age, or culture. The researcher is a co-worker, rather than the sole "expert." The entire process is cooperative, aimed at problem-solving, prevention, development, and empowering the client to assume responsibility for his/her role in the process and putting his/her weaknesses and strengths into perspective (Savickas, 1993). Storytelling is an example of a naturally occurring phenomenon in Africa that can be used to facilitate a changed approach to counseling.

Storytelling

One of the proudest talents of Africans is their ability to tell stories (Maree & Molepo, 2005). It is common practice to have a family gathering, after supper, for instance, to listen to stories told by elders, with the younger people also participating in the jokes and discussions. The principle of *Ubuntu* is to share whatever is eaten, enjoyed, and experienced, whether sorrowful or joyous. Such a practice may constitute one of the ways in which a storied approach to counseling may be introduced. Each client may be requested to tell his/her story in a group context, while the counselor facilitates the direction of these stories. This code of *Ubuntu* may be utilized by counselors as a means through which clients can reveal their experiences in order to build on and map out their future.

The importance of storytelling in an African context was demonstrated in the process and activities of the Truth and Reconciliation Commission (TRC), which is, broadly speaking, one of South Africa's post-1994 success stories after the transition from apartheid to a full and free democracy. Despite some flaws and much criticism, both valid and unfounded, it is generally regarded as an example of the salience of the opportunity afforded victims to tell their stories and to experience some measure of validation (SA History Online, 2008). The TRC was a court-like body assembled in South Africa after the end of apartheid, and any individual who felt that he or she had been a victim of aggression or abuse could come forward and be heard at the TRC. The perpetrators of violence were also given the opportunity to bear testimony and request amnesty from prosecution. The TRC was set up in terms of the *Promotion of National Unity and Reconciliation Act* No. 34 of 1995, and the mandate of the commission was to afford individuals the opportunity to "tell their story," and to bear witness to, have the offences recorded, and experience, where possible, some restitution regarding human rights violations. In all, more than 20,000 individuals made use of the Commission to tell their stories. Criticisms were various, ranging from the lack of sufficient funds to recompense victims, to the more philosophical one of defining the "real truth" and distinguishing it from the individual and emotional "truths." However, the salience of the TRC rested on the opportunity for individuals to recount their stories and have them enter the public domain. This opportunity, in the words of the Reverend Desmond Tutu (1999b, quoted in Matthews, 2001, p. 1), helped validate the experiences of ordinary people and "aided the healing of a nation," creating "a painful yet clean window into South Africa's past" and enabling the nation to "attain perspective, and where possible, forgiveness" to the benefit of both victim and perpetrator. Therefore, despite the risk of opening themselves to vulnerability and the trauma of reliving violations and aggression, the honest sharing of experiences proved to have helped individuals validate painful experiences and have "some balm ... poured on them" (Tutu, quoted in Matthews, 2001, p. 1) so that a healing process can start.

Cultural singing and dancing

Throughout the ages, indigenous African experiences have been expressed through cultural singing and dancing. Simply put, as Malobola (2001, p. 1) describes it, "singing is a way of life; there is no ceremony that is not accompanied by singing... It is also a means to express the experiences of the important turning points in the life of an individual." Whether their stories carry great import, such as descriptions of decisive battles or tribal contracts, or whether they accompany more mundane affairs such as harvesting, building the kraal or soil filling, singing, recitation, and dancing, with the accompaniment of drums, marimba, horns, and other musical instruments, have given African people communal pride, self-esteem, and a sense of belonging. Clearly, when other approaches fail, an invitation to engage in song or recitation will facilitate counseling with some clients of African descent, if only to help create a relaxed mood, or by stirring up old memories. The refrains of the following songs are quoted to illustrate the simplicity of expression, but also hint at a depth of feeling that is experienced during stressful encounters with problems:

Ngesab' ukwenda nje mina gesab' unosokana
Ngesag' unosokana unamezw' ahlabahlabako

(I fear for I am afraid of the mother-in-law
I fear the mother-in-law she uses thorny words).

Translated: Malobola (2001, p. 54)

Maye! Ubuntandani bubuhlungu
Ubuntudandani obungaka
Maye! Ngitlhoge ababelethi
Bengitlhoge nonosakana
Ngitlhoge nabodadwethu

(Being an orphan is painful!
Such orphanhood!
Alas! I do not have parents
I don't even have a mother-in-law
I do not have sisters) ...

Translated: Malobola (2001, p. 54)

Traditionally, songs and recitations have afforded women and children one of the few opportunities to express their experiences and views openly with impunity. Furthermore, singing and dancing are also used to instruct and entertain, and have therefore been a powerful vehicle for shaping the behavior of the youth and ultimately carrying the cultural capital of a tribe.

Exploiting African Clients' Natural Affinity for Group Work

Counselors trained in a Euro-American counseling tradition may need to make some adjustments first when they wish to facilitate a group of clients from African descent. It may be a good idea to start dialogues by proceeding from a group or game context in which clients may gradually become used to the concept of sharing experiences. This may encourage clients to take counselors into their confidence and become able to share their life experiences, as the latter are regarded as confidential (*ke khupamarama*) and the group members may have been conditioned not to share experiences randomly with just anyone. More often than not, a lengthy process is necessary to facilitate entry to the inner feelings of individuals in the African context. The introduction of a topic through a fable or the retelling of a folktale is a nonthreatening approach that can help the individual to gain confidence first and feel safe in the situation.

The Need to Show Consideration for Values and a Different World View in Counseling

To be able to function effectively in a diverse context, counselors need at least to acquire the following skills (Hickson & Christie, 1989, p. 167):

- An understanding of their own values and assumptions, as well as assumptions about human behavior, to become able to identify and accept differing values
- Becoming aware of generic characteristics of counseling, as well as its relation to matters such as class and culture
- Being willing to act on the basis of a critical analysis of their own conditioning, as well as that of their clients, and the sociopolitical system in which they find themselves
- Becoming culturally aware in order to understand the bases for world views and to accept world views that differ from theirs
- Being willing to be eclectic in administering counseling, as well as striving to create the widest possible array of microcounseling skills, which may have relevance for the idiosyncratic lifestyles of individual clients

Diverse sociocultural groups (societies) value different types of skills and expertise, with the result that members of distinct social groups do not develop along uniform lines (Curran, 1988). According to Hickson and Christie (1989), the outcome of any therapeutic intervention depends, to some extent, on the combined influence of the values of the client, the therapist, and the cultural milieu in which they function. Nell and Bodibe (cited in Tlali, 1999), and Hickson, Christie, and Shmukler (1990) argue conclusively that a sound understanding of the client's world views is essential, since this helps counselors to understand themselves and their clients. In addition, this understanding makes explicit both parties' values, beliefs, suppositions, and attributions, facilitates mutually accepted and agreed-on therapeutic goals and processes, and helps counselors to access clients' subjective realities. The potential impact of cultural forces/influences and of the acculturation process (including the influence of the environment on clients, such as the effect of urbanization on sociocultural factors like the language they use), as well as the impact of lifestyle and levels of education should be considered when any measuring strategy is designed and developed.

Exploiting the oral tradition to facilitate the telling of life stories enables counselors to gauge the world views of clients, which is a critical facet of cross-cultural counseling. Hickson and Christie (1989) explain that Western psychology has in the past been dominated by Eurocentric psychoanalytic, behaviorist, and humanist paradigms, and that each of these is based on an idiosyncratic world view (or "cosmological foundation"), which, in turn, defines, explains, and predicts cause and effect, human behavior, and psychopathology. A world view is defined as the way in which people perceive their relationship to "nature, institutions, other people and things" (Sue, in Hickson, Christie & Shmukler, 1990, p. 171) and it co-determines the way in which persons think, make decisions, and define matters. Atkinson, Morten, and Sue (in Hickson & Christie, 1989) explain that a person's world view includes a dynamic interaction between matters such as race, ethnicity, age, life stage, gender, lifestyle, social class, degree of acculturation, level of education, ordinal family position, marital status, and geographical situation.

Counseling Clients Whose Language Differs from that of the Counselor

Clients whose language and culture differ from that of the test developer and counselor often experience a number of linguistic and cultural problems if subjected to a cross-cultural counseling situation. Rural African clients, in particular, find themselves in a situation where they first have to understand the concepts or items in their own language and culture before they can respond to or internalize a situation. The next step would then be to equate or relate their understanding of the concept to what the counselor wants. Major confusion often develops, because a client's understanding of the item may be totally different from the Eurocentric meaning of the concept as expected by the tester, or the context in which and for which the tester had formulated the test. It thus can be said that the context is challenged by the syntax.

Culture and language frame the individual's symbolic world to which meaning and sense are ascribed (Savickas, 1993; Van Niekerk, 1996). Adequate language usage should help to ensure that individuals express themselves effectively in terms of their feelings and the directions they may wish to pursue in their lives (Herr, 1997). The language of the counselor, or the inability to speak the language of the client, can therefore become one of the main prohibitive factors in facilitating counseling. Ideally speaking, counselors need to master the mother tongue of a client in the most possible and basic way. Of course, code-switching will minimize many of the problems accompanying idiomatic expressions and other forms of expression, but it is simply not possible to expect a counselor to learn a new language, as mastery of a language takes many years to attain. Because no simple solution is advanced, it is best to warn that if language is not taken seriously, distrust may jeopardize the well-intended suggestions of counselors and, consequently, great care must be taken to find common ground and explicate terms as much as possible.

Helpful Strategies in a Diverse Setting

Chen (2001, p. 318) proposes the following guidelines or "helping strategies" for development professionals, which take on special significance in a diverse setting (Chen, pp. 326–328):

- The need to facilitate subjectivity. Counselors need to engage clients in becoming subjectively involved in the counseling process, with a special emphasis on the question: "What do these results mean to me?"
- Clients need to develop a personal intention, that is, personal goals, objectives, and outcomes. To do this, clients first have to internalize the meaning of their personal life journey experiences.
- Clients and counselors need to develop a keen understanding of the counseling or development context. For this to occur, counselors should keep in mind the need to remind themselves consistently to put clients' narratives into perspective (i.e., interpret and perceive clients' expressions) in "the very experiential context in which such meaning exists" (Chen, 2001, p. 327). Furthermore, counselors need to help clients clarify and make sense of the context during counseling.
- Counselors need to support clients in making sense of their experiences, that is, promoting and facilitating a sense of flexibility and creativity in their perception of meaning. Amundson (in Chen, 2001) stresses the fact that clients can reconstruct the meaning of events.
- Counselors need to help clients construct meanings for planning for the future. In this sense, the counseling process becomes a possible opportunity for "active engagement" (Amundson, in Chen, 2001).

As indicated before, a folktale can also be used as a *memorate* or as a tool and an introduction during a counseling session.

Interventive Use of Folktales: Diagnosis, Well-being, and Development

The trained therapist can ask the client to recount a story. Chances are that the person will tell a story from memory, or failing that, devise a narrative along the lines of a remembered story. The two folktales in Case Study 2.2 and 2.3 serve as examples of stories for use in a session.

COUNSELING PROCEDURES WITH PEOPLE OF AFRICAN ANCESTRY

Jung (1959) preferred analyzing folktales to dreams, because he believed that they exemplify the archetypes in the human psyche in that folktales are universal, but dreams are more individualized. Because the oral tradition is a naïve and spontaneous product of the psyche, a folktale cannot represent anything else but that which is already present in the psyche. Personal symbols are connected to an individual's personal past, or they are confronted by suprapersonal symbols that represent archetypal content. Archetypal symbols are considered to be "healthy signs", although archetypes per se are not classified as healthy or unhealthy, good or bad, because they function outside such assertions. The enhancement of the unconscious has a healing effect on the psyche when, as in folk and fairy tales, it is articulated as the pain and suffering that appears as a problem in the beginning of the tale and that is resolved in the end.

In both tales presented here, a specific problem is addressed. However, whereas the first tale follows the traditional structure of an African folktale, the second tale is an extended aphorism, and in its simple moralizing, it more simply exemplifies a homily and translates into various guises. For instance, in Knappert's version (1970), it is given as a Swahili legend, with the ruler a Sultan and the tone reminiscent of *1001 Arabian Nights*. In this version, a king rules from a palace, but in another account, it is a "great chief" who rules from a "rich kraal" and whose wife is "happy and fat." In its present form, the lesson in *The Meat of Tongues* is patently obvious, and despite a certain charm, has fewer folkloric aspects. The second tale, despite its simple allure and the sound marital advice it offers, lacks potential as a *memorate* (Hollis et al., 1993, p. xi) and is therefore less useful as a therapeutic tool.

Regarding the first tale, its more enigmatic character confirms Von Franz's (1978) notion that although myth and legend center on the basic patterns of the human psyche, they are immersed in the cultural fabric. Because folktales contain less conscious cultural-specific material than myth and legend, Von Franz favors them as a therapeutic tool. The folktale more succinctly mirrors the basic patterns of the human psyche and appeals, in its universal language, to people of all ages, races, and cultures. According to Von Franz, because folktales transcend cultural and racial differences, they can also more effortlessly transfer to different contexts. As a representation of human universality, therefore, folktales are especially valuable when a therapist is required to work across cultural barriers. No therapist can have a profound knowledge of the cultural discourse of all ethnic groups, but when a therapist understands quintessential human characteristics, meaningful contact with a member from another social group can be established. The telling of a folktale in therapy can be an indication of the individual's own psychic projections or potential for development. When personal problems are thus connected to collective archetypal processes as represented in folktales, individuals feel that, as their problems are universal enough to be the focus of a folktale, there is hope that such problems can be resolved. After all, the realization that other people experience the same problems and have found some resolution is one of

Case Study 2.2: Litokotoko

There was a little child called Litokotoko. Her mother had many children, but they died, being killed by their grandmother. After a time that woman again gave birth to a child, a girl; she was born with hands and feet. One day, the mother said to the grandmother: "Stay here with my child; I go to the fountain." She went; the grandmother remained with the child. When she was alone, she took a knife, and cut off the hands and feet of that child. She went and hid them in her hut. When she saw the mother of the child coming from the fountain, she also came back.

The mother of the child arrived and put her pitcher down.

The child cried. The grandmother went to her and said: Oh! Who has taken away the hands and feet of my grandchild? The mother asked: What has happened to my child? I told you to stay with her. Who has taken away her hands and feet? The grandmother said: I do not know. The mother asked: Who has cut off the hands and the feet of my child? I told you to stay with her. Then she wept. The people came, saw the child, and wondered who could have cut off her hands and feet.

The child grew up, having neither hands nor feet, till she was a grown-up girl; she used to lie on the ground. One day the people went to the gardens. Her grandmother said: Litokotoko, my grandchild, why do you not give me food? Litokotoko said: Grandmother, how can I give you food, since I have neither feet nor hands? Her grandmother said: If I give you hands and feet, will you give me some food? She answered: Yes, grandmother, I shall give you some food, if you give me hands and feet.

She, the grandmother, brought them, the feet and the hands; she put them in, she put them in, she put them in, she put them in. Litokotoko stood up and walked, and gave her food. Litokotoko took a pitcher and went to the fountain, she put the millstone straight, and ground the grain, the people being still in the gardens. Then, she cooked the porridge, stirred it, swept the floor, and removed the ashes.

When the people were coming back in the evening, her grandmother took back her hands and feet, and went to hide them in her hut. Litokotoko, who has been sweeping here? She said: It was grandmother. Her mother was silent; she went to sleep.

The next morning they went to the gardens. The grandmother said: Litokotoko? She answered: Grandmother? She said: Are you not going to give me food? She answered: Since I have neither hands not feet, grandmother, how can I give you food?

Shall I lend you feet and hands? She said: Yes, grandmother.

She lent them to her. Litokotoko gave her food; the grandmother ate it, she ate it. Litokotoko took a pitcher, went to the fountain, swept the floor, removed the ashes.

Litokotoko said to herself: This time, today, grandmother shall not take back my hands and feet again. The grandmother vainly called: Litokotoko! Litokotoko! The girl remained silent and answered not, till the working companies came back from the gardens. When her father arrived, Litokotoko showed herself, having her hands and feet. The father wondered. The mother arrived and wondered too.

Her father asked her: Litokotoko, where did you get your feet and hands from? She said: I got them from grandmother. When the people were gone to the gardens, grandmother used to call me and tell me to give her food. I used to answer grandmother: Since I have neither hands nor feet, how can I give you food? Then, grandmother used to give me these hands and these feet. Then, I give her food. I grind grain, I sweep the floor, I remove the ashes, and I go to the fountain. When the working companies come back, grandmother cuts my feet and my hands. Today, I have hidden myself. The father said: These are really the hands and the feet of my child. They went to sleep.

The next morning he went to the chief's court. He arrived there and told the chief. The chief called a great assembly. That woman was called and placed there. She was asked about her deeds. She confessed and said that these were indeed the hands and feet of Litokotoko. Then, she was put to death.

This is the end of the tale.

the basic principles for successful group therapy. It is usually with this note of hopefulness that problems can be solved that most folktales end.

In Jungian terms, although certain archetypes, such as the Earth Mother, are supra-ordinate personalities that represent the individual in its totality, a single facet of the personality is also a dichotomous entity that can transform itself from one personality to its polar opposite, depending on its positive or negative qualities. The Mother can therefore appear as either a nurturing or a destructive entity. This is clearly the role played by the grandmother in *Litokotoko*.

Litokotoko

Litokotoko is, according to De Vos (2001), a BaSotho folktale first published in 1908 by a French missionary, Jacottet. Although the destructive symbol of the brutal grandmother is the most remarkable facet of this tale, it is by no means an isolated one in world literature. The

Case Study 2.3: The Meat of Tongues

A great king lived with his wife in a beautiful palace, but the queen was unhappy. She grew thinner and sadder and more listless every day. In the town, there lived a poor man whose wife was healthy and happy and strong. When the king heard about the lovely wife of the poor man, he asked him to come to his palace. "What is your secret? Why is your wife healthy and happy and strong? You must have a secret, what is it?"

The poor man said: "I feed my wife the meat of the tongue".

The great king called the farmer and told him to sell him all the tongues of all the cattle that he could find in town. And the tongues of sheep too. The king ordered him not to sell tongues to anyone else.

Every day farmer slaughtered cattle and sheep and brought the tongues of the cattle and sheep to the palace and the king's cook baked and roasted and cooked, and baked and roasted and cooked all the tongues and then brought the tasty tongues to the king.

The king called his wife and watched her eat the tasty tongues, three times a day, then four times a day, then five times a day. But the king's wife grew even thinner and sadder and more listless.

The king called the poor man and told him that they were going to change wives. The poor man didn't want his happy wife to go to the king's palace, but he had no choice.

The poor man took the king's thin, sad wife home with him and sent his happy and healthy wife to the king's palace. The happy wife then started to grow thinner and sad, although she was eating the tongues of many sheep and cattle three times, four times, five times a day.

The poor man went home to the king's thin wife at night, and would greet her, telling her about things he had done and seen during the day. And they would laugh at his stories. The poor man would take his old guitar and sing songs for the king's thin wife. Every night he will play for her and make her laugh.

Within a month the king's wife grew happy and lovely to look at with her skin gleaming and her cheeks round. And during the day when the poor man was away she was still laughing, thinking about his stories and his songs while she ground the grain and swept his hut.

Then the king came to take his wife back. He found her happy and healthy and strong, and she didn't want to go back to the king's palace. The king asked her what the poor man had fed her on, and she told him. Only then did he understand the meaning of the meat of the tongue.

role of the hag or witch is also a very prominent one in European folktales, ranging from the witch who fattens Hansel to become a succulent morsel, to the series of tales in Russian oral tradition featuring the murderous and cannibalistic grandmother/witch, the Baba Yaga.

As stated previously, when discussing this tale, the client's historical situation will influence her interpretation of the grandmother's cutting off of her grandchild's hands. Traditionally, in an African context, the role of the grandmother is a nurturing one. Even – or especially in the light of the HIV/AIDS pandemic – in twenty-first century Africa, the relationship with the grandmother is a particularly close bond, with grandchildren more often than not residing with the grandmother owing to parents' work (which is also the case in *Litokotoko* with the regular absence of both parents) or death.

The crucial aspect in *Litokotoko*, namely the relationship of grandmother–granddaughter, is the fact that the mother archetype here is a flawed and abusive one. This is a contradiction of the traditional nurturing aspect of the mother, not only in Jungian terms, but certainly in an African context, in which grandparent–grandchild interaction is characterized by mutual respect (*ukuhlonipha*, in Xhosa) and affectionate bantering (*ukufekethisa*, in Xhosa). The negative face of the archetype is manifested in the destructive force of evil witches and embittered hags – whether in the figure of the Baba Yaga, Hansel and Gretel's witch, or Litokotoko's brutal grandmother. In the case of the latter, Jung (1959) would argue that the ego consciousness of the daughter here is disempowered by the viciousness of the grandmother. In the telling or shared experience of this story, a female client will subconsciously identify with the motif of fragmentation, disenfranchisement, or dysfunction with regard to a mother figure. The symbol of the amputation of hands and feet clearly exemplifies feelings of helplessness and despair. Litokotoko, after all, cannot function as other young girls in her tribe. Her social interaction is restricted, and her future outlook hopeless. However, in the grand tradition of a Jack (of Beanstalk fame), a clever little pig, and Hansel's sister Gretel, Litokotoko cleverly uses the only opportunity afforded her when her grandmother is too lazy (or incapacitated herself) to fetch her own food. In other words, Litokotoko is rescued from her passive existence by her grandmother's need, with the requirement and ritual of food playing a central role in her deliverance. Litokotoko is transformed from a disabled maiden to a nurturing entity, and her integration becomes complete when she takes charge of her own situation.

During counseling, the immobilization a client experiences through a negative mother complex can be resolved. The feeling of helplessness, the symbolic experience of

Research Box 2.1: Story Telling as Therapy

Schwartz, S., & Melzak, S. (2007). Using storytelling in psychotherapeutic group work with young refugees. *Group Analysis*, *38*, 293–306.

Objective: Many young asylum seekers and refugees from across the globe, who have been separated from their parents and communities, travel to Britain to seek asylum, either alone or accompanied by unsupportive parents or strangers who cannot care for them. These children are all survivors of political violence; adolescents who suffer from the devastating after-effects and impact of, for example, separation, loss, and internal disruption. At the Medical Foundation for the Care of Victims of Torture, a Human Rights organisation, professionals strive to provide psychotherapy to these adolescents in an attempt to help them recall and reconnect with positive and formative aspects of their personal history, including mythology and culture, on the one hand, and to help them understand and deal with the conflicting dualities (e.g., vulnerability and resilience, inhibition and creativity, as well as feelings that they either deserve to be alive or are dispensable).

Method: A case study is presented in which an integrated model that combines, for example, psychodynamic principles, developmental thinking, storytelling, drama therapy and group psychotherapy, was used by the authors in a group context (fifteen adolescents between fifteen and twenty-one years of age attended) at the Foundation with displaced adolescents to reconnect them with their past and deal with their dualist emotions.

Results: Participants are firstly invited to reflect on their week and everyone gets an opportunity to talk. By carefully listening for subjects and themes to emerge from these reflections, adolescents are encouraged to share (their stories) and listen (to others). By discussing stories and carefully clarifying questions, confidence is instilled in participants to share not only their own, personal stories, but also traditional stories. Results reveal that it is advisable to begin with a general discussion on the uses and effects of tradition, folklore, and magic in the adolescents' traditional societies. Therapists could keep to a discussion of the vicissitudes of daily life, and proceed to test ideas from magical or traditional thinking to help adolescents deal with unresolved issues. Lowered resistance to mother cultures often facilitates discussions about individual cultures' folk characters, heroes and heroines, myths, and fables, until a story or folk tale is remembered, after which the storytelling session commences. Subconscious messages are identified by paying attention to diverse facets of adolescents' communication, including body language, observing them, listening for finer nuances, deconstructing language, and so forth. Whether therapists subsequently work with the group or with an individual person only, depends on a number of factors, but it seems plausible to work with individual adolescents and their stories first and to share these stories with the group at a later stage. Participants clearly feel safer after these sessions and readily express their ideas and views; however, it takes somewhat longer to reflect on their emotions. Sessions are ended by performing a ritual in which adolescents are helped to step out of the roles they have adopted in their stories. This is done to help adolescents disengage from the characters in their stories and re-establish reality orientation.

Conclusion: The approach adopted here will need to be revisited and adapted to suit the needs of different populations in different settings. Nonetheless, findings seem to suggest that the use of storytelling in group therapy with displaced adolescent refugees is a viable strategy to help these victims deal with feelings of rejection and anxiety, to help them view the world more positively and deal with dualist emotions. By incorporating folklore, myth, magical stories, and tradition to assist and facilitate healing, inappropriate coping mechanisms, for example, denial, are unlearned and replaced with healthy ones. Over time, the painful traumatic story is rewritten and a new story, built on acceptance of the past but also on hope for the future, is gradually written and lived.

Questions

1. What are the authors' two specific therapeutic aims in their work with displaced adolescent refugees?
2. What is the role of myth and folk tale in the therapeutic process with displaced adolescent refugees?
3. What are the core episodes in group therapy with these adolescents?

"having one's hands cut off at the elbow," can be overpowering, leading to incapacity and depression. Confronting the negative can facilitate acceptance and begin a process of healing.

The second tale, albeit charming in its aphoristic brevity, clearly lacks the potential for therapy. The traditional African folktale's power clearly lies in its symbolism and archetypal complexity, and it can serve both client and counselor well in therapeutic sessions.

SUMMARY AND CONCLUSIONS

In this chapter, we discussed some of the different forms the oral tradition in an African context may assume. We analyzed the meaning and significance of the oral tradition and some of its constituent genres, such as myth, legend, and fable in an African context, and we introduced the concept of the oral tradition in counseling with clients of African ancestry. We critiqued the unwarranted emphasis on a positivist approach to counseling in an African context, still holding sway in a largely Euro-American counseling paradigm, and we emphasized the importance of exploiting the oral tradition. Finally, we analyzed two folktales to exemplify the interventive use of folktales (diagnosis, well-being, and development) in counseling.

EPILOGUE

This chapter would be incomplete without some reference to milestone events in South Africa, in particular, over the past two decades, and possibly their link with the implementation of the oral tradition in counseling.

First, the authors believe that events at the macro (national) level are curiously synchronous with developments at the micro level; in other words, what occurs at the national level is mirrored in psychologists' consulting rooms. Second, counseling theories reveal a historic development that to a high degree agrees with parallel scientific and societal values that are given preference during a particular period in a particular country. Although neither the specific values nor the climate in which most of the counseling theories developed in the Euro-American tradition can be imposed directly on the South African situation, this has mostly been the case. Given that theories do not continue to develop in isolation but in interaction with one another, we believe that generalized counseling theories must necessarily have an effect on the local development of counseling as a science. These counseling theories provide psychologists with the theoretical foundation for establishing a practice with the final objective an acceptable practice that is in the best interests of their clients. With this in mind, the working assumption that will guide our elucidation is first the fact that a culture of sharing and a focus on the collectivistic needs (of the group) rather than individualistic needs characterize roughly 90% of the South African society (Watson et al., 2009). Second, South Africa is currently in a state of flux and turbulence, with poverty, exacerbated by xenophobia, unemployment rates that hover in the region of 40%, spiralling crime levels, ever-increasing socioeconomic inequality, immigration, lack of political leadership, and political instability, characterizing our society.

Against this frame of reference, we postulate that numerous workshops, at various levels, have shown conclusively that the collective and individual stories of South Africa have not been told as yet. In fact, we believe that we have not even begun to scratch the surface of this capacity. We firmly believe, with the Reverend Desmond Tutu, that unless the many individual stories of people of African ancestry are eventually told and the storytellers listened to with empathy and understanding, our collective psyche will remain scarred and hurt and the South African nation deeply divided. It is for this reason that we plead for a storied approach, as a salient facet of the oral tradition, to be introduced into schools and classrooms, thereby facilitating open discussion. and, indeed, healing of the pain that is manifesting in various unwanted forms in our country. We have a feeling this might very well be the case in many other parts of Africa as well.

REFERENCES

Abdi, Y. O. (1975). The problems and prospects of psychology in Africa. *International Journal of Psychology*, *10*(3), 227–34.

Amundson, N. E. (2003). *Active engagement: Enhancing the career counselling process* (2nd ed.). Richmond, B.C.: Ergon Communications.

Amundson, N. E. (2006, August). *Bridge over troubled waters: Guidance crosses*. Keynote presented at the IAEVG Conference, Denmark.

Amundson, N. E., Niles, S. G., & Harris-Bowlsbey, J. (2004). *Essential elements of career counselling.* Vancouver: Merrill Prentice-Hall.

Ben-Amos, D. (1971). Toward a definition of folklore in context. *The Journal of American Folklore*, *84*(331), 3–15.

Bettelheim, B. (1976). *The uses of enchantment*. London: Thames and Hudson.

Carney, S. (2006) *Folktales: What are they?* Retrieved January, 23, 2009 from http://falcon.dmu.edu/~ramseyil/tradcarney.htm.

Chen, C. P. (2001). On exploring meanings: Combining humanistic and career psychology theories in counselling. *Counselling Psychology Quarterly*, *14*(4), 317–30.

Curran, H. V. (1988). Relative universals: Perspectives on culture and cognition. In G. Claxton (Ed.), *Growth points in cognition* (pp.173–192). London: Routledge.

Dasen, P. R. (1993). Theoretical/conceptual issues in developmental research in Africa. *Journal of Psychology in Africa*, *1*(5), 151–8.

De Vos, E. (2001). *Die moederargetipe in Afrikasprokies. (The mother archetype in African falk tales.)* Unpublished master's thesis, University of Pretoria, Pretoria, South Africa.

Ebersöhn, L., & Eloff, I. (2006). Identifying asset-based trends in sustainable programmes, which support vulnerable children. *South African Journal of Education*, *26*(3), 457–68.

Finnegan, R. (1970). *Oral literature in Africa*. Nairobi: Oxford University Press.

Herr, E. L. (1997). Career counselling: A process in process. *British Journal of Guidance and Counselling*, *25*, 81–93.

Hickson, J., & Christie, G. (1989). Research on cross-cultural counselling and psychotherapy: Implications for the South African context. *South African Journal of Psychology*, *19*(3), 162–71.

Hickson, J., Christie, G., & Shmukler, D. (1990). A pilot study of worldview of black and white South African adolescent pupils: Implications for cross-cultural counselling. *South African Journal of Psychology*, *20*(3), 170–7.

Hollis, S. T., Pershing, L., & Young, M. J. (1993). *Feminist theory and the study of folklore*. Urbana & Chicago: University of Illinois Press.

Jordan, A. C. (Ed.). (2004). *Tales from Southern Africa*. Johannesburg: AD Donker.

Jung, C. G. (1959). *The archetypes and the collective unconscious*. London: Routledge & Kegan Paul.

Knappert, J. (1970). *Myths and legends of the Swahili*. Johannesburg: Heinemann.

Leach, M. M., Akhurst, J., & Basson, C. (2003). Counselling psychology in South Africa: Current political and professional challenges and future promise. *The Counselling Psychologist, 31*(5), 619–40.

Leong, T. L., & Ponterotto, J. G. (2003). A proposal for internationalizing counselling psychology in the United States: Rationale, recommendations, and challenges. *The Counselling Psychologist, 31*(4), 381–95.

Levers, L. L. (1997). Cross-cultural training in Southern Africa: A call for psychoecological pluralism. *International Journal of Intercultural Relations, 21*(2), 249–77.

Lewis-Williams, J. D. (Ed.) (2002). *Stories that float from afar: Ancestral folklore of the San of Southern Africa*. Kenilworth, South Africa: David Philip.

Lynch-Brown, C., & Tomlinson, C. (1993). *Essentials of children's literature*. Boston: Allyn & Bacon.

Malimabe-Ramagoshi, R. M., Maree, J. G., Molepo, M., & Alexander, D. (2007). Child abuse in Setswana folktales. *Early Child Development and Care, 177*(4), 433–48.

Malobola, J. N. (2001). *Performance and structure of Southern Ndebele female folk songs: experiences of womanhood*. Unpublished master's dissertation, University of Pretoria, Pretoria, South Africa.

Malott, K. M. (2008). Achieving cultural competency: Assessment of US-based counselor educators instructing internationally. *International Journal for the Advancement of Counselling, 30*(1), 25–37.

Maree, J. G. (2005). Bending the neck to the yoke or getting up on one's hind legs? Getting to grips with bullying. *South African Journal of Criminology, 18*(2), 15–33.

Maree, J. G., Bester, S. E., Lubbe, C., & Beck, C. (2001). Postmodern career counselling to a gifted black youth: A case study. *Gifted Education International, 15*(3), 324–38.

Maree, J. G., & Ebersöhn, L. (Eds.) (2002). *Lifeskills and career counselling*. Pretoria: Heinemann.

Maree, J. G., & Ebersöhn, L. (2006). Administering narrative career counselling in a diverse setting: Trimming the sails to the wind. *South African Journal of Education, 26*(1), 49–60.

Maree, J. G., & Ebersöhn, L. (2008). Applying positive psychology to career development interventions with disadvantaged adolescents. In V. Skorikov & W. Patton (Eds.), *Theorising children's and adolescents' career development*. Sydney: Sense Publishers.

Maree, J. G., & Molepo, J. M. (2005). The use of narratives in cross-cultural career counselling. In M. McMahon & W. Patton (Eds.), *Career counselling: Constructivist approaches* (pp.69–82). New York: Routledge.

Maree, J. G., & Molepo, J. M. (2006). *Narrative career counselling: facilitating a storied approach to counselling in four provinces in South Africa*. Unpublished research report. Pretoria: University of Pretoria.

Mathews, S. (2001). Problems in learning from traumatic history. *Safundi, 2*(2), 1–6.

Mkhize, N. (2004). Social transformation and career marginalisation: Theoretical and research implications. Paper read at the 10th Anniversary South African Congress of Psychology: Democratising the psyche, Durban, September 20–23, 2004.

Mpofu, E. (2003). Conduct disorder: Presentation, treatment options and cultural efficacy in an African setting. Retrieved February, 16, 2009 from *International Journal of Disability, Community and Rehabilitation, 2*(1), http://www.ijdcr.ca/VOL02_01_CAN/articles/mpofu.shtml

Nicholas, L., Naidoo, A. V., & Pretorius, T. B. (2006). A historical perspective of career psychology in South Africa. In G.B. Stead & M.B. Watson (Eds.), *Career psychology in the South African context* (2nd ed., pp. 1–10). Pretoria, South Africa: Van Schaik.

Niles, S. G., & Harris-Bowlsbey, J. (2002). *Career development interventions in the 21st century*. Upper Saddle River, NJ: Merrill Prentice-Hall.

SA History Online. (2008). *On the road to democracy: The Truth & Reconciliation Commission*. Retrieved February, 10 2009 from http://www.sahistory.org.za.

Sanchez, G. (2006). *Social communication through fairy tales*. Retrieved January, 6, 2009 from http://www.unm.edu/~abqteach/fairy_tales/02-03-12.htm.

Savickas, M. L. (1993). Career counselling in the post-modern era. *Journal of Cognitive Psychotherapy: An International Quarterly, 7*(3), 205–15.

Savickas, M. L. (2007a). Internationalisation of counselling psychology: Constructing cross-national consensus and collaboration. *Applied Psychology: An International Review, 5691*, 182–8.

Savickas, M. L. (2007b). Reshaping the story of career counselling. In J. G. Maree (Ed.), *Shaping the story – a guide to facilitate narrative counselling* (pp. 1–3). Pretoria: Van Schaik.

Schwartz, S., & Melzak, S. (2005). Using storytelling in psychotherapeutic work with young refugees. *Group Analysis, 38*, 293–306. Retrieved February, 9, 2009 from http://gaq.sagepub.com.

Skovholt, T., Hansen, S., Goh, M., Romano, J., & Thomas, K. (2005). The Minnesota International Counseling Institute (MICI) 1989 – Present: History, joyful moments, and lessons learned. *International Journal for the Advancement of Counseling, 27*(1), 17–33.

Stead, G. B., & Watson, M. B. (2006). Indigenisation of career psychology in South Africa. In G.B. Stead & M.B. Watson (Eds.), *Career psychology in the South African context* (pp. 181–90). Pretoria, South Africa: Van Schaik.

Straker, G. (1988). Child abuse, counselling and apartheid: The work of the Sanctuary Counselling Team. *Free Associations, 10*, 7–38.

Tlali, M. T. (1999). A review of the mono-cultural approach to psychology and various criticisms of cross-cultural counselling and psychotherapy in the South African context. *Vital, 13*(1), 33–9.

Tutu, D. M. (1999a). Foreword by Archbishop Emeritus Desmond Tutu to the Truth and Reconciliation Commission of South Africa Report. Cape Town: Grove Dictionaries, Inc.

Tutu, D. M. (1999b). Foreword by the most reverend Desmond M TUTU Archbishop Emeritus, Chairperson of the South African Truth and Reconciliation Commission. Retrieved January, 9, 2009 from http://www.sahistory.org.za.

UN Integrated Regional Networks. (2002). Folktales to address modern problems. Retrieved January 7, 2009 from http://www.aegis.com/news/irin/2002/IR020715.html.

Van Niekerk, E. J. (1996). Enkele aspekte van die postmodernistiese kritiek teen die modernisme en die relevansie daarvan vir die opvoedkunde.(Some facets of postmodern critique against modernism and its relevance.). *South African Journal of Education, 16*(4),210–15.

Von Franz, M-L. (1978). *Projection and re-collection in Jungian psychology: Reflections of the soul*. La Salle, IL: Open Court.

Watson, M. B., & Fouche, P. (2007). Transforming a past into a future: Counselling psychology in South Africa. *Applied Psychology: An International Review*, *56*(1), 152–64.

Watson, M. B., & McMahon, M. (2004). Postmodern (narrative) career counselling and education. *Perspectives in Education*, *22*(1), 169–70.

Watson, M., McMahon, M., Mkhize, N., Schweitzer, R., & Mpofu, E. (2010). Career counseling people of African ancestry. In E Mpofu (Ed.), *Counseling people of African ancestry*. New York: Cambridge University Press.

Watson, M. B., & Stead, G. B. (2002). Career psychology in South Africa: Moral perspectives on present and future directions. *South African Journal of Psychology*, *32*(1), 26–31.

Windling, T. (1995). *Introduction*. In T. Windling (Ed.), *The armless maiden and other tales for childhood's survivors* (pp. 13–16). New York: Ton Associates.

Winslade, J. (2007). Constructing a career narrative through the care of the self. In J. G. Maree (Ed.), *Shaping the story – a guide to facilitate narrative counselling* (pp. 52–62). Pretoria: Van Schaik.

SELF-CHECK EXERCISES

1. Examine some of the different forms the oral tradition in an African context may assume.
2. Explain the potential role of the oral tradition in counseling clients of African ancestry.
3. Analyze the meaning and significance of the oral tradition and some of its constituent genres, such as myth, legend, and fable in an African context.
4. Critique the unwarranted emphasis on a positivist approach to counseling in an African context in relation to the importance to utilize the oral tradition in the counseling of people of African ancestry.
5. Reflect on the interventive use of folklore (diagnosis, well-being, and development) in counseling.

FIELD-BASED EXPERIENTIAL EXERCISES

1. Read a number of African folk tales and try to grasp the symbolism involved.
2. Interview clients of African ancestry and invite them to share their stories with you.
3. Interview counselors who work with clients of an African ancestry and ask these colleagues to explain how they use folktales in counseling with their clients.
4. Now obtain permission and observe this counselor actually applying theory in practice.

MULTIPLE-CHOICE QUESTIONS

1. Circle the *correct* answer. In attempting to investigate the value of continuing traditional elements in a modern, largely urban, de-Africanized setting, we maintain that the traditional African oral tradition:
   a. Has been almost unrecognizably transformed through globalization, technocratization, and urbanization.
   b. Has retained its power to provide a means through which people can attain some understanding of aspects that affect their lives.
   c. Cannot be considered potentially relevant in a postmodern society.
   d. Has no place in counseling of African ancestry.
2. Circle the *incorrect* answer. In the course of a previous study on the oral tradition (Malimabe-Ramagoshi, Maree, Molepo, & Alexander, 2007), we:
   a. Confirmed the belief that the majority of oral tradition constituents are meant to have a moral message.
   b. Found that the hero in folktales is often flawed.
   c. Did not encounter many instances of good behavior.
   d. Found that very few folktales, of the ones that we read, dealt with *Ubuntu/Botho*.
3. Circle the *incorrect* answer. The use of storytelling in counseling with clients of African ancestry seems like a viable concept, for the following reasons:
   a. One of the proudest talents of Africans is their ability to tell stories (Maree & Molepo, 2005).
   b. It is not common practice to have a family gathering, after supper, to listen to stories told by elders, with the younger people also participating in the jokes and discussions.
   c. The principle of *Ubuntu* is to share whatever is eaten, enjoyed, and experienced, whether sorrowful or joyous.
   d. Such a practice may constitute one of the ways in which a storied approach to counseling may be introduced. Each client may be requested to tell his/her story in a group context, while the counselor facilitates the direction of these stories.
   e. This code of *Ubuntu* may be utilized by counselors as a means through which clients can reveal their experiences in order to build on and map out their future.
4. Circle the *incorrect* answer. The interventive use of folktales in counseling with clients of African ancestry (including diagnosis, well-being, and development) may include the following elements:
   a. The therapist can ask the client to recount a story.
   b. The client will probably tell a story from memory.
   c. Failing to tell a story from memory, the client may devise a narrative along the lines of a remembered story.
   d. Clients automatically enter a trance-like state when they tell stories.
5. Circle the *correct* answer. Against the frame of reference outlined in this chapter, we postulate that:
   a. Numerous workshops, at various levels, have shown conclusively that the collective and

individual stories of South Africa have already been told.

b. There is little need to focus our attention on this matter in the twenty-first century.

c. The Reverend Desmond Tutu is probably correct in saying that unless the many individual stories of people of African ancestry are eventually told and the storytellers listened to with empathy and understanding, our collective psyche will remain scarred and hurt and the South African nation deeply divided.

d. The introduction of a storied approach (as a salient facet of the oral tradition) into schools and classrooms is bound to be a time-consuming and potentially futile exercise.

Answers to the multiple-choice questions are provided at the back of the book

3 Assessment for Counseling Intervention

Lynne Radomsky, Sofoh Hassane, Michelle Hoy-Watkins, and Chiwoza Bandawe

OVERVIEW. A key concept in any psychological process is the assessment of the appropriateness of the need for any intervention. As such, the application of assessment criteria in the psychological milieu requires an in-depth understanding of inter- and intrapersonal aspects, as well as the broader social, economic, political, and multicultural phenomena. To this end, this chapter explores the development of assessment techniques and the complex and unique approach required of the culturally intentional counselor. The adaptation of Western-based techniques in such a context, as well as the development of culturally specific assessment tools, requires that special attention is given to assessor competency, as well as ethical and legislative considerations. In this chapter, we seek to locate the process of assessment within a multicultural context. A brief history of the development of psychological assessment is presented. The concept of a multicultural approach to assessment, as well as assessor competency, highlights the need for assessor efficacy and training. Ethical implications of a multicultural assessment approach are discussed. The chapter concludes with suggestions for future research.

LEARNING OBJECTIVES

By the end of the chapter, the reader should be able to:

1. Identify the main criteria for a culturally intentional counselor.
2. Examine the cross-cultural applicability of assessment instruments.
3. Outline the criteria required for the assessment of people of African ancestry.
4. Outline the criteria required for assessor competency.
5. Discuss the legislative and ethical considerations necessary for the assessment of people of African ancestry.

INTRODUCTION

The diverse complexity that characterizes today's postmodern world has a direct impact on the approach adopted by psychological counselors. Historically, Western-based or Eurocentric approaches were used by most counselors to govern how counselors understood the problems experienced by clients, as well as the types of assessment strategies, interventions, and management plans employed to treat what was perceived as deviant patterns of behavior. However, Western-based approaches may be inadequate in addressing the counseling needs of the culturally diverse societies comprising people of African ancestry. There is, at present, a growing appreciation of the different ways that clients may construct their realities, hence their counseling needs. Historically, methods of assessment for counseling were based on the Western cultural values and belief systems. Little attention was given to the possibility that what may be considered pathological or deviant in one culture, and thus in need of remediation, may be a reflection of a spiritual calling in another culture and in need of amplification and integration.

IMPORTANCE, KEY CONCEPTS, AND A BRIEF HISTORY OF ASSESSMENT PROCEDURES

Psychological assessment is an important aspect of professional decision making in various multidisciplinary fields. Assessment procedures often form the basis of data collection for research purposes. Sir Francis Galton first coined the term "mental test," and most well known assessment batteries were further developed within the Western based or Eurocentric context. Hysamen (1983, p. 9) noted that assessment procedures were essentially measurements that consisted of the "assignment, according to fixed rules, of numbers to indicate differences in the magnitude of some attribute of persons or objects."

This procedure required proficiency with written tasks, and the testee's performance was assessed according to a predetermined standard. Assessment instruments were based predominantly on a "hypothetico-deductive model," which essentially supported a "context of justification" framework. That is, the results were used to justify a preexisting standard (Terre Blanche & Durrheim, 2002, p. 4).

In South Africa, particularly, the development of psychological assessment tools was characterized by the collation of tests for separate cultural and language groups (Foxcroft, 2004). Although some attention was paid to the different cultural groups that comprised the South African society, little effort was made to determine the cross-cultural applicability of these procedures.

Information Box 3.1: The Culturally Intentional Counselor

The task of assessing a client's need for a counseling intervention requires that the counselor adopts a culturally intentional stance (Ivey, D'Andrea, Ivey, & Simke-Morgan, 2002, p. 2). The literature identifies five factors as defining the culturally intentional counselor:

1. World view: This factor relates to the idea of how the client and the counselor distill meaning from their individual experiences.
2. Cultural intentionality: This factor refers to the ability to communicate awareness of diverse issues such as racial identity, spiritual awareness, linguistic understanding, family values, and socioeconomic history within a cultural context.
3. The scientist-practitioner: The ability to translate scientific knowledge into practice within a multicultural context.
4. Ethics: The understanding of the diversity inherent in ethical practice where different cultures may subscribe to different moral bases and the counselor's ability to understand and respect such differences.
5. The community genogram: A practical method to aid the exploration of each client's interface with his or her culture and personal experiences.

Current shifts in awareness require that the researcher and practitioner remain sensitive to the broader social, economic, political, and cultural phenomena. Draguns (1977) notes that despite the fact that some attention to a transcultural psychiatric endeavor was attempted by Kraepelin as early as 1904, advances have been slow. Research that attempts to investigate naturalistic clinical accounts outside of the Western paradigm, as well as the informal accounts of treatment of psychiatric disorders in different countries, still focuses on the representation of recognized diagnostic categories.

The methodologies employed in these attempts were characterized by a lack of self-consciousness of the observer and the assumption that observational characteristics were similar across cultures. Thus, transcultural psychiatry was etic in nature, in that it was accepted that similar phenomena could and would be observed across different cultures, and that different cultures used the same frame of reference to understand so-called psychiatric deviance (Draguns, 1977).

Recent Developments in Assessment Procedures

The inadequacies of these traditional approaches have been recently recognized, and more attention is given to cross-cultural comparisons of psychopathological criteria. Assessment instruments have to change to accommodate this different focus. Greater cognizance is given to the context in which data are gathered and to the instruments used to gather such data. For example, greater use is made of symptom rating scales, interview schedules, and qualitative research methodologies. Most importantly, recent trends in the development, formulation, and implementation of assessment processes focus on the multicultural approach.

Examples of recent developments are depicted by the culturally specific assessment tools that have been developed for use with Black or African American populations (Jones, 1996). These tests were written from the perspective of the daily experiences of Blacks, because many of the tests being used with this population failed to consider a cultural approach. For example, the common thread between these culturally specific tests for Blacks is that they were created within an African-centered conceptual framework that considers racial identity, historical political factors, socioeconomic factors, personality traits, family values, and so forth (Jones, 1996).

Culturally Specific Assessment Techniques

There are several theoretical models that support the need to develop and use culturally specific techniques with people of African descent. Perhaps one of the most relevant theories is indigenous psychology. Kim, Yang, and Hwang (2006) discuss the need to conceptualize individuals within a cultural context. They define indigenous psychology as the integration of specific beliefs, practices, and values of the individuals being studied or treated. Kim et al. note that "indigenous psychology emphasizes examining of psychological phenomena in context: familial, social, political, philosophical, historical, religious, cultural, and ecological context" (p. 6).

Another approach is the contextualist model, which emphasizes a range of diversity among individual cultures. According to the contextualist theory, understanding individual cultural traditions and sociopolitical practices should be foremost (Harley, 2005). Finally, the integrationist approach focuses on the importance of blending indigenous-based practices and cross-cultural models of psychological assessment to develop a mainstream level of understanding of the individual (Harley, 2005).

The influence of Black psychology on assessment procedures

Theories of Black psychology suggest the need for an Africentric approach to or a culturally specific perspective

Discussion Box 3.1: The Cross-cultural Dilemma

The purpose of this exercise is to help you be aware of the dilemma of professional counselors in Ghana and Niger, where clients believe that they have psychological problems because they have offended the spirits of their ancestors. It will also enhance your awareness of how culture and belief systems play a major role in the entire helping relationship.

Professional helpers are required by several codes of ethics and standards for testing and assessment to demonstrate competence (education, training, and experience) in assessing all clients' problems. Professional helpers in Ghana and Niger are trained to do so; but they do not have the education, training, and experience to holistically assess African clients who believe that their psychological problems are connected to their ancestors' spirits. These professionals are well aware that using Western psychological instruments that focus only on the psychological aspect of human functioning may lead to an inaccurate assessment. Yet, they are required to assess all clients' problems regardless of age, race, ethnicity, gender, disability, national origin, religion, sexual orientation, linguistic background, or other personal characteristics.

Questions

1. As a professional helper, in using a Western psychological instrument to assess an African client for counseling intervention, what variables might affect your work?
2. How will your training and the Western instrument you are using influence your assessment?
3. What precautions will you take that will help you better assess your client?
4. Consider the following four critical areas: selection of instrument, administration of instrument, scoring, and interpreting results. Discuss likely opportunities and challenges with people of African ancestry.

on understanding individuals of African descent (Baldwin, 1991). Known to many as the father of Black psychology, Joseph White notes that the essential focus of any attempts to understand people of African descent should be to examine the Black experience as a whole (Baldwin, 1991). Specifically, concepts such as communication, oral tradition, or the importance of language should be considered. A focus on family values (i.e., extended family, matriarchy, community, neighbors) is also important to understanding people of African ancestry, because these traditions help to shape individualism. White also notes the importance of acknowledging and having respect for the level of generalized paranoia that many people of African ancestry hold as a result of their historically based persecutory experiences in America. This type of paranoia, if understood from a cultural perspective, would not be regarded as pathological.

African or Black Psychology, as defined by Wade Nobles (as cited in Baldwin, 1991), posits that its culture rests on indigenous or African theoretical foundations. Further, Nobles states that Black Psychology encompasses oral traditions, spirituality, communal existence, and extended family that can be traced to the historical values, beliefs, and traditions of West African people. Similar to White (1991), Nobles discusses the prevalence of oral tradition, religion, community, and kinship or collective unity in African psychology.

Many psychologists began to question the reliability and validity of traditional psychological test instruments being used with people of African ancestry that had not been normed or validated with relevant populations. According to White (1991), such a practice does not allow the examiner or practitioner to consider the lifestyles of the African people when formulating clinical opinions that can be detrimental to the client. Failure to recognize and incorporate a cultural perspective when assessing people of African ancestry can lead to misinterpretation of responses, misdiagnosis, and failure to conceptualize appropriately the needs of the client.

Multicultural Approaches to Assessment

Psychological assessment has always played, and continues to play, a very important role in counseling. It is essential for all professional counselors to have basic knowledge and skills in assessment. It is important that counselors demonstrate competency in assessment, because proficiency in assessment is directly related to effectiveness in counseling intervention. According to Zytowski (as cited in Schafer, 1996), assessment guides and motivates a professional toward seeking additional information for decision making. Juhnke (1996) emphasized that assessment provides counselors with direction for treatment.

The ever increasing diversity in our society and the idea of ensuring fair and equitable treatment for individuals regardless of race, ethnicity, culture, language, age, gender, sexual orientation, religion, or physical ability, emphasizes the need for skills in the choice and application of appropriate assessment strategies. In every respect, these skills enable professional counselors in a multicultural setting to facilitate and choose the right counseling strategies to meet the diversity of client needs (The Association for Assessment in Counseling [AAC], 2003).

Definitions of multiculturalism

Multiculturalism is a complex, diverse, and layered phenomenon that is accordingly difficult to define in a precise manner. Bekker and Leilde (2003) note that the term *multiculturalism* is used in three distinct ways:

1. A description of cultural diversity within a society;
2. An ideological concept legitimizing the incorporation of ethnic diversity in the societal structure; and
3. A public policy designed to create national unity in a diverse population.

Multiculturalism is not exclusively applicable to the realm of psychology and has its roots in the political arena. For example, in South Africa, multiculturalism is particularly relevant, as previously disadvantaged groups demand recognition and the accommodation of their differences. The idea of a multicultural society permeates most areas of South African life, including policy making and socioeconomic and political strata. This influence is strongly felt in the field of psychological assessment. As noted previously, psychological assessment forms the bedrock of most counseling interventions. Counselors interview clients and administer assessment instruments with the view of determining their clients' readiness for interventions. As further noted, these assessments are intrinsically flawed, as multicultural factors often are not given precedence. Factors that are pertinent to the management of the case may be lost when a predominantly Eurocentric assessment measure is applied within a multicultural setting.

Current trends in multicultural assessment

The cultural understanding of psychological distress in countries with people of African ancestry such as South Africa, Ghana, and Niger has historically been based mainly on a spiritual model. The spiritual model of assessing psychological disorders still is used widely, even though the influence of Western education has encouraged a more Western approach. Families, religious leaders, and traditional healers are consulted to assess and resolve social and psychological distress (Hsiao-Wen & Dzokoto, 2005).

It is no longer enough for the counselor to be technically and theoretically proficient or competent. Cultural, spiritual, and social dimensions often influence the results obtained. A multicultural approach has become important for client retention and treatment. Most cultures have complex and multilayered ways of understanding, managing, and treating mental health issues. As such, to assess the need for counseling in an ethical and congruent way, an understanding of what constitutes "deviant" behavior within a particular cultural context is essential.

Multicultural Factors in Diagnosis

Kirmayer (1989) reflected on the idea that cultural differences affect the diagnosis and interpretation of deviant behavior. Theories of emotion, as well as the cultural concept of the individual in society, have an impact on the identification of behavior as deviant, as well as on the understanding of symptoms as either symbolic expressions of cultural processes or meaningless dysfunctional acts.

Western psychiatric nosology is based mostly on diagnostic criteria that fit predetermined distinct categories of disorders. The identification of these categories was based on the observation, documentation, and clustering of symptoms that emerged from a predominantly Eurocentric concept of normal versus deviant behaviors. Little consideration was given to the possible effect of cultural differences in the understanding, assessment, classification, and treatment of psychological disorders.

Ethnopsychological theories of the self, emotion, and the expression of distress all influence the response to deviant behavior within a specific culture, as well as the assessment of such behavior as actually deviant and requiring labeling and remediation (White & Kirkpatrick, 1986). Within many multicultural societies, such as South Africa, the concept of labeling is a sensitive one that requires an awareness of the political implications embedded in such a process (Foxcroft, 1997). As such, any procedure that assesses the need for counseling within a culturally diverse society or population with African ancestry ideally would combine an etic and emic approach (Van de Vijver & Rothman, 2004). This combination would require an approach that is both methodologically sound and culturally sensitive.

Cross-cultural Applicability of Assessment Instruments

White and Kirkpatrick (1986) note that the attention given to the cultural concept of the individual being assessed offers an approach that moves beyond the narrow parochial assumptions of Western psychological theory. Kirmeyer (1989) and Florsheim (1990) identify three prominent phenomena that influence the reliability, validity, and applicability of assessment instruments across cultures. These include self-knowledge and behavior, the location of deviant behavior, and the meaning of symptoms.

Self-knowledge and behavior

In the West, self-authenticity is prized, and many psychological interventions focus on self-actualization, individuation, and self-knowledge. However, in many indigenous cultures, self-development may be sacrificed in favor of the broader community ethos. Florsheim (1990) maintains that the concept of the self underlies the essence of the difference between Western and indigenous assessment procedures.

In Western ethos, the self is autonomous, and differentiation is a measure of health, maturity, and well-being. Within the indigenous cosmology, the concept of the self is more relational and interdependent. Life stages such as birth, marriage, and death are community affairs.

Information Box 3.2: Sources of Bias in Cross-cultural Assessment (Van de Vijver & Rothman, 2004, p. 3)

1. Construct bias

This bias occurs when there is a partial overlap in the definitions of the construct across cultures, skills do not belong to all cultural groups, there has been poor sampling of relevant behavior, and not all the domains of the construct are sampled.

2. Method bias

This bias occurs when samples cannot be compared because of differences in, for example, education; there are differences in environmental conditions; there is ambiguity in the instructions given; the expertise levels of the administrators differ; there are communication and language incompatibilities; and there are differences in the familiarity with the stimulus material, response procedures, and response styles.

3. Item bias

This bias occurs when there has been poor item translation, and items may assess different traits or abilities, and culturally specific meanings or nuances of meaning.

Definitions of the self have a direct impact on the formulation of illness, health, assessment, and treatment modalities. Within a Western paradigm, the restoration of health is geared toward the restoration of the individual's autonomy, independence, and self-sufficiency. Within traditional cultures, health is about the reestablishment of harmonious relationships among the individual, the family, the community, and the ancestors. As such, assessment criteria will be influenced by the culturally specific epistemology in which the assessment instrument is developed and implemented.

The location of deviant behavior

The assessment and diagnosis of deviant behavior within the Western approach tends to locate the cause of the deviance within the individual, that is, intrapsychically. Assessment criteria for counseling are based on the individual's ability to change. In indigenous cultures, symptomatic behavior is attributed to an external agent and treatment focuses on the rectification of a perceived imbalance located within the individual's family, community, or spiritual frame of reference. The ability to change and to restore well-being is not solely the responsibility of the individual.

The meaning of symptoms

Western-based diagnostic and assessment approaches generally view symptoms as meaningless, arbitrary deviations from a preestablished norm. Assessment criteria entail establishing or quantifying how far from the norm the behavior deviates: mild, moderate, or severe deviations. In direct contrast, traditional cultures view symptomatic behaviors as inseparable from the cultural fabric from which they emerge. Symptoms are imbued with a symbolic meaning that can be traced back to a cultural foundation. Becoming ill is thus not an arbitrary event in the individual's life, but is understood in relation to a broader cultural patterning.

Littlewood (1990) asserts that a multicultural assessment should be aware that Western concepts do not migrate easily into the realm of traditional cultures. What is regarded as disease in the West may carry a different meaning for different cultures.

> The meaning of illness for an individual is grounded in – though not reducible to – the network of meanings an illness has in a particular culture: The metaphors associated with a disease, the ethnomedical theories, the basic values and conceptual forms and the core patterns that shape the experience of the illness and the social reactions to the sufferer (Good & Good, 1982).

For any assessment process to be considered as valid and reliable within different cultures, there needs to be a good fit among the practitioner, the client, the diagnostic and therapeutic system, and the sociocultural context.

CRITERIA FOR ASSESSMENT FOR PEOPLE OF AFRICAN ANCESTRY

A number of researchers cite the following five criteria as forming the foundation of a multicultural assessment approach that is applicable for people of African ancestry (Craig & Beishuizen, 2002; Draguns, 1977; Foxcroft, 2004): (1) conceptualization and classification of illness, (2) linguistic equivalence, (3) appropriateness of content, (4) type of measurement, and (5) cultural relevance of the test design.

Conceptualization and Classification of Illness

Western models of psychiatric illness make clear distinctions between symptom and syndrome, etiology and prognosis, disease and classification. These classifications are

Research Box 3.1: Test Development and Validation

Durrheim, K., Baillee, K., & Johnstone, L. (2008). The development and validation of a measure of racial justice perceptions (study 1). *South African Journal of Psychology*, *38*(4), 615–632.

Objective: This study aimed to develop an understanding of racial attitudes by means of a pincer movement, comparing themes expressed in existing indices of racism with the opinions expressed by ordinary South Africans in the media.

Method: The study developed a pool of items that had currency as everyday expressions of racial opinion in the current South African context.

Thematic analyses were performed to survey themes in debates about racism. This source contained a random sample of 3,800 newspaper articles that were coded under the themes "racism" or "discrimination" by the South African Media Archive. These articles appeared in different newspapers and magazines published in South Africa. Each article was described qualitatively by means of two comments that described the context within which the event occurred and the manifestation of racism that the article described.

Examples of statements provided by context and manifestation

Context category	Manifestation category
Editor gives his views on the fact that matrics are obliged to fill in their race on exam papers.	"They call it affirmative action, but I think it is prejudice."
ANC document urges an intensified campaign to combat racism.	The de-racialization of the working class consciousness still has to emerge in the country.

Results: Dominant themes emerged from the analyses. Debates about racial desegregation, racial policy, and affirmative action featured prominently.

Conclusion: Commonalities between the ranges of themes characterizing racism in the racial attitude literature and the local media were identified.

Questions

1. Discuss whether or not a measure of racial justice perceptions is relevant for your particular social context.
2. Administer Duckitt's Subtle Racism Scale to a group of participants.
3. Conduct a thematic analysis of fifty statements obtained from current media publications such as newspapers and magazines.
4. Compare the results of the thematic analysis to the results obtained in the Duckitt's Subtle Racism Scale.

imposed on the experience of the illness, and the main focus is in understanding the "how" of the disease and not the "why." Within a multicultural context, this approach is inadequate, and the applicability of a classification system is valid only when all the meanings of the symptoms are linked to the context and culture of the affected person.

Linguistic Equivalence

A multicultural context demands that attention is given to the language of the culture, the assessor, the assessed, and the assessment instrument. Draguns (1977) points out that the development of equivalent measures of the same instrument in different languages requires more than a mere mechanical translation of the measurement criteria. The development of a linguistically reliable measurement instrument also must include the nuances of linguistic understanding and cultural applicability. Meanings can be lost or changed during the translation process and, as such, invalidate the reliability of the assessment tool. In addition, a further difficulty is encountered in that in the comparison of the tool across different languages, reliability must be applicable not only to the parent language, such as English, but between all the subsequent translations as well. In South Africa, this presents a particular challenge in that the country has eleven official languages. A standardized assessment tool must be comparable across all of these languages and their associated cultural groups.

Appropriateness of Content

It has been noted previously that most existing assessment tools were developed within the Western or Eurocentric contexts. As such, these tools reflect the context in which they originated. To have cross-cultural validity, an

Discussion Box 3.2: The RESPECTFUL model of Counseling

D'Andrea and Daniels (in Ivey et al., 2002, p. xvii) propose the RESPECTFUL model of counseling and development, which addresses the need for a comprehensive model of human diversity. This framework attempts to incorporate the following factors that impact human development and relationships:

R – Religious or spiritual identity
E – Economic status
S – Sexual identity
P – Psychological maturity
E – Ethnic identity
C – Chronological and developmental challenges
T – Trauma and threats to well-being
F – Family background
U – Unique physical characteristics
L – Language

Conduct at least three interviews with individuals from diverse communities with respect to how these factors impact their development and well-being.

Questions

1. How do these ten factors influence development in diverse communities?
2. How could specific counseling and psychotherapeutic interventions incorporate the RESPECTFUL model?
3. Critically discuss the ten factors with respect to the cross-cultural applicability of each.

assessment tool must reflect the content and represent the behavior that is familiar to the particular culture in which the assessment tool is to be used. In addition, cross-cultural applicability would be required in order to allow for comparative studies. The format of the tool requires further attention. Self-reporting and paper-and-pencil formats are not necessarily reflective of many multicultural societies.

Type of Measurement

The Western-based approach is one that is familiar with the idea of the symptom as the unit of investigation or assessment. Within many other cultures, the symptom is not necessarily an exhaustive criterion when understanding deviant behavior. Phenomenological studies reveal the importance of the subjective experience of the symptoms, as well as the effect of the culture on the understanding of the symptomatology.

Cultural Relevance of the Test Design

Foxcroft (2004) notes, in addressing the relevance of psychological assessment in the multicultural society of South Africa, that the purpose of the assessment instrument must reflect the constructs that are unique to each cultural group, as well as reflect a cross-cultural validity. Related to this is the educational status of the tested. For example, in South Africa, the quality of education across cultural groups varies greatly, and this has a direct impact on the ability of the individual to cope with the assessment process. Results may thus be biased toward proficiency with educational criteria, rather than cognitive ability.

ASSESSMENT FOR COUNSELING WITHIN THE AFRICAN CONTEXT

Within the South African context of the Traditional Healing paradigm, distinctions are made between culturally mediated deviant behavior and conventional psychiatric disorders. Kirmayer (1989) notes that culturally mediated deviant behaviors receive more familial and social support, do not disrupt socially appropriate and adaptive functioning, do not result in the loss of social standing, and are linked to culturally congruent content. As such, indigenous patterns of behavior do not easily fit the narrow point-based criteria that characterize a Western-based diagnostic classification system such as the *DSM-IV –TR*. Such a classification system typically reflects the biomedical paradigm of the mind–body split. The traditional healer does not make such distinctions, and there is an understanding of the continuity and interrelatedness among mind, body, and spirit.

Africans perceive psychological distress to be related to the spirits, and they believe that healers can cure a variety of problems, including psychological disorders, infertility, impotence, and bad dreams. As such, the need for helpers with a similar world view continues to exist. In addition, the lack of appropriately trained psychiatrists and other helping professionals such as counselors and psychologists in Africa, as well as the poor proximity to existing services, is another reason why Africans continue to seek help from traditional healers (Lamb, 1983; Mbiti, 1989; Sylla, 1988; Vontress, 1991).

According to several theorists (Diallo & Hall, 1989; Hegba, 1979; Keharo & Bouquet, 1950; Retel-Laurentin, 1969; Spence, 1988 as cited in Vontress, 1991), traditional healers use a variety of methods to diagnose clients' problems. Some of these methods include taking a medical history, including physical, psychological, and spiritual; evoking spirits of ancestors to get needed answers; evoking mental images of the client's problem; anthroposcopy (looking at clients and telling them who they are and what their problems are); lithomancy (throwing bones on the ground and telling patients what is wrong with them simply by the landed configuration of the bones); shell-listening; crystal-gazing; botanomancy (reading of leaves); and, cartomancy (reading of cards).

THE INTERFACE BETWEEN WESTERN AND INDIGENOUS APPROACHES

Although many Africans still use traditional healers for resolving their psychological problems, more and more helping professionals, in South Africa, Niger, and Ghana, are being trained nationally and abroad to meet their needs. These helping professionals receive training in the use of Western psychological instruments in the various categories such as career/vocational, cognitive/ability, interests/attitudes, motivation, and personality.

Even though psychological instruments may be used to understand a presenting concern, it is not clear how such data alone are useful in assessing the client's problem, as Africans believe that their problems are linked to their ancestors. Therefore, counselors must feel comfortable in exploring the traditional beliefs African clients have about their psychological distress (Vontress, 1991).

Mental health counseling is becoming more and more popular worldwide. It is important to look seriously at the appropriateness of direct introduction of Western psychological interventions into non-Western countries. The roles that culture and religion play in assessment, case conceptualization, and treatment need to be examined.

Qualified assessors should have appropriate education, training, and experience in using tools, which includes the highest degree of ethical codes, laws, and standards that guide professional counselors. Anything short of this can lead to mistakes that eventually may harm the client (Association for Assessment in Counseling, 2003).

Adapting Western-based Assessment Methods

The psychological tools helping professionals use are developed predominantly in the West and are not standardized for clients of African ancestry. The tools' reliability, validity, appropriateness, and applicability for the culture of the client are thus questionable. Hence, for example, many counselors in Ghana and Niger modify the Western tools to suit the culture of their clients and meet their assessment needs, and they rely mostly on clinical interviews to develop effective client conceptualization and treatment plans.

One example of the adaptation of Western-based assessment methods can be found in Ghana. The Cape Coast University in Ghana is developing career interest inventories, and the University of Ghana, Legon is currently testing the effectiveness of a personality inventory that they have adapted from one developed in the West. Such examples emphasize the need for changes in assessment approaches and techniques. It is important for counselors who practice in any multicultural context to be proficient in different assessment procedures.

NARRATIVE APPROACHES TO COUNSELING

Not all counseling approaches utilize formalized assessment techniques. One approach that provides an alternative to this is known as narrative counseling. Narrative counseling is a world view strategy, theoretically located in a postmodern critical approach framework (see also Chapter 2, this volume). Although it originates and has been developed in Australia, it is an approach that is very conducive to counseling people of African ancestry.

Narrative counseling works in ways that transform communities, recognizing that the community ethos is very strong in Africa. The strength of the approach is its effectiveness in context. It operates within the idiosyncrasies of each population group. It is therefore a contextual approach to counseling that works from the premise that people are the experts of their own lives, and as such, there is no formal assessment for counseling. This is a reaction to the assumption that the assessor is placed in the role and position of an expert. Narrative counseling holds a negative view of the role of experts, seeing them as taking away power in people's lives – potentially diminishing the ability to make changes, centralizing people's knowledge experience. The key issue relies upon what is really going on for the client and not for the therapist as the expert.

The Issue of Power in Counseling

The narrative approach addresses the issue of power in counseling. It alerts the therapist to the fact that power is everywhere and there is need to be sensitive to it. Counselors tend to marginalize people and centralize things, for example; it could be that the counselor is centralizing pathology as opposed to potential and strengths. The counselor could also be centralizing Western approaches in handling problems that preclude cultural factors. Narrative counseling, therefore, seeks to shift the distribution of power, in order to establish a power-sharing dialogue (Winslade & Monk, 1998). It is this dialogue that produces the effectiveness of the counseling.

There are several processes the counselor will engage in when negotiating this power-sharing dialogue, for

Information Box 3.3: Future Research: Where Narrative Counseling Can Go

Narrative counseling has much potential for future research. Storytelling is part of people's life experience, and this approach could be used to help people who are going through challenging life experiences such as HIV/AIDS. HIV-positive people can share their stories and research could focus on how the telling of such stories could give them agency and emotional support. Generally, there has been much focus on the difficulties and negative aspects of the African experience and too little attention given to the positive and successful elements of people's life experiences and stories. A narrative approach can open such doors. Because narrative focuses on unique outcomes, it can bring these stories and successes to light. Every person living in any community has his or her life story as well as various experiences that have a reflection on his or her social and mental well-being. People's experiences differ depending on age, sex, and the nature of the community in which they have been brought up. Thus, for example, the challenges that a 30-year-old woman has faced differs from that of an elderly man of 80 years of age. As such, experiences of triumph over the challenging realities of daily life in Africa need to be highlighted. Future research can explore common themes in these stories of triumph and thus provide tools for counseling that strengthen people's resilience to the daily challenges faced on the continent. Counseling needs to learn from people's lived experience.

example, asking the client for permission to ask questions or take notes (instead of assuming this right by virtue of being the counselor). In the course of the session, the counselor refers back to the client to ask if the session is helpful. The client is further asked to share his or her ideas about what he or she thinks might be helpful in dealing with the situation. Throughout, the client is treated as worthy of professional respect and as an expert in his or her own life.

The Narrative Approach to Assessment

The assessment is not a separate part of the history-gathering process. The counseling begins right away. The counselor is on the alert for strengths the client has. The client may be focused on what is absent, on weaknesses, and what he or she lacks. Such thinking leads to distress. The therapist looks instead for the unique outcomes, the places or events of strength the client has, and problems the client has overcome. The therapist will make a note of this. Examples of unique outcome questions include (Morgan, 2000):

1. How have you managed to stop the problem from getting worse?
2. Are there times when the problem is not as bad as usual?
3. Are there times when it is less dominating and bossy?
4. Can you think of a time when the problem could have stopped you or got in the way but didn't? What happened?
5. Is there a story you can tell me about a time when you resisted the problem and did what you wanted to do instead?

The narrative counselor listens for areas of competence and abilities and tries to highlight the successes and strengths in the stories people tell. If there is any "assessment" involved, this is what the counselor assesses to identify the strengths and resources that the client has, as reflected from the story being presented. The assessment is not a separate part of the history-gathering process.

The point of this process is not to determine whether the client is suitable for counseling or the extent to which the client can cope with counseling, but rather, the counselor stores up this information for later use when it is time to work with the client in constructing a preferred and more helpful storyline (Winslade & Monk, 1998).

The Primary Focus of the Narrative Approach

The founder of this approach, Michael White (2008, p. 1), writes that "the primary focus of a narrative approach is people's expressions of their experiences of life." The basic premise of a narrative approach is that people's lives are storied. It is through these interpretive acts that people give meaning to their experiences of the world. These interpretive acts render people's experiences of life sensible to themselves and to others. Meaning does not predate the interpretation of experience. This approach therefore has a clear link to the strong oral traditions of Africans, whereby storytelling is an integral part of life.

Narrative counseling is a positive approach to counseling, a way that respects the *Ubuntu* – the summation of African life, the strength, potential, and humanity of the person. In that way, it is an approach that is linked to African values. Despite the heterogeneity and dynamism of the African continent, there are commonalities that unite the African experience. This communal embeddedness and connectedness of a person to other persons is illuminated by the idea that the individual is affected by what happens to the whole group, as indeed the whole group is affected by what happens to the individual. In African philosophy, the African view of persons oscillates around this pivotal point (Bandawe, 2005). A narrative therapeutic approach recognizes and respects this ethos, as it recognizes that the stories people live operate in context.

CULTURALLY SPECIFIC TESTS FOR PEOPLE OF AFRICAN ANCESTRY

Recognizing the importance of developing culturally specific tests for people of African ancestry, Robert Williams was one of the first psychologists to develop psychological assessment instruments from an African/Black perspective. Drawing from an Afrocentric theoretical paradigm or theory of Black psychology, Williams (1972) created several tests including a projective test: the Themes Concerning Blacks Test (TCB). The TCB was an original test that was created in response to the use of the Thematic Apperception Test (TAT) with people of African ancestry. The TCB consists of twenty charcoal drawings that feature images, characteristics, and day-to-day experiences of people of African ancestry.

Several researchers have studied the cultural and cross-cultural relevance of the TCB (Matthews-Evans, 1992; Squire, 1985; Weaver, 1978, White, Olivieira, Strube, & Meertens, 1995). Several of these scholars compared the stories told by African Americans in response to the Thematic Apperception Test (TAT) and the TCB. The TAT contains images of individuals of European descent and does not incorporate the cultural experiences of people of African ancestry. The studies that examined the cultural relevance of the TAT in comparison to the TCB found that the participants told longer stories, attributed a greater degree of positive stories, or projected racial attribution in response to the TCB.

White et al. (1995) compared responses from the TCB among African Dutch, African Surinamers, and African Americans. They found that there was little variance in the responses between groups with regard to the emotional tone projected and the Afrocentric themes attributed to the cards. That is, the participants attributed similar socio-cultural and historical experiences (Hoy, 1997). White et al. (1995) hypothesized that the responses elicited common cultural themes, because people of African descent share a common history of ancestry, oppression, race, and psychological experiences.

The Contemporized-Themes Concerning Blacks Test

The development of the Contemporized-Themes Concerning Blacks Test (C-TCB) (Hoy, 1997; Hoy-Watkins, 2008) was twofold. The first goal was to update the original version of the Themes Concerning Blacks Test (TCB) (Williams, 1972). The TCB is a projective test that was developed to provide an alternative to the use of Thematic Apperception Test (TAT) with people of African ancestry. Each of the TCB cards was illustrated in charcoal and depicts imagery of people of African ancestry in various situations. The cultural specificity of the TCB cards is clearly portrayed, as each card captures the lifestyles, physical characteristics, and values of Blacks (Hoy-Watkins & Jenkins-Monroe, 2008).

The TCB was created during an era of economic strife, political warfare, and overt racial oppression in America. While people of African ancestry continue to face many of the same hardships consistent with some of the original themes depicted in the TCB, Blacks and African Americans face additional sociopolitical issues that have become equally prevalent in the African community. These issues include teenage pregnancy, single parenting, institutionalized racism (e.g., racial disparity in the workplace, the legal system, etc.), the prevalence of HIV/AIDS, and media portrayal (which is typically negative) of people of African ancestry. The thematic cards of the C-TCB illustrate these social and political concerns. Other issues portrayed in the C-TCB test are autonomy/individual motivation, political leadership, Black pride (or cultural identification/unification), and extended family/kinship (Hoy-Watkins, 2008).

In addition to including new themes, the C-TCB also includes new imagery. The cards were produced in color, and the pictures portray diverse physical characteristics (i.e., skin tone, facial features, hair texture, hair styles, physical build, and clothing, etc.) of members of African descent (Hoy, 1997).

The second goal of the C-TCB was to create a test that continued the legacy of approaching assessment from a cultural perspective for people of African ancestry. That is, the C-TCB was created from an Afrocentric perspective that incorporates sociopolitical issues; addresses the importance of family, kinship, and group dynamics; and allows for ethnic/cultural identification. In addition, the scoring system includes items (personality traits) that are African-centered. The personality traits that are measured include group needs, interpersonal relations, Black pride, family unity, self-concept, autonomy, and goal-setting/motivation (Hoy-Watkins, 2008).

The twenty-seven projective cards of the C-TCB portray nine central themes that are measured by storytelling. The themes include teenage pregnancy, political leadership/Black pride, extended family/family unity, single parenting, safe sex and drug use (implications of HIV/AIDS), media portrayal of people of African ancestry, institutionalized racism, individual motivation/autonomy, and academic motivation/achievement (Hoy-Watkins & Jenkins-Monroe, 2008). Based on the results of the standardization of the C-TCB with college-aged African American men and women ages eighteen to thirty-two, the themes portrayed are culturally relevant and elicited more positive affective stories than negative ones (Hoy, 1997). The general relevance of the social, political, educational, familial, and economic themes portrayed are applicable to Blacks across many different cultures (e.g., age, race, gender, sex, etc.). Furthermore, C-TCB can be used in multiple clinical and counseling settings including hospitals, community mental health, counseling centers, and forensic/correctional environments.

Duzant (2006) compared the use of the C-TCB to the Thematic Apperception Test with thirty-two African

Research Box 3.2: Culturally Relevant Assessments

Hoy, M. (1997). Contemporizing the themes concerning blacks test (C-TCB). Unpublished Doctoral dissertation. The California School of Professional Psychology-Alameda.

Objective: This study aimed to develop a revised version of the Themes Concerning Blacks Test (Williams, 1972). First, new thematic cards were created that included chromatic images. Second, with regard to the individuals portrayed in the pictures, the main objective was to create images that embody the unique features of individuals of Black or African descent. That is, each card depicts the diversity of physical characteristics (i.e., facial features, skin tone, hair styles, hair texture, attire, etc.) represented within this diverse community. Third, the aim was to represent common day-to-day situations experienced primarily by African Americans, as well as members of other African groups, by focusing on the following themes: single parenting, kinship/extended family, individual motivation/autonomy, teenage pregnancy, media portrayal of Blacks or African Americans, institutionalized racism, substance abuse, and the implications of HIV/AIDS. The fourth objective was to develop a culturally relevant scoring system that would assess the test-taker's attribution of culturally based personality functioning, as well as mood states in response to each card (Hoy-Watkins, 2008). That is, the C-TCB is conceptually based upon African-centered principles (i.e., kinship, culture, spirituality, and community) (Hoy-Watkins, 2008).

Method: The study entailed the administration of all twenty-seven thematic C-TCB cards to 100 African Americans. Participants included fifty African American females and fifty African American men between the ages of eighteen and thirty-two. Each individual was asked to tell a story based upon structured interview questions.

Results: Each participant's responses were rated to assess construct validity and to determine agreement between raters (e.g., inter-rater reliability). In addition, the participants' attribution of culturally relevant personality functioning and affective states was scored by each rater. Construct validity was established in that nine of the expected themes emerged. The C-TCB Manual provides the history of the C-TCB, user qualifications, administration procedures, scoring process, test limitations, conceptual framework, and practice scoring (Hoy-Watkins, 2008).

Conclusions: Given the Afrocentric theoretical basis of the C-TCB, and the strong degree of cultural identification attributed to the cards, there are promising implications for the cross-cultural use of the test within the African Diaspora. Given the diverse thematic content attributed to the cards (i.e., teen pregnancy, parenting, kinship, academic achievement, etc.), the C-TCB can be used within a number of counseling and clinical settings (e.g., outpatient, school-based, inpatient, college counseling, correctional, etc.).

Questions

1. Discuss whether or not the C-TCB would be relevant in assessing the mental health needs of the population you work with or aspire to work with.
2. What cultural relevance do you think the C-TCB would have with the individuals whom you provide treatment?
3. What clinical or counseling setting do you think the C-TCB should be piloted and studied?

Americans. Specifically, the word length of each story and emotional tone elicited by participants were compared with the use of both tests. The results revealed that participants told lengthier stories on the C-TCB as compared to the TAT. Additionally, greater emotional tone was elicited on the C-TCB than with the TAT. The results imply that participants identify greater with the use of culturally relevant tests.

Regarding future research, administration of the C-TCB with other African cultures is needed. The C-TCB has been administered to a sample of college-aged Ghanaian males. The stories told by the Ghanaian males will be compared to the stories told by a sample of college-aged African American men. The goal of this research is to assess for cross-cultural relevance (i.e., similarity of personality traits, racial identification, commonalities in affective states, and recognition of similar sociopolitical factors).

ISSUES FOR RESEARCH AND OTHER FORMS OF SCHOLARSHIP

We discuss only three of these: assessor competency and ethical, and legal issues. We addressed several other related issues in previous sections and will not repeat them here.

Assessor Competency

As assessment directs counselors in the treatment of clients, it is essential that professional counselors and other helping professionals have competency in assessment, because assessor competency has an impact on the counseling intervention. Culturally competent assessors are aware of and understand the effects of race, culture, and ethnicity on the clients' personality development, career choices, manifestation of psychological disorders,

Discussion Box 3.3: Implications for Counselor Education Programs

The Council for Accreditation of Counseling Related Educational Programs (CACREP), American Psychological Association (APA), American Counseling Association (ACA), American School Counselor Association (ASCA), and all other counseling-related professional associations in their code of ethics and standards of practice require counselors to be culturally competent in both the assessment and treatment of clients from diverse cultural backgrounds. Counselor education programs, therefore, should offer courses and field experiences that will enable counselors to achieve competence in assessing clients of African ancestry.

Academic courses should include a wider range of models. Through intensive and well organized individual and group supervision by experienced mentors, counselor education programs can ensure that practicum or internship experiences are consistent with their program's model of training. Coursework and practicum should be integrated and taught in a coherent and cumulative manner. (Cohen, Van de Creek, & Krishnamurthy, 2004).

According to Dana, Aguilar-Kitibuti, Diaz-Vivar, & Vetter (2002), offering culturally focused specialized assessment courses in counselor education programs will enhance counselors' knowledge of specific cultures, inapplicability of available norms, and interpretation issues.

Counselor education programs need to increase diversity in assessment training that incorporates appropriate technology. There is also the need to recognize and encourage diverse methods for teaching assessment that will help make counselors who work with clients of African ancestry culturally competent assessors. All these can be done in the cultural context of the client.

Question

1. Consider how these processes could be researched within your particular multicultural and educational context.

help-seeking behavior, and appropriateness of intervention strategies (AAC, 2003). Counselors assessing clients of African ancestry for intervention need to be competent in the selection of assessment instruments. Care should be taken to select instruments that are culturally relevant and appropriate. The norms, reliability, and validity of the instrument also are important in helping counselors to be fair and equitable in assessing their clients who come from a different cultural background.

Effective counselors have skills and techniques needed for administering, interpreting, and scoring instruments, as well as communicating results. When interpreting and reporting the meaning of assessment results, the client's cultural background should be taken into account. Where assessment results are influenced by age, gender, socioeconomic status, color, disability, religion, sexual orientation, ethnicity, or culture, the information may be invalid and could be harmful to clients. Specifically, assessors should evaluate how culture has an impact on assessment results. Culturally competent counselors have knowledge about potential bias in assessment instruments and, therefore, use procedures and interpret findings keeping in mind the culture and linguistic characteristics of the clients (AAC, 2003; AACE, 1998).

Assessment should take place in a cultural context, so that counselors can provide effective treatment using relevant and appropriate intervention strategies. Good assessors are competent counselors who possess effective counseling skills. The AAC (2003) stated in its document, *Standards for Multicultural Assessment*, that for counselors to achieve competency in assessing clients from different cultural backgrounds, they have to be competent in the following areas:

1. Selection of Assessment Instruments: Content and Purpose.
2. Selection of Assessment Instruments: Norms, Reliability, and Validity.
3. Administration and Scoring of Assessment Instruments.
4. Interpretation and Application of Assessment Results.

Legislative Implications

The growing understanding of multicultural factors that define various diverse communities requires a reworking of relevant legislation and ethical considerations (Foxcroft, 1997; Van de Vijver & Rothman, 2004). The promulgation of the New Employment Equity Act 55 of 1998, Section 8 (Government Gazette, 1998) of South Africa stipulates that "psychological testing and other similar assessments are prohibited, unless the test or assessment being used – (a) has been scientifically shown to be valid and reliable, (b) can be applied fairly to all employees; and (c) is not biased against any employee or group." In other words, under South African law, psychologists are bound to ensure actively that all assessment instruments are fair and unbiased. In Niger and Ghana, there is no legislation that guides the use of psychological instruments. Instruments used by counselors, psychologists, psychiatrists, and other helping professionals are all developed in the West. There are concerns regarding the relevance and

Information Box 3.4: Characteristics of Ethical Practice for Assessment of People with African Ancestry (Foxcroft, 1997, p. 232)

Ethical practice includes:

1. An awareness of the test-takers world
2. The appropriate use of the assessment instrument
3. The implementation of the correct protocol for gaining permission and consent
4. Choosing suitable venues and times for assessment
5. An awareness of the effect of the administrator
6. Ensuring that instructions are clearly understood
7. The use of appropriate normative data
8. An awareness of background factors such as educational level, literary levels, and familiarity with the assessment activity

appropriateness of the instruments in use. They are not culturally and linguistically appropriate for the clients.

There are professional organizations in Niger, such as the Association of Niger Psychologists and Psychiatrists (ANPP), and in Ghana there is the National Guidance and Counseling Association (NGCA) and the Ghana Psychological Association (GPA). However, because there is no legislation that governs professional counselors in Niger and Ghana, very few legal issues are reported.

Counselors and other helping professionals are well aware of the issues regarding the content, purpose, norming, reliability, and validity of testing and assessment instruments. They are also aware of the instruments' different forms of bias, including construct bias and item bias. Because assessment is an essential function of the counselor, which paves the way for effective intervention, counselors in Niger and Ghana cautiously select, adapt, and administer instruments taking into consideration the culture, language, and religion or spirituality of their clients. They complement formal assessment instruments, such as the Beck Depression Inventory, with clinical interviews and observations.

Instruments developed in the West are adapted to suit the culture and religion or spirituality of each client by substituting words or phrases in original instruments with culturally and religiously appropriate ones. Counselors try to ensure that the language used is not offensive to their clients and that the instruments will be relevant and appropriate for their clients; however, they base their instruments on Western developed instruments.

Ethical Considerations

The core ethical edict of any psychological intervention is that nothing is done that would harm the client. This applies to assessment procedures as well. The International Test Commission (ITC, 2001) determines ethical practice in assessing clients. According to the ITC (2001, p. 7), the practitioner must endeavor to "use tests appropriately, professionally and in an ethical manner, paying due regard to the needs and rights of those involved in the testing process and the broader context in which the testing takes place."

Korman (1973) asserts that the provision of services to individuals from diverse backgrounds by professionals who are not well versed in the cultural practices of the client is unethical. It is also unethical to deny these services to clients in need because of a lack of competently trained and informed professionals. The onus is on the relevant professionals to develop assessment instruments that address the multidimensional milieu of a culturally diverse population and to ensure that all potential sources of bias are at the very least minimized or at best eradicated.

SUMMARY AND CONCLUSIONS

This chapter presented a discussion of the complex challenges that the professional counselor faces practicing in a multicultural context, in general, and with people of African ancestry, in particular. The existing assessment instruments were developed predominantly within a Western-based environment that is characterized by trends toward acculturation and the reduction of difference to a predetermined norm. It is clear that such processes are intrinsically flawed for application in a multicultural society and cannot be summarily applied to people of African ancestry.

The use of assessment tools remains a prominent part of the counselor's professional diagnostic battery, and obtained results are highly influential today. Relevant, reliable, and valid tools have the potential to enhance the counselor's insight into the client's world. However, until there is recognition of the need to use more processes that do not rely heavily on normative data, such as the narrative approach, results elicited from assessment tools, which are not valid for a multicultural realm, have the potential to perpetuate racially discriminatory myths and stereotypes.

There is a growing awareness of the need to factor in cultural criteria in the assessment process. However, reliable, bias-free, and culturally valid instruments are not readily available. Much is being done to meet this need, such as the development of the TCB. However, the scope for future research and development in this domain remains an urgent and dire need.

REFERENCES

Association for Assessment in Counseling (AAC). (2003). *Responsibilities of users of standardized tests*. Alexandria, VA: Author.

Association for Assessment in Counseling (AAC). (2003). *Standards for multicultural assessment*. Alexandria, VA: Author.

Association for Assessment in Counseling and Education. (AACE). (1998). *Competencies in assessment and evaluation for school counselors*. Alexandria, VA: Author.

Baldwin, J. A. (1991). African (Black) psychology: Issues and synthesis. In R. L. Jones (Ed.), *Black psychology* (pp. 125–33). Berkeley: Cobb & Henry.

Bandawe, C. R. (2005). Psychology brewed in an African pot: Indigenous philosophies and the quest for relevance. *Higher Education Policy*, *18*, 289–300.

Bekker, S., & Leilde, A. (2003). Is multiculturalism a workable policy in South Africa? *International Journal on Multicultural Societies*, *5*(2), 119–34.

Cohen, R. J., Van de Creek, L., & Krishnamurthy, R. (2004). Psychological assessment: Process and outcomes in defining competence. *Journal of Clinical Psychology*, *60*, 725–39.

Craig, A. P., & Beishuizen, J. J. (2002). Psychological testing in a multicultural society: Universal or particular competencies? *Intercultural Education*, *13*(2), 201–11.

Dana, R. H., Aguilar-Kitibuti, A., Diaz-Vivar, N., & Vetter, H. (2002). A teaching method for multicultural assessment: Psychological reports contents and cultural competence. *Journal of Personality Assessment*, *79*, 207–15.

Diallo, Y., & Hall, M. (1989). The healing drum: African wisdom teachings. In Vontress, C. E. (1991). Traditional healing in Africa: Implications for cross-cultural counseling. *Journal of Counseling and Development*, *70*, 242–9.

Draguns, J. G. (1977). Advances in the methodology of cross-cultural psychiatric assessment. *Transcultural Psychiatric Research Review*, *14*, 125–43.

Durrheim, K., Baillie, K., & Johnstone, L. (2008). The development and validation of a measure of racial justice perceptions. *South African Journal of Psychology*, *38*(4), 615–32.

Duzant, R. (2005). *Differences of emotional tone and story length of African American respondents when administered the Contemporized Themes Concerning Black Test versus the Thematic Apperception Test*. Unpublished doctoral dissertation, The Chicago School of Professional Psychology, Chicago.

Florsheim, P. (1990). Cross cultural views of self in the treatment of mental illness: Disentangling the curative aspects of the myth from the mythic aspects of the cure. *Psychiatry*, *53*, 304–15.

Foxcroft, C. D. (1997). Psychological testing in South Africa: Perspectives regarding ethical and fair practices. *European Journal of Psychological Assessment*, *13*, 229–35.

Foxcroft, C. D. (2004). Planning a psychological test in the multicultural South African context. *South African Journal of Industrial Psychology*, *30*(4), 8–15.

Good, B. J., & Good, M.-J. D. (1982). Towards a meaning centered analysis of popular illness categories: 'Fright-illness' and 'heat-distress' in Iran. In A. J. Marsella & G. M. White (Eds.), *Cultural conceptions of mental health and therapy* (pp. 141–66). Dordrecht: Reidel.

Government Gazette. (1988). *Republic of South Africa*, 400, 19370. Cape Town, October 19, 1988.

Harley, D. A. (2005). African American and indigenous counseling. In D. A. Harley & J.M. Dillard (Eds.), *Contemporary mental health among African Americans* (pp. 293–307). Alexandria, VA: American Counseling Association.

Hegba, M. P. (1979). Sorcellerie: Chemere dangereuse? [Sorcery: Dangerous myth?]. In Vontress, C. E. (1991). Traditional healing in Africa: Implications for cross-cultural counseling. *Journal of Counseling and Development*, *70*, 242–9.

Hoy, M. (1997). Contemporizing of the themes concerning blacks test (c-tcb). Unpublished doctoral dissertation, The California School of Professional Psychology, Alameda, CA.

Hoy-Watkins, M. (2008). Manual for the Contemporized-Themes Concerning Blacks test (C-TCB). In S. R. Jenkins (Ed.), *A handbook of clinical scoring systems for Thematic Apperceptive techniques* (pp. 685–95). Hillsdale, NJ: Lawrence Erlbaum Associates.

Hoy-Watkins, M., & Jenkins-Monroe, V. (2008). The Contemporized-Themes Concerning Blacks test (C-TCB). In S. R. Jenkins (Ed.), *A handbook of clinical scoring systems for Thematic Apperceptive techniques* (pp. 659–84). Hillsdale, NJ: Lawrence Erlbaum Associates.

Hsiao-Wen, L., & Dzokoto, V. (2005). Talking to the master: Intersections of religion, culture, and counseling in Taiwan and Ghana. *Journal of Mental Health Counseling*, *27*(2), 117–28.

Huysamen, G. K. (1983). *Psychological measurement. An introduction with South African examples*. Pretoria: Academia.

International Test Commission (ITC). (2001). International guidelines for test use. *International Journal of Testing*, *1*(2), 93–114.

Ivey, A. E., D'Andrea, M., Ivey, M. B., & Simek-Morgan, L. (2002). *Theories of counseling and psychotherapy: A multicultural perspective*. Boston: Allyn & Bacon.

Jones, R. (1996). Handbook of tests and measurements for Black populations: Introduction and overview. In R. L. Jones (Ed.), *Handbook of tests and measurements for Black populations* (pp. 3–15). Hampton, VA: Cobb & Henry.

Juhnke, G. A. (1996). Mental health counseling assessment: Broadening one's understanding of the client and the clients' presenting concerns. Eric Digest. Retrieved June 10, 2007 from http://www.ercidigests.org/1996–3/mental.html

Kerharo, J., & Bouquet, A. (1950). Sorciers, feticheurs et guerisseurs da la Cote d'lvoire-Haute Volte: les hommes, les croyances, les practiques, pharmacopee, et therapeutique. [Sorcerers, fetish men and healers of Ivory Coast-Upper Volta: Men, beliefs, practices, pharmacopoeia and therapeutics]. In Vontress, C. E. (1991). Traditional healing in Africa: Implications for cross-cultural counseling. *Journal of Counseling and Development*, *70*, 242–9.

Kim, U., Yang., K., & Hwang, K. (2006). Contributions to indigenous and cultural psychology: Understanding people in context. In U. Kim, K-S Yang, & K. Hwang (Eds.), *Indigenous and cultural psychology* (pp. 3–25). New York: Springer.

Kirmayer, L. J. (1989). Cultural variation in response to psychiatric disorders and emotional distress. *Social Science and Medicine*, *29*, 327–39.

Korman, M. (1973). *Levels and patterns of training in psychology*. Washington, DC: American Psychological Association.

Lamb, D. (1983). *The Africans*. New York: Vintage Books.

Littlewood, R. (1990). From categories of contexts: A decade of the new cross-cultural psychiatry. *British Journal of Psychiatry, 156*, 308–27.

Matthews-Evans, D. (1992). *Psychological responses of Black Americans to the TCB and TAT projective techniques (culturally specific tests)*. Unpublished doctoral dissertation, The George Washington University, St. Louis.

Mbiti, J. S. (1989). *African religions and philosophy* (2nd ed). Oxford: Heinemann.

Morgan, A. (2000). *What is narrative therapy? An easy to read introduction*. Adelaide: Duluich Publications.

Retel-Laurentin, A. (1969). Oracles et ordalies chez les Nzakara. [Oracles and trails among the Nzakara]. In Vontress, C. E. (1991). Traditional healing in Africa: Implications for cross-cultural counseling. *Journal of Counseling and Development, 70*, 242–9.

Schafer, W. D. (1996). Assessment skills for school counselors. Eric Digest. Retrieved June 10, 2007 from http://www.ercidigests.org/1996–2/school.html

Spence, L. (1988). The encyclopedia of the occult. In Vontress, C. E. (1991). Traditional healing in Africa: Implications for cross-cultural counseling. *Journal of Counseling and Development, 70*, 242–9.

Squire, L. H. (1985). *Race differences in responses to thematic apperception test stimuli material*. Unpublished doctoral dissertation, The California School of Professional Psychology, Berkeley/Alameda.

Sylla, Y. (1988, June 21). Sante: A Dabakala, les guerisseurs ont pignon sur rue. [Health: At Dabakala, the traditional healers have the upper hand]. In Vontress, C. E. (1991). Traditional healing in Africa: Implications for cross-cultural counseling. *Journal of Counseling and Development, 70*, 242–9.

Terre Blanche, M., & Durrheim, K. (Eds.). (2002). *Research in practice*. Cape Town: University of Cape Town Press.

Van de Vijver, A. J. R., & Rothman, S. (2004). Assessment in multicultural groups: The South African case. *SA Journal of Industrial Psychology, 30*(4), 1–7.

Vontress, C. E. (1991). Traditional healing in Africa: Implications for cross-cultural counseling. *Journal of Counseling and Development, 70*, 242–9.

Weaver, V. (1978). *A study of the response of Black males ages 9–12 to two thematic apperception tests: TCB and TAT*. Unpublished master's thesis, University of Cincinnati.

White, A. M., Olivieira, D. F., Strub, M. J., & Meertens, R. H. (1995). The themes concerning blacks (TCB) projective techniques as a measure of racial identity: An exploratory cross-cultural study. *Journal of Black Psychology, 21*(2), 104–23.

White, G., & Kirkpatrick, J. (1986). *Person, self and experience: Explaining Pacific ethnopsychologies*. Berkeley: University of California Press.

White, J. (1991). Toward a Black psychology. In R. L. Jones (Ed.), *Black psychology* (3rd ed., pp. 5–15). Berkeley: Cobb & Henry.

White, M. (2008, September). Narrative therapy by Michael White. Pratiques Narratives. Retrieved November 3, 2008 from http://www.pratiquesnarratives.com/English-articles-Narrative-Therapy-by-Michael-White.html

Williams, R. (1972). *Themes concerning Blacks test*. St. Louis, MO: Washington University.

Winslade, J., & Monk, G. (1998). *Narrative counselling in schools: Powerful and brief*. Thousand Oaks, CA: Corwin Press.

SELF-CHECK EXERCISES

1. List and explain the five criteria of a culturally intentional counselor.
2. Discuss the idea of multiculturalism
3. Explain the three prominent phenomena influencing the reliability, validity, and applicability of assessment instruments cross-culturally.
4. List the criteria for assessment of people from African ancestry.
5. What are the ethical considerations for assessing people of African ancestry?
6. How does culture and spirituality influence assessment of the African client's problem? Discuss.
7. Some theoretical perspectives of counseling tend to abstain from assessment and diagnosis because they promote wrong and harmful labels. Discuss your opinion of this point of view.
8. Discuss how professional counselors can enhance awareness of their own cultural values and biases and their clients' world views.

FIELD-BASED EXPERIENTIAL EXERCISES

1. Select an instrument for assessment and rate according to issues of cultural fairness and cultural bias in assessment instruments, spiritual, professional, ethical, and legal problems counselors encounter in assessment.
2. Assess the competency of counselors in administering, scoring, interpreting, reporting, and applying assessment results. Comment on the possible direction for the development of assessment tools that are relevant and appropriate for clients with an African ancestral background.
3. Use the narrative counseling approach to understand people who are experiencing life challenges such as HIV/AIDS. Explore common themes in these stories and discuss how this approach could provide tools for counseling that strengthen people's resilience to the daily challenges faced on the African continent.

MULTIPLE-CHOICE QUESTIONS

1. Multiculturalism is a factor in assessment because:
   a. Factors that are important to the management of a case may be lost where a Eurocentric assessment measure is applied.
   b. Multiculturalism allows for many languages to be used in assessments.
   c. Multiculturalism is a specific assessment tool.
2. The main criteria that influence the reliability, validity, and applicability of assessment instruments cross-culturally include:
   a. The language of the assessment tool.

b. The number of people from different cultural groups who use the assessment tool.
c. Self-knowledge and behavior; the location of deviant behavior and the meaning of symptoms.

3. The difference between Western approaches to assessment and that of the traditional approaches is:
a. The traditional healer is well known to the client.
b. The traditional healer does not make a distinction among mind, body, and spirit.
c. The traditional healer does not use any assessment tools.

4. The culturally competent assessor is someone who:
a. Speaks many languages and who can communicate with different cultural groups.
b. Is aware of the effects of race, culture, and ethnicity on the client's behavior.
c. Has been trained in a multicultural country.

5. The core ethical edict of any psychological intervention is that nothing is done that would harm the client. This means that:
a. Only assessors who are from the same cultural group as their clients can do assessments.
b. Assessors must have an awareness of the clients' world views.
c. As long as the assessor is qualified, no harm can be done to the client.

Answers to the multiple-choice questions are provided at the back of the book

4 Research on Counseling in African Settings

Lisa Lopez Levers, Michelle May, and Gwen Vogel

OVERVIEW. This chapter focuses on current research that illuminates counseling practices in African settings. The aim of this focus is first to examine and critique historic and current counseling practices in sub-Saharan Africa, and second, to provide an analysis of the available research that has been conducted on these practices. A recurrent theme in this chapter is an emphasis on the importance of empirically investigating counseling practices and how they are applied in African settings; such rigorous inquiry includes both quantitative and qualitative methods.

In the first part of the chapter, we examine specific constructs, offering working definitions that are contextually relevant to research on counseling in African settings. In the second part, we discuss relevant historical and cultural issues that anchor an understanding of counseling-related research in Africa. In the third part, we offer a look at current counseling practices and related research in African settings. In the fourth part, we provide an evidence-based discussion concerning the efficacy of counseling practices and research, as these are applied in African settings. In the following three parts of the chapter, we examine the cultural legacy of counseling practices in Africa, identify related disciplines, and discuss comparative indigenous practices. We conclude the chapter by identifying the implications for future research in African settings. Supplemental instructional features follow, which can serve as the basis for classroom discussion or as a means for helping the individual reader respond to the material.

LEARNING OBJECTIVES

By the end of the chapter, the reader should be able to:

1. Explain the relevance of indigenous culture to contemporary counseling practices and related research.
2. Identify the major counseling approaches used in African settings and the research endeavors associated with each.
3. Recognize gaps in the research related to counseling in African settings.
4. Justify the need for culturally relevant research endeavors that can yield results leading to more Afrocentric approaches to counseling interventions in Africa.
5. Identify potential areas for future research that are relevant to counseling in African settings.

INTRODUCTION

The context for counseling in African settings, as well as for counseling-related research, is a complicated one. The ethnocultural milieu of contemporary Africa is highly heterogeneous, contrary to the stereotypes held by many Westerners, and the social outcomes of various historical epochs are manifested in cultural overlays that have contributed to additional levels of social and cultural complexity. For example, the mores of colonizers and early Christian missionaries have had a strong, usually imposed, impact upon traditional African culture and its indigenous knowledge base. A central feature of this impact, spanning at least the past four centuries, has related to the inherent differences between African and Western world views.

The conduct of "research" is complex and influenced by the world views and priorities of the participants (see also Chapter 5, this volume). In this chapter, we identify the ways in which counseling in African settings has been examined, so that we can then identify the gaps in this research.

IMPORTANCE, DEFINITION, AND SCOPE OF KEY CONCEPTS

The following subsections offer brief discussions of essential contextual concepts that are important to understanding the context of research on counseling in African settings. These include world view, indigenous knowledge, and counseling.

World View

World view, from the German *Weltanschauung*, is taken as the essential paradigm or framework that comprehensively explains a person's place in the world or the universe, and by extension, the particular structure of reality that is shared by members of the person's group (tribe, society, etc.). A definitive world view is represented by the values, social behaviors, myths, lore, and ceremonies of the particular society. While Western societies tend to be marked by individualism and competitiveness, with a rather rigid dualistic world view, indigenous societies tend to be more collectivist and cooperative in nature, with a more relativistic perspective of the universe. African cosmology, in general, is representative of the latter.

Indigenous Knowledge

The term *indigenous* simply refers to having origins in a particular region. Obviously, modernity has had an impact on indigenous peoples throughout the world, as well as upon the ways in which they have or have not continued traditional practices. Indigenous knowledge is described by Theis et al. (2000) as a useful concept, coined in the 1980s, which provides a stronger case for knowledge generation, especially in synthesizing modern with traditional or local understandings. They assert that the construct allows for "partnerships between academics and 'communities'... which were based on closer dialogue between the parties involved" (Theis et al., 2000, Annex 5, p. 4). They further elaborate that "Participatory approaches between scientists and 'communities' led to a greater adoption of new ideas....[and that] 'Indigenous knowledge' transfer was more successful in answering local cultural needs" (Annex 5, p. 4). In her discussion of African traditional healing as a primary example of indigenous knowledge that has contemporary application, Levers (2006c, p. 87) argues that it is "particularly important for African counsellors to engage the cultural relevance of this indigenous knowledge system, especially in the face of the HIV/AIDS pandemic and the reality that many Africans continue to seek health care services from traditional healers."

Counseling

Counseling is typically defined in terms of process and relationship (Levers, 1997a); for example, Patterson and Welfel (1999, p. 21) define counseling as "an interactive process characterized by a unique relationship between counselor and client that leads to change in the client." Levers emphasizes the importance of client meaning making and client empowerment, while acknowledging the determinedly Western slant of the structures that underlie the contemporary counseling enterprise.

In traditional African cultures, people historically have sought advice, guidance, and healing from village chiefs, village elders, traditional healers, and the ancestors; in other words, these were the traditional "counselors." However, unlike Western dualism, African cosmology does not separate mind and body, science and religion. The notion of seeking guidance or healing from a professional counselor – usually a stranger, or at least someone who is not a member of the indigenous community – is foreign to many Africans. So the term *counseling*, here, has a connotation of modernity and implies the professional or paraprofessional activity of someone who has received Westernized training in counseling. Even at African universities, where advanced degrees in mental health fields are conferred, mostly Westernized theories are taught. Much of what is known about counseling in Africa, relative to practice, research, and application, is based upon Western models and interpretations. Levers (1999) has advocated for designing a counselor education model that is grounded in the context of Africa, and as we suggest throughout this chapter, there continues to be a strong call to conduct culturally sensitive and culturally relevant research so that Africans can construct Afrocentric models of training and intervention.

HISTORY OF COUNSELING-RELATED RESEARCH IN AFRICAN SETTINGS

Areas of research and development have included studies on healing, the transportability of Western practices into African settings, and influences of funding bodies. We consider these next.

African Indigenous Healing

African traditional healing is based on *indigenous* knowledge systems (see also Chapter 1, this volume). These indigenous knowledge systems are diverse and have developed over centuries in interaction with specific contexts. Furthermore, these knowledge systems are constantly adapting and changing in response to their contexts (Barnhardt & Kawagley, 2005; Cardinal, 2001; Horsthemke, 2004). Indigenous knowledge is relational and shared collectively. Another important aspect of indigenous knowledge is that it includes revealed knowledge through dreams, visions, intuition, and revelation through the connection with nature. Dialoguing among different role-players is another important method of knowledge creation in African settings; for example, oral records of indigenous knowledge are shared in the present and transmitted across generations (Barnhardt & Kawagley, 2005; Steinhauer, 2002). The intersection between indigenous and Western knowledge systems, as well as aspects mainly relevant to Western knowledge systems, are highlighted in Discussion Box 4.1.

Traditional and faith healers are considered to be credible and held in high regard, because they can use the forces of nature and can make contact with the spirit world (MacLachlan, 2000; Peltzer, 2001; Vontress, 1999b; Yeh, Hunter, Madan-Bahel, Chiang, & Arora, 2004). Traditional healers are considered to be holistic healers, that is, priest-physician-psychologists (Levers & Maki, 1994, 1995). Traditional healers use various methods, including divination, to diagnose and discover information about their clients. For example, a graduate student from Liberia studying in the United States reported that he knows a healer who throws bones and tells the client what is wrong with him or her by reading the configuration of the bones (M. May, personal communication, September 22, 2008). Importantly, traditional healers focus on deeper roots of clients' problems, work toward preventing repetition of problems, and provide holistic interventions (Peltzer, 2001). In the healing relationship, the traditional healers create a climate of trust, acceptance, positive regard, and empathetic understanding when interacting with their clients. Traditional healers also use several healing techniques to address their clients' problems (Vontress,

Discussion Box 4.1: Differences and Similarities between Indigenous and Western Knowledge Systems

Barnhardt and Kawagley (2005, p. 16) have identified qualities that have been associated with traditional or indigenous knowledge and with Western science; they further extrapolated some of what they call the "common ground" principles. They view indigenous knowledge systems as reflecting a more holistic perspective, with trust in traditional knowledge and respect for all living things; whereas, they view Western science as consumed with reductionism and a tendency toward compartmentalization, with understanding of the world as limited to a particular type of evidence and marked by skepticism. Consider what you know about the differences in traditional versus modern world views, try to tease out what might be seen as common ground between them, and address the following questions in your discussions.

Questions

1. Critically discuss the qualities of traditional, indigenous knowledge systems. Illustrate your answer with examples from your community setting.
2. Critically discuss the qualities of Western knowledge systems. Illustrate your answer with examples from your community setting.
3. Discuss the similarities and differences between the qualities of traditional/indigenous and Western knowledge systems.
4. A young Zulu boy, Mpho, growing up in Kwazulu-Natal in South Africa, goes to a Catholic school where he becomes a very good friend of an Indian boy and a Chinese girl. They spend most of their time together at school, as well as after school. Mpho often visits his friends and participates in their social and cultural activities. What world view do you think Mpho will adhere to when he grows up? Substantiate your answer.

1999b). In their research in the southern region of Africa, Levers and Maki have drawn parallels between aspects of traditional healing and modern counseling practices, especially within the purview of those involving existential variations of counseling.

Transportability of Western Approaches

Modern counseling practices in Africa primarily have been based on Western forms of talk counseling. Globally and regionally, in the past twenty years, there has been an increase in research focusing on culturally sensitive counseling that acknowledges traditional assumptions, beliefs, and practices. Several researchers have encouraged an Afrocentric approach to counseling in which they explicate counseling methods based on the assumptions of indigenous knowledge systems and practices (Bakker & Mokwena, 1999; Levers, 1997b, 1999, 2006b, 2006c; MacLachlan, 2000; Peltzer, 2001; Vontress, 1999a, 1999b).

Modern research practices in Africa, until recent times, typically have emphasized positivistic research methods, indicating a lack of naturalistic research methods and culturally sensitive practice by focusing on Westernized counseling practices. According to Reviere (2001), the traditional Eurocentric research criteria, based mainly on positivistic paradigms of objectivity, reliability, and validity, are inadequate, especially for research involving human experiences. Consequently, she argues for new research orientations to the creation and interpretations of data based on an Afrocentric world view.

Multiple stakeholders – including members of society, academics, independent researchers, government entities, international donor agencies, and the nongovernmental organization (NGO) sectors – are beneficiaries, but not necessarily equal beneficiaries, of counseling and research in Africa. For sociohistorical and geopolitical reasons, although universities in Africa were included within the colonialist framework, they were designed to be teaching universities rather than research universities; for specific examples, one can review the development of tertiary education in Malawi (Zeleza, 2002) and South Africa (Pityana, 2005). Thus, the participation of African academics in research endeavors has been influenced by how the universities within African countries have developed, as well as by their relationships with the government of the day. In the period immediately following colonialism, working relationships developed in many countries between the academy and the government; however, as the university sector grew exponentially, the relationships between academic researchers and their governments sometimes deteriorated. This occurrence has been due mainly to political and economic developments in the different African countries. Furthermore, some researchers who have been educated and trained in sub-Saharan Africa have migrated to Euro-American countries because of a lack of favorable working conditions (Hassan, 2008). Those who have remained have found themselves involved in consultancy and other work, at the expense of their research endeavors, to maintain their socioeconomic status (Zeleza, 2002).

Influences and Priorities of Funding Bodies

International donor agencies constitute another important category of stakeholders in research in Africa, and their influences have grown since the1980s, to the extent that their contributions have become indispensable. The relationship between the donor and the recipient of research grants seems to be inherently unequal, insofar as the donors can set the research agenda, and the recipients are required to follow the terms of reference (Crossley & Holmes, 2001; Okolie, 2003; Zeleza, 2002). The NGO sector, representing independent research centers, has been more successful in conducting research that has been of benefit to civil society, in that they have had a different working relationship with government, civil society, and the international donor organizations (Zeleza, 2002).

Skinner's (1998) study illuminates the overlap between research and counseling processes. The knowledge, insights, and skills from counseling can be of value to an investigator and the ensuing research process. However, it does not mean that researchers necessarily should be counselors, but rather that the inquiry process can be enhanced through additional training in relevant counseling skills. Furthermore, counseling by counselors embedded in African settings during the last twenty years has provided practical opportunities for the creation of knowledge and practices, especially relative to culturally sensitive research and counseling (Bakker & Mokwena, 1999; Levers, 1997b, 1999, 2002, 2003a, 2003b, 2006a, 2006b, 2006c; MacLachlan, 2000; Peltzer, 2000, 2001; Vontress, 1999a, 1999b).

CURRENT COUNSELING PRACTICES AND COUNSELING-RELATED RESEARCH IN AFRICAN SETTINGS

Counseling services have a vital role to play in many settings across the globe. Effective responses to disaster situations, for example, have involved the whole of government, NGOs, and community members. At any given phase in a country's development (postconflict, recovery, poverty reduction, government establishment, industrialization, education/technological advancement, etc.), mental health/counseling services can play a key role in supporting necessary community stabilization and expansion. Counseling services have been proven to help reduce the severity of traumatic reactions, for example, and to facilitate peace-building activities; they also have been used to improve medication compliance in the health sector. In addition, counseling has served to help support national and civic development in many countries and to incorporate sustainable economic and employment opportunities into community practices after stabilization after a disaster event.

Reasons for Counseling

In an industrialized context, it is not unusual for people to seek counseling to improve self-esteem, to explore issues related to quality of life, or simply to promote self-development. However, in an African context, it is usually more the case that individuals enter into counseling in response to some cataclysmic life event. Although this may not *always* be true, it usually has been true, because the reality is that most Africans do not have the luxury of engaging in counseling services. Perhaps the major exception to this is guidance counseling and career counseling, as it is offered in schools. For these reasons, we have elected to focus on the following sectors of counseling and counseling-related research that seem to have grown recently or are emerging: disaster mental health responses, HIV/AIDS counseling, health counseling, rehabilitation counseling, trauma counseling, orphans and other vulnerable children (OVC) counseling, and psychoeducational counseling. In each of the following subsections, we briefly describe the area of counseling practice, identify the applications relevant to African settings, and review the associated research literature.

Disaster Mental Health Responses

Epidemiological studies show that disaster is not a rare event. Even if only a few individuals are primarily affected, disasters can have a widespread and devastating impact on health and on national and community stability. In recent years, African countries have been faced with such natural disasters as massive floods, earthquakes, and famines due to environmental conditions; African countries also have been faced with man-made disasters such as genocide, war, and forced migrations.

Less developed countries have greater morbidity and mortality from disasters than do more developed countries, even when population density is controlled. Many of these developing countries are situated in Africa. Between 1967 and 1991, disasters around the world killed 7 million people and affected 3 billion (Cater, Revel, Sapir, & Walker, 1993). During this period, an average 117 million people living in developing countries were affected by disasters each year, as compared to about 700,000 in developed countries, a striking ratio of 166:1. In recognition of the human cost of disasters, the United Nations General Assembly designated the 1990s as the decade of natural disaster reduction (United Nations, 1989).

In recent years, disaster research has seen dramatic increases in the study of psychological and social effects of disaster. In general, this developing literature suggests that mild to moderate stress reactions in the emergency and acute phases of disaster are highly prevalent, but that the majority of people affected by disasters recover fully within six to sixteen months (Baum & Fleming, 1993; Green & Lindy, 1994; Steinglass & Gerrity, 1990). Of the people who develop symptoms consistent with a disorder, the most common have been identified as acute stress disorder, posttraumatic stress disorder, major depression, generalized anxiety disorder, substance abuse, somatization disorders, adjustment disorder, complications of bereavement, family violence, and child or spouse abuse.

While the continent of Africa experiences a plethora of natural disasters, many countries are lacking adequate infrastructures for dealing with even the most blatant after effects. In areas where people do not have access to safe shelter, clean water, or enough to eat, counseling is naturally low on the list of priorities. Research regarding counseling interventions is an even lower urgency. Placing mental health low on the list of priorities unfortunately is based on the now-entrenched misunderstanding that individuals have an established hierarchy of needs (i.e., Maslow's hierarchy of needs) that must be met in chronological order.

Contemporary research suggests that mental health and adequate coping are not mutually exclusive from or secondary to basic shelter and security needs. In other words, safe shelter and food need to be offered simultaneously with psychosocial support, just as baseline levels of cognitive and behavioral functioning need to be restabilized before individuals can benefit from other interventions. For example, an acutely traumatized person, left unsupported at a disaster site, has a difficult time multitasking and getting organized enough to advocate for or utilize basic resources (e.g., accessing food programs, finding clean water, using available social services). If emotional support systems are not put in place, individuals are at risk of missing opportunities to access other support services and resources.

Mental Health Outcomes

There is an emerging body of research on mental health outcomes following disasters (e.g., de Jong et al., 2001; Mollica et al.; 1993; Shore, Vollmer, & Tatum, 1989). However, aside from some of these widely sited epidemiological studies of affected communities, selected methodologies have varied widely, as have the samples assessed and measures used. Reports of high rates of post-disaster morbidity may therefore accurately reflect higher rates of mental health problems, or they could reflect selected samples, unreliable measures, or secondary stress reactions. Because of the chaos resulting from disaster, the disruption and displacement of the populations, and the overriding need to respond to human distress, research is frequently opportunistic, and the generalizability of such findings is subsequently limited.

Indigenous peoples may be more adversely affected by disasters than other groups, because the disaster frequently is superimposed on the fact that these communities have been enduring ongoing social marginalization, poor physical health with few treatment options, socioeconomic constraints, and oppression. Disasters not only bring about additional distress and trauma, but the displacement that results from the disaster event also can cause indigenous peoples to be dislocated from traditional places of importance and safe places to practice traditional ceremonies. History further indicates that it is not uncommon for indigenous peoples to be cast as scapegoats in the post-disaster period, reflecting ongoing community discrimination and, all too often, racism.

Raphael (1996, 1997) emphasizes that it is critical that, where indigenous communities are affected by disaster, their leaders are involved in the development of culturally appropriate recovery and support processes. Of particular significance is the support that can be provided to these communities and the recognition that there may be premorbid effects of past trauma, which may add to difficulties of adaptation. In addition, the importance of family and community networks, both in the reaction to disaster and particularly in the recovery process, should be acknowledged.

Needs of communities vary, depending on contextual factors and also on current socioeconomic disadvantage, demoralization, and adverse health circumstances. A community's role in its own response and recovery is particularly important, because the situation of disaster may inadvertently lead to both neglect and overcontrol of already marginalized groups. The added adversity of disaster is that its occurrence may turn into a critical risk factor for developing psychopathology for individuals already experiencing the most adverse outcomes of marginalization.

HIV/AIDS Counseling

It is common knowledge that the HIV/AIDS pandemic has been devastating to sub-Saharan Africa, particularly in the southern region (see also Chapter 16, this volume). While sub-Saharan Africa has approximately 10% of the world's population, recent statistics indicate that it bears the burden of 64% of all HIV infections globally; UNAID (2006) has estimated that 21.6 million to 27.4 million people there are HIV infected. Based on shear numbers, we know that there are multitudes of people affected by the HIV and AIDS pandemic; of these, many are in need of counseling for various reasons. Of course, this includes the psychosocial needs of those who are HIV positive and those who are living with AIDS; but it also includes the mental health of family members and their issues of fear, stigma, grief, and loss, as well as the mental health of friends, caregivers, children, and community members. The pandemic affects every sector of living, from the most personal to the most public, and each sphere has its associated set of problems. Levers (2006a) has illuminated the need for identifying pertinent psychoeducational HIV and AIDS interventions, especially those that are culturally relevant and based on research.

Unfortunately, the pendulum of prevention-based programming has swung from the free flow of condoms to funding limited solely to abstinence; although both approaches are necessary pieces of the larger picture, neither is sufficient to serve fully the public health need for preventing transmission of the virus. The most prevalent counseling responses have entered around VCT (voluntary counseling and testing) and medication compliance.

Studies increasingly point to the value of voluntary HIV counseling and testing (VCT) as a HIV prevention tool (Painter, 2001). Studies in Africa frequently report that VCT is associated with reduced risk behaviors and lower rates of seroconversion among HIV serodiscordant couples. Many of these studies point out that VCT has considerable potential for HIV prevention among other heterosexual couples and recommend that VCT for couples be practiced more widely in Africa. However, follow-up regarding the long-term efficacy of VCT has been extremely limited. Thus, current understandings from social/behavioral research on how individuals and couples in sub-Saharan Africa manage HIV risks, as well as HIV prevention interventions to support HIV prevention efforts, have remained underdeveloped.

Health Counseling

The importance of examining health behaviors and other health outcomes cannot be overemphasized anywhere in the world. Behavioral responses to stressful events include changes in sleep, eating patterns, and use of addictive substances, as well as changes in exercise patterns. Physiological effects at the hormonal level have been suggested to result in increased visits to medical and mental health facilities, and disaster survivors may evidence a range of symptoms and complaints that cause them to seek help in places other than the mental health sector (Green & Lindy, 1994). Thus, it is important that nurses and other frontline medical providers in urban and rural African settings be aware of and respond to the range of somatic complaints and health behaviors that may appear in post-disaster periods. Assessments need to include the possibility of stressor effects on physical health as well as underlying psychological reactions. Recognizing and responding to both health and mental health needs, and dealing with them appropriately, can be essential to achieving optimal health outcomes.

In reality, many Africans consult with traditional healers regarding health concerns, and thereby receive de facto counseling services from the healers. In terms of modern health counseling interventions, the impetus for such service may be found in the participatory mechanisms that are a part of the structure of the primary health care or district health systems found throughout much of sub-Saharan Africa. Examples of such counseling practices in health sectors in Africa include HIV and AIDS, social safety nets for vulnerable populations, hunger, and malaria and tuberculosis prevention.

In their hermeneutic translational research, Levers, Magweva, and Mpofu (2007) reviewed the structure of district health systems in eastern and southern Africa. In their examination of the facilitators for and barriers against participation in health care, they emphasized that "health care in Africa is a complex and multi-faceted issue" (Levers et al., 2007, p. 3). Their report explicated the power relations that remain interwoven throughout the district health systems, underscoring the need for expanded health literacy among ordinary African citizens. Within the current system, the key actors who are best positioned to facilitate the delivery of health counseling services are the village health workers. Unfortunately, "[L]ittle use has been made of local health education committees or the trained expertise of village health workers or their supervisors" (Levers et al., 2007, p. 20).

Trauma Counseling

The experience of traumatic life events has been increasing in war-affected populations in Africa as civilians increasingly are exposed to war, torture, and forced migration. African refugees, who have fled from war regions, often report a number of extremely stressful experiences such as physical and psychological torture, shelling, sexual violence, and other atrocities (see also Chapters 12 and 15, this volume). As a consequence, a high prevalence of posttraumatic stress disorder (PTSD) has been reported in these populations (de Jong et al., 2001; Mollica et al., 1993).

Within the past decade, empirical knowledge about effective psychotherapeutic treatment for PTSD has rapidly increased (Foa, Keane, & Friedman, 2000). Treatment for PTSD is well studied in civilian populations with victims of traumatic events who live in industrialized counties such as the United States, Europe, or Australia. In contrast, the knowledge about effective treatment of PTSD in Africa, especially areas affected by war, remains scarce. In spite of the considerable attention that war-torn populations have received from psychosocial organizations in recent years, little clinical research has been conducted on how adequately to support and treat these groups.

The need for trauma-related counseling interventions is as widespread in African countries as it is anywhere in the world, and different types of counseling approaches have been utilized by different psychosocial organizations all over the world (Van der Veer, 1998). These types of treatment, often referred to as "trauma counseling" or "cross-cultural counseling," encompass a large variety of approaches, such as problem-solving techniques (Amani Trust, 1997), trauma support groups, and individualized assistance, including variants of exposure therapy (World Health Organization/United Nations High Commissioner for Refugees [WHO/UNHCR], 1996).

Unfortunately, the infrastructure for supporting trauma-related services is minimal, as is the human resource capacity. For example, Life Line International has centers, in various southern African countries, that are staffed by paraprofessionals. They are able to offer as much crisis intervention as human resources allow, but workers at such centers frequently find themselves dealing with cases of interpersonal violence – such as sexual assault, homicide, suicide, incest, and domestic violence – for which their paraprofessional training has not adequately prepared them and for which referral is not possible. Levers,

Research Box 4.1: Constructing Indigenous Models of Counseling

Peltzer, K. (1999). A process model of ethnocultural counselling for African survivors of organized violence. *Counselling Psychology Quarterly*, *12*(4), 335–51.

Objective: The study investigated indigenous counseling concepts for victims of traumas in Uganda. The study aimed at developing a heuristic framework for constructing a process model of ethnocultural counseling for survivors of organized crime.

Method: Interviews with about 500 counseling and psychotherapy cases of survivors of organized violence collected over a 10-year period were analyzed. Data were examined using qualitative inquiry methods.

Results: A counseling model that encompassed African counselors' indigenous concepts resulted from the study.

Conclusion: Indigenous models of counseling are possible from interviews with members of African cultural communities.

Questions

1. How is indigenous knowledge related to ethnocultural counseling?
2. How would you evaluate the extent to which the findings of the research represent insider versus outsider perspectives?

Kamanzi, Mukamana, Pells, and Bhusumane (2006) report that even in post-genocide Rwanda the effort toward systemic trauma counseling for an entire population largely suffering from posttraumatic stress disorder (PTSD) is slow in coming; the reasons are complex, but this is at least partly due to the need to build sustainable training programs.

There is a very large body of literature on the relationship between traumatic events and mental health outcomes, but research focused exclusively on counseling practices and outcomes studies in African settings is much more limited. Although it is acknowledged that research in the disaster areas, refugee settings, and remote African settings can be difficult to conduct, many of the existing findings are limited by a shortage of psychometrically sound studies. Methodological limitations include small sample sizes, biased convenience samples, treatment seekers or compensation seekers, and great variability in the use of measures and assessment time points. Furthermore, the vast majority of studies have focused chiefly on assessing PTSD and ignored other more prevalent outcomes such as depression and other anxiety disorders. In most cases, the counseling procedures and duration of treatment are not rigorously standardized. This lack of standardization poses a serious constraint for the evaluation of counseling practices, and as of yet, there is no clinical trial that examined the efficacy of counseling approaches for traumatized refugees.

There are, however, a few exceptions to the lack of adaptation of scientific knowledge from PTSD research to the conditions in sub-Saharan Africa. Paunovi and Ost (2001) showed that exposure treatment is a promising treatment approach for refugees who had fled to Sweden. A limitation of this study was the rather rigid inclusion criteria. These findings can be applied only to the minority of refugees who manage to flee to Western countries and adapt to the new culture. Furthermore, there was no control group in this study that would control for spontaneous remission and unspecific effects.

In general, there continues to be a dearth of research regarding traumatized refugees who continue to live in dangerous situations, and even less is known about the efficacy of psychotherapeutic approaches for this population, especially in Africa (see also Chapter 12, this volume). Neuner, Schauer, Elbert, and Roth (2002) studied the use of narrative exposure therapy (NET), a short-term approach based on cognitive-behavioral therapy and testimony therapy, with Sudanese refugees who fled from the civil war to Northern Uganda. In a refugee camp setting, they compared the efficacy of three treatment conditions in a randomized controlled trial. The control group received psychoeducation only. A second group received four sessions of supportive counseling in addition to psychoeducation, and the third group was offered four sessions of narrative exposure therapy that also included a psychoeducation component. A significant difference between narrative exposure therapy and supportive counseling was found, but not between narrative exposure therapy and psychoeducation (Neuner et al., 2002). Limitations in the cited studies indicate an urgent need for further studies in this field.

Similarly, Neuner, Schauer, Klaschik, Karunakara, and Elbert (2004) examined the efficacy of NET in a randomized controlled trial involving Sudanese refugees living in a Ugandan refugee settlement. There were forty-three participants diagnosed with PTSD, and they either received four sessions of NET, four sessions of supportive counseling, or a psychoeducational intervention that consisted of only one session. The results of the study indicated that NET is a promising approach for treating PTSD among refugees still living in unsafe conditions. However, one limitation of the study relates to the abbreviated nature of the psychoeducational intervention; it is typical that such interventions occur over the course of at least several sessions. Additional research is needed in this sensitive area of trauma recovery to ascertain whether psychoeducational interventions might be efficacious in human-resource scarce areas.

Levers (2002) examined the effects of violence, gender, disability, and poverty on the development of young children in Northern Namibia. In this ethnographic appraisal, the children's teachers were interviewed, because the children were still too affected by recent conflict in the area. Levers identified the ameliorative effects of school-based countermeasures on the deleterious experiences of the children. Especially helpful to the children were social support and persistent teacher attention. Although limited by sample size and direct accessibility to young children's experiences of trauma (they were too traumatized to serve as participants), the study "provides an initial framework for understanding the educational effects of violence, gender bias, disability, poverty, and privation on children's development and offers a potential structure for examining associated resiliencies as well" (Levers, 2002, p. 40).

Counseling for Orphans and Other Vulnerable Children

As an extension of the situations resulting from both the HIV and AIDS pandemic and the frequency of trauma-related experiences such as genocide, war, and forced migrations, the psychosocial concerns of orphans and other vulnerable children (OVC) have emerged as extremely important (see also Chapter 19, this volume). Any children affected by HIV and AIDS may be traumatized by extreme situations such as an ill, dying, or deceased parent, but African children are even more vulnerable owing to the cultural taboos in many African societies that prohibit discussion of illness and death with children. Likewise, many African survivors of trauma may have the added burden of being expected to suffer in silence because of social taboos.

Most African countries have some version of Child Line, a crisis intervention/hotline type of community service that a child may call if he or she is being abused. However, there are obvious infrastructural and capacity problems associated with this, as with any type of community-based service, especially in developing contexts. Even in the countries that have signed the International Child Rights Declaration, many children continue to be traumatized by maltreatment and abuse. In spite of capacity problems, designated professionals, such as pediatricians and teachers, could be signified as the "first line of defense" for recognizing children who have been traumatized, neglected, abused, or maltreated; guidance and counseling teachers in the schools could be positioned to mitigate some of the worst situations, if given the systemic permission and empowerment to do so.

Levers (2003b) conducted qualitative research with guidance and counseling teachers to ascertain their knowledge about orphans in their schools. When provided with relevant information about the bio-ecological model of development, concomitant with information about the effects of trauma on child development, the teachers were able to articulate clear interventions that could be carried out in their schools and classrooms for low or no cost. Malema (2006) conducted qualitative research with the caregivers of children infected by HIV and affected by HIV and AIDS. She demonstrated that culturally appropriate training interventions could ease the social taboos surrounding caregiver discussion of illness with infected children and of death with children who lost parents. Roos, Potgieter, Coetzee, and Lehobye (2003) examined the use of a specific psychoeducation program to integrate homeless South African children into a children's residential facility.

Rehabilitation Counseling

A focus on the psychosocial effects of disability is relatively recent in African countries; therefore, the field of rehabilitation counseling is still emerging. Yet the environmental causes of disability are high in developing contexts. In earlier discussions (e.g., Levers, 1999; Sebatane, Levers, & Ralebitso, 1993) about the utility of rehabilitation counseling in sub-Saharan countries, a general impression evolved that the need for rehabilitation counseling in African countries has a strong link with health counseling, especially concerning issues of HIV and AIDS, along with health promotion, disease prevention, substance abuse, and disability management issues.

Mpofu et al. (2007) offered an examination of rehabilitation personnel training and education in seven sub-Saharan countries and their relevance to advocacy for counseling interventions. Consistent with the dearth of literature pertaining to disability issues in African countries, this examination found that disability still is emerging as a human rights issue. Hopefully the need for counseling interventions, identification of best practices, and evidence-based investigations of efficacy are soon to follow. Examples of rehabilitation counseling in African countries are found mainly within the NGO and international donor sectors. Although it is not unusual for Ministries of Health to have rehabilitation units, financial and human resource constraints prohibit much priority being placed on the provision of psychosocial counseling for persons living with a disability. A similar situation exists in the disability-related units housed within Ministries of Education.

There is a dearth of scholarly research related to rehabilitation counseling in African countries (Mpofu et al., 2007). The disability-related literature tends to focus on interventions associated with medical, prosthetic, and pharmacological aspects of disability rather than the psychosocial implications of living with a disability; hence, there is little focus on counseling. Some governments have had a history of providing resources to accommodate the needs of persons living with disabilities, for example, Zimbabwe at the end of the twentieth century (Mpofu, 2000, 2002; Mpofu & Harley, 2002). Recent research concerning the need for rehabilitation counseling can be found in some governmental evaluation reports (e.g., Levers & Magweva, 2005; Levers, Magweva, Maundanei, & Mpofu, 2008).

Psychoeducational Practices

The use of awareness campaigns, prevention programs, and other community-based interventions has introduced the Western social-service practice of conducting psychoeducational interventions to mitigate problems within a delimited population. Psychoeducational interventions often have been used in tandem with personal counseling sessions within the Western social-service delivery system. However, considering capacity issues within the health and mental health care sectors in developing countries, individual counseling may, at least at the present time, be considered a luxury in most African countries. If group psychoeducational interventions are found to be efficacious, this may be a way of delivering counseling-based services to larger numbers of people, as well as a means for educating consumers of services and their families.

Psychoeducational interventions have been effective particularly in arenas like HIV and AIDS, alcoholism and substance abuse, and youth development ventures. Psychoeducation also has been used within the health care sector, specifically to promote awareness about the impact of conditions like malaria, tuberculosis, and sexually transmitted infections. Because psychoeducational interventions target not only the consumer of services, but also family members, significant others, close friends, and community members, its use can have a powerful effect.

Olley (2006) evaluated the efficacy of an individualized psychoeducation (PE) program aimed at reducing psychological distress and risky sexual behavior and enhancing self-disclosure associated with an HIV diagnosis. Study participants were ninety-four consecutive attendees at a walk-in nongovernmental voluntary counseling and testing (VCT) center in Nigeria. According to the author, the participants were asked to complete a precounseling, baseline questionnaire detailing their sociodemographic characteristics, psychopathology, sexual practices, self-disclosure intention, and coping behaviors. Screening for HIV was completed for each, and posttest counseling was offered. Those who tested positive were assigned randomly to either a PE or a waitlist control group. Psychometric inventories and self-reports were used as major outcome measures. Significant reductions on all measures were observed at four weeks after the intervention, along with reduced risky sexual practices. The investigation indicated "efficacy of a manual-driven PE program for self-disclosure, reduction of depression and improvement in safe sexual practices" (Olley, 2006, p. 1025).

Fonchingong, Mbuagbo, and Abong (2004) examined barriers to counseling for HIV and AIDS patients in Cameroon and explicated the roles of state and church in facilitating support counseling across multiple dimensions of existence. Based on their findings, they promote the use of psychosocial interventions similar to psychoeducational strategies.

CURRENT TRENDS IN COUNSELING RESEARCH IN AFRICA

One current trend, which is of academic significance, is the relatively new interest shown by African graduate students in conducting naturalistic inquiry into culturally relevant themes of counseling in African settings. This trend has been occurring regardless of whether the student is studying abroad or in a home African country. A recent example is Bhusmane's (2007) doctoral dissertation that investigated mechanisms of indigenous counseling in one southern African country. Another example is Msimanga- Ramatebele's (2008) doctoral dissertation, an inquiry into the lived experiences of African widows; she examined the cultural rituals associated with death, loss, grief, and bereavement, teasing out their implications for and applications to modern professional counseling. Both of these students graduated from an American university, but returned to their African homes to collect data and sort through the layers of cultural significance.

Some master's students at African universities likewise are looking to traditional values and indigenous knowledge for data collection projects. For example, Malema (2006) based her master's thesis on her investigation of the challenges and adjustment strategies that face the caregivers of children living with HIV and AIDS. The results of the study arose from culturally sensitive interventions with the caregivers to explore ways of having important discussions with children while still not fracturing cultural taboos. The resulting synergy illuminated pathways for conducting new ways of proceeding that were culturally conducive to the desired effect.

The AIDS and Society Research Unit (ASRU) at the University of Cape Town has made a concerted effort to support "innovative research into the social dimensions of AIDS in South Africa, and explores the interface between qualitative and quantitative research" (ASRU, 2006, para. 1). The site lists a completed dissertation (Wienand, n.d.) regarding "The Potential of Visual and Participatory Approaches to HIV Literacy in South Africa," for example. The site also lists a number of ongoing dissertations, and these include the following counseling-related works: biopsychosocial dynamics of HIV-disclosure (Almelah, n.d.); using music to promote HIV/AIDS education and to challenge stigma (Chidanyika, n.d.); the impact of highly active antiretroviral therapy (HAART) on labor market participation by people on AIDS treatment for more than three years (Coetzee, n.d.) and the impact

Research Box 4.2: Psychoeducational Intervention in Botswana

Levers, L. L. (2006a). Focus groups and related rapid assessment methods: Identifying psycho-educational HIV/AIDS interventions in Botswana. In C. Fischer (Ed.), *Qualitative research methods for the psychological professions* (pp. 377–410). New York: Elsevier.

Objective: The study designed and tested the efficacy of culturally relevant HIV and AIDS psychoeducational and prevention interventions for camp workers in Botswana.

Method: Rapid Appraisal Methods (RAMs) were used in this qualitative investigation. The main method used for data collection was a series of focus groups with camp administrators and camp workers. These were supplemented by key informant interviews and participant observation (the researcher lived at the main camp, in a tent, for three weeks; she previously had spent time at the camp on numerous occasions, and was therefore familiar to many of the workers).

Results: Three major themes arose from the data analysis: (1) the need for accurate information, (2) the need for culturally relevant training, and (3) the identification of relevant psychosocial and cultural issues. The last theme is particularly germane to the topic of the present chapter. It became evident that many of the employees retained traditional beliefs regarding the etiology of AIDS. For example, constructs such as *thokolosi* (a disembodied spirit, often thought to be sent by traditional doctors for the purpose of magic or sorcery) and *boswagadi* (a condition associated with death and mourning when a widow has not performed certain traditional cleansing rituals) were essential to their ethnomedical understandings about HIV and AIDS.

Conclusions: The need for culturally informed counseling and psychoeducational interventions associated with mitigating the spread of HIV and AIDS was apparent throughout the results of the study. Interestingly, while the inquiry was being conducted, it was not unusual for participants to stop by the researcher's tent, "just to talk." It was in these informal talk sessions that numerous issues related to the need for counseling, within the context of the research topic, were identified.

Questions

1. Using the example of HIV and AIDS, how is cultural relevance essential to counseling and related activities that are conducted in African settings?
2. Identify a public counseling-related HIV and AIDS project that does not seem to be meeting its goals. Examine the situation from a culturally sensitive perspective. Can you identify ways of reshaping the project, from a cultural perspective, so that it would be more effective for and responsive to the intended population?

of HAART on HIV Testing in South Africa (Lane, n.d.); media representation of "highest level" AIDS and denial in South Africa (Kallon, n.d.); women's experiences of HIV (Kane, n.d.); and HIV/AIDS-related stigma in Cape Town (Maughan-Brown, n.d.).

A second current trend is the extent to which academics, both African and Euro-American, have begun to initiate respectful research projects that illuminate the richness of indigenous knowledge through naturalistic and phenomenological inquiry. One example is the interest in how traditional healing practice links with counseling practice (e.g., Levers, 2006b, 2006c; Levers & Maki, 1994, 1995; Marks, 2006; Mngqundaniso & Peltzer, 2008; Peltzer, Mngqundaniso, & Petros, 2006a, 2006b).

ISSUES FOR RESEARCH AND OTHER FORMS OF SCHOLARSHIP

Many lacunae exist in both the theoretical and research literatures concerning counseling in African settings. We know little about traditional African counseling needs in reference to counseling; we also know little about the interaction of traditional cultures with modern and post-colonial cultural overlays and the concomitant need for counseling interventions. Many of our assumptions about psychosocial aspects of counseling interventions, indeed, about the dynamics of the counseling process itself, are based upon our understandings of positivist paradigms of epistemology and ontology. The Cartesian slant of modern counseling does not dovetail easily with indigenous ways of knowing and helping. We need to be creative in constructing inquiry that addresses this.

To enhance the delivery of counseling services in African settings, methods of naturalistic inquiry need to be adopted in tandem with relevant positivist methods of research. Culturally relevant examinations of the lived experiences of Africans can set the stage for more informed understandings of the day-to-day psychosocial aspects of interpersonal concerns in Africa. Along with standard qualitative and quantitative research designs, researchers need to construct culturally sensitive and culturally relevant program evaluations, community-based research strategies, and symptom-reduction research inquiries.

Discussion Box 4.2: Principles of the Research Partnership

The Swiss Commission for Research Partnerships with Developing countries ([KFPE], 1998, and cited in Crossley and Holmes, 2001, p. 402) has identified eleven principles of research partnership. These principles have appeared throughout the development literature and include the following: (1) decide on the objectives together; (2) build up mutual trust; (3) share information and develop networks; (4) share responsibility; (5) create transparency; (6) monitor and evaluate the collaboration; (7) disseminate the results; (8) apply the results; (9) share profits equitably; (10) increase research capacity; and (11) build on the achievements. Consider the KFPE principles in your discussion of the following.

Questions

1. Critically discuss the principles that govern the research partnership in a counseling setting. Draw on the different sections in this chapter to explain the principles, and where possible, illustrate the principles with examples from your community setting.
2. How are some of these principles parallel to the dynamics of the counseling process?

Evidence of Efficacy

A considerable body of scientific research is now available to guide the formulation of appropriate mental health responses and to help in the identification of those who may require ongoing support; however, the analysis of the efficacy of this research is still in its infancy. Research has shown that a majority of individuals and communities show considerable resilience and strength in the face of disaster, yet there is much to learn from those who adapt, as well as from those who fail to adapt, to such difficult and stressful circumstances. In addition, so much of the research that has been conducted has used exclusively Western theories and models, and has thus not always rendered results that are efficacious in African settings. To ensure the efficacy of counseling and research in African settings, it is important to consider counseling and research practices that are based on the principles of multicultural counseling and research (Humphrey, 2001; MacLachlan, 2000; Menzies, 2001; Smith, 2005; Steinhauer, 2002; Yeh et al., 2004); these are highlighted within the following sections on interdisciplinary approaches, emic (insider) versus etic (outsider) perspectives, and folk-oriented research.

Interdisciplinary Approaches

The disciplines that have looked at the indigenization of research practices have been anthropology, education, history, medical studies, philosophy, sociology, and social work (Hortshemke, 2004; Kanuha, 2000; Smith, 2005; Steinhauer, 2002). The themes within these different areas of study and global contexts include the importance of understanding indigenous knowledge systems and the awareness of the impact of the assumptions of different world views within counseling and research contexts. For example, Smith (2005), through her research endeavors in education, built a research agenda that uses indigenous epistemologies to explore the experiences of indigenous people. This research has resulted in an ability to facilitate new outcomes and to pose new research questions in education in particular, and for research in general, in indigenous contexts across the world. Such contemporary cross-disciplinary inquiry parallels the historical–political overview of and the challenges for research in Africa that have been offered and identified throughout this chapter.

Another area that contributes to indigenization of counseling and research is the culturally sensitive research conducted in American, Asian, Australian, and other non-African contexts with indigenous people. Crossley and Holmes (2001) remind us of how research in African settings occurs within a global context; they make useful suggestions about the nature of relationships with national agencies to strengthen national and local African research, and consequently, counseling endeavors. Such relationships highlight the importance of fostering research partnerships and emphasizing the working alliance between external and insider experts; they also encourage collective knowledge creation, as well as inspiring research that is mutually beneficial to all actors through the implementation and dissemination of the outcomes of the research process (Crossley & Holmes, 2001; Humphrey, 2001; Menzies, 2001; Okolie, 2003).

Emic versus Etic Perspectives

The role of cultural issues in counseling and research practices has been examined by researchers who either have been embedded in the African context (MacLachlan, 2000, Peltzer, 1999, 2001, 2002; Vontress, 1999a, 1999b) or were insiders (Bakker & Mokwena, 1999; Kanuha, 2000; Nwachuku & Ivey, 1991). Counselors also have shown varying awareness of the impact of their world views on the counseling experiences of their clients; the extent to which and how this cultural awareness has been implemented in counseling and counseling research requires further exploration. However, the need for developing working relationships with different stakeholders in the counseling/research context, especially with traditional and faith healers, requires urgent attention (Humphrey, 2001; MacLachlan, 2000; Peltzer, 2001). It also is important to bear in mind that the cultural context cannot be separated

Case Study 4.1: Facilitating Research and Conducting Interviews

Conducting ethnographic research relies upon building trust with local informants who participate in interviews with the researchers. In preparation for their research with African traditional healers, Levers and Maki (1994) made contact with local African academic experts to begin to ascertain who possessed knowledge about indigenous healers in the three southern African countries in which they conducted their inquiry. They identified healers who were highly respected in their communities, and they always made sure that their contacts could present their research quest in a way that they would be *invited in* by the healers, rather than imposing upon them. Even though most of the healers knew English, Levers' and Maki's native language, the researchers always took a translator with them, so that the healers could choose whether or when to use English or the local language. In all cases, the healers preferred to speak about healing practices in their own languages, so the translators translated into English for the researchers. Levers and Maki asked their questions in English to the translator, who in turn translated the questions into the local language. The interviews typically lasted for several hours, and sometimes for the entire day. Several healers invited Levers and Maki back for more information on another day. One healer invited the researchers to an all-day initiation of one of her students. The researchers traveled to a remote and rural area to attend the initiation. They spent the entire day and evening; they participated in some parts of the event, as culturally appropriate, with the other attendees.

Questions

1. Critically discuss the steps that the researchers took to work with insiders to secure interviews with the traditional healers.
2. What other steps would you have followed to ensure that you could interview a traditional healer about the healing relationship with his or her clients?

from the demands of the political context and that this has an impact on counseling and research practices.

It is essential to note that cultural issues and indigenous knowledge have not remained static. For example Peltzer (2002, p. 84) identified the following three distinctive categories of people living in sub-Saharan Africa: the traditional persons, who are little affected by modernization and functioning within the framework or theory of their cultures; the transitional persons, who move between two cultures, that is, the traditional culture and a contemporary, industrial, or postindustrial world, with regard to their daily activities; and, the modern persons, who fully participate in the activities of the contemporary, industrial, or postindustrial world. Furthermore, the definition and nature of indigenous knowledge indicates that it changes over time to deal with the demands of ever-changing sociopolitical contexts having an impact on counseling and research practices.

As the reader may be aware by now, the assumptions of the African world view have had an impact on counseling and research practices. For example, the psychosocial unit with which indigenous healers have worked within interdependent cultures is the group, focusing on the extended family, elders, and community members, rather than the individual or the nuclear family (Nwachuku & Ivey, 1991; Yeh et al., 2004). Subsequently, this group emphasis has had an impact on counseling and counseling-related research in African cultures, which has led to implications for the unit of study in the research process. The types of research methods used in African settings are also influenced by an African world view; quantitative or experimental methods, which focus on cause-and-effect relationships and do not go beyond the physical, cognitive, and emotional realms of human existence, are not appropriate in an indigenous context that values circular causality and includes the spiritual and metaphysical realms of human existence (Nwachuku & Ivey, 1991; Steinhauer, 2002; Yeh et al., 2004). Qualitative research methodologies such as ethnography, narrative inquiry, phenomenology, and case studies have focused on entering and understanding the lived experiences of the research participants, and in so doing, have come closer to addressing the needs of research participants and their communities. However, these methodologies have not necessarily been informed by indigenous knowledge systems and the African world view. By being aware of assumptions of African world view, we have access to a variety of research methods, tools, and techniques that can enhance quantitative research, qualitative research, and mixed methods alike (Steinhauer, 2002; Yeh et al., 2004).

The *ethical considerations*, in counseling and research, are important in the context of unequal power relationships, which require mindfulness of the need for greater equity between the counselor/researcher and the counseling/research participant. This greater equity can be established through ethical guidelines and methods that include decreasing the dependence and increasing the efficacy of participants, through counseling and research that focuses on the participants' coping skills and strengths (LaFromboise, Foster, & James, 1996). Ethical considerations in multicultural counseling also are challenged by the involvement of the extended family and members of

Discussion Box 4.3: The Two-headed Snake

Schoffeleers and Roscoe (1985) recorded an old African folk tale about a two-headed snake, which was so long that its beginning and end spanned two nations. But the snake's heads were very different. One head was rich, with guards and servants; and he wanted everyone to know that he was the master, the Chief. The other head had very little worldly goods. The Chief composed a song about the land being his alone. After singing it aloud, he heard someone in the distance repeating his song, and he became livid. He demanded to know who this was; he sent his guards to find and kill him. While the guards searched, the Chief continued to sing the song so that the guards could find the culprit, and the other voice continued to echo the song.

After a very long journey, following the other voice, the guards finally found that it was just the head at the other end of the snake. But they also realized that it was the body of their Chief; they were fearful even to touch what belonged to him, so they reported back to him. The Chief declared that this was nonsense, and ordered them to go back and kill the other. The guards obeyed, they went off to slay the other; and they returned to tell the Chief that they had carried out his orders. The Chief sang aloud, to test whether or not there would be an answer; of course there was not, so he felt confident that in defeating his rival, he now possessed all the land. Within a few days, the dead head decomposed, which spread through the snake's whole body, right to the Chief. As his demise was upon him, he tried to sing his song, but as he uttered the first line about the land being his alone, he collapsed and was dead.

Questions

1. What do you think about this story? Do you think that the counseling profession can learn from this African story?
2. Now imagine that the snake has multiple heads, with each head representing the different stakeholders in counseling and research in Africa. Now reconsider the question again. Do you think that researchers and counselors in African settings can learn from this African story?

the community (Yeh et al., 2004), as well as the definition and the intervention of the problem. Should research practices in counseling become more community oriented, issues pertaining to the nature of the research problems, the ownership of the data, confidentiality of the data, and dissemination of results take on a different nature than in the counseling and research practices that are embedded in individualistic societies and based on middle-class values (Humphrey, 2001; LaFromboise et al., 1996).

Folk-oriented Research

Several areas of research based on the impact of culture on counseling and research can be suggested. It is important to explore the experiences of clients who use indigenous healing services. It also is important to realize that clients may explore the benefits of different healing services resulting in the need for comparing clients' experiences of the different healing systems, that is, indigenous and Western systems. Counselors should enhance their understanding and knowledge of indigenous forms of healing, indigenous healing practices, and the healers who provide these methods of healing. It also would be beneficial to investigate how both Western and African ways of healing could be integrated to provide optimal psychological services. Examining how clients' cultural background and sociodemographic variables are related to their responsiveness to, and preferences for, different healing methods would assist practitioners in providing relevant services for clients (Yeh et al., 2004). These research areas are not exhaustive, but rather, they focus on enhancing counselors' understanding of indigenous healing systems and developing a relationship with indigenous healers that can have an impact on the provision of counseling services in the different mental health areas.

SUMMARY AND CONCLUSIONS

In this chapter, we have addressed the complexity of current research that illuminates counseling practices in African settings, especially as these modern practices are situated within traditional indigenous contexts. We explored the contextual considerations for examining counseling and research in African settings, with an emphasis on the need for cultural relevance, cultural sensitivity, and cultural appropriateness across all decisions relative to selecting theories, techniques, strategies, interventions, and methods associated with both counseling and research activities. We explicated the significance of considering such constructs as world view and indigenous knowledge when examining contemporary counseling and research endeavors in African settings. We offered a brief history of counseling-related research, as well as a discussion of current counseling practices and counseling-related research. Based upon our review of the literature, we identified several specific counseling-relevant areas upon which to focus our discussion, and these included the following: disaster mental health responses, HIV/AIDS counseling, health counseling, trauma counseling, counseling for orphans and other vulnerable children (OVC), rehabilitation counseling, and psychoeducational practices. For each of these topical areas, we organized and reported the evidence-based information, which we had gleaned from our review of the professional literature, according to (1) a brief description of the topical area, (2) current applications of the strategies and techniques being described, and (3) related counseling research.

We identified two current trends in research, as these are relevant to African settings. The first involved the increase of African graduate students conducting original naturalistic inquiry into culturally relevant themes of counseling in African settings. A second involved the extent to which African and non-African researchers have begun to follow more culturally respectful trajectories of inquiry that are informed by indigenous knowledge. We identified gaps in the theoretical and research literature, as well as future research needs. We discussed the evidence of efficacy, as it pertains to counseling and research in African settings, and we delineated the related disciplines affected by this discourse. Finally, we provided an overview of the implications for research, particularly illuminating the role of cultural issues in counseling and research practices in African settings. Clearly, the way forward, in regard to current research on counseling in African settings, is to honor the indigenous knowledge that preceded modern counseling; this can be accomplished through the use of naturalistic inquiry, as a strategy that is parallel to the use of modern research methods, in understanding the modern psychosocial complexities that overlay traditional concerns.

REFERENCES

AIDS and Society Research Unit (ASRU). Haiku: hiv/aids coordination. University of Cape Town. Retrieved November 3, 2008 from http://www.hivaids.uct.ac.za/cms/index.php?Itemid=0&id=31&option=com_content&task=view

Almelah, C. (n.d.). *The bio-psychosocial dynamics of HIV-disclosure in the South African context*. Unpublished doctoral dissertation, University of Cape Town, Cape Town, South Africa.

Amani Trust. (1997). Assessment of the consequences of torture and organised violence: A manual for field workers (revised). Harare, Zimbabwe: Author.

Bakker, T. M., & Mokwena, M. L. E. (1999). African perspectives on behaviour. In P. Avis, A. Pauw, & I. Van der Spuy (Eds.), *Psychological perspectives: An introductory workbook* (pp. 193–207). Cape Town: Pearson Education South Africa.

Barnhardt, R., & Kawagley, A. O. (2005). Indigenous knowledge systems and Alaskan native ways of knowing. *Anthropology and Education Quarterly*, *36*(1), 8–23.

Baum, A., & Fleming, I. (1993). Implications of psychological research on stress and technological accidents. *American Psychologist*, *48*, 665–72.

Bhusmane, D-B. (2007). *Mechanisms of indigenous counseling in Botswana*. Unpublished doctoral dissertation, Duquesne University, Pittsburgh, PA.

Cardinal, L. (2001). What is an Indigenous perspective? *Canadian Journal of Nature Education*, *25*(2), 180–2.

Cater, N., Revel, J., Sapir, D., & Walker, P. (1993). *World Disasters Report 1993*. Geneva: The International Federation of Red Cross (IFRC) and Red Crescent Societies (RCS).

Chidanyika, T. (n.d.). *Healing the nation: An exploration of the role of musicians in promoting HIV/AIDS education and challenging HIV-related stigma in Masvingo, Zimbabwe*. Unpublished master's thesis, University of Cape Town, Cape Town, South Africa.

Coetzee, C. (n.d.). *Having the HAART to live: The impact of HAART on labour market participation for patients in Khayelitsha who have been on treatment for more than three years*. Unpublished doctoral dissertation, University of Cape Town, Cape Town, South Africa.

Crossley, M., & Holmes, K. (2001). Challenges for educational research: International development, partnership and capacity building in small states. *Oxford Review of Education*, *27*(3), 395–409.

de Jong, J. T. V. M., Komproe, I. H., Van Ommeren, M., El Masri, M., Araya, M., Khaled, N., van de Put, W., & Somasundaram, D. (2001). Lifetime events and posttraumatic stress disorder in four postconflict settings. *JAMA*, *286*(5), 555–62.

Foa, E. B., Keane, T. M., & Friedman, M. J. (2000). *Effective treatments for PTSD*. New York: Guilford Press.

Fonchingong, C. C., Mbuagbo, T. O., & Abong, J. T. (2004). Barriers to counselling support for HIV/AIDS patients in south-western Cameroon. *African Journal of Aids Research*, *3*(2), 157–65.

Green, B. L., & Lindy, J. D. (1994). Posttraumatic stress disorder in victims of disasters. *Psychiatric Clinics of North America*, *17*, 301–9.

Hassan, M. H. A. (2008). Global science gaps need global action. *Issues in Science and Technology*, *24*(2), 57–64.

Horsthemke, K. (2004). 'Indigenoius knowledge', truth and reconciliation in South African higher education. *South African Journal of Higher Education*, *18*(3), 65–81.

Humphrey, K. (2001). Dirty questions: Indigenous health and 'Western research.' *Australian and New Zealand Journal of Public Health*, *25*(3), 197–202.

Kallon, I. (n.d.). *The print media's representation of "highest level" AIDS denialism in South Africa: Distortion or dictum?* Unpublished thesis, University of Cape Town, Cape Town, South Africa.

Kane, D. (n.d.). *Women's experiences of HIV, unemployment, and motherhood in Site B, Khayelitsha*. Unpublished master's thesis, University of Cape Town, Cape Town, South Africa.

Kanuha, V. K. (2000). "Being" native versus "going native": Conducting social work research as an insider. *Social Work*, *45*(5), 439–49.

LaFromboise, T. D., Foster, S., & James, A. (1996). Ethics in multicultural counselling. In P. B. Pedersen, J. G. Draguns, W. J. Lonner, & J. E. Timble (Eds.), *Counselling across cultures* (4th ed., pp. 47–72). London: SAGE Publications

Lane, H. (n.d.). *The impact of HAART on HIV testing in South Africa*. Unpublished master's thesis, University of Cape Town, Cape Town, South Africa.

Levers, L. L. (1997a). Counselling as a recursive dynamic: Relationship and process, meaning-making and empowerment. In T. F. Riggar & D. R. Maki (Eds.), *Rehabilitation counselling: Profession and practice* (2nd ed., pp. 170–82). New York: Springer.

Levers, L. L. (1997b). Cross-cultural training in southern Africa: A call for psychoecological pluralism. *International Journal of Intercultural Relations*, *21*, 249–277.

Levers, L. L. (1999). Designing counsellor education in a developing context: A prospectus for a southern African regional counsellor training and resource center. *Journal of Sustainable*

Development in Africa, *1*(1), 26 pp. Retrieved October 25, 2008 from http://www.jsd-africa.com/Jsda/Winter%201999/articlespdf/ARC-designing%20counsellor%20education.pdf

Levers, L. L. (2002). Northern Namibian teachers on the effects of violence, poverty, and privation on young children's development: School-based countermeasures. *Journal of Children and Poverty*, *8*(1), 5–44.

Levers, L. L. (2003a). Sustainable HIV/AIDS abatement in Botswana: Contextual factors & cultural relevance. Paper presented at the National HIV/AIDS/STI/Other Related Infectious Diseases Research Conference 2003, sponsored by the National AIDS Coordinating Agency (NACA), Gaborone, Botswana.

Levers, L. L. (2003b). The consultative workshop as a qualitative method of inquiry: The case of teachers and counsellors working with AIDS orphans in Botswana. Monograph of papers presented at the Ethnographic and Qualitative Research in Education 2003 Annual Conference, June 6, 2003, Pittsburgh, PA. Retrieved from http://www.education.duq.edu/institutes/PDF/papers2003/Levers1.pdf

Levers, L. L. (2006a). Identifying psychoeducational HIV/AIDS interventions in Botswana: Focus groups and related rapid assessment methods. In C. Fischer (Ed.), *Qualitative research methods for the psychological professions* (pp. 377–410). New York: Elsevier Press.

Levers, L. L. (2006b). Samples of indigenous healing: The path of good medicine. *International Journal of Disability, Development and Education*, *54*, 479–88.

Levers, L. L. (2006c). Traditional healing as indigenous knowledge: Its relevance to HIV/AIDS in southern Africa and the implications for counsellors. *Journal of Psychology in Africa*, *16*, 87–100.

Levers, L. L., Kamanzi, D., Mukamana, D., Pells, K., & Bhusumane, D-B. (2006). Addressing urgent community mental health needs in Rwanda: Culturally sensitive training interventions. *Journal of Psychology in Africa*, *16*, 261–72.

Levers, L. L., & Magweva, F. I. (2005, March). *Report on a national rehabilitation plan and training programme*. Windhoek, Namibia: Ministry of Lands, Resettlement, and Rehabilitation, Government of the Republic of Namibia.

Levers, L. L., Magweva, F. I., Maundanei, T., & Mpofu, E. (2008). *A report on a comprehensive study of social safety nets for people with disabilities in Botswana*. A study sponsored by the Botswana Ministry of Health, at the request of the Botswana Office of the President. Gaborone, Botswana: Ministry of Health.

Levers, L. L., Magweva, F. I., & Mpofu, E. (2007). *Discussion paper 40: A review of district health systems in east and southern Africa: Facilitators and barriers to participation in health*. Published online by Regional Network for Equity in Health in east and southern Africa (EQUINET) as an EQUINET Discussion Paper. Retrieved March 19, 2007 from http://www.equinetafrica.org/bibl/docs/DIS40ehsLOPEZ.pdf

Levers, L. L., & Maki, D. R. (1994). *An ethnographic analysis of traditional healing and rehabilitation services in southern Africa: Crosscultural implications*. A report prepared for the World Rehabilitation Fund, National Institute on Disability and Rehabilitation Research, U.S. Department of Education. Stillwater, OK: National Clearing House for Rehabilitation Training Materials, Oklahoma State University.

Levers, L. L., & Maki, D. R. (1995). African indigenous healing, cosmology, and existential implications: Toward a philosophy of ethnorehabilitation. *Rehabilitation Education*, *9*, 127–45.

MacLachlan, M. (2000). Cultivating pluralism in health psychology. *Journal of Health Psychology*, *5*(3), 372–82.

Malema, N. (2006). *Challenges and adjustment strategies facing caregivers of children living with HIV and AIDS*. Unpublished master's thesis, University of Botswana, Gaborone, Botswana.

Marks, L. M. (2006). Global Health Crisis: Can indigenous healing practices offer a valuable resource? *International Journal of Disability, Development and Education*, *53*(4), 471–8.

Maughan-Brown, B. (n.d.). *HIV/AIDS-related stigma in Cape Town, South Africa*. Unpublished doctoral dissertation, University of Cape Town, Cape Town, South Africa.

Menzies, C. R. (2001). Reflections on research with, for, and among indigenous peoples. *Canadian Journal of Native Education*, *25*(1), 19–36.

Mngqundaniso, N., & Peltzer, K. (2008). Traditional healers and nurses: A qualitative study on their role on sexually transmitted infections including HIV and AIDS in KwaZulu-Natal, South Africa. *African Journal of Traditional, Complementary and Alternative Medicines*. *5*, 380–6.

Mollica, R. F., Donelan, K., Tor, S., Lavelle, J., Elias, C., Frankel, M., & Blendon, R. J. (1993). The effect of trauma and confinement on functional health and mental health status of Cambodians living in Thailand-Cambodia border camps. *JAMA*, *270*(5), 581–6.

Mpofu, E. (2000). Rehabilitation in international perspective: A Zimbabwean experience. *Disability and Rehabilitation*, *23*, 481–9.

Mpofu, E. (2002). Disability and rehabilitation in Zimbabwe: Lessons and implications for rehabilitation practice in the U.S. *Journal of Rehabilitation*, *68*(4), 20–5.

Mpofu, E., & Harley, D. A. (2002). Disability and rehabilitation in Zimbabwe: Lessons and implications for rehabilitation practice in the U.S – Disability and Rehabilitation in Zimbabwe. *Journal of Rehabilitation*, *68*(4), 26–33.

Mpofu, E., Jelsma, J., Maart, S., Levers, L. L., Montsi, M. M. R., Thlabiwe, P., Mwamwenda, T., Ngoma, M. S., & Tchombe, T. M. S. (2007). Rehabilitation in seven sub-Saharan African countries: Policies, personnel, training, and education. *Rehabilitation Education*, *21*, 223–30.

Msimanga-Ramatebele, S. H. (2008). *Lived experiences of widows in Botswana: An ethnographic examination of cultural rituals of death, loss, grief, and bereavement – implications for professional counseling*. Unpublished doctoral dissertation, Duquesne University, Pittsburgh, PA.

Neuner, F., Schauer, M., Elbert, T., & Roth, W. T. (2002). A narrative exposure treatment as intervention in a Macedonia's refugee camp: A case report. *Journal of Behavioural and Cognitive Psychotherapy*, *30*, 205–9.

Neuner, F., Schauer, M., Klaschik, C., Karunakara, U., & Elbert, T. (2004). A comparison of narrative exposure therapy, supportive counseling, and psychoeducation for treating posttraumatic stress disorder in an African refugee settlement. *Journal of Consulting and Clinical Psychology*, *72*, 579–87.

Nwachuku, U. T., & Ivey, A. E. (1991). Culture-specific counselling: An alternative training model. *Journal of Counseling and Development*, *70*(1), 106–11.

Okolie, A. C. (2003). Producing knowledge for sustainable development in Africa: Implications for higher education. *Higher Education*, *46*, 235–60.

Olley, B. O. (2006). Improving well-being through psycho-education among voluntary counseling and testing seekers in Nigeria: A controlled study. *AIDS Care*, *18*, 1025–31.

Painter, T. M. (2001). Voluntary counseling and testing for couples: A high-leverage intervention for HIV/AIDS prevention in sub-Saharan Africa. *Social Science & Medicine, 53*, 1397–1411.

Patterson, L. E., & Welfel, E. R. (1999). *The counselling process* (5th ed.). Pacific Grove, CA: Brooks/Cole.

Paunovi, N., & Ost, L. G. (2001). Cognitive-behavior therapy vs exposure therapy in the treatment of PTSD in refugees. *Behaviour Research and Therapy, 39*, 1183–97.

Peltzer, K. (1999). A process model of ethnocultural counselling for African survivors of organized violence. *Counselling Psychology Quarterly, 12*(4), 335–51.

Peltzer, K. (2001). Traditional mechanisms for cultivating health in Africa. In M. MacLachlan (Ed.), *Cultivating health: Cultivating perspectives on promoting health* (pp. 157–75). New York: John Wiley & Sons.

Peltzer, K. (2002). Personality and person perception in Africa. *Social Behaviour and Personality, 30*(1), 83–94.

Peltzer, K., Mngqundaniso, N., & Petros, G. (2006a). A controlled study of an HIV/AIDS/STI/TB intervention with traditional healers in KwaZulu-Natal, South Africa. *AIDS Behavior, 10*(6), 683–90.

Peltzer, K., Mngqundaniso, N., & Petros, G. (2006b, August). HIV/AIDS/STI/TB knowledge, beliefs and practices of traditional healers in KwaZulu-Natal, South Africa. *AIDS Care, 18*(6), 608–13.

Pityana, N. B. (2005). *On higher education policy in contemporary South Africa*. UNISA. Retrieved November 3, 2008 from http://www.unisa.ac.za/default.asp?Cmd=ViewContent&ContentID=16926

Raphael, B. (1996). Social re-integration and political action. In E.L. Giller & L. Weisæth (Eds.), *Post-traumatic stress disorder*. London: Baillière Tindall.

Raphael, B. (1997). The interaction of trauma and grief. In D. Black, M. Newman, J. Harris-Hendriks & Mezey, G. (Eds.), *Psychological trauma. A developmental approach*. London: Gaskell.

Reviere, R. (2001). Toward an Afrocentric research methodology. *Journal of Black Studies, 31*(6), 709–28.

Roos, V., Potgieter, E., Coetzee, M., & Lehobye, K. (2003). The process of developing a psycho-education programme to promote the integration of homeless children into a children's home. *The Social Work Practitioner-Researcher, 15*(1), 61–75.

Schoffeleers, J. M., & Roscoe, A. A. (1985). *Land of fire: Oral literature from Malawi*. Limbe, Malawi: Popular Press.

Sebatane, E. M., Levers, L. L., & Ralebitso, M. (1993, July). A participatory action research inquiry into the need for short-term/intensive counselor training and train-the-trainers in Lesotho. Paper presented at the *BOLESWA Education Symposium*, Maseru, Lesotho.

Shore, J. H., Vollmer, W., & Tatum, E. L. (1989). Community patterns of posttraumatic stress disorders. *Journal of Nervous & Mental Disease, 177*(11), 681–5.

Skinner, J. (1998). Research as a counselling activity? A discussion of some uses of counselling within the context of research on sensitive issues. *British Journal of Guidance and Counselling, 26*(4), 535–40.

Smith, L. T. (2005). Building a research agenda for indigenous epistemologies and education. *Anthropology and Education Quarterly, 36*(1), 93–5.

Steinglass, P., & Gerrity, E. (1990). Natural disasters and posttraumatic stress disorder short-term versus long-term recovery in two disaster-affected communities. *Journal of Applied Social Psychology, 20*, 1746–65.

Steinhauer, E. (2002). Thoughts on indigenous research methodology. *Canadian Journal of Native Education, 26*(2), 69–81.

Swiss Commission for Research Partnerships with Developing Countries (KFPE). (2001). *Enhancing research capacity in developing and transition countries*. Berne: Author.

Theis, M., Erickson, W., Lloyd-Jones, T, Gandelsonas, C., Kalra, R., Khiabany, G., & Vallejo, L. (2000). *Improving research knowledge technical transfer*, DFID Research Project R 7171. London: Max Lock Centre, University of Westminster and Water Engineering Development Centre, Loughborough University.

UNAIDS. (2006). *2006 Report on the global AIDS epidemic*. Retrieved December 27, 2007 from http://www.unaids.org/en/KnowledgeCentre/HIVData/GlobalReport/Default.asp

United Nations. (1989, December 22). *International decade for natural disaster Reduction United Nations General Assembly*. Retrieved November 3, 2008 from http://www.un.org/documents/ga/res/44/a44r236.htm

Van der Veer, G. (1998). *Counseling and therapy with refugees and victims of trauma* (2nd ed.). West Sussex, England: John Wiley & Sons.

Vontress, C. E. (1999a). Interview with a traditional African healer. *Journal of Mental Health Counselling, 21*(4), 326–36.

Vontress, C. E. (1999b). Traditional healing in Africa: Implications for cross-cultural counselling. *Journal of Counselling and Development, 70*(1), 242–9.

Wienand, A. (n.d.). *The potential of visual and participatory approaches to HIV Literacy in South Africa*. Unpublished master's thesis, University of Cape Town, Cape Town, South Africa.

World Health Organization/United Nations High Commissioner for Refugees. (1996). *Mental health of refugees*. Geneva: World Health Organization.

Yeh, C. J., Hunter, C. D., Madan-Bahel, A., Chiang, L., & Arora, A. K. (2004). Indigenous and interdependent perspectives of healing: Implications for counseling and research. *Journal of Counseling and Development, 82*(4), 410–19.

Zeleza, P. T. (2002). The politics of historical and social science research in Africa. *Journal of Southern African Studies, 28*(1), 9–23.

SELF-CHECK EXERCISES

1. Define indigenous knowledge. Discuss how indigenous knowledge arises from indigenous culture. How is this important to professional counselors, especially in the process of conducting culturally relevant counseling research?
2. Interview several African counselors working with indigenous populations to find out the prevailing culturally appropriate counseling approaches being used. What types of research questions can you formulate that would contribute to the research literature involving counseling in African settings?
3. Find two research articles in your library that deal with counseling in African settings. Read each article for the pertinent information that it provides, but also read each article to assess the research gaps surrounding the particular topic.
4. After studying this chapter and completing the different exercises, reflect on how the learning experience about counseling and research has changed

or enhanced your assumptions about research and counseling in your context. Also, reflect on how these assumptions may have an impact upon your research practices within counseling settings. How do your reflections relate to the need for culturally relevant research in African settings? Identify some of the issues that may lead to more Afrocentric perspectives and approaches to counseling.

5. Critically discuss the different stakeholders in counseling and research settings by referring to the individual, group, community, national, and international contexts. How does this apply to counseling in African settings? In examining the needs of stakeholders in African settings, generate a list of areas that need research to practice culturally sensitive and culturally relevant counseling.
6. For counseling to develop and address the psychological needs of Africans, African psychologists, counselors, and others have to struggle with the following two questions: (1) Should counselors and others in Africa develop a localized, indigenous psychology to address specifically the circumstances and the requirements of the different peoples of Africa? (2) Should counselors and others in Africa work toward a universal theory of counseling? What is your position regarding these two questions? Substantiate your answer.

FIELD-BASED EXPERIENTIAL EXERCISES

1. Interview a traditional or faith healer to determine his or her area of expertise and perceptions of how knowledge is created and transferred about the helping relationships in his or her context.
2. Interview a lay counselor to determine his or her area of expertise and perceptions of how knowledge is created and transferred about the helping relationships in his or her context.
3. Interview a counselor to determine his or her area of expertise and perceptions of how knowledge is created and transferred about the helping relationships in his or her context.
4. Approach five learners at a school nearby, and conduct individual interviews with them to determine
   a. Whether they have received psychoeducational counseling about HIV/AIDS
   b. What information they found most useful
   c. What information they found least useful
   d. From which other sources in their community they received information about HIV/AIDS
   e. Which of the sources, including the psychoeducational counseling, they have found to be the most useful
5. Approach three members of the community and conduct individual interviews with them to determine
   a. Whether they have been approached by other field workers
   b. What were the research project/questions
   c. How did they feel about being approached by field workers
   d. Whether they were informed about the outcomes of the research project/questions

MULTIPLE-CHOICE QUESTIONS

1. Fill in the blanks. Western societies tend to be more __________ in nature, with a rather rigid dualistic world view, while indigenous societies tend to be more __________ in nature, with a more relativistic perspective of the universe.
   a. individualistic/competitive
   b. individualistic/collectivist
   c. collectivist/competitive
   d. collectivist/cooperative
   e. cooperative/competitive
2. Fill in the blank. Traditional healers use various methods, including ______________, to diagnose and discover information about their clients.
   a. divination
   b. formal reports
   c. conversations with researchers
   d. conversations with doctors
   e. looking at the stars
3. In the indigenous paradigm, how is knowledge revealed?
   a. In dreams, visions, and intuition
   b. In conversations between role players
   c. In conversations between traditional healers and clients
   d. In dialogue between traditional healers and counselors
   e. In rigid quantitative methods of knowledge creation
4. Which of the following situations relates to Raphael's (1996, 1997) emphasis that intervention is critical when indigenous communities are affected by disaster?
   a. That their leaders are involved in the development of culturally appropriate recovery and support processes
   b. That counselors implement appropriate recovery and support processes without collaboration with traditional leaders
   c. That counselors implement appropriate recovery and support processes using lay counselors in the community
   d. That their leaders are not interested in negotiating with agencies that can provide assistance in dealing with the disasters
   e. That international agencies implement appropriate recovery and support processes without collaboration with traditional leaders
5. Why are quantitative experimental research methods not the best research approach to use in a traditional African setting?
   a. These methods value circular causality of the indigenous context.

b. These methods include the metaphysical realms of human existence.
c. These methods include the spiritual realms of human existence.
d. These methods primarily focus on cause-and-effect relationships.
e. These methods go beyond the physical and cognitive realms of human existence.

6. What, according to research done by Painter (2001), is considered to be of value as a HIV prevention tool?
   a. Programs encouraging abstinence amongst teenagers
   b. Free flow of condoms in public areas
   c. Voluntary HIV counseling and testing
   d. Media drives about HIV prevention targeting teenagers
   e. Psychoeducational programs aimed at HIV prevention
7. The knowledge about effective treatment of PTSD in Africa or areas affected by war remains scarce. Although war-torn populations have received considerable attention from psychosocial organizations in recent years, little clinical research has been conducted on which of the following?
   a. How psychoeducational interventions can benefit these groups
   b. How adequately to support and treat these groups
   c. How narrative inquiry can be used to treat these groups
   d. How narrative exposure therapy can be used to support these groups
   e. How rehabilitation counseling can be used to treat these groups
8. What psychosocial unit(s) do indigenous healers typically work with in interdependent cultures?
   a. The individual
   b. The nuclear family
   c. The individual and nuclear family
   d. The extended family and community
   e. The elders and the nuclear family
9. Which of the following best completes this sentence? Another area that contributes to indigenization of counseling and research practices is:____________.
   a. culturally sensitive research conducted in American, Asian, Australian, and other non-African contexts with indigenous peoples
   b. research only in African contexts
   c. research only on local settings within African contexts
   d. research only in Asian contexts
   e. research only in local settings within American contexts
10. Which of the following best completes this sentence? Ethical considerations in an indigenous African context ________________________.
   a. increase the dependence of the participants in the research process
   b. have to reconsider the ownership and confidentiality of data collected during research
   c. have not been mindful of greater equity among the stakeholders
   d. have not been challenged by the involvement of the extended family
   e. have not been challenged by the involvement of the members of the community

Answers to the multiple-choice questions are provided at the back of the book

5 Deconstructing Counseling Psychology for the African Context

Anbanithi Muthukrishna and David Lackland Sam

OVERVIEW. In this chapter, we examine how counseling psychology theory, practice, and research may be deconstructed and transformed to make them more relevant for the African context. "Deconstruction" refers to ways in which one can expand the limits of accepted conceptual meanings in counseling psychology and in the process show that those meanings are complex and unstable. The aim, in this chapter, is to deconstruct ideological biases and traditional assumptions that have influenced counseling psychology in African contexts. The chapter shows that in deconstructing traditional psychology, the need for transformation becomes an important imperative, that is, change in the nature of counseling psychology in African contexts, the counseling psychology community, its social institutions, the theories that influence the field, its research agendas, and its practice.

LEARNING OBJECTIVES

By the end of the chapter, the reader should be able to:

1. Explain why it is necessary to transform counseling psychology for the African context.
2. Discuss the hegemonic influences of counseling psychology theory and practices in Africa.
3. Outline ways in which we can begin to make counseling psychology theory, practice, and training more relevant to the cultural–sociopolitical contexts in Africa.
4. Suggest what can be considered relevant research for the discipline of counseling psychology in Africa.

INTRODUCTION

In African contexts, Western theories, concepts, and methods, which have emanated largely from high-income countries, still influence psychological science and practice, including counseling psychology, despite the fact that African scholars have over the years questioned their applicability and relevance (e.g., De la Rey & Ipser; 2004; Nsamensamg, 1995; Painter and Terre Blanche, 2004; Stead & Watson, 2006). Scholars have drawn attention to the colonizing impacts of Western ways of knowing and knowledge production on more developing contexts (Bulhan, 1985; Holdstock, 2000; Nsamensamg, 1995). They have challenged the taken-for-granted ways of knowledge production and have called for different methodologies and approaches. Mkhize (2008) explains that counseling psychology has been accused of excluding others' ways of being in the world. Regarding the training of counseling psychologists, it is well known that most training in African contexts is biased toward Western models of psychology, as most psychologists in Africa have been educated in Western colleges and universities. African psychologists internalize and practice these Western models of psychology with its Eurocentric bias.

These debates suggest that the discipline of counseling psychology, including concepts, methods, and interpretations, has emanated from one cultural region of the world (the European-American). Allwood and Berry (2006) suggest that this can be conceived as the significant impact of one indigenous psychology – that of Western societies. A major criticism of this trend has been the fact that Western psychology is "culture-bound" and not universal. In reality, it should be viewed as one of many possible indigenous psychologies, and should be questioned in more developing contexts on grounds that it is ethnocentric.

There is, therefore, a compelling need to develop alternate paradigms and models to understand the realities in African contexts (Holdstock, 2000). As the globalization movement is rapidly emerging, it is important to examine other world views different from those with which one is familiar, and in so doing reassess one's own reality. Nsamenang (2006) explains, for example, that there are significant differences in the values and practices that inform and guide the nurturing of children throughout the world as individuals develop in a huge variety of ecological and sociopolitical circumstances. Nsamenang further argues there is a need to explore, first, how this understanding informs theory, research, practice, and pedagogy of international psychology, and second, how these insights can be theorized to explain the wide variety of global developmental trajectories. It is therefore important that in the counseling profession we evaluate the theories we use, how we practice psychology, and how we undertake research in Africa. There is a need to develop alternate lenses to investigate the unique research questions that emanate from an African context.

African scholars have argued for the development of psychology, including counseling psychology, that is socially, contextually, and culturally valid (e.g., Durojaiye, 1993; Mkhize, 2008; Nsamensamg, 1995, 2006). There has been a movement toward exploring an Afrocentric paradigm to contest the Eurocentric counseling and its focus on universality (e.g., Naidoo, Olowu, Gilbert, & Akotia, 1999). Bulhan (1985) has pointed to the oppressive imperialism in psychology. According to Macleod (2004), the challenges for counseling psychology in Africa include (1) theory building that can provide insights into the unique sociohistorical (2) alternate lenses to investigate unique research questions that emanate from an African context, and (3) expansion of traditional research approaches, topics, and participants so that they inform the sociopolitical concerns of Africa.

IMPORTANCE, DEFINITION, AND SCOPE OF KEY TERMS AND CONCEPTS

To examine the hegemony of counseling practices in Africa critically, one needs to examine the assumptions underlying current theory, research, and practice upon which traditional Western psychology has had an impact. In their attempts to engage with this, Owusu-Bempah and Howitt (2000), Burr (2002), and Hayes (2002) argue that Eurocentric psychology has been derived from a value system that is individualistic in its orientation, training, and application. In addition, it is viewed as a psychology relevant largely for people who hold the values of an industrialized society. Thus, current counseling practices may be considered as culturally inappropriate, as they have neglected the social and mental health concerns in diverse African sociopolitical contexts. We now examine some of the ways in which current paradigms and models fail to represent the lived realities in African contexts.

Conceptualization of the Self

Eurocentric conceptions of "self" have been embedded in the training of many psychologists in Africa, and this has led to contradictions and dilemmas for their practice. For example, the Western conception of the self values individual autonomy and responsibility and stresses the independence of the self from the social world (Owusu-Bempah & Howitt, 2000). In contrast, most African cultures view the individual as intertwined and constantly interacting with the sociocultural environment (Holdstock, 2000). A view of the person as an independent unit of the social system entrenches the idea that the psyche and consciousness are embedded within the individual. Holdstock argues that in African culture the psyche is not independent of culture and social context, and that they in fact include each other. Furthermore, the psyche is not fixed and universal, but *in process* as it interacts with the social world. It changes, depending on time and context. In other words, our values, beliefs, and behavioral patterns are contextually bound. Holdstock (2000, p. 201) suggests that one of the reasons that psychology has not progressed in Africa is that "the ideologies and methodologies of contemporary psychology do not fit into the inclusive value system of African people."

The Notion of "Culture"

In psychology, debates around the concept of "culture" have been multifaceted and laden with varying assumptions, ranging from views that "culture" is bounded, timeless, and unchanging, to "culture" being linked to macroprocesses, historically shaped, and contested (Taylor, 2007).

In mainstream psychology, the notion of culture in psychology has been linked to exotic, essentialist references to "the African" personhood. In recent debates, many researchers have argued that the concept of "culture" is a dynamic concept, constantly changing and evolving. An individual is embedded within a variety of sociocultural contexts or cultures (e.g., country or region of origin, ethnicity, religion, gender, family, birth cohort, profession). Holdstock (2000), for example, argues that each of these cultural contexts influences an individual and is associated with a set of ideas and practices, that is, a cultural framework or schema. Cultural meanings are the views individuals hold of the world and of themselves, and also of their beliefs, values, norms of conduct, myths, and conceptions of the spiritual. In other words, culture is a system of meanings. Holdstock explains that, according to social constructionists, cultural beliefs are shared understandings, the values of everyday life, and the everyday practices that express and construct those values. He argues that Western psychology has entrenched a mistaken perception of an homogeneous, so-called African, perspective. Maree, Ebersöhn, and Molepo (2006) point out that faulty inferences occur especially when researchers assume that sociocultural situations are static rather than dynamic. For example, it must be understood that although traditions may form the basis of people's beliefs and values, traditional culture is not the everyday reality for most contemporary indigenous people, in particular, in the face of increasing globalization. There is a need for a shift from the narrow view of particularism in understanding culture and to acknowledge heterogeneity and contradictions in cultural systems.

Conceptions of the "African Personality"

According to Lassiter (1999), culture and personality studies have been criticized by social scientists and social advocates. The argument made is that many of these studies have resulted in unscientific stereotyping and have entrenched cultural relativism. In addition, findings have been that many of these studies have had a particularistic focus on specific populations and topics (Nsamenang, 2005). A further criticism is made that culture and personality studies do not examine the uniqueness of the individual, nor do they take into account the impact of particular social structures and functions on the individual. Lassiter points out that focusing on broad cultural patterns can conceal the impact of racism and classism, for example. He warns that such findings can be misused to oppress or persecute a particular group.

Many African scholars have conceded that there are broad psychological and cultural themes and patterns that are unique to Africa, but they also contend that these broad cultural patterns are in the process of constant change (Nyasani, 1997; Nsamenang, 2005, 2008). They stress that research therefore needs to ask what it means to be African and what is "Africanness" in the face of increasing globalization. Lassiter (1999) argues that particularist studies impede an understanding of ongoing global cultural processes. The concept of the African personality is an ever-changing concept that that needs constantly to be redefined by Africans themselves. African personality studies do not have to exclude the exploration of traditional cultural belief systems and behavioral patterns. A key reason, as elucidated by Holdstock (2000), is that many individuals have exhibited the ability to function effectively in the contexts of traditional African and modern technological frameworks. This often results in two complementary and mutually exclusive meanings of the same reality. The focus of research should be on studying the broader core values, cultural themes, and adaptive responses of Africans to indigenous sociocultural circumstances and changing external influences.

Conceptions of "Youth" in Africa

Recent debates have suggested that in counseling psychology theory and practice it is necessary to supplement static psychological accounts of growth and development of adolescence and youth with more sociological accounts. Chigunta (2002), in his analysis, seems to support postmodern approaches that reject objectivist accounts of youth as a universal life stage. He explains that, in much of Africa, there is the tendency to extend the category of youth to thirty years and beyond. This occurs because of the emerging phenomenon of the prolonged period of youth *dependence* in African contexts that results from the inability of youth, because of poverty and underdevelopment, to pursue independent and sustainable livelihoods. The concept of "youth" in African contexts, therefore, has meaning only if it is seen in relation to the specific circumstances of social, political, and economic conditions. Chigunta (2002) explains that the category youth involves a complex continuum of problems with a range of characteristics and behaviors that cut across age segments in different contexts. Durham (2001) suggests that the notion of "youth" is both relational and socially and culturally constructed. It even may be the social effect of power.

This discussion suggests that psychology needs to perceive the value of postmodern accounts of the subjective, as well as to ascertain how things are experienced rather than being viewed as objective reality. The reason for this is that objective reality is unknowable or inaccessible to the human mind in the context of social reality. The challenge in rethinking the concept of "youth," in the African context, is to maintain a balance between recognizing the importance of physical and psychological changes that occur in the lives of young people and recognizing the extent to which these are constructed by contextual factors and negotiated by individuals who do have agency. A postmodern perspective holds that the self is social.

In the same vein, postmodern approaches reflect a shift from seeing adolescence as a universal, natural, ahistorical stage of growing up with immutable characteristics. The argument is that such a focus neglects to factor in the social processes that construct the notion of "adolescence." A postmodern view stresses the sociocultural processes of constructing adolescence and identity through the agency that the adolescent can exhibit (Lesko, 1996). In counseling psychology, a valuable research focus could be conducting ethnographic studies of youth culture in a variety of African contexts.

The Notion of "Family"

The concept of "family" in African contexts is complex. On the one hand, African families often include an extended "kin network" and their relationships and connections, and could include individuals who do not fit into the conception of the Western "nuclear family." On the other hand, the notion of "the family" in Africa is not static and has been changing in many African contexts for many reasons including political, economic, and social.

In the arena of HIV and AIDS, in African contexts, there is evidence of multiple configurations of "family" that often include child-headed households, female-headed households, and grandmother as main caregiver (Harley, 2006; Muthukrishna & Ebrahim, 2006). In addition, women and girls have significant caring responsibilities, for example, caring for multiple family members from three or four generations in very complex situations. This includes caring for the elderly, people with disabilities, those with mental illness, and a range of chronic illnesses and conditions that frequently are exacerbated by substance abuse, family violence, and premature death (Harley, 2006). Research needs to explore the intricacies of what it means to provide family care within different African communities.

The preceding discussion suggests the critical need for counseling psychology, in African contexts, to examine the knowledge, skills, and beliefs people have about themselves, and how people function in the familial, community, social, cultural, and ecological contexts.

Universalism versus Particularism

Many researchers have cautioned that research in counseling psychology cannot be located in terms of only one interpretative theory or model (see also Chapter 4, this volume). This argument relates to the issue of universalism

Discussion Box 5.1: The African Personality

The Senegalese psychiatrist Sow (1977, 1978) portrays individuals and in particular Africans as having a personality comprising of four concentric layers. These concentric layers consist of an outer layer made up of the body and a second layer made up of the physiological functioning of the individual, which is the physiological vitality principle. The third layer, the psychological vitality principle, is essentially the psychological functioning of the individual. The innermost layer, where the person's soul or spirit can be found, is the spiritual principle. The different concentric layers of personality are linked to different aspects of the person's environment: The spiritual principle links the individual to the world of ancestors. The psychological vitality principle is linked to the individual and to his extended family, and the physiological vitality principle is linked to the community. Figure 5.1 is a schematic illustration of the different layers making up the African personality.

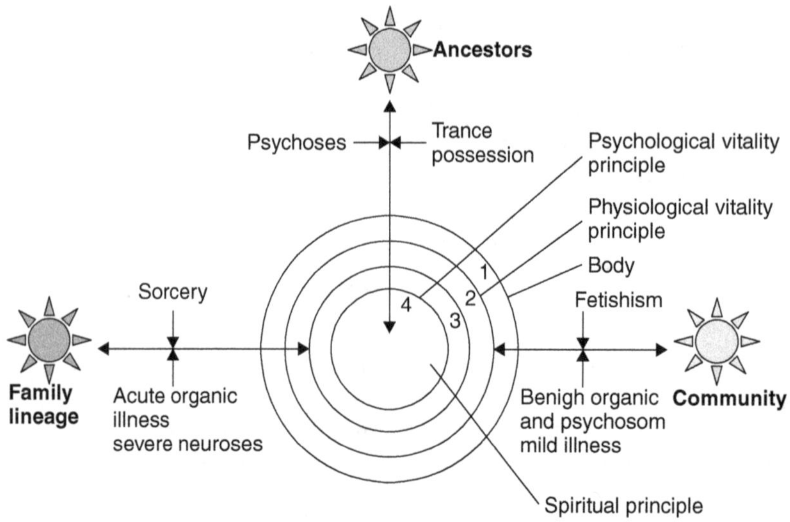

Figure 5.1. The African personality. (From Berry et al. [2002]. *Cross-cultural psychology: Research and applications*, 2nd ed., Figure 4.1. Reprinted with permission of Cambridge University Press.)

For a normal functioning African, the different principles should be in equilibrium. According to Sow, the traditional African interpretation of illness and mental disorders, and their treatments, can be understood in terms of this personality theory. A disorder occurs when the equilibrium is disturbed on one or the other of the axes; diagnosis consists of discovering which axis has been disturbed, and therapy will attempt to reestablish the equilibrium. A disturbance in the first axis – the spiritual principle – would result in serious chronic psychotic illness. Such a disturbance is interpreted as spirits transmitting messages from the ancestors. Disequilibrium in the second axis – the psychological vitality principle – would lead to organic illness, acute anxiety states, severe neuroses, and wasting away. A disturbance in the equilibrium with the community – the third axis or the physiological vitality principle – would result in benign organic and psychosomatic illnesses as well as neurotic states. As a general rule, healing requires the resolution of conflict (with the community, family, or ancestors) and the consequent restitution of equilibrium

Questions

1. Is there an African personality? Support your answer with reasons.
2. Using Sow's theoretical model, discuss functioning in an African cultural context you are familiar.
3. Discuss the perceived influences of ancestors, family and community on health and wellbeing.
4. What principles based on the model by Sow would be relevant to counseling a tradition-led person of African cultural heritage?

versus particularism. Holdstock (2000) argues that particularism needs to be counterbalanced, by studies that emphasize cross-cultural similarities, to avoid the danger that such research may lead to stereotypical and ethnocentric conclusions and analyses. He explains that analyses should examine sociocultural uniqueness, which is necessary to understand individual identity, sociopolitical goals, and social cohesion. In addition to this, and in keeping with the universalist perspective, the search for general laws underlying the behavior of people needs to be pursued. In other words, we need to explore what is common to different sociocultural groups. The argument is that these two levels of inquiry, the particular and general, are important if researchers are to contribute to more informed international discourse.

Emic versus Etic Research Strategies

As explained, a key feature of counseling practice and research from an indigenous psychology perspective is that it becomes a way of generating locally relevant knowledge and practice by privileging the input of local people, by doing research *with* rather than *on* people. Kim and Berry (1993) explain that the development of indigenous psychologies results from emic strategies of research. The concept of emic was used by Pike (1967) to signify an approach from within a cultural system – one that provides insight into indigenous phenomena, and in which meaning derives from understanding phenomena in their own terms. The aim is to learn from (rather than to study) members of a cultural group and to understand their world view as they define it. According to Lett (1996), emic constructs are accounts, descriptions, and analyses expressed in terms of the conceptual schemes and categories that are regarded as meaningful and appropriate by the members of the culture under study.

The etic approach is the outsider's interpretation of the experiences of that culture (Laws & McLeod, 2004; McInerney, 1992). Etic constructs are accounts, descriptions, and analyses expressed in terms of the conceptual schemes and categories that are regarded as meaningful and appropriate by the community of scientific observers. Etic refers to the search for universal laws of behavior. Morris, Kwok Leung, Ames, and Lickel (1991) suggest that each approach has its advantages and disadvantages. The distinction between emic and etic, or indigenous and imported, should not be viewed as being at odds, but rather, as complementary and as an integrative framework representing different levels of indigenization.

EXPLORING CONTEXTUALLY APPROPRIATE PRACTICES

The literature on indigenous psychologies over the years has offered the possibilities of various research methods and approaches (see, e.g., Enriquez, 1997; Gabrenya et al., 2006; Holdstock, 2000; see also Chapters 2 and 3, this volume). A challenge for the researcher is the development of indigenous instruments and research methods. There are various data collection methods and techniques, for example, storytelling, community dialogue, narrative research, and participative methods that may be useful in gaining insight into the various nuances of interactions. The advantage is that these methods value the story and storytelling, which are important communicative tools in African contexts with oral traditions. Allwood and Berry (2006), on the basis of their study, point to the importance of investigating psychological phenomena by means of the local language and of using samples of genuine local cultural material, including video recordings or vignettes in questionnaires. In studies of very young children and children in vulnerable circumstances, for example, children in poverty and children affected by HIV/AIDS and other social and health risks, researchers have shown the value of in-depth individual interviews, participant observation, focus group interviews, and case studies in understanding the children's subjective experiences (Ebrahim, 2007; Muthukrishna, 2006; Muthukrishna & Ebrahim, 2006; Muthukrishna & Ramsuran, 2007; Van der Riet, Hough, & Killian, 2005). Qualitative research methods such as interviewing, focus groups, and participant observation are relevant to the oral traditions and personal interactions in the African context. Interviews and focus groups involve person-to-person interaction and enable the collection of data directly from the source, from people as they live the issue being studied. Furthermore, qualitative research methods have an added advantage, in that participants feel more valued, because they are in control of meaning making in the research process.

A participatory research approach to data collection enables the production of knowledge in an active partnership with the participants who are affected by that knowledge (Babbie, 2002; Francis, Muthukrishna, & Ramsuran, 2006). Participatory approaches, according to Babbie, produce grounded knowledge through collaborative relationships between participants and researchers and by locating the research in a community. Participation does not simply imply the mechanical application of a "technique" or method, but instead, a part of a process of dialogue, action, analysis, and change. The successful use of participatory techniques lies in the process, rather than simply the techniques used. Thus, the genuine use of participatory techniques requires a commitment to ongoing processes of information sharing, dialogue, reflection, and action (Theis & Grady, 1991).

HISTORICAL INFLUENCES AND CONTEXTS OF COUNSELING IN AFRICA

The preceding discussion on the hegemony of dominant paradigms and theories in psychology suggests the need for a contextualist perspective in counseling psychology, which gives recognition to the interaction between individual and context (Gifford & Hayes, 1999; Morris, 1993). All phenomena are viewed as acts-in-context. Contextualist theories stress the construction of behavior and development within a fluid and changing interplay of social and political factors in specific cultural contexts. For this reason, contextualism refers to both the current and historical context of an act, and the historical situatedness of the meaning and function of behavior. In addition, Nsamenang (2006) argues that recognition must be

Research Box 5.1: Alternative Participatory Approaches

Jacobs, S. & Harley, A. (2008). Finding voice: The photovoice method of data collection in HIV and AIDS-related research. *Journal of Psychology in Africa*, 18(3), 431–438.

In a study[1] conducted in an African context, photovoice as a research technique (Wang, 1999) was used to explore the lives of children and families living in the context of HIV and AIDS. Participants in the study who were involved in photovoice were members of a community support group consisting of People Living with AIDS. Participants took photographs to depict their work in the community. Photographs were presented and discussed in a workshop arranged by the researcher.

Below is the text from interactions between a participant and the researcher during the workshop.

R: What did you say is not right about this place?

P: What I can say? This is where more men will be infected with the virus. This is the popular bottle store where people sit and drink alcohol.

R: Why did you feel it was important to take this photograph?

P: I took this photo because it is important to talk about this place because this is not a right place you want to be at. More people need to know about what happens here and to avoid the place, especially the stupid men who get drunk and don't know that their lives will be over soon. You see, the men come and drink, but what is wrong about this place is that we, the females, wait for them outside. If they are drunk, we can sell our body to them easily to make money.

R: Does this happen on a daily basis?

P: Yes, it happens every day after hours. So if there is someone that comes with a partner, they will come and sit inside to drink, but those who don't have partners, the girls just wait outside until those men inside are drunk and then we wait for them.

R: Do lots of girls come to this place?

P: Yes, there are people that I know. Some of the girls I know are positive; but they still go there. No one even thinks about using a condom. So, HIV/AIDS is happening in Linhill and when the drunk men step outside this bar, the virus is waiting to catch them. I don't want this type of life for my sister.

(*Text from audio tape of the photovoice workshop*)

Questions

Engage with the questions below in relation to the research project described above.

1. Would you consider photovoice to be a contextually relevant research method? Explain.
2. Would you describe it as a participatory research tool? Give reasons.
3. Do you think the technique of photovoice has elements of an indigenous research paradigm and methodology? Explain why.
4. To what extent does this research technique help one understand the complexities of life in this particular community? Explain.
5. Discuss ethical issues that might emanate from the use of photovoice in African contexts.

[1] These data are based on work supported by the National Research Foundation (NRF) under grant no. 2054168. Any opinion, findings, and conclusions or recommendations expressed in this article are those of the authors, and, therefore, NRF does not accept any liability in regard thereto.

given to the changing national and global circumstances in which individual development takes place.

The Relational and Contextual Basis of Counseling

These debates have serious implication for training issues in African contexts. Counseling psychology must be seen as relational and contextual. The focus has to be on the promotion of well-being, prevention, transformation of social mechanisms and structures, and the emancipation of people. In many African countries, wracked by civil war and political strife, psychologists need to assist in creating communities and cultures of peace, social justice, and advocacy. Larty (2001) stresses that counseling psychology should reflect social engagement, that is it should be a strength-based and emancipatory practice. Thus, we need to be locating psychological theory, training, research, and practice within the social, historical, and cultural realities of communities. The question to engage with is: What is the context of counseling in African contexts? The discussion that follows points to key contextual issues that have an impact on the work of African psychologists.

The HIV Challenge

The HIV/AIDS pandemic has generated new needs in communities as it affects adults and children in various ways (e.g., Kaaya & Fawzi, 1999; Simbayi, Kalichman, Strebel, Cloete, Henda, & Mqeketo, 2007; Watson & Fouche, 2007). Many children have become orphans and live in extremely vulnerable situations. Girls are often the caregivers for dying parents and siblings. Watson and Fouche (2007) draw attention to the various cultural issues that may have an impact on counseling, in relation to HIV/AIDS, such as the economic and emotional aspects of sexual relationships, the strong cultural links between women's status in society and childbearing, fear of rejection and stigmatization surrounding disclosure of HIV status, and fatalistic acceptance of misfortune (Watson & Fouche, 2007). Awareness and understanding of the psychological well-being of families are critical for counselors. For example, with the HIV/AIDS pandemic, the cycle of grief and loss and the feelings of powerlessness and hopelessness are ever present in families in many African countries. The significance placed on attending funerals of family and community members is evident in various social institutions such as schools and universities. There is a tremendous impact on aspects of people's lives including children's school attendance, finances, and emotional upheaval.

Watson and Fouche (2007) call for a new framework for counseling services for individuals and families affected by the pandemic to ensure well-being in the face of the pandemic. Larty (2001) suggests that there is a need for a kind of pluralism with complex interactions between lay, traditional (such as spiritist beliefs, traditional healing arts, and various forms of religious rituals), and mainstream counseling approaches. Watson and Fouche argue for the need for client-centered counseling in the African setting. The provision of factual information needs to be balanced with a person-centered approach, exploring the client's conception of the problem and helping the client identify persons in their network who can give further psychosocial support. Chaava (1990) described a counseling approach with a strong educational component where complex issues were simplified to content that could be understood. This is an important factor in encouraging persons with HIV and their communities to take a proactive approach in decreasing the spread of HIV/AIDS. Watson and Fouche stress that counseling models need to shift beyond the individual to the family and wider community to ensure development of sustainable support for persons and families affected by HIV. The authors explain that the inclusion of families in the counseling process will be valuable as it draws on and strengthens traditional systems and patterns of support and care. It also has the potential to change attitudes and practices regarding sexual behavior and dealing with issues of stigma. However, in involving families, psychologists will need to engage with the ethical issues of confidentiality and the fear of stigma among persons with HIV. Watson and Fouche point out that the knowledge and skills required in counseling families are quite different and will present different psychological challenges for the psychologist than those that occur at a more individual level.

The Effects of Modernization

Stead and Watson (2006) have explained a further contextual issue in the African context, which is the fact that the priorities and concerns of African people have changed in the face of modernization. We agree with Stead and Watson's analysis that in many African contexts, adults have become more focused on earning money and are thereby less occupied with many of the traditional practices that formerly influenced the upbringing of young people. The impact of media access has resulted in aspirations among young people that cannot be satisfied in their own environment. Various new choices have to be made, and young people must acquire the skills to assess situations and make informed decisions. There is no longer a natural, predictable order from birth to adulthood for the African child. However, it must be borne in mind that although social and cultural changes are taking place in Africa as a result of globalization, there are some practices that continue, such as initiation of young people. Initiation of adolescents is a milestone in their development that marks the transition to adulthood. We believe that gradually African counselors are accepting that these practices cannot be ignored or completely abandoned, as they are part of the changing world views of people. Already, in some contexts, progress is being made to formalize some of the practices and organize them as part of the children's official education. These trends suggest that psychologists have to learn about and understand diverse contexts and the changing frames of reference and world views of people.

Racism

The experience of racism in African contexts and for African people in many countries internationally is an issue important to counseling psychology theory, training, and practice. However, the subject of race and racism is often silenced, denied, and minimized in political discourses in Africa and the West. Duncan, Stevens, and Bowman (2004) explain that racism is an ideology that legitimizes the power of one racial group and justifies it viewing all other groups as inherently inferior. It is an active and powerful social category that frames and shapes identities and social hierarchies. They explain that it involves systematically unequal relations of power in all the major spheres of society, as it is linked to processes of social, political, and economic domination and marginalization. Racist ideology exists at individual, institutional or systemic, and societal level. It produces and reproduces systematic inequalities between racialized groups. Racism

Discussion Box 5.2: The Question of Race in Counseling

Some form of racism should be assumed to be present in any form of client–counselor relationship where racial difference exists (Lago & Thompson, 2002), such as in the case between a Black African and a white Euro-American. Two client–counselor contexts where racism may be an issue of concern are *White client and Black counselor* and *White counselor* and *Black client*. Some central elements in these racial contexts may include, but are not limited to: superiority and inferiority complex on the part of the White and Black, respectively; the Black counselor most likely to have studied in a White middle-class institution, trained in Euro-American theories, with middle-class Euro-American white lecturers; or the Black may have experienced some racisms and racial slurs in the course of his or her life.

Questions

1. Describe and discuss in concrete terms how racism may play out in these contexts, bearing in mind the issues highlighted.
2. How will you as a counselor deal with racism during a counseling session, and ensure that it will not hamper your work?
3. It has been argued that it is important for counselors, both Black and White, to confront their own internal and external racism. Suggest pedagogical approaches, for example, experiential learning methods, that could enhance training programs for counselors.

is pervasive and complex embedded in the institutions and conventions of everyday lives. The World Conference on Racism, Racial Discrimination, Xenophobia and Related Intolerance (2001), in its final report noted "with concern the continued and violent occurrence of racism, racial discrimination, xenophobia and related intolerance, and that theories of superiority of certain races and cultures over others, promoted and practiced during the colonial era, continue to be propounded in one form or another even today" (Office of the Commissioner on Human Rights, 2001, p. 5).

Racism in Africa is a serious social issue impacting human lives, national prosperity, and social cohesion. Severe economic inequalities and the marginalization of persons from access to basic economic and social conditions result in tensions among groups. Racism has resulted in the emergence of xenophobia (an attitudinal orientation of hostility against non-natives in a given population) and armed conflicts, with appalling human rights violations committed by various racial and ethnic groups. Within any one country, there are diverse groups protecting tribal traditions, cultures, religions, social classes and resources, and political power. In the United States, it is well documented that racism, as an ideology, has played a critical role in the past and current psychological oppression of African Americans (Lumumba, 2005; Plous & Williams, 1995).

Poverty and Underdevelopment

In African contexts, psychologists cannot ignore compelling social realities such as poverty, underdevelopment, and various social injustices and oppression, including gender violence (see also Chapters 12, 13, 15, and 18, this volume). Traditionally, scientific discourse has medicalized and psychologized individuals, families, and communities wracked by social problems such as teenage pregnancy; poverty and under development; violence, death, loss, and grief; poor school attendance; low academic performance; high dropout rates for girls; gender violence in school, home, and community; and crime. Counseling psychology needs to be located within an inclusionary, social justice and health promotion orientation.

Career Counseling

An important area in counseling is career counseling (see also Chapter 18, this volume). In the same vein, career counseling has to be framed in the context of social and historical factors that present career challenges to individuals (Maree et al., 2006). The lack of employment opportunities for young people in developing countries, including African countries, demands that career counseling takes on new emphases such as community capacity building and wealth generation. In the current socioeconomic climate, in most African countries, young people need to develop multiple skills, for example, decision making, dealing with change, entrepreneurship, reassessing their natural resources, income generation, and creating and maintaining markets, as suggested by Maree et al. (2006). In other words, counseling psychology would need to develop skills that will promote job creation and not merely the process of employment seeking.

INDIGENOUS COUNSELING: APPROACHES AND PRACTICES

For a vibrant counseling program in Africa, there is a critical need to move away from individualistic and decontexualized models of understanding human behavior and to engage at different interfaces and sites. Research and counseling strategies need to foreground the lived experiences of individuals, families, and their communities. Lumumba (2005) argued that practicing counseling from a Euro-centered approach has serious limitations for most African American clients. She stressed that counselors have an important role in helping African Americans "break the psychological shackles of racism" (p. 126). An important process is that counselors would have to rethink and reevaluate their views about Africa, Africans, and African Americans, and educate themselves on African history, customs and culture. They would also have to confront racism and examine their own internalized racism.

Counselors have to acknowledge and understand the embeddedness of their practice in sociopolitical realities at individual, interpersonal, and institutional levels. This process suggests a vision of a counseling psychology practice that is located in social advocacy.

Examining Indigenous Approaches

So far, our discussion alludes to the fact that counseling theories and methods have been, to a large extent, a Western enterprise, and these cannot be applied indiscriminately to Africans or people of African ancestry. This implies either the development of methods and approaches that are relevant and applicable to Africans, or the modification of existing Western approaches. While the first approach entails indigenous African counseling practices, the latter approach entails adapting existing methods to suit the African situation. Much already has been written about the indigenous African approaches (see Chapters 1 and 4, this volume), and these are not reiterated here. However, we note that African contexts use time-tested alternative and complementary health care systems.

Alternative and complementary approaches

From a medical, anthropological view point, African indigenous counseling approaches fall under the folk sector of the health care systems (Kleinman, 1980; see also Chapter 2, this volume). This sector includes individuals specialized in forms of counseling, healing practices that are either sacred or secular, or a mixture of the two. They include such people as spiritual or indigenous healers, traditional doctors, clairvoyants, and herbalists (see also Chapter 1, this volume). In the African context, this group of counselors has collectively and commonly been referred to by the derogatory term *witch doctors*, although some researchers argue that most of these practitioners belong to the same group of people referred to as *shaman*. These are counselors, medicine men/women, and healers who use traditional practices to communicate with the spirit world. In southern Africa, these are referred to as *sangomas*. Precisely who shaman, sangoma, or traditional doctors are and how they conduct their practice varies from community to community. In the Zulu community of South Africa, for instance, these individuals include sacred divination carried out by female *isangomas*, or male herbalists – *inyangas* – and fetish priests – such as *Komfo* – among the Akans in Ghana (Helman, 2000).

The activities of these people actually cover a wide range of practices. If the healing practice is closely linked to religion, it may be called "religious healing practice" or a "healing ceremony." If this involves the mediation of spirit, it may be called *shamanism* or *divination* or *fortune-telling*. Under each of these, different forms of practices have been identified (see Winkelman, 1992 for a discussion).

Spirit mediumship refers, in the broadest sense a situation, to a healer, a client, or both, experiencing an altered state of consciousness, in the form of dissociation or possession at the time of the healing ritual. Depending on who is dissociated or possessed, three patterns can be recognized (Tseng, 2002). In true shamanism, it is the healer who is dissociated or possessed. Here, the specialist (shaman) as a medium is considered to be possessed by a spirit and to serve as a means of communication. The proven authority of the shaman with the supernatural power is the basis for the therapeutic process. The *zar* healing ceremony involves both the client and the healer entering into altered states of consciousness. Prince (1980) has indicated that *zar* is common in Muslim societies, including Muslims in Africa. In some cases, instead of the shaman dissociating, it is the client who enters into a trance. This trance is achieved with the help of the "shaman," or more correctly the healer. The patient, in a trance-like state, gains insights into his or her sickness from the spirit world.

Divination is the act of trying to foretell future events by occult or magical and religious means. A shaman may be able to carry out divination through insights gained from his or her communication with spirits. Divination may take forms that do not include the help of spirits, such as the positioning of seeds or nuts, which the diviner throws on the ground. It also could involve, for instance, the shaking of the diviner's hands, and through this, it is suggested that the diviner receives information by supernatural means about events that are yet to happen, and how these can be offset. In a number of instances, this divination can be achieved by appeasing a wanton spirit (Winkelman, 2002).

The philosophy of shamanism is based on a belief in (ancestral) spirits. As was pointed out, belief and reverence of ancestors is central to the African personality. Both men and women may be called by spirits to take up the shamanic role. This role may involve an initiation through an illness or another form of mishap of close death experience. It is suggested that during the illness or near-death experience, the prospective shaman is informed by the spirits of his or her new role. During this encounter, the individual may acquire the necessary skills. In some other societies, shaman powers are thought to be inherited, while in some other places, they are thought to be "called" and have to go through lengthy training (Levers & Maki, 1995).

Research Box 5.2: Contextually Sensitive Approaches

Maree, J. G., & Beck, G. (2004). Using various approaches in career counselling for traditionally disadvantaged (and other) learners: Some limitations of a new frontier. *South African Journal of Education*, *24*(1), 80–7.

Objective: This study compared the traditional and postmodern career-counseling approaches toward traditionally disadvantaged learners in South Africa, focusing specifically on the practical implementation of both approaches. It also explored whether narrative career counseling could be successful for learners from traditionally disadvantaged cultural backgrounds in South Africa.

Method: A qualitative case study approach was used because it has a strong contextual function, and is able to provide a rich description of the unique facets of the two approaches to career counseling. The unit of analysis or subject of this case study was a seventeen-year-old, Zulu-speaking girl whose parents had no access to the unaffordable career counseling services available.

Results: A postmodern approach to career counseling addresses a number of flaws in the traditional approach, especially with respect to disadvantaged learners. Career counseling, in a postmodern South Africa, needs to shift from an objective approach to a more interpretative process. New and creative ways of assessment need to be developed. Counselors need to be facilitators rather than experts in career counseling and career choices who do all the thinking and decision making. They should allow their clients to speak, act, think, and choose for themselves, that is, clients must be led to accept responsibility for their own choices and development.

Conclusion: Career counseling in a South African context needs to move away from the almost sole use of psychometric tests to an approach that recognizes the individual's social and historical background.

Questions

1. What do you think would be some shortcomings of traditional career counseling for a South African and African context?
2. What are the characteristics of a postmodern approach to career counseling?
3. Describe some creative assessment approaches that could be used to address the flaws in traditional approaches to career counseling.
4. What do you see as some limitations of a postmodern approach to career counseling for an African context?

Participatory Methods

Regarding specific participatory approaches, Seidel and Coleman (1999) have made effective use of narratives and story lines in "envoicing" HIV-positive men and women in rural KwaZulu-Natal, a province in South Africa. Huber and Gould (2003) have used children's drawings, including maps and time lines, to investigate school nonattendance of orphans in Tanzania. Other research involving participatory techniques illustrates different ways in which to establish effective communication with children by allowing children and young people to shape the agenda, by focusing upon real life and concrete events, and by involving children in "handling things" rather than "just talking" (Steiner, 1993; Thomas & O'Kane, 1998). In recent studies, methods that have proved valuable included photovoice, drawings, mapping, flow diagrams, play, matrices, transect, drama, stories, and songs (Ebrahim, 2007; Harley, 2006; Jacobs & Harley, 2008; Van der Riet et al., 2005).

ISSUES FOR RESEARCH AND OTHER FORMS OF SCHOLARSHIP

The relevance and appropriateness of theoretical frameworks, and how these inform research within the counseling psychology profession, have been consistently criticized in the literature. The preceding discussion stresses that counseling psychology practice needs to address the indifference of mainstream psychology to extrinsic factors such as culture, society, meaning, and context. Researchers and professionals need to realize that differential forms of consciousness occur as a function of the historical and sociocultural locations of individuals (Gabrenya, Kung, & Chen, 2006; Nsamenang, 2005, 2006; Serpell & Jere-Folotiya, 2008).

Reflexive Practice and Methodology

A number of researchers have called for a generative reflexive practice and research methodology based on contextualism (e.g., Bishop 2007; Bishop, Sonn, Drew, & Contos, 2002; Bishop, Sonn, Fisher, & Drew, 2001). This kind of practice and methodology is considered relational where multiple contexts such as history, culture, and social class are acknowledged as sources that give meaning to social and psychological experiences and influence social realities. These researchers argue that such practices can recognize the multiple ways in which meanings are negotiated and constructed in relations. They argue that emphasis needs to be placed on interrogating power, and being vigilant to how power is expressed and reproduced in ideologies and discourse. Professionals need to reflect on their own role in colonizing practices, and avoid assumptions about the origin of a social problem, for example, the phenomena of teenage pregnancy viewed in terms of personal deficits. Bishop argues that persons, behaviors, processes, and environments need to be viewed as aspects of a whole, not as independent components. This would require an interdisciplinary approach exploring how related disciplines such as gender studies, social justice education, and peace education may influence counseling approaches.

We would agree that caution needs to be taken with respect to emphasizing cultural dichotomies. However, the exclusion of a focus on cultural realities poses a serious problem for research and practice in African contexts. Nsamenang (2008) makes the point that consciousness develops through interacting with multiple cultural realities. Therefore, to intervene appropriately is to ground theory, research, and practice in the local culture and context. Maree et al. (2006) draws attention to a problem in South African psychology that has resulted in ignorance, on the part of therapists, of the rich diversity of African indigenous methods of healing.

Indigenizing Psychology

There is little doubt that an in-depth understanding of context is a prerequisite for socially relevant research and intervention related to social and psychological issues in African contexts. Nsamenang (2008, p. 77) warns that a failure to do this can "misdirect research and programmatic efforts" and further entrench misconceptions about African contexts.

The recent development of indigenous psychologies in their many forms presents both a challenge to, and the possibility for renewal of counseling psychology in Africa. Sinha (1997) identified four "threads" of indigenous psychology. He suggests that psychological knowledge should (1) arise from within the culture, (2) reflect local behaviors, (3) be interpreted within a local frame of reference, and (4) yield results that are locally relevant. This means that the approaches, methods, tests, concepts, and theories have to change to make the discipline more relevant to context.

On the other hand, Sinha (1997), Holdstock (2000), and Church and Katigbak, (2002), in their analyses, point to four aspects of the indigenization of psychology: first, *theoretical and conceptual indigenization* – development of indigenous concepts and theoretical frameworks; second, *methodological indigenization* – development of instruments and methods that are socioculturally sensitive; third, *topical indigenization* – the extent to which the topics under study are relevant to the concerns of the society and people; and fourth, *institutional indigenization* – the extent to which institutional and organizational structures and processes support the creation and dissemination of indigenous psychological knowledge.

These definitions stress that the goal of indigenous psychology is to generate a local psychology within a specific cultural context of shared meanings and values. Sonn (2004) explains that indigenous psychology is about locating psychological research and practice within the social, political, historical, and cultural realities of communities.

There have been minimal attempts to develop indigenous counseling theories or frameworks in Africa. Holdstock (2000) argues that when theoretical frameworks have been referred to, they often have been Western frameworks and have drawn on imported theories. He explains that an indigenous theory can be considered a theory if the assumptions, constructs, operational definitions, and predicted phenomena of the theory are rooted in a particular setting – historical, political, ecological, and cultural, or if they have a culturally relevant conceptual and empirical basis. By this definition, Holdstock (2000) argues one can conclude that theoretical development has proceeded only to the point of specifying constructs, for example, the concept *Ubuntu* in the South African context. This kind of theorizing has been conceptual rather than linked to empirical data. Many researchers have argued that theory building in indigenous psychology, as opposed to Western psychology, involves building theories from a bottom-up approach on the basis of local phenomena, findings, and experiences. In contrast, Western psychology has aimed to discover decontextualized, mechanical, universal principles. Indigenous psychology questions the universality of existing psychological theories and attempts to discover psychological universals in social, political, cultural, and ecological contexts.

Combining Indigenous Practices with Western Approaches

The larger majority of Africans live in rural areas, and it is within these settings that indigenous counseling methods prevail. In urban areas, it is normal that ailing individuals first consult with a professional, who invariably has been trained within the Western approach. Often times, the expected help may not be achieved, because the client's belief system is rooted in a traditional African world view, and the approaches used by the counselor may be based on different tradition. There may therefore be the need to "indigenize" the Western approaches in order to accommodate African belief and traditional systems. Moreover, globalization is placing more and more pressure on Africa to "modernize" its health care system, that is, to become more biomedical in orientation. Unfortunately, the larger part of sub-Saharan Africa still lacks trained professionals to take up this challenge. For instance, in 2000, there were only 18 psychiatrists in Ghana for its population of 18 million (Roberts, 2001). Meanwhile, there were about 45,000 traditional healers. The ubiquity of traditional healers in the country underscores the need for the Western professionals to infuse some of their methods with traditional beliefs and practices. This issue is well illustrated in the example

Discussion Box 5.3: Indigenizing Western Marriage Therapy for Sub-Saharan Africa[2]

Objective: To adapt Western marriage therapy for contemporary West and East Africa by drawing upon indigenous beliefs on marriage.

Theoretical Framework: Important for marriage therapy, in these regions of Africa, is the role of theory: obligations and privileges are taken to be linked to the occupancy of social positions. Marriage conflicts arise when the individuals occupying the different roles fail to perform their expected roles.

The traditional African marriage therapy is one of mediation, where the mediators are two or more elders, acting as jury, while the conflicting couple comprises the litigants. Settling marriage disputes involves the drama of claim (by one spouse), counter claim (by the other spouse), and the pronouncement of judgment (by the elders), involving what has to be done by the spouse more at fault. In the contemporary marriage therapy, the counselor takes the role of the elder, and serves both as the mediator and mentor (advocate) for the couple in conflict.

Therapeutic Sessions: In the Western approach, sessions normally take place in the therapist's office, and in the traditional African approach, sessions would normally take place in the wife's father's home. In contemporary African settings, this can be the home of the therapist. Whereas sessions in the Western approach are normally an hour long with weekly meetings, which may go on for months, in traditional African approaches, the entire therapy may take place in the course of a day, including the pronouncement of "judgment." In contemporary Africa, this process also may take several days, but sessions can be every other day, and the duration of a session is not limited to an hour, but rather as long as it takes a litigant to lay forward his or her case, which could take several hours. Unlike the Western approach, where joint couple sessions may take place, the traditional African approach may begin with individual sessions, in order to avoid interruptions when one of the couple is putting forward his or her side of the conflict. In the contemporary African approach, the couple initially may be met jointly, and on alternate days individually shifting between the husband and the wife. This ideally begins with the husband, as the traditional head of the family. The therapist infuses the sessions with indigenous beliefs and traditions through the use of metaphors and proverbs that are based on the culture. Many cultural beliefs and traditions are enshrined in proverbs and metaphors, partly as a result of the long oral tradition that characterizes these regions of the world.

Reconciliation and Reenactment: The therapeutic sessions end jointly, when a pronouncement is made of who has been more at fault, and how the wronging partner has to appease the wronged spouse. During the sessions, the idea is to help the couple to discover meaning in their marriage and a new appreciation of one another. The entire process is aimed at offering the couple alterations of their perceptions and change in expectations, attitudes, and misunderstandings about marriage.

Once a verdict is passed, the partner more at fault is expected to make up for "damages" to the offended spouse for appeasement purposes. Within the African context, "I'm sorry" is not seen as enough. A material (rather than a monetary) compensation of an appeasement gift is the norm. In the traditional African setting, as part of the reconciliation, the couple may be expected to take a traditional drink such as the "palm wine" together. The drinking most often takes place after a libation has been offered to the ancestors. In contemporary Africa, another form of drink may be offered, and rather than libation, a prayer may be offered.

[2] Source: Nwoye, A. (2000). Building on the indigenous: Theory and method of marriage therapy in contemporary Eastern and West Africa. *Journal of Family Therapy, 22*, 347–59.

of a sixteen-year-old girl with schizophrenia, as identified by Roberts (2001). This girl's village believed that she was sick because her mother did not adhere to the traditions of the village. In addition to medication, the attending psychiatrist asked the girl to go to the shrine, where the chief priestess offered few chickens on her behalf to pacify the gods. With this, the mother, the daughter, and the entire village believed that the girl was healed, and they then related to her as a normal girl.

It is difficult to prescribe a specific method or methods when it comes to indigenizing Western approaches, except to provide an illustrative example (see Discussion Boxes 5.3 and 5.4 for such an illustrative example on marriage therapy and counseling clients with mental health problems). Relevant knowledge of the cultural traditions and beliefs of the client is a major prerequisite in providing "indigenized counseling."

Research Focus

Research emanating from the field of psychology, including counseling psychology, in the African context has been criticized because it is rooted in a different ontology, epistemology, and cultural framework. Adair (1999) points out that many psychologists who are trained in Western models of psychology locate the focus of their research in problems highlighted in Western literature and fail to research issues that arise from their own contexts. There

Discussion Box 5.4: Case Studies

Read the two cases below and answer the questions that follow

Somewhere in Western Europe, a man, who until recently has been normal, suddenly began to behave in a bizarre way. His relatives suspected that he was sick, so they took him to psychiatrist at the nearby hospital. Upon careful examination, the psychiatrist declared that the man was indeed sick. Soon afterwards, the man received lots of sympathy and was exempted from his usual social duties and work. Even though his behavior was seen as bizarre, he was not sanctioned because he was not seen as directly responsible for his strange behavior, but the sickness. After further careful examination, including detailed medical history, psychological test results, and interviews, the psychiatrist came up with the diagnosis, and outlined the method for his treatment. Methods included different forms of therapy and the use of some medications from the nearby pharmacy shop. While the man had to take the drug medication himself, the psychiatrist undertook the psychotherapy. The man also had to make some changes in some of his daily routines (e.g., being admitted in the hospital for some few days for closer observation). Once the psychiatrist correctly diagnosed the sickness and the prescribed therapy and drugs were carefully administered for a couple of months, the sickness was eventually eliminated and the man got well again.

Somewhere in West Africa, a man who, until recently has been normal, suddenly began to behave in a bizarre way. His relatives suspected that an evil spirit possessed him, so they took him to the shrine of the local witch doctor. Upon careful examination, the witch doctor declared that the man was indeed possessed. Soon afterwards, the man received lots of sympathy and was exempted from his usual social duties and work. Even though his behavior was seen as bizarre, he was not sanctioned because he was not seen as directly responsible for his strange behavior, but the evil spirit. After further careful examination and interviews with close family members and friends, the witch doctor identified the evil spirit. He then gave instructions as to how the evil spirit should be exorcised. This exorcism involved different forms of rites and rituals, such as the drinking of different kinds of herbs from a nearby forest. Some of the rites involving animal sacrifices were performed by the man himself, and others on his behalf by his relatives. The man also had to make some changes in some of his daily routines (e.g., being kept in the shrine for some few days for closer observation). Once the witch doctor correctly identified the evil spirit and the prescribed rites and rituals were conscientiously followed for a couple of months, the evil spirit was eventually exorcised, and the man got well again.

Based on the two cases above, discuss:

a. What are the similarities and differences in the family's response to the bizarre behavior of the man and the manner of treatment?
b. Are we dealing with the same or different phenomena?
c. From your background and perspective, can any one approach taken to deal with the man's bizarre behavior be more justified than the other, and if so, which one?
d. Can you think of reasons why "spirits" play such a dominant role in the West African case? To what extent are "sprits" responsible for one's "bizarre behavior" in your native society?
e. What is the role of culture in the different approaches taken here?
g. How will the man's bizarre behavior be explained and treated in an imaginary society that does not have culture?

The case material has been adapted from:
Sam, D. L. & Moreira, V. (2002). The mutual embeddedness of culture and mental illness. In W. J. Lonner, D. L. Dinnel, S. A. Hayes, & D. N. Sattler (Eds.). Online Readings in Psychology and Culture. Western Washington University, Department of Psychology, Center for Cross-Cultural Research. Website: http://www.wwu.edu/~culture.

have been calls for attention to be given to topical indigenization, that is, research on applied topics that address societal needs and problems. Western research topics often appear disconnected from local cultural and material conditions. In addition, many Western trained psychologists have pointed to the mismatch between the cultural values and ideology that inform Western research, in which they have been trained, and those of their home societies (e.g., Sinha, 1997).

Many scholars have called for non-elite research that reflects realities of more developing contexts (e.g., Enriquez, 1997; Kim & Berry, 1993; Naidoo et al., 1999). Local psychologists are urged to use local cultural sources to study the lives and concerns of people in their local contexts and to use appropriate research methods. Smith (1999) has critiqued the taken-for-granted ways of knowledge production and the colonizing impacts of "Western" ways of knowledge production for African contexts, suggesting the need for different methodologies and approaches that ensure that research with local peoples can be more ethical, relevant, and useful.

The pursuit of the goal of decolonization of research requires the critical evaluation of theories, concepts, methods, and tools to ensure that they are compatible with the social and psychological phenomena being studied and with their embeddedness in their ecological, economic, social, cultural, and historical contexts. Hayes (2002) explains that researchers need to explore frameworks other than positivism upon which to base their methodologies. What is required is that scholars be willing to be innovative and to commit to breaking the barriers to new ways of knowledge production, new forms of theory, and alternative ways of interpreting research findings. One characteristic of emerging indigenous psychologies is a shift toward qualitative research methods for studying different cultural contexts (Gabrenya et al., 2006).

Indigenizing Theory, Research, and Practice

As previously noted, indigenous psychology represents an approach in which the content of a culture (meaning, values, and beliefs) and the context (family, social, cultural, community, and ecological) are integral to research design. There have been calls for a more critical, contextual adoption of theories, along with a questioning of their applicability and limitations (Watson & Fouche, 2007). This would mean that the field of counseling psychology would have to consider how theory and research translates into the reality of its practice. Watson and Fouche suggest that psychologists and researchers must see this as an opportunity for innovation in theory development. Macleod (2004) explains that this would enable psychologists to contribute toward theory development, not only in their own country, but at a more global level as well (Macleod, 2004). De la Rey and Ipser (2004) suggest the need for interdisciplinary studies in counseling psychology, as cross discipline knowledge and theory building provide an opportunity to understand and be more responsive to sociopolitical and contextual factors in African contexts.

One feature of indigenous research is a questioning of the utility and appropriateness of positivist epistemology. Positivism has been a guiding principle of Western social science, particularly of psychology. Positivism, as an epistemological approach, emphasizes universalism, quantitative empiricism, deductive hypothesis testing, value-free science, and determinism (Gabrenya et al., 2006; Sham & Hwang, 2005). The goal of an indigenous psychology is to develop a psychology that is appropriate for the culture and the context. This approach would imply making the research more culturally and contextually sensitive and appropriate, and making the discipline autochthonous (Adair, 1999). By autochthonous, Adair means a psychology that is independent of its Western origins and can make an impact on addressing local problems by engaging in its own local practice, training, research, and discipline development.

SUMMARY AND CONCLUSIONS

In this chapter, we argue that counseling psychology has a critical role to play in dealing with issues of social justice and human rights, for example, in contexts of violence, educational systems that are failing children, social and political oppression, social and institutional barriers, stigma arising from HIV/AIDS, and poverty. In fact, counseling psychologists have to be change agents and advocates for social change.

The pursuit of an indigenous counseling psychology, in the African context, can be enhanced in various ways. One of the dangers of indigenous counseling theories is a shift to insularity and cultural specificity, and an uncritical exclusion of Western psychology theories from debates and analyses. Indigenous counseling insights need to be related to those in other cultures as part of a cross-indigenous approach. This comparison will help to address premature generalizations about cultures and contexts, and provide more authentic understandings of the psychology of a particular group. Researchers and counseling psychology professionals have to commit to the sustained development and validation of indigenous counseling strategies and approaches, and research paradigms, theories, methodologies, and techniques.

From our experience in the field, it is evident that there is limited information on culturally sensitive approaches, with rich African cultural and contextual components, that are available to counselors and other health service providers. There is no doubt that, as practitioners and researchers in the field, we need to take into account the social, political, and cultural characters of peoples in African contexts. Over the years, the view has been that Western models in African contexts have not been effective in engaging with local social problems.

REFERENCES

Adair, J. G. (1999). Indigenization of psychology: The concept and its practical implementation. *Applied Psychology: An International Review*, *48*, 403–18.

Allwood, C. M., & Berry, J. W. (2006). Origins and development of indigenous psychologies: An international analysis. *International Journal of Psychology*, *41*, 243–68.

Babbie, E. (2002). *Social research*. Belmont, CA: Wadsworth Group.

Bishop, B. J. (2007). Methodology, values and quantitative world views in qualitative research in community psychology. *The Australian Community Psychologist*, *19*(1), 9–18.

Bishop, B. J., Sonn, C. S., Drew, N. M., & Contos, N. E. (2002). The evolution of epistemology and concepts in an iterative generative reflective practice. The importance of small differences. *American Journal of Community Psychology*, *30*, 493–510.

Bishop, B. J., Sonn, C. C, Fisher, A. F., & Drew, N. M. (2001). Community based community psychology: Perspectives from Australia. In M. Seedat (Ed.), *Community psychology in Southern Africa*. Cape Town, South Africa: Oxford University Press.

Bulhan, H. A. (1985). *Frantz Fanon and the psychology of oppression*. New York: Plenum Press.

Burr, V. (2002). *The person in social psychology*. Hove, East Sussex: Psychology Press.

Chigunta, F. (2002). The socio-economic situation of youth in Africa: Problems, prospects and options. Retrieved May 20, 2008 from http://www.yesweb.org/gkr/res/bg.africa.reg.doc

Church, A. T., & Katigbak, M. S. (2002). Indigenization of psychology in the Philippines. *International Journal of Psychology, 37*(3), 129–48.

De la Rey, C., & Ipser, J. (2004). The call for relevance: South Africa psychology ten years into democracy. *South African Journal of Psychology, 3*, 544–52.

Durham, D. (2001). Youth and the social imagination in Africa: Introduction to parts 1 and 2. Retrieved May 10, 2008 from http://muse.jhu.edu/demo/anthropological_quarterly/v073/73.3durham.pdf

Durojaiye, M. O. A. (1993). Indigenous psychology in Africa: The search for meaning. In U. Kim & J. W. Berry (Eds.), *Indigenous psychologies: Research and experience in cultural context* (pp. 211–220). Newbury Park, CA: SAGE Publications.

Ebrahim, H. B. (2007). *The social construction of childhood within the cultures of two Early Childhood Centres (ECD) in KwaZulu-Natal: An ethnographic study*. Unpublished doctoral dissertation, University of KwaZulu-Natal, Durban, South Africa.

Enriquez, V. G. (1997). Filipino psychology: Concepts and methods. In H. S. R. Kao & D. Sinha (Eds.), *Asian perspectives on psychology* (pp. 40–53). Thousand Oaks, CA: SAGE Publications.

Francis, D., Muthukrishna, N., & Ramsuran, A. (2006). Deconstructing participatory research in an HIV/AIDS context. *Journal of Education, 38*, 139–63.

Gabrenya, W. K., Kung, M., & Chen, L. (2006). Understanding the Taiwan indigenous psychology movement: A sociology of science approach. *Journal of Cross-Cultural Psychology, 37*, 597–622.

Gifford, E. V., & Hayes, S. C. (1999). Functional contextualism: A pragmatic philosophy for behavioral science. In W. O'Donohue & R. Kitchener (Eds.), *Handbook of behaviorism* (pp. 285–327). San Diego: Academic Press.

Harley, A. (2006). Life is hard: Community perspectives on barriers to basic education. In N. Muthukrishna (Ed.), *Mapping barriers to basic education in the context of HIV and AIDS: A report on research conducted in the Richmond District, KwaZulu-Natal* (pp. 194–230). Pietermaritzburg, South Africa: School of Education and Development, University of KwaZulu-Natal.

Hayes, N. (2002). *Psychology in perspective* (2nd ed.). London: SAGE Publications.

Helman, C. G. (2000). *Culture, health and illness* (4th ed.). London: Arnold.

Holdstock, T. L. (2000). *Re-examining psychology: Critical perspectives and African insights*. London: Routledge.

Huber, U., & Gould, W. (2003). The effect of orphanhood on primary school attendance reconsidered: The power of female-headed households in Tanzania. HIV/AIDS impact on education. Clearinghouse. Retrieved on June 10, 2008 from http://iiep.tomoye.com/ev.php

Jacobs, S. & Harley, A. (2008). Finding voice: The photovoice method of data collection in HIV and AIDS-related research. *Journal of Psychology in Africa, 18*(3), 385–92.

Kaaya, S. F., & Fawzi, M. C. (1999). HIV counseling in sub-Saharan Africa. *AIDS, 13*(12), 1577–9.

Kim, U., & Berry, J. W. (1993). *Indigenous psychologies*. Thousand Oaks, CA: SAGE Publications.

Kleinman, A. (1980). *Patients and healers in the context of culture*. Berkeley, CA: University of California.

Lago, C., & Thompson, J. (2002). Counselling and race. In S. Palmer (Ed.), *Multicultural counseling: A reader* (pp 3–20): London: SAGE Publications.

Larty, E. Y. (July, 2001). *Global views for pastoral care and counseling: Post-modern, post- colonial, post-Christian, post-human, post-pastoral*. Paper presented at the 7th Asia-Pacific Congress on Pastoral Care and Counseling, Perth, Western Australia.

Lassiter, J. E. (1999). African culture and personality: Bad social science, effective social activism, or a call to reinvent ethnology? Retrieved January, 10, 2007 from http://web.africa.ufl.edu/asq/v3/v3i2a1.htm

Laws, K., & McLeod, R. (2004). Case study and grounded theory: Sharing some alternative qualitative research with systems professionals. Retrieved December 10, 2010 from http://www.systemdynamics.org/conferences/2004/SDS_2004/PAPERS/220MCLEO.pdf

Lesko, N. (1996). Past, present, future conceptions of adolescence. *Educational Theory, 46*, 453–71.

Lett, J. (1996). Emic/etic distinctions. Retrieved December, 12, 2007 from http://faculty.ircc.cc.fl.us/faculty/jlett/Article%20on%20Emics%20and%20Etics.htm

Levers, L. L., & Maki, D. R. (1995). African indigenous healing, cosmology, and existential implications: Toward a philosophy of ethnorehabilitation. *Rehabilitation Education, 9*, 127–45.

Lumumba, H. (2005). Breaking the psychological shackles of racism: Implications for empowering African American clients. Retrieved June 10, 2008 from http://counselingoutfitters.com/vistas/vistas05/Vistas05.art26.pdf

Macleod, C. (2004). Position paper: Critical research issues in psychology. Unpublished paper, Department of Psychology, University of Fort Hare, Alice, Eastern Cape, South Africa.

Maree, K., Ebersöhn, L., & Molepo, M. (2006). Administering narrative career counseling in a diverse setting: Trimming the sails to the wind. *South African Journal of Education, 26*(1), 49–60.

McInerney, D. M. (1992, November). Indigenous educational research: Can it be psychometric? Paper presented at the *AARE/NZARE Conference Educational research: Discipline and Diversity*, Geelong, Victoria, Australia.

Mkhize, N. (2008, March). Incorporating indigenous perspectives in counselling psychology – speaking together. Keynote address at the *2008 International Counseling Psychology Conference*, Chicago.

Morris, E. K. (1993). Contextualism, historiography, and the history of behavior analysis. In S. C. Hayes, L. J. Hayes, H. W. Reese, & T. R. Sarbin (Eds.), *Varieties of scientific contextualism* (pp. 137–65). Reno, NV: Context Press.

Morris, M. W., Kwok Leung, K., Ames, D., & Lickel, B. (1991). Views from inside and outside: Integrating emic and etic insights about culture and justice judgment. *The Academy of Management Review, 24*, 781–96.

Muthukrishna, N. (Ed.). (2006). *Mapping barriers to basic education in the context of HIV and AIDS: A report on research conducted in the Richmond District KwaZulu-Natal*. Pietermaritzburg, South Africa: School of Education and Development, University of KwaZulu-Natal.

Muthukrishna, N., & Ebrahim, H. (2006). Experiencing education and care in the early years. In N. Muthukrishna (Ed.), *Mapping barriers to basic education in the context of HIV and AIDS: A report on research conducted in the Richmond District KwaZulu-Natal* (pp. 145–61). Pietermaritzburg, South Africa: School of Education and Development, University of KwaZulu-Natal.

Muthukrishna, N., & Ramsuran, A. (2007). Layers of oppression and exclusion in the context of HIV and AIDS: The case of adult and child learners in the Richmond District, KwaZulu-Natal. *International Journal of Inclusive Education*, *11*, 401–16.

Naidoo, J. C., Olowu, A., Gilbert, A., & Akotia, C. (1999). Challenging Euro American-centered psychology: The voices of African psychologists. In W. J. Lonner & D. L. Dinnel (Eds.), *Merging past, present, and future in cross-cultural psychology: Selected papers from the Fourteenth International Congress of the International Association for Cross-Cultural Psychology* (pp. 124–134). Lisse, the Netherlands: Swets & Zeitlinger.

Nsamenang, A. B. (1995). Factors influencing the development of psychology in Sub- Saharan Africa. *International Journal of Psychology*, *30*, 729–38.

Nsamenang, A. B. (2005). Educational development and knowledge flow: Local and global forces in human development in Africa. *Higher Education Policy*, *18*, 275–88.

Nsamenang, A. B. (2006). Human ontogenesis: An indigenous African view on development and intelligence. *International Journal of Psychology*, *41*, 293–7.

Nsamenang, A. B. (2008). Culture and development. *International Journal of Psychology*, *43*(2), 73–7.

Nyasani, J. M. (1997). *The African psyche*. Nairobi, Kenya: University of Nairobi and Theological Printing Press.

Office of the Commissioner on Human Rights. (2001). Final report: World Conference on Racism, Racial Discrimination, Xenophobia and Related Intolerance. Retrieved May 2, 2009 from http://www.unhchr.ch/pdf/Durban.pdf

Owusu-Bempah, J., & Howitt, D. (2000). *Psychology beyond Western perspectives*. Leicester, England: BPS Books.

Painter, D., & Terre Blanche, M. (2004). Critical psychology in South Africa: Looking back and looking forwards. Retrieved May 20, 2008 from http://www.criticalmethods.org/collab/critpsy.htm

Pike, K. L. (1967). *Language in relation to a unified theory of the structure of human behavior*. The Hague: Mouton.

Plous, S., & Williams, T. (1995). Racial stereotypes from the days of American slavery: A continuing legacy. *Journal of Applied Social Psychology*, *25*(9), 795–817.

Prince, R. (1980). Variations in psychotherapy procedures. In H. C. Triandis & J. G. Draguns (Eds.), *Handbook of cross-cultural psychology* (Vol. 6, pp. 291–349). Boston: Allyn & Bacon.

Roberts, H. (2001). A way forward for mental health in Accra? *Lancet*, *357*, 1859.

Seale, C., Gobo, G., Gubrium, J. F., & Silverman, D. (2004). *Qualitative research practice*. London: SAGE Publications.

Seidel, J., & Coleman, R. (1999). Gender, disclosure, care and decision-making in KwaZulu-Natal, South Africa. In P. Aggleton, G. Hart, & G, Davies (Eds.), *Families and communities responding to AIDS* (pp. 53–66). London: UCL Press.

Serpell, R., & Jere-Folotiya, J. (2008). Developmental assessment, cultural context, gender and schooling in Zambia. *International Journal of Psychology*, *43*, 88–96.

Sham, M., & Hwang, K. K. (2005). Special issue on responses to the epistemological challenges to indigenous psychologies. *Asian Journal of Social Psychology*, *8*(1), 3–4.

Simbayi, L. C., Kalichman, S., Strebel, A., Cloete, A., Henda, N., & Mqeketo, A. (2007). Internalized stigma, discrimination, and depression among men and women living with HIV/AIDS in Cape Town, South Africa. *Social Science & Medicine*. *64*,1823–31.

Sinha, D. (1997). Indigenizing psychology. In J. W. Berry, Y. H. Poortinga, & J. Panday (Eds.), *Handbook of cross-cultural psychology* (pp. 130–69). Boston: Allyn & Bacon.

Smith, L. T. (1999). *Decolonizing methodologies: Research and indigenous peoples*. London: ZED Books.

Sonn, C. C. (2004). Reflecting on practice: Negotiating challenges to ways of working. *Journal of Community & Applied Social Psychology*, *14*, 305–13.

Sow, I. (1977). *Psychiatrie dynamique africaine* [African dynamic psychiatry]. Paris: Payot.

Sow, I. (1978). *Les structures anthropologiques de la folie en Afrique noire*. The anthropological structures of madness in black Africa]. Paris: Payot.

Stead, G. B., & Watson, M. B. (2006). Indigenisation of career psychology in South Africa. In G. B. Stead & M. B. Watson (Eds.), *Career psychology in the South African context* (2nd ed., pp. 181–90). Hatfield, Pretoria, South Africa: Van Schaik.

Steiner, M. (1993). *Learning from experience: World studies in the primary curriculum*. Stoke on Trent, Staffordshire: Trentham Books Limited.

Taylor, J. J. (2007). Assisting or compromising intervention? The concept of 'culture' in biomedical and social research on HIV/AIDS. *Social Science and Medicine*, *64*, 965–75.

Theis, J., & Grady, H. M. (1991). *Participatory rapid appraisal for community development: A training manual based on experiences in the Middle East and North Africa*. London: Save the Children Federation and IIED.

Thomas, N., & O' Kane, C. (1998). The ethics of participatory research with children. *Child and Society*, *12*, 336–48.

Tseng, W. (2002). *Handbook of cultural psychiatry*. San Diego: Academic Press.

Van der Riet M., Hough, A., & Killian, B. (2005). Mapping HIV & AIDS as a barrier to education: A reflection on the methodological and ethical challenges to child participation. *Journal of Education*, *35*, 75–98.

Wang, C. C. (1999). Photovoice: A participatory action research strategy applied to women's health. *Journal of Women's Health*, *8*(2), 185–92.

Watson, M. B., & Fouche, P. (2007). Transforming a past into a future: Counseling psychology in South Africa. *Applied Psychology: An International Review*, *56*(1), 152–64.

Winkelman, M. (1992). Shamans, priests and witches. A cross-cultural study of magico-religious practitioners: Anthropological Research Papers No. 44. Tempe, AZ: Arizona State University Press.

Winkelman, M. (2002). Shamanism as neurotheology and evolutionary psychology. *American Behavioral Scientist*, *45*, 1873–85.

SELF-CHECK EXERCISES

1. What have been some of the criticisms and limitations of traditional psychology, including counseling psychology, as practiced in African contexts?
2. What are the key challenges for the transformation of counseling psychology in Africa?
3. Why are Eurocentric conceptions of the notion of "self" problematic for the African context?
4. What are some of the misconceptions surrounding the notion of "culture" that have been entrenched in African contexts by mainstream psychology?

5. Discuss the debates around conceptions of "youth" in African contexts?

FIELD-BASED EXPERIENTIAL EXERCISES

1. Bearing in mind the contextual realities of Africa, how will you indigenize your favorite counseling method/approach for an African? Identify and discuss the problems you may face in the indigenization process.
2. Undertake a small-scale research project to explore the complexities around the notion of "family" or "youth" in your context.
3. Use ONE participatory research technique to explore a social issue in your context. Critique its effectiveness in conducting socially just research.

MULTIPLE-CHOICE QUESTIONS

1. The hegemony of dominant counseling psychology in African contexts can be seen in thinking such as:
   a. Counseling psychology is individualistic in orientation.
   b. Counseling practitioners do not have to pay attention to the social and mental health concerns in African contexts.
   c. The "self" is viewed as striving for individual autonomy.
   d. The self is viewed as independent of culture and context.
   e. All of the above.
2. From an indigenous psychology perspective, the notion of "culture" means:
   a. Culture is unchanging and static.
   b. There is no heterogeneity in cultural systems.
   c. Culture is historically shaped and a contested notion.
   d. There is a single homogeneous African perspective.
   e. All of the above.
3. Personality studies in counseling psychology can be made more relevant for the African context if:
   a. They do not examine the influence of social structures on the individual.
   b. They exclude completely the exploration of traditional cultural beliefs and behavioral patterns.
   c. They emphasize cultural relativism.
   d. They have, as a starting point, the position that personality is a changing concept that needs to be constantly redefined by Africans.
   e. All of the above.
4. An indigenous psychology perspective would argue that conceptions of "youth" need to be revisited and should include the view that:
   a. It is possible to hold objective conceptions of "youth."
   b. The concept "youth" is not relational.
   c. The concept "youth" is knowable and universal.
   d. The concept "youth" has meaning only if it is embedded in social, political, and economic conditions.
   e. All of the above.
5. The counseling psychology profession in Africa needs to break away from dominant paradigms and see psychological phenomena as:
   a. Processes in context
   b. Socially constructed within a fluid interplay of sociopolitical factors
   c. Historically situated
   d. Impacted by the global and local circumstances in which development takes place
   e. All of the above
6. A generative contextualist counseling perspective can be distinguished in the following way:
   a. Persons, behaviors, and environments are independent.
   b. There is only one way in which meaning making happens.
   c. There is no need to examine how power is expressed and the issue of power relations.
   d. There are multiple ways in which meanings are negotiated and constructed in social relations.
   e. All of the above.
7. Research frameworks within an indigenous African psychology will emphasize:
   a. There is a need to decolonize research in counseling psychology.
   b. The content of a culture and the context are crucial components of a research design.
   c. Interdisciplinary studies are important for theory building.
   d. Two levels of inquiry, the general and the particular, should inform theory building.
   e. All of the above.
8. A transactional approach to counseling psychology theory and research emphasizes that:
   a. There are intricate links between context, temporal factors, and physical and psychological phenomena.
   b. Individuals do not have agency.
   c. Individuals are agents of their own actions and collective agents of their culture.
   e. Psychological phenomena are not impacted by context.
   d. All of the above.
9. In order to indigenize research paradigms, which of the following beliefs, processes, and practices are critical?
   a. Research must be seen as a sociopolitical project with the goal of social justice at the center.
   b. Research must be conducted on people.

c. There must be no community participation in research.
d. Research can uncover one central truth.
e. All of the above.

10. Participatory research methods are useful, because:
   a. The researcher decides on the research question(s).
   b. They can help understand people's world views as defined by the researcher.
   c. They reduce power imbalances between the research and the participants.
   d. Predetermined theoretical issues always determine the research questions.
   e. All of the above.

Answers to the multiple-choice questions are provided at the back of the book

6 Racial Oppression, Colonization, and Identity: Toward an Empowerment Model for People of African Heritage

Alex L. Pieterse, Dennis Howitt, and Anthony V. Naidoo

The most powerful tool in the hands of the oppressor is the mind of the oppressed.

—Steve Biko (1946–1977), speech given in Cape Town, 1971

OVERVIEW. The psychological experiences of people of African heritage have been shaped and influenced by the enduring legacy of European colonization and the Atlantic slave trade. As such, counselors who seek to promote health and healing for Africans and those impacted by the African Diaspora need to understand the psychological antecedents of·oppression as experienced by individuals of African descent. Furthermore, counselors and healers can draw on models of psychological liberation in an attempt to promote a healthy racial identity and to establish models of community empowerment. This chapter reviews the literature addressing the psychological impact of racism and racial oppression and provides a case illustration of the principles of psychological liberation for people of African heritage.

LEARNING OBJECTIVES

By the end of the chapter, the reader should be able to:

1. Identify key historical events associated with psychological oppression.
2. Summarize research findings describing the relationship between racism and psychological functioning.
3. Outline key aspects of "mental colonization" and describe steps toward "decolonization of the mind."
4. Describe elements of a community intervention designed to promote liberation and empowerment.

INTRODUCTION

Within the United States, in June 2006, the total number of Black/African American inmates in state or federal institutions accounted for 40 percent of the entire prison population (U.S. Department of Justice, June 2007), even though they are just 16 percent of the total population. At present, nearly 20 percent of the population of South Africa between the ages of fifteen and forty-nine years are living with HIV/AIDS, representing one of the highest rates of infection in the world (UNAIDS/WHO, 2006). Indeed, it is salutary to note that, irrespective of South Africa's economic resources, the incidence of HIV/AIDS in South Africa rivals that of other African countries lacking comparable economic resources. Possibly, the most cogent common denominator between these two sets of troubling statistics is the history of race relations in both countries, a history in which the ideology of white supremacy laid the foundation for generations of racial subordination and oppression, effects that continue to be maintained and felt into the twenty-first century (Hook, 2004; Smedley, 1999), and that extend far beyond the borders of South Africa and the United States.

Irrespective of attempts to provide a more balanced perspective of African history (Asante, 2007), the prevailing view of Africa continues to be one of war, social upheaval, and political dysfunction (Meredith, 2006). As a result, African nations continue to be confronted with much of the same paternalistic response from the West as they were when Africa was systematically divided up by European colonial powers. In most respects, in this postcolonial world, neo-colonialism persists through such vehicles as international trade, financial institutions, and tourism. Alien Western culture has made invasive inroads into many parts of Africa, while, at the same time, the establishment of international market–controlled economies have led to a growing spiral of poverty (Hooks, 2004). Thus, given the ongoing oppression and marginalization experienced by African nations and people of African descent, the psychological antecedents of this oppression are considered to be an important and urgent area of inquiry.

IMPORTANCE, DEFINITION, AND SCOPE OF KEY TERMS AND CONCEPTS

In recent decades, psychologists have increasingly emphasized the influence of contextual variables on human development and psychological health. Consequently, a growing project in the psychological literature has been to investigate the impact of experiences of racism, racial harassment, and racial trauma on a variety of psychological outcomes such as traumatic stress, psychiatric symptomatology, and psychological well-being (Bryant-Davis & Ocampo, 2005; Carter, 2007; Paradies, 2006; Pieterse & Carter, 2007; Williams & Williams-Morris, 2000). Early indications suggest that experiences of racism can result in psychological distress and adverse effects on psychological well-being (Williams, Neighbors, & Jackson, 2003). Some have viewed the legacy of the trans-Atlantic slave trade as having a critical influence on the current psychological processes of Africans, both on the continent and via the Diaspora. In this regard, contemporary scholars refer to the psychological effects of slavery as akin to a type of intergenerational trauma (Cross, 1998; Leary, 2005). However, we recognize the need to be cautious about what is being said, lest we replicate the oppressive and intentional view that has sought to depict people of African descent as pathogenic. On the contrary, there is plenty of evidence that people of African origin are typically psychologically healthy, and in no way should they be routinely construed as psychologically damaged. To illustrate, Owusu-Bempah and Howitt (1999) document instances in which problems of Black children are construed as problems broadly to do with their race, when there are very obvious nonracial factors involved, but ignored in counseling and therapy. Nevertheless, in the context of a discussion on counseling people of African descent, it is essential to explicate current knowledge of racial oppression and psychological functioning among Africans and individuals of African descent. To facilitate the discussion, a historical perspective has been adopted. As such, the current discussion must begin with a contextualization of European colonialism in Africa and trans-Atlantic slavery (Carter & Pieterse, 2005; Foster, 1993; Simone, 1993).

HISTORICAL ASPECTS: COLONIZATION AND RACIAL OPPRESSION IN CONTEXT

The coastal areas of West Africa are littered with the remnants of European involvement dating back from the fifteenth century. In places such as the coast of Ghana, a fort or its remnants can be found on bays just a few miles apart. They were built and rebuilt by competing European nations – the Swedish, the Portuguese, the Dutch, the British, and many others. Their purpose was, clearly, to protect and secure the "interests" of these European nations, and, of course, their function sometimes changed over time. Initially, the European interest in the African continent was in the indigenous resources. Wealth was always the objective, but this might have been from gold, palm oil, rubber, and, most notoriously, wealth from slavery. Full-blown colonization of Africa came late compared to the colonization of the rest of the world. The rush to colonize Africa largely followed the abolition of the slave trade early in the nineteenth century and continued until the process of decolonization began in the 1950s, when the United Kingdom "gave" Ghana its "independence." Many colonial nations followed suit in the next few years. Of course, the postcolonial period of European involvement in Africa has been dubbed the era of neo-colonialism and effectively describes the modern situation. Neo-colonialism refers to the financial, trade, and similar arrangements that work to the advantage of former colonizing countries, as well as other powerful nations, to the continued disadvantage of the economically, if not militarily, subjugated African nations. Third-world debt is just one debilitating manifestation of neo-colonialism. A very concrete example of neo-colonialism at work can be seen in the events following the decolonization of the Belgian Congo (now known as the Democratic Republic of the Congo [DRC]) in 1960. After decolonization, more than two thirds of the economy of the "liberated" colony was under Belgian control, through the operations of a commercial company – the Société Générale de Belgique. Historically, the Société had been the major force in Belgian colonies. (The role of commercial companies in the colonization process, in general, should not be underestimated.)

It should come as no surprise, then, to find that the DRC is currently one of the world's poorest countries. According to the World Bank Developmental Indicators (2006), the country is 186th out of 187 countries in terms of gross national product, which refers to the total value of the goods and services produced by a country. Belgium, in contrast, is ranked fifteenth in the world. It is also of relevance that the largest proportion of slaves taken to the Americas was from the area that now includes the DRC, as well as the Republic of the Congo, which was a former French colony. Approximately 40 percent of slaves originated from this area (Lovejoy, 2000).

The migration, free or forced, of Africans began long before the fifteenth century and the beginnings of Black slavery to other European colonies. The details of African migration are substantially different for different parts of the world and at different times. In the case of the United States, for example, the slave trade was responsible for the transportation of the majority of the ancestors of current African Americans from Africa. However, this transportation is only part of the story. At present, there are substantial numbers of Black people migrating directly to the United States from African countries, especially Nigeria, Ethiopia, and Ghana. Of the estimated 35 million African Americans currently in the United States, about one million were actually born in Africa. Generally, these modern migrants have a high school education, and include upwardly mobile professionals admitted into the United States via the lottery visa system. Of course, some are asylum seekers or refugees, although only 10 percent of refugees to the United States are of African origin.

In general, the situation is, of course, historically different in Great Britain and Europe. It is known that there were African people in Europe from as early as the second century. Only in modern times have there been substantial numbers of people of African origin in Europe. Historically, Black Africans had a presence in Europe as sailors, merchants, and domestic workers. Despite the centrality of Europeans in the slave trade, few Africans were transported to Europe as slaves during slavery times. In the United Kingdom, for example, the

Discussion Box 6.1: The Myth of Black Family Pathology

Awareness of the appalling history of African colonization and slavery, in itself, does not ensure that appropriate assessments will be made by counselors. Take the analogy of the controversy variously known as the recovered memories/false memories debate. The crux of this was that, based on the relationship between child sexual abuse and various adult psychological problems, some therapists overgeneralized to make the assumption that the likely root cause of adult problems is sexual abuse in childhood. This assumption is fallacious. There is no doubt that colonialism and slavery profoundly affected the capacity of Black peoples to fulfill themselves psychologically, socially, and economically. As can be seen from this chapter, this impaired capacity was precisely the colonialists' intent. Nevertheless, there has been a long history of ideological assaults on the cultures of Black people based on this intent. Social policy defines some matters as social issues, which may be the result of key events. For Black families, the publication of the Moynihan Report (1965) in the United States typified Black single-parent families as a "tangle of pathology." Lobo (1978), a pediatrician of Indian origin, described Black families in London in the following terms:

There is a distinct lack of a warm, intimate, continuous relationship between the children and their mothers from which both would get satisfaction and enjoyment. (p. 36)

The truth of this statement is regarded as self-evident, and no research evidence accompanies the claim.

Questions

1. How do Western theories of family development and family cohesion contribute to the perception of Black families as being pathological?
2. What cultural world view can a counselor draw on to identify and emphasize the strengths of the Black family structure?

arrival of substantial numbers of people of slave descent began only in the period of decolonization following the Second World War. So, in the 1950s, migrant workers from the Caribbean area, a prime location of slavery because of the sugar plantations, were able to travel to Britain. At that time, citizens of ex-colonies held British passports, but they also were encouraged, financially and by other means, to travel to Britain to work in the health and transport services, where there was a chronic shortage of workers. At the same time, exploitative encouragement was given in British (ex-) colonies to African people to migrate to Britain. Much the same applied in other European countries.

CURRENT IMPLICATIONS OF HISTORICAL LEGACIES

The importance does not lie in the detail, as such, but in the many historical routes by which people of African descent reached the Western world. While not all share a family history of slavery, they all have in common the impact of European colonization. Not only can people of African descent bring different needs to the counseling environment, but they differ widely in terms of their cultural backgrounds. This difference may have a profound bearing on what social (support) resources are available to them. If one spends just a short period of time in a sub-Saharan African country, he or she becomes acutely aware that the family structures are very different from those of Western nations. In particular, it is obvious that the extended family structure still dominates, despite invasive Western influences, such as international media. The nuclear family is simply not the norm. More broadly, sub-Saharan African countries remain relatively collectivist (rather than individualist) cultures despite the pressures of modernization. For the Western observer, this collectivist culture initially can appear very confusing; child-rearing patterns, as an example, are very complex to the Western mind, because a child may move from one place to another and away from his or her biological parents in ways uncharacteristic of the Western child. Grandparents, aunts and uncles, and more distant relatives may take over prime responsibilities, at different stages in ways that are now virtually unknown in the West. Furthermore, the incapacity of biological parents to bring up a child is not inevitably a matter for state (social work) intervention but part of how the family ensures that its children prosper, even in adverse circumstances. Indeed, the children may be in one country and the biological parents in another. To a Western observer, these may seem odd circumstances, but this is a function of the perspective of modern Western values, rather than anything intrinsically problematic or troublesome.

Other non-White communities are subject to varied assumptions to explain the problems of their children. For example, Indian families in the West, are characterized as being overprotective, which is held to have its own adverse consequences on a family's offspring (Howitt, 1992). Such ideas may have profound influences on the way professionals interact with members of Black and other ethnic minority communities. There is evidence that child-care placement decisions are racially biased; that Black children are characterized as manifesting behavioral problems, by the school system, and differentially responded to as a consequence; and, that throughout the care system, differential treatment is common (Owusu-Bempah & Howitt, 2000). A study by Owusu-Bempah (1994) employed a social work case study of a boy who manifested a number of problems. Social workers in training read one of two versions of the case study. In one case, the boy was described as being White and in the other case he was described as being Black. Eighty-five percent of the social workers mentioned identity crises as the cause of the Black boy's problems, but only 25 percent did so when the boy was described as White. In other words, the race of the boy profoundly influenced the explanatory framework deployed, despite the otherwise identical descriptions of the boy.

While neo-colonialism, colonialism, and slavery continue to have immense negative consequences for Black nations, it is faulty reasoning to assume that all problems of Black people can be traced back to the history of colonialism and slavery. For this reason, careful assessment is required.

Collectivist cultures have been identified as having four distinctive attributes (Markus & Kitayama, 1991; Triandis, 1995):

1. *Conceptions of self*: Self-identity is defined in relation to the group and involves the interdependence between the individual and their group or community. In individualistic cultures, the self is largely what differentiates the individual from others. It is more autonomous and independent.
2. *Setting goals*: The goals of the group are more important than those of the individual. In individualist cultures, priority is given the individual's personal goals.
3. *Norms and attitude*: Cultural or group values determine behavior, whereas, in individualist cultures, the priority is given to the attitudes or personal standards that distinguish the individual from others.
4. *Meeting needs*: The interest of the community predominates in collectivist cultures. So, the family may be very influential on whether a couple stays together. In contrast, in an individualistic culture, families often believe that it is inappropriate to intervene in what it regards as the affairs of the individuals involved.

It seems likely, therefore, that the survival of collectivist cultures in colonized nations is indicative of the power of the family and community in resistance to the worst excesses of colonialism. This idea is not to suggest that the pressures of modernization are not affecting collectivist cultures – they are – but there remain vast areas of Africa where the collectivist culture is hegemonic and apparent. Of course, these differences between collectivist and individualistic cultures will be represented in clients of African origins, but in very different variations. Some new migrants will most certainly demonstrate some collectivist characteristics, whereas African Americans, whose ancestors were enslaved in the United States, might be more likely to exhibit elements of individualism, having assimilated individualistic Americanism over generations. Yet, as typified in the Black church and the structure of Black families, there still remains clear evidence of the collectivist aspects of their heritage (Boyd-Franklin, 2006).

An example of the collectivist culture, as exhibited in modern migrants from Africa (as do those from other parts of the world), is seen in how money is regularly sent back to their families and communities. These are known as remittances and can constitute a sizeable contribution to the gross national products of some African countries. Of course, these remittances provide a tangible example of collectivism at work and may be misunderstood, from the perspective of individualism, as merely representing exploitation of the host nation.

Slavery, Colonialism, and Imperialism

Despite the intimate association of slavery with the history of the United States, it is important for several reasons to understand that, irrespective of their relatively large absolute numbers, proportionately few of the slaves taken from Africa ended up in what is now the United States. While figures continue to be debated, it is estimated that about two thirds of a million African slaves went to the United States, which constituted probably about 4 percent of the totality of slaves (Thomas, 1997). Slavery was most associated with the sugar trade, and something like 35 percent of slaves went to the Caribbean (West Indies) and about the same proportion to Brazil. It should not be forgotten that before African slavery, the indigenous peoples of the Americas had been subject to slavery until practicalities meant that the source of slaves had to change. Nevertheless, the general image of the slave trade is primarily one with the United States at the center of the New World activity. One might also pause for thought when he or she notes that the worst history of racism in countries built on immigrant slave labor is probably associated with the United States, rather than any of the other countries that received larger numbers of slaves.

While the servitude of slavery is an easily recognizable consequence of racial oppression, the practical power of colonialist nations to ensure that Black peoples were held in their position of subservience to their colonial masters was immense and extensive. For example, the Agricultural Survey Commission for European Settlement in Northern Rhodesia (now Zambia) recommended in 1932 that land with poor water supplies, soil, and nutritional value be given to Africans, as it was unsuitable for European livestock (Allan, 1965). Thus, it is important to note that the machinations of colonialism not only provided the direct force to subjugate nations, but also ensured that an army of academics, scientists, and others contributed the academic and scientific justification for the actions of the colonialists. So intellectuals made claims of intellectual deficiencies of Black peoples, which may have seemed

Discussion Box 6.2: The Gate of Return

The slave-fort at Cape Coast in Ghana is now a World Heritage Site. One of the things that guidebooks point out about this fort is the sign over the exit, which reads "The Gate of No Return," where the enslaved Africans went out to the ships. A few years ago, Black tourists from the United States were instrumental in getting a sign erected on the other side of the gate, which reads "The Gate of Return," in recognition of Black Americans who were beginning to return to West Africa. Of course, this begs the philosophical question of whether American tourists could really return socially and culturally to Africa. This return is unlikely for the vast majority of Black people living outside of Africa. Physically, as Black people, they may go through the "Gate of Return." However, culturally, what do they bring that is African, and what do they bring that is American or Western? Furthermore, the notion of a contemporary "Gate of Return" disregards the attempts of the American Colonization Society (The Society for the Colonization of Free People of Color of America) in 1822 to return free people of African descent back to a colony that a few years later became Liberia.

Questions

1. Review the history of Liberia and describe ways in which this country represents aspects of a "Gate of Return," that is, a return to sovereignty, empowerment, and aspects of a "Gate of No Return," that is, the loss of sovereignty and cultural identity.
2. In which ways is the process of racial identity among Africans and individuals in the African Diaspora similar and different?

erudite to some, but in reality were mere prejudices serving the interests of imperialist nations (Howitt & Owusu-Bempah, 1994). This debate on cultural and genetic factors in intelligence dominated much of psychology, for example, from the late nineteenth century to the end of the twentieth century. One purpose of this construction of intelligence was simply to make Black people feel inferior and inadequate by promoting the view that they simply lack the educational potential of White people. Only by abandoning their culture could Black nations make progress in a world dominated by the power and economies of Western nations.

Racism

Frequently, it is argued that racism was an essential concomitant of colonialism and slavery, in that it provided justification for treating human beings worse than animals (see also Chapter 5, this volume). The history of racist thinking closely parallels the emergence of the slave trade and colonialism. Further, the intellectualization of racism, in the writings of leading thinkers, including putative scientists, is often seen as crucial to the process of psychological imperialism, which sought to define subservient peoples as psychologically inept and incapable of self-direction.

The definition of the "other," in the imperialist and colonialist mentality, was a crucial part of the ideology buttressing the appalling treatment meted out to those made subservient. A simple example is the change in the meaning of the word "barbarian." The original ancient Greek meaning of the word essentially identified non-Greeks, whose language or attempts to speak Greek sounded much like "bar-bar" (or babble). In other words, the word referred essentially to all non-Greeks. However, during the centuries of slavery and colonialism, the word took on the meaning of uncivilized savagery and barbarity – that is, the most extreme forms of cruelty.

Travelers and others drew on a repertoire of descriptive terms that portrayed Africans and others as inhumane and savage. Furthermore, the use of the term "tribes" categorized complex and effective African nations as little different from groupings of wild animals to which exactly the same term would be applied. The problem is not particularly in the term, but rather in the way in which the term is applied. If it were applied universally to similar groupings, then any objections would be effectively neutralized. However, it is not applied to Western nations, but largely to African peoples and a few other indigenous groups. There is more to it than that, however, as exemplified by Howitt and Owusu-Bempah's (1994) analysis of the use of the term "tribe" and similar terms in an American psychology textbook considered to be a classic, namely, *Introduction to Psychology* (Atkinson, Atkinson, Smith, & Hildard, 1993), still available in a modified form. This textbook was among the most commonly used in the teaching of psychology in the second part of twentieth century. Nevertheless, when attempting to write about African peoples, the term "tribe" was used even in the 1990s; whereas the only other use of the term is to refer to tribes of primates. As observed by Howitt and Owusu-Bempah (1994):

> [T]he term *tribe* is reserved for monkeys and black people to convey much the same meanings as primitive, savage or undeveloped. Through arguments, repetitions and juxtapositions, the text is fastidious in representing non-North American black people as (a) strange and other than Westerners, (b) an undifferentiated mass, and (c) primitive. (pp. 72–73)

Psychological Imperialism

The concept of psychological imperialism refers to the onslaught upon colonized peoples with the tacit intent of making them both vulnerable and manipulable (Owusu-Bempah & Howitt, 2000). As a consequence, even today, some African leaders doubt their own ability and doubt the ability of citizens to be anything but mere followers (Ogungbamila, 2005). As a result of psychological imperialism, African people accord high esteem to all things Western that the colonialists left as their bequest – language, religion, custom, and style of dressing. The Western way of life is the standard by which things are judged as acceptable or unacceptable – and, all too often, a life in the West is the ultimate ambition of African youth. Africans, as a consequence of both slavery and colonialism, were prized away from their African roots, but never properly replanted in Western culture. According to the Nigerian scholar Bolanle Ogungbamila, the deadweight of their European cultural influences leaves Africans incompletely committed to African cultures and African values. Furthermore, Ogungbamila points out that imperialism and colonialism are distinguished in the following way: Imperialism refers to the variety of different ways in which a nation achieves power over others (e.g., propaganda, military power, animosity between groups within the country, and so forth), whereas colonialism involves the physical occupation of the other country. Consequently, when colonialism came to an end, there remained a great deal of opportunity for other imperialist tendencies to hold sway. Thus, aspects of colonialism that were superficially viewed as benign were in actuality more malignant in nature. This colonialism is illustrated by the educational systems employed in the British colonies, the objectives of which were not the emancipation of the indigenous peoples, but rather (1) to ensure that communications between Africans and the European colonists would be easier; (2) to ensure a supply of interpreters and clerks capable of being part of the colonial workforce, yet subservient; and (3) to indoctrinate the colonized people with European culture.

Thus, the historical legacy of nation building, colonization, and subjugation has been identified as having important ramifications for people of African descent, particularly in relation to those associated with identity, agency, and conflicting world views. Hence, we now turn to a more detailed examination of psychological correlates of racial oppression and points of intervention in the process of counseling.

PSYCHOLOGICAL MANIFESTATIONS OF RACIAL OPPRESSION

The psychological impact of colonization on Africans has been identified as a crucial issue for many years (Fanon, 1952; Mannoni, 1964). Early work, largely undertaken by European and American psychoanalysts, viewed the African psyche from the perspective of deficiency, a legacy of colonialist thinking about those who are subjugated. McCulloch (1995) has documented the approach taken by colonial psychiatry and highlights the underlying thread of viewing the African as "abnormal" based on "observed" deficits in personality, morality, and intellect. Thus, in the *Psychology of Colonization*, Mannoni would describe the colonized personality of the Madagascans as characterized by inferiority and dependence, a stance similar to Kardiner and Ovesy's (1951) view, following the psychoanalytic evaluations of twenty-five "Negroes" in New York, that their personalities were marked by low self-esteem and aggression.

African American psychologists also have focused on the psychological response to oppression, highlighting models associated with racial identity, negative self-concept, and internalized racism (Landrum-Brown, 1990; White, 1984). Recently, the literature has turned to empirical examinations of psychological reactions to racism and racial oppression. Driven by the development of a range of instruments designed to assess the frequency and stressfulness of racism-related experiences (Utsey, 1998), there is now a fairly robust body of scholarship examining the psychological correlates of racism and racial oppression, as well as the role of moderating and mediating variables such as spirituality, social support, and racial socialization (Carter, 2007; Williams & Williams-Norris, 2000). In sum, the literature has indicated that experiences of racial oppression and trauma can be associated with adverse mental health outcomes. One criticism of the current thinking, however, is that the focus has primarily been on individual psychological processes, with a tendency to examine only psychological distress and adverse physiological outcomes such as hypertension (Paradies, 2006; Williams et al., 2003).

However, this literature fails to recognize that such individualized psychologies ignore the basic collectivism of the African personality with the family, community, society, and culture. In other words, it continues the imperialist strategy of removing people of African descent from those psychological and cultural world views that represent an important part of their identity. In this regard, liberation psychology offers a contextualized framework in which to understand both the antecedents of psychological distress and the path toward empowerment, thereby a restoring of the true self. A narrow reading of the history of colonialism tends to ignore the fact that resistance to colonization was as much a part of the history of colonized nations as was subjugation. For example, the Ashanti aligned themselves politically with the Dutch in their resistance against the British; it took from 1823 to 1900 for the British finally to overcome the resistance of the Ashanti through a series of wars.

Liberation Psychology

Liberation psychology emphasizes the transformation of psychological processes associated with oppression, as well as the need to challenge and transform those social

Research Box 6.1: Perceived Discrimination

Williams, D. R., Gonzalez, H. M., Williams, S., Mohammed, S. A., Moomal, H., & Stein, D. J. (2008). Perceived discrimination, race and health in South Africa. *Social Science Medicine*, *67*, 441–52.

Objective: This research explored the influence of racial difference in perceived discrimination and the extent to which perceptions of discrimination were associated with psychological distress

Method: Data were drawn from the South African Stress and Health Survey, a nationally derived sample of 4,351 South African Adults. The survey included measures on discrimination, general life stress, mental health, and self-esteem. Data was analyzed using multiple regression procedures and the model tested the mediating effects of racial difference on the relationship between perceived discrimination and psychological health.

Findings: Blacks (Africans, Indians, and Coloreds) were two to four times more likely to report discrimination than Whites. Blacks reported higher levels of psychological distress, and perceived discrimination was positively associated with ill health for Blacks and not for Whites

Questions

1. How may these findings be translated to counseling interventions and prevention practices by counselors working with individuals of African descent?
2. What other research methodologies might be used to assess the impact of racial discrimination of physical and mental health?
3. For historically oppressed and marginalized groups, is it possible to differentiate between race-related stress and general life stress, or are these two types of stressors significantly correlated?

conditions producing the oppression (Moane, 2003). Thus, Martin-Baro (1994) states that liberation "involves breaking the chains of personal oppression as much as the chains of social oppression" (p. 27). Foster (2004) offers a definition of liberation psychology as "involving questions of the psychological processes, dynamics, capacities, and practices through which people may achieve emancipation, freedom, liberation and escape particular power structures of oppression and exploitation" (p. 560). A final and important aspect of liberation psychology is the emphasis it places on the collective communities that share a collective history of oppression and, as such, articulates communal healing and collective empowerment (Moane, 2003). Thereby, liberation psychology, provides an important and conceptually consistent framework to review the psychological manifestations of colonization and to describe aspects of empowerment designed to reestablish individual and collective self-efficacy.

Mental Colonization

A central theme, in the literature focusing on the psychological processes associated with oppression, is the manner in which the oppressed come to internalize the beliefs and assumptions held about them by the oppressor, both in regard to inferiority of the oppressed and superiority of the oppressor. Perhaps nowhere is this "bind" more graphically illustrated than in Fanon's *Black Skin /White Masks* (1952).Employing a psychoanalytic lens, Fanon carefully illustrates the "neurosis of Blackness," that is, wanting to be White. Of importance here is that the neurosis does not represent a repudiation of Blackness; rather, it entails a wish to be in a position of power, as is the White man. As Hook (2004) emphasizes, the "neurosis of Blackness" can be understood only in the context of the colonial encounter, that is, "It is an outcome of a specific configuration of power, of real material, economic, cultural and sociopolitical conditions that continually celebrate and empower the white subject and continually denigrate and dispossess the black man or women" (p. 117).

Perhaps Dubois's (1903) contribution of "double consciousness," the process by which Black Americans negotiated being American *and* "Negro," provides an important framework in which to appreciate the process of negotiating this "configuration of power." The picture as painted by Dubois was dynamic, tumultuous, and self-preserving:

> The Negro even feels his two-ness – An American, a Negro: two souls, two thoughts, two unreconciled strivings...two warring ideals in one dark body whose dogged strength alone keeps it from being torn asunder. (p. 3)

So here in the phenomenon of *Double Consciousness* and the condition of a *Neurosis of Blackness*, we have captured the core constructs, which are repeated in the literature addressing the psychological response to racial oppression, as illustrated through colonization and the ideology of White supremacy. We can see it in Chinweizu's (1987) call for a *Decolonization of the African Mind*, in Nobles' (1986) description of a *conceptual incarceration* experienced by individuals of African descent who have accepted Eurocentric systems of belief and knowledge. We see it in the state of internalized racism (Speight, 2007). Again, it is important to emphasize that what we are describing here are those psychological processes associated with the colonial encounter, the process of being de-empowered as a function of race.

Discussion Box 6.3: Barack Obama, Africa, and the African Diaspora

In an historic election, in November 2008, Barack Obama was elected as the first non-White president of the United States. President Obama, a biracial individual who identifies as Black, garnered an incredible 96 percent of the African American vote. Obama's election was greeted with great enthusiasm and joy in Africa, with the BBC noting that "Obama's election was being celebrated across the continent" (http://news.bbc.co.uk/2/hi/africa/7710394.stm). Yet, it is interesting to note that policies associated with the African continent were largely missing from President Obama's election campaign; furthermore, it was widely noted that as a candidate, President Obama chose to run a race-neutral campaign, largely presenting himself as a symbol of postracial America. Some have argued that issues germane to the African American community such as health disparities, reparations for slavery, affirmative action, and disproportionate rates of incarceration and poverty, gained little attention during President Obama's presidential campaign. While race was downplayed during the 2008 U.S. presidential election campaign, President Obama's election was greeted as evidence that the United States had finally dealt with the legacy of racism and slavery as encapsulated in the following heading from the *New York Times*: Racial Barriers Erased as Voters Embrace a Call for Change.

Questions

1. Given the apparent lack of attention to issues specifically affecting Africans and African Americans by candidate Obama, from a psychological perspective, how might one understand the generally positive response to President Barack Obama's election by individuals of African descent?

TOWARD A DECOLONIZATION OF THE MIND

Facilitating a shedding of the colonial mentality, while continuously experiencing the colonial encounter, is perhaps the greatest challenge for mental health professionals working with people of African descent, Hook (2005), drawing on Fanon, captured the essence of this challenge when noting that Fanon understood colonialism as " a means of not only appropriating land and territory, but of appropriating culture and history themselves, that is a way of appropriating the means and resources of identity, and hence affecting powerful forms of psychical distress and damage" (p. 482). The psychological antecedents of this appropriation has taken many forms. African American psychologists have written about the experience of invisibility (Franklin, 1999), the constant exposure to microaggressions (Pierce, 1995), the intergenerational transmission of trauma associated with slavery, and the deculturalization of Africans (Leary, 2005). While referring to this experience of enslavement and colonization as the "Maafa" of "great disaster" (Hotep & Hotep, 2003), indeed the "Maafa" can be viewed as an ongoing phenomenon, particularly as it relates to the intergenerational transmission of trauma (Cross, 1998; Gagné, 1998).

Mental health professionals are at a critical juncture both to facilitate a more adaptive and healthier response to the ongoing experience of racial oppression for individuals of African descent and to build on cultural strengths and forms of resilience. Consistent with a liberation approach, the counselor is charged with responding to the racial trauma and challenging the ongoing system of oppression. One quickly realizes, therefore, that dominant Western models of psychological intervention, with a focus on individual intrapsychic processes and an accompanying lack of attention to social structures of oppression, provide a challenging framework in which to practice the psychology of liberation (Hook, 2005; Watts & Abdul-Adil, 1994). Thus, the mental health practitioner begins with a self-assessment and inventory of their level of preparation to participate in the practice of liberation. We propose that an effective model of intervention for psychological decolonization would include the following facets:

1. A confrontation of false consciousness through an examination of an individual's belief system, that is, the extent to which it reflects elements of the colonial mentality and the extent to which it embraces African-centered philosophical principles of identity such as collectivism, spirituality, intersubjectivity, and historical connectivity (Nobles, 1984).
2. An appreciation of the postcolonial nature of racial oppression. Watts and Abduli-Adil (1994) argue that a process of empowerment includes the act of educating the oppressed as to the nature of their oppression, the tools associated with their subjugation, and the patterns of psychological responses typically ascribed to the experience of racial oppression. To illustrate, the notion of having gained independence is a powerful tool of postcolonial oppression. Here Fanon's observation, articulated in the *Wretched of the Earth* (1963), is particularly apt, noting the colonists' response to the request or demand of independence: "Since you want independence, take it and starve" (p. 97). Thus, while Africa has collectively gained the status of independence, the social hierarchies and distributions of wealth represent not only vestiges of colonial rule, but are patterned on the very systems of oppression that have resulted in staggering disparities between Africa and the West. The point of emphasis here is that in addressing a

decolonization of the mind, the mental health professional has to acknowledge and incorporate the notion that personal subjectivities can be understood only in the context of those linkages among social structures, political ideologies, and collective identities (Foster, 2004). Thus, one cannot facilitate psychological empowerment without appreciating the political context within which the psychological intervention takes place (Hook, 2005).

3. The process of decolonization involves a process of grief. Here the work of African American psychologist Barbara Wallace (2006) is particularly appealing. By providing communal spaces for collective grief, she positions African Americans, in such a manner whereby the generational trauma associated with the Maafa can start to be validated and legitimized by the collective community. By waiting for or relying on the oppressor to provide validation of generational trauma, the power dynamic associated with the ideology of White supremacy is reified, and thus, the colonial mentality maintained (Buck, 2004).
4. The act of reclaiming a true self requires reeducation and resistance.

African American James Jones (2003) has described a cultural orientation among persons of African descent identified by the acronym TRIOS. For Jones, the TRIOS cultural orientation consists of five domains: (1) a past–present orientation to time; (2) rhythm, recurring patterns of behavior associated with an attempt to provide psychological structure to external realities; (3) improvisation, a mechanism of establishing structure to social interaction; (4) orality, the oral tradition via music, story telling of connecting the past to the present; and (5) spirituality, the most central aspect of African culture, which recognizes a belief in the immaterial and locates causality within forces beyond human beings. Therefore, in order to implement effectively notions of resistance and reparation of the self, counselors need to be knowledgeable about African cultural patterns and world views and accept these orientations as valid and as legitimate as the traditional Eurocentric notions of individualism, objectivity, and a focus on the future.

Further, scholars, such as Graham (2005), have identified the concept of Maat as a philosophical system that undergirds both resistance and healing within the African Diaspora. Specifically, Maat, as embodied in African-centered world views, provides an understanding of the human condition and a prescription for remedy that is located in three guiding principles: (1) the spiritual nature of human beings; (2) the interconnectedness of all things; and, (3) one of mind, body, and spirit. Therefore, counselors working with peoples of African descent, particularly in relation to the experience of oppression and racial trauma, are encouraged to incorporate an African-centered approach that emphasizes this spirituality and interconnectivity. Of note, this emphasis runs contrary to European notions of individualism and serves to explain, in part, the history of racism in psychology that has spanned several centuries (Graham, 2005; Howitt & Owusu-Bempah, 1994). In summary, the process of decolonization is essential as persons of African descent seek to reclaim identity and resist ongoing racial oppression. As Fanon (1963) noted:

> Decolonization ... influences individuals and modifies them fundamentally ... It brings a natural rhythm into existence with a new language and humanity. Decolonization is the veritable creation of a new humanity. But this creation owes nothing of its legitimacy to any supernatural power: the "thing" which has been colonized becomes human during the same process by which it frees itself. (pp. 36–7)

The preceding sections have provided a historical context in which to appreciate the psychological response to racial oppression among persons of African descent. In addition, liberation psychology has been described as a conceptual framework for counseling those who have experienced racial oppression. Finally, specific guidelines have been offered that incorporate African-centered cultural orientations and that provide a critical platform for healing and resistance. The following section, therefore, shows how ideas of liberation and empowerment may be applied.

LIBERATION AND EMPOWERMENT: A COMMUNITY INTERVENTION

The scenic town of Stellenbosch lies thirty miles northeast of Cape Town, and was the second to be settled by European people in South Africa. It is renowned as one of the premier wine-producing areas of the world and is arguably one of the wealthiest agricultural regions in the country. The wealth of Stellenbosch, however, draws not only from the legacy of expertise, knowledge, and industry of the Dutch and French Huguenot descendent farmers, who were granted lease hold by the Dutch East India Company, but also from the blood, sweat, and exploitation of slaves, whose labor was used to toil the earth to ultimately produce the wine and the wealth. The legacy of colonial slavery and apartheid is manifest still in the stark socioeconomic disparity between rich and poor, following racial lines, as the majority of the Black and mixed-parentage communities continue to be disadvantaged, impoverished, marginalized, and disaffected in comparison to the White residents who live in affluent communities.

Up until the end of the apartheid era (South Africa's first democratic elections took place in April 1994), farmers in the Stellenbosch region were notorious for using the dop-system (tot system) to pay their workers, in part, with daily or weekend rations of cheap wine (from the residue of the wine-making process) for their labor (London, Saunders, & Te Water Naude, 1998). Although slavery was formally abolished in 1834, the coercive practices developed to constrain emancipated slaves – and to continue the economic viability of the Cape's wine farms – have left oppressive legacies for rural social relations in South Africa. The lives of farm laborers continued to be dominated by exploitation, control, and paternalism. The antecedents of this system continue to manifest in the form of a high alcoholism rate, fetal alcohol syndrome prevalence, high unemployment, low income, low educational levels, domestic violence, child abuse, and other correlates and consequences of oppressive poverty. One alarming correlate is that the Western Cape region, of which Stellenbosch is a part, has the highest fetal alcohol syndrome prevalence rate of 60 to 70 per 1,000 children reported in any community worldwide (Viljoen et al., 2005).

Many farm workers have been living on farms for many generations, trapped in difficult social conditions that perpetuate the cycle of poverty. These conditions readily translate into negative social behavior among the young people in the community: alcohol and drug abuse, teenage pregnancy, sexually transmitted diseases, school truancy and attrition, delinquent behavior, and a heightened susceptibility to gangs. Within this context, a request was received for a psychological intervention at a health facility predominantly serving farmer workers. The following section describes the process in which this request was transformed into an empowering liberatory intervention for youth from these communities.

The Genesis of the Project

The project evolved initially from a letter to the Psychology Department of Stellenbosch University, at the beginning of 2000, requesting assistance with psychological services at the newly opened primary health care facility in the Jamestown community. The facility provided basic health care not only to the residents of Jamestown but also to many seasonal workers living in informal settlements on the outskirts of the town and to farm workers living on neighboring wine estates. Using a community psychology model as a frame of reference (Nelson & Prilleltensky 2005) – one that emphasizes understanding the embedded systems in the context, the need for empowerment, and liberational and social justice awareness as seminal values of praxis – a process of engagement was set up that initially included a series of contact visits and consultation meetings with the clinic staff and other relevant community role-players and organizations. These included the primary and high school principals, local clergy, local governance representatives, community elders, and the local municipality. These consultation processes permitted the third author and a team of eight Master's students in counseling psychology to gauge local community opinion and perceptions of the nature of the issues requiring attention, thus gaining a broader understanding of the local context of this community (e.g., its history, socioeconomic conditions, psycho-social needs, risk and protective factors, and aspirations, among others). The consultation served as a platform upon which to establish formal links and personal and working relationships between the project team and community role-players. The consultation discussions also helped to identify potential partners and resources and created space for community input and participation from the onset of the project (Naidoo & Van Wyk, 2003). The voices and involvement of local residents are crucial to the success and sustainability of community-based endeavors (Petersen & Ramsay, 1993; Prilleltensky, 2001).

At a community forum meeting involving community role-players and staff and students from the Psychology Department, community leaders presented the sociohistorical background and contextual features of Jamestown, the clinic nursing staff presented an overview of the major health concerns of residents, and the university role-players provided input on possible resources and intervention options. It was significant to hear the residents speak proudly of how the community had survived the ravages of apartheid and retained a strong collective identity, a strong indication of the resilience in the community. The community leaders, however, expressed a common concern about the difficulties the youth of Jamestown were facing, namely, the high school dropout rate, increasing levels of alcohol and substance abuse, teenage pregnancies, violent behavior, and gang-related activity. Subsequent research in the Stellenbosch district, undertaken two years later, indicated homicide as the major cause of non-natural death in the fifteen- to forty-nine-year age cohort, thereby justifying the concern of the community leaders (Marais, Naidoo, Donson, & Nortje, 2007).

At the conclusion of the meeting, the Jamestown Community Project (JCP) was initiated, with the community leaders formally inviting the university role-players to work in their community. Relevant partnerships were established to address the identified concerns (Naidoo & Van Wyk, 2003). The community forum discussions helped to counter the disempowering victim-blaming discourse that frequently reduces negative structural and sociopolitical conditions to intrapsychic pathologies (Albee, 1982, 1986; Felner, Felner, & Silverman, 2000) and emphasized the need to focus on a broader systemic understanding of what was happening in the community to bring about changes at the macro level (Orford, 1992). This community challenged the team to engage beyond the narrow prescripts of mainstream psychology, with its emphasis on individual behavior. Foundational premises of the JCP were: (1) effective interventions needed to be based on a thorough contextual analysis and at multiple levels; (2) community participation was central to defining the needs and to identifying and formulating interventions; (3) a multilevel approach, organized around consensually defined curative, preventive, developmental, and advocacy objectives, was essential; and (4) a coalition of partners was needed to deliver effectively on planned interventions (Naidoo & Van Wyk, 2003).

An action-research methodology was used to design the different activities that began to constitute the Jamestown community project. The implementation of the JCP has been previously described in several publications to which readers can refer for more detail (Marais et al., 2007; Naidoo & Van Wyk, 2003; Van Wyk & Naidoo, 2006). Initially, individual counseling services were introduced at the health clinic, with referrals coming from the health staff, as well as the two schools in the area. Group-based interventions were initiated at the school in response to developmental needs identified by the school staff. Consultations also were rendered to address the needs of the nursing and school staff. By the second year, a full-time counseling psychology internship was established in the Jamestown community to sustain these interventions, but using a community psychology rather than a traditional mainstream counseling psychology orientation (Van Wyk & Naidoo, 2006).

In response to the community leaders' expressed concern about the disaffected youth in the community, a youth project was initiated in partnership with a nonprofit organization called Usiko at the local high school. Usiko's mission to create and implement programs for youth-at-risk and youth in conflict with the law, based on rites of passage, mentoring, and the use of wilderness, was a good fit for the youth project. However, the challenge was to translate these concepts into the local context. A team of thirteen adult male mentors were initially recruited from the local community. Using this collective as a circle of wisdom and power, reminiscent of indigenous cultures, the Usiko model and its concepts were debated and gradually shaped into the nuts and bolts (structure, content, and processes) of the actual program. Formative and summative processes further helped to consolidate the evolving program. Notwithstanding, the mandate from the project funders for a focus on "93 male delinquents," the program was initiated at a high school with a preventative objective and used a rites-of-passage approach to assist adolescents from high-risk backgrounds with the challenges they face. While the program initially was focused on adolescent male participants, a parallel program was introduced two years subsequently, at the request of the community.

According to Naidoo and Van Wyk (2003), prevention programs are more effective and better enhanced when they are comprehensive, target multiple ecological levels, and utilize combined approaches that facilitate enhancement/promotion and prevention/risk reduction (Felner et al., 2000). In adopting a prevention approach, the program endeavored to preclude the inefficient victim-blaming models that frequently reduce negative structural sociopolitical conditions to intrapsychic pathologies (Albee, 1982, 1986; Felner et al., 2000; Hook, 2002). Adopting a rites-of-passage approach became very instrumental and empowering for the project, as the apartheid political system had severely eroded the transfer of cultural traditions and rituals. The rites-of-passage approach permitted the mentors to engage with the young participants, not only regarding the transitional challenges of their journey from adolescence to adulthood, but also to raise their awareness of the sociopolitical contexts of their lives. The program activities supported by the mentoring relationship guided the participants to explore their own senses of self and life circumstances and to develop dreams or visions for their future. The use of wilderness settings for these reflective activities proved very facilitative. Several joint activities also were convened for the mentors and mentees to bond and interact in a group context. In one such activity, the mentors and young participants journey to Robben Island and engage directly with their colonial history. The mentees are challenged by the symbolic significance of the experience of being on the island where Nelson Mandela and other political activists against apartheid were imprisoned for many years. This experience allows for a reflection on their own history, their own contexts, to inspire to rise beyond the adversities that might currently imprison or limit them (poverty, adverse family circumstances, being stigmatized as farm children, racism) and, in the vein of Martin Luther King, to dare to dream, to set their own vision for their future. This powerful experience provides rich personal material for many subsequent discussions about identity, context, and emancipation.

RESEARCH CONSIDERATIONS

We have noted that when dealing with individuals from African descent, the range of psychotherapeutic interventions might include approaches not emphasized in the more accepted Western models of counseling and psychotherapy. Therefore, it would be important to examine the extent to which these alternative approaches are effective. Furthermore, the applicability of traditional research methodologies when seeking to establish the efficacy of culturally appropriate interventions among individuals of African descent needs to be considered.

Historically, the emphasis of psychology has been on individual intrapsychic processes. It is clear that when employing elements of liberation psychology, the focus becomes one of community-based interventions that emphasize strengths and resources as opposed to pathology and dysfunction. Research approaches that include qualitative methodologies such as ethnography and phenomenology might be particularly useful when seeking to examine the efficacy of interventions such as the Usiko project. Furthermore, quantitative methodologies that emphasize objective quantification of psychological/behavioral processes might fail to capture the subjective nature of individual responses to racial oppression and mental colonization. In this regard, we would encourage the use of qualitative methodologies when seeking to understand the psychological response to racial oppression, and would suggest that Critical Psychology (Hook, 2005; Nelson & Prillentensky, 2005) and Liberation Psychology (Thompson & Alfred, 2009) offer important theoretical frameworks for this type of inquiry.

With regard to specific research foci, here we suggest a shift away from the emphasis on psychological distress and adverse health outcomes (Williams & Mohammed, 2009)

Case Study 6.1: The Usiko Program

Phase 1 – Rites of Passage and Leadership Program for Boys and Girls

In the first year, participants are supported in their journey to adulthood through weekly group sessions, two intensive wilderness-based excursions, and other interventions focusing on developing self-esteem, personal growth and identity, leadership development, and life planning. Hiking and camping in a natural wilderness setting is used to access the healing and restorative powers of nature and, in concert with structured rites-of-passage rituals, youth are supported to engage therapeutically with their personal histories and circumstances and to develop alternative stories and visions for their lives. During this phase, mentors are recruited from the community and participate in a series of training workshops and activities to develop their understanding of the mentor role. The participants receive individual mentoring from these older men and women from their communities. Where needed, participants and their families receive individual or family counseling and support. The focus of this phase is on exploration, restoration, and healing. To help the participants prepare for crossing the threshold to adulthood, the pain and the struggles of childhood and adolescence (and the historical context) first have to be engaged.

Phase 2 – Life Skills Programs at School

In the second year, activities during this phase are directed at identifying the potential and developing the skills of the participants. Weekly group activities are conducted with the participants to assist with developmental issues of adolescence in their context such as sex and sexuality, HIV awareness, relationships, dealing with feelings, peer pressure, substance abuse, world of work issues (career choice and career planning, interviewing, and CV writing), study skills, community involvement, and school-related concerns (study skills, remedial assistance, and exam preparation). Topics more germane to the needs and interests of individual participants also are accommodated. These activities provide a supportive climate in which the participants can develop alternative ways of coping.

Additional activities include a visit with the mentors to Robben Island, a road trip for which the participants raise funds, participation in their own community project, and a culminating Crossing of the Threshold program, in which the young participants are supported by a group of adult men with the challenges facing adult men. Given the multiracial composition of this gathering, many issues are stirred and brought to the surface for the young participants and the adult mentors alike.

Phase 3 – Livelihood and Skills Development Program

The main purpose of this phase is to provide continued support to the participants during the vulnerable transition from school to work. The activities are geared to assist the graduates of the school-based program gain access to work and further training opportunities. Participants who have dropped out of school also are assisted with alternative educational and training options. Activities include assistance with job applications, career counseling, job-hunting skills, computer skills training, driver's license training, basic business skills, and arranging learnerships and internships. Individualized assistance is given, commensurate with the needs of the young person.

Evaluation of the Program: The Usiko Program has succeeded at multiple levels, with examples of young men and women moving beyond the shadows of their past and their contexts, going on to assume leadership positions in their schools and communities, asserting their talents in terms of arts, crafts, and music; several go on to be first-generation college and university students in their families and farm communities. Two young men were awarded leadership scholarships to Canada. Significantly, several of the program graduates have returned to become mentors in the project, wanting to invest in the development and liberation of their peers. Recently, the project achieved a significant milestone in becoming an independent community organization, constituted by the very men and women who have dared to unshackle their minds and be involved in the creation of a new reality for the young people from their community.

Questions

1. Imagine you are describing the Usiko program to someone who is unfamiliar with it. Provide a brief description of the program, including the goals and interventions.
2. How does the Usiko program reflect elements of Liberation psychology and community empowerment?
3. In which ways does the Usiko program differ from Western notions of counseling and psychotherapy?
4. How might you adapt the Usiko program to your work environment or cultural context?

Research Box 6.2: Ethnic Identity in African Americans

McMahon, S. D., & Watts, R. J. (2002). Ethnic identity in urban African American youth: Exploring links with self-worth, aggression and other psychosocial variables. *Journal of Community Psychology*, *30*, 411–31.

Objective: To explore the influence of ethnic/racial identity on feelings of self-worth and aspects of mental health.

Method: Self-report surveys were administered to 209 African American adolescents, both male and female. The surveys included measures of Ethnic identity, Depression, Self-worth, Anxiety, Coping, and Aggression. Data were analyzed using correlation-based procedures.

Results: The findings indicated that ethnic/racial identity was associated with greater levels of self-worth and lower levels of depression and anxiety. Additional ethnic/racial identity was positively associated with healthy coping and less aggression.

Conclusion: For African American youth, ethnic identity might be an important consideration when seeking to implement preventive interventions designed to decrease aggression and facilitate mental health.

Questions

1. Explain how a positive sense of racial identity might be protective against feelings of depression and anxiety for individuals of African descent.
2. What are the cultural implications for professional counselors who offer services to adolescents?

and more a focus on the effects of activism and resistance to oppression. The work of Watts and colleagues (1994, 1999, 2007) offers important insights into the psychological benefits of actively resisting racial oppression. In addition, while the concept of intergenerational transmission of trauma is now widely accepted, the points at which the cycle of trauma can be interrupted are not well known. In this regard, community/collective grieving (Wallace, 2006) and rites of passage programs (Harvey & Hill, 2004) could be important areas of research to understand those process elements associated with self-efficacy and well-being, in the context of ongoing racial oppression among individuals of African descent. Finally, Speight (2007) has directed our attention to the role of internalized racism and the need to further explore, among individuals of African descent, the psychosocial correlates associated with seeing oneself through the eyes of the oppressor, that is, incorporating within one's self-concept the attributes of inferiority projected onto individuals of African descent by such processes as colonization, racial oppression, and institutionalized racism.

SUMMARY AND CONCLUSIONS

Colonialism and other forms of racial oppression are manifestations of the ideology of dominance based on the belief in White racial superiority. The preceding discussion has located racial oppression within a historical context of colonial occupation and slavery. Here we have seen how racial categorization was closely associated with the emerging scientific approach of grouping phenomena, according to observable differences. Furthermore, the idea of race was well suited to a process of domination, where indigenous peoples were viewed as primitive and deficient, both scientifically and theologically, and Europeans were regarded as enlightened and civilized. Given the enduring nature of the racial oppression that grew out of this ideology, the growing body of literature examining psychological aspects of racial oppression has been reviewed to show how racism-related stress has been implicated in such psychological states as depression, anxiety, and traumatic stress and that cultural variables such as spirituality, rhythm, and orality are viewed as important determinants of coping with racial oppression (Jones, 2003). Liberation psychology, with its grounding in the works of Fanon (1952, 1963) and Martin-Baro (1994), is proposed as a critical framework for the amelioration of the psychological effects of racial oppression. Finally, a case illustration was provided that highlights a community intervention as one approach to applying the principles of liberation psychology. This community-centered intervention involved a process of collective empowerment, stemming out of its collective ownership and engagement by the community.

It is our hope that by situating racial oppression in a historical context, by highlighting the psychological processes associated with racism, and by illustrating the principles of a liberation psychology, we have added to the needed knowledge base of those psychological healers committed to the work of restoring human dignity in the face of historical and ongoing oppression.

REFERENCES

Albee, G. W. (1982). Preventing psychopathology and promoting human potential. *American Psychologist*, *37*, 1043–50.

Albee, G. W. (1986). Towards a just society. Lessons from observations on the primary prevention of psychopathology. *American Psychologist*, *48*, 891–8.

Allan, W. (1965). *The African husbandman*. Edinburgh: Oliver and Boyd.

Asante, M. (2007). *The history of Africa: The quest for eternal harmony*. New York: Routledge.

Atkinson, R. L., Atkinson, R. C., Smith, E. E., & Bem, D. J. (1993). *Introduction to psychology* (11th ed.). New York: Harcourt Brace Jovanovich

Boyd-Franklin, N. (2006). *Black families in therapy* (2nd ed.). New York: Guilford Press.

Bryant-Davis, T., & Ocampo, C. (2005). Racist incident–based trauma. *The Counseling Psychologist, 33*(4), 479–500.

Buck, C. (2004). Sartre, Fanon, and the case for slavery reparations. *Sartre Studies International, 10*, 123–38.

Carter, R. T. (2007). Racism and psychological and emotional injury: Recognizing and assessing race-based traumatic stress. *The Counseling Psychologist, 35*, 13–105.

Carter, R. T., & Pieterse, A. L. (2005). Race: A social and psychological analysis of the term and its meaning. In R. T. Carter (Ed.), *Handbook of racial-cultural psychology and counseling: Theory and research* (Vol. 1, pp. 41–63). Hoboken, NJ: John Wiley & Sons.

Chinweizu. (1987). *Decolonising the African mind*. Lagos: Pero Publishers.

Cross, W. E. (1998). Black psychological functioning and the legacy of slavery: Myths and realities. In Y. Danieli (Ed.), *International handbook of multigenerational legacies of trauma* (pp. 387–400). New York: Plenum Press.

Dubois, W. E. B. (1903). *The souls of Black folk*. New York: Penguin Press

Fanon, F. (1952). *Black skin/White masks*. New York: Grove Press.

Fanon, F. (1963). *The wretched of the Earth*. New York: Grove Press

Felner, R. D., Felner, T. Y., & Silverman, M. M. (2000). Prevention in mental health and social intervention. In J. Rappaport & E. Seidman (Eds.), *Handbook of community psychology* (pp. 9–42). New York: Kluwer Academic/Plenum Press.

Foster, D. (1993). The mark of oppressions? Racism and psychology reconsidered. In L. J. Nicholas (Ed.), *Psychology and oppressions: Critiques and proposals* (pp. 128–41). Johannesburg, RSA: Skotaville Publishers.

Foster, D. (2004). Liberation psychology. In D. Hook (Ed.), *Critical psychology* (pp. 559–602). Cape Town: UCT Press.

Franklin, A. J. (1999). Invisibility syndrome and racial identity development in psychotherapy and counseling African American. *Counseling Psychologist, 27*, 761–93.

Gagné, M-A. (1998). The role of dependency and colonialism in generating trauma in first nations citizens. In Y. Danieli (Ed.), *International handbook of multigenerational legacies of trauma* (pp. 341–54). New York: Plenum Press.

Graham, M. (2005). Maat: An African-centered paradigm for psychological and spiritual healing. In R. Moodley & W. West (Eds.), *Integrating traditional healing practices into counseling and psychotherapy* (pp. 210–19). Thousand Oaks, CA: SAGE Publications.

Harvey, A. R., & Hill, R. B. (2004). Afrocentric youth and family rites of passage program: Promoting resilience among at-risk African American youths. *Social Work, 49*, 65–74.

Hook, D. (2002). Psychotherapy, discourse and the production of psychopathology. In D. Hook, & G. Eagle (Eds.), *Psychopathology and social prejudice* (pp. 20–54). Cape Town: University of Cape Town Press.

Hook, D. (2004). *Critical psychology*. Cape Town: University of Cape Town Press.

Hook, D. (2005). A critical psychology of the postcolonial. *Theory and Psychology, 15*, 475–503.

Hotep, U., & Hotep, T. (2003). *Dictionary of African centered knowledge*. Pittsburgh, PA: KTYLI.

Howitt, D. (1992). *Child abuse errors: When good intentions go wrong*. Hemel Hempstead, UK: Harvester-Wheatsheaf.

Howitt, D., & Owusu-Bempah, J. (1994). *The racism of psychology: Time for change*. Hemel Hempstead, UK: Harvester Wheatsheaf.

Jones, J. (2003). TRIOS: A psychological theory of the African legacy in American culture. *Journal of Social Issues, 59*, 217–42.

Kardiner, A., & Ovesy, L. (1951). *The mark of oppression: A psychological study of the American Negro*. Cleveland, OH: World Press.

Landrum-Brown, J. (1990). Black mental health and racial oppression. In D. Ruiz & J. P. Conners (Eds.), *Handbook on mental health and mental disorder among Black Americans* (pp. 113–32). New York: Greenwood Press.

Leary, J. D. (2005). *Post-traumatic slave syndrome: America's legacy of enduring injury and healing*. New York: Uptone Press.

Lobo, E. (1978). *Children of immigrants to Britain Their health and social problems*. London: Allen & Unwin.

London L., Sanders, D., & Te Water Naude, J. (1998). Farm workers in South Africa – the challenge of eradicating alcohol abuse and the legacy of the "dop" system. *South African Medical Journal, 88*, 1093–5.

Lovejoy, P. E. (2000). *Transformations in slavery*. Cambridge: Cambridge University Press.

Mannoni, O. (1964). *Prospero and Caliban: The psychology of colonization*. New York: Prager Press.

Marais, S., Naidoo, A., Donson, H., & Nortje, C. (2007). Strategic violence prevention partnerships in a peri-urban South African town: The case of the Jamestown community project. *African Safety Promotion Journal, 5*(1), 19–30.

Markus, H. R., & Kitayama, S. (1991). Culture and the self: Implications for cognition, emotion, and motivation. *Psychological Review, 98*, 224–53.

Martin-Baro, I. (1994). *Writings for a liberation psychology*. Cambridge, MA: Harvard University Press.

McCulloch, J. (1995). *Colonial psychiatry and the "African mind."* New York: Cambridge University Press.

McMahon, S. D., & Watts, R. J. (2002). Ethnic Identity in urban African American youth: Exploring links with self-worth, aggression and other psychosocial variables. *Journal of Community Psychology, 30*, 411–31.

Meredith, M. (2006). *The state of Africa*. London: The Free Press.

Moane, G. (2003). Bridging the personal and the political: Practices for a liberation psychology. *American Journal of Community Psychology, 31*, 91–102.

Moynihan, D. (1965). The *Negro family in the United States: The case for action*. Washington, DC: U.S. Government Printing Office.

Naidoo, A. V., & Van Wyk, S. B. (2003). Intervening in communities: Combining curative and preventive interventions. In V. E. Franchi & N. Duncan (Eds.), *Prevention and intervention practice in post-apartheid South Africa* (pp. 65–80). Binghamton, NY: Haworth Publishers.

Nelson, G., & Prilleltensky, I. (Eds.) (2005). *Community psychology: In pursuit of liberation and well-being*. London: Palgrave Macmillan.

Nobles, W. (1986). *African psychology: Toward its reclamation, revitalization and reascension*. Oakland, CA: Black Family Institute.

Ogungbamila, B. (2005). A psychological re-appraisal of the impacts of colonialism and imperialism on African development. *Ife Psychologia, 13*(1), 113–22.

Orford, J. (1992). *Community psychology: Theory and practice*. Chichester, England: John Wiley & Sons.

Owusu-Bempah, K. (1994). Race, self-identity and social work. *British Journal of Social Work, 24*, 123–36.

Owusu-Bempah, K., & Howitt, D. (1999). Even their soul is defective. *The Psychologist, 12*, 126–30.

Owusu-Bempah, K., & Howitt, D. (2000). *Psychology beyond Western perspectives*. Leicester, England: BPS Books.

Paradies, Y. (2006). A systematic review of empirical research on self-reported racism and health. *International Journal of Epidemiology, 35*, 888–901.

Petersen, I., & Ramsay, S. (1993). Mental health and development in a shack settlement: The case of Bhambayi. *Psychology in Society, 17*, 35–50.

Pierce, C. M. (1995). Stress analogs of racism and sexism: Terrorism, torture, and disaster. In C.V.Willie., P. P. Rieker., B. M. Kramer., & B. S. Brown (Eds.), *Mental health, racism, and sexism*. Pittsburgh, PA: University of Pittsburgh Press.

Pieterse, A. L., & Carter, R. T. (2007). An examination of the relationship between general life stress, racism-related stress, and psychological health among Black men. *Journal of Counseling Psychology, 54*, 101–9.

Prilleltensky, I. (2001). Value-based praxis in community psychology: Moving toward social justice and social action. *American Journal of Community Psychology, 29*, 747–78.

Simone, M. (1993). Western war machines: Contextualizing psychology in Africa. In L. J. Nicholas (Ed.). *Psychology and oppressions: Critiques and proposals* (pp. 81–127). Johannesburg, RSA: Skotaville Publishers.

Smedley, A. (1999). *Race in North America: Origin and evolution of a worldview* (2nd ed.). Boulder, CO: Westview Press.

Speight, S. L. (2007). Internalized racism: One more piece of the puzzle. *The Counseling Psychologist, 35*, 126–34.

Thomas, H. (1997). *The slave trade: The story of the Atlantic slave trade, 1440–1870*. New York: Simon & Schuster.

Thompson, C. E., & Alfred, D. M. (2009). Black liberation psychology and practice. In H. A. Neville, B. M. Tynes, & S. O. Utsey (Eds.), *Handbook of African American psychology* (pp. 483–94). Thousand Oaks, CA: SAGE Publications.

Triandis, H. C. (1995). The self and social behavior in differing cultural contexts. In N. R. Goldberger, & J. B. Veroff (Eds.), *The culture and psychology reader* (pp. 326–65). New York: New York University Press.

UNAIDS/WHO. (2006). *UNAIDS 2006 Report on the global AIDS epidemic*. Geneva: Author.

U.S. Department of Justice. (2007). *Bureau of Justice Statistics, Bulletin*, NCJ 219416

Utsey, S. O. (1998). Assessing the stressful effects of racism: A review of instrumentation. *Journal of Black Psychology, 24*, 269–88.

Van Wyk, S. B., & Naidoo, A. V. (2006). Broadening mental health services to disadvantaged communities in South Africa. *Journal of Psychology in Africa, 2*, 273–82.

Viljoen, D. L., Gossage, J. P., Adams, C., Jones, K. L., Robinson, L. K., Hoyme, H. E., Snell, C., et al. (2005). The epidemiological characteristics of fetal alcohol syndrome in a South African community of the Western Cape Province. *Journal of Studies on Alcohol, 66*, 593–604.

Wallace, B. C. (2006). Healing collective wounds from racism: The community forum model. In M. C. Constantine & D. W. Sue (Eds.), *Addressing racism: Facilitating cultural competence in mental health and educational settings* (pp. 105–23.) Hoboken, NJ: John Wiley & Sons.

Watts, R. J., & Abdul-Adil, J. (1994). Psychological aspects of oppression and socio-political development: Building young warriors. In R. Newby & T. Manley (Eds.), *The poverty of inclusion, innovation and interventions: The dilemma of the African American underclass*. New Brunswick, NJ: Rutgers University Press.

Watts, R., Griffith, D., & Abdul-Adil, J. (1999). Sociopolitical development as an antidote for oppression: Theory and action. *American Journal of Community Psychology, 27*, 255–72.

Watts, R., & Flanagan, C. (2007). Pushing the envelope on youth civic engagement: A developmental and Liberation Psychology perspective. *Journal of Community Psychology, 35*, 1–14.

White, J. L. (1984). *The psychology of Blacks: An Afro-American perspective*. Englewood Cliffs, NJ: Prentice-Hall.

Williams, D. R., Gonzalez, H. M., Williams, S., Mohammed, S. A., Moomal, H., & Stein, D. J. (2008). Perceived discrimination, race and health in South Africa. *Social Science Medicine, 67*, 441–52.

Williams, D. R., & Mohammed, S. A. (2009). Discrimination and racial disparities in health: Evidence and needed research. *Journal of Behavioral Health, 32*, 20–47.

Williams, D. R., Neighbors, H. W., & Jackson, J. S. (2003). Racial/ethnic discrimination and health: Findings from community studies. *American Journal of Public Health, 93*, 200–8.

Williams, D. R., & Williams-Morris, R. (2000). Racism and mental health: The African-American experience. *Ethnicity and Health, 5*, 243–68.

World Bank Development Group. (2006). '06 World Development indicators. Retrieved May 2, 2008 from http://devdata.worldbank.org/wdi2006/contents/cover.htm

SELF-CHECK EXERCISES

1. Describe the relationship between colonization and the current status of African nations.
2. Outline the four identifying factors of collectivistic cultures. Identify aspects of African culture that would be considered consistent with collectivism.
3. What was Fanon's core idea in relation to the psychological impact of colonization?
4. Define "internalized racism."
5. Why is "Liberation Psychology" an important consideration when working with individuals of African descent?
6. How does the Jamestown Project reflect principles of liberation and empowerment?

FIELD-BASED EXPERIENTIAL EXERCISES

1. Interview individuals living on the continent, Africans who have immigrated to European countries, and individuals of African descent living in the United States or the United Kingdom. Focus the interview on their experience of racism and racial oppression and how they view their racial identity. For example, how does the salience of being Black vary across

these individuals? How does the experience of racism vary across these individuals?

2. Arrange for a group viewing of "500 years later." This film, directed by Owen Alik Shadadah, documents the ongoing impact of the "African holocaust of enslavement and colonialism." Discuss your reactions to the video.
3. Observe a "rites of passage" ceremony and document how this ceremony draws on aspects of African culture that could serve as a model for community empowerment.

MULTIPLE-CHOICE QUESTIONS

1. Scholars see the psychological impact of slavery as:
   a. A healthy adjustment process
   b. A form of intergenerational trauma
   c. Dependent on how many generations the descendents have been in the host country
   d. A function of ego strengths of the individual
   e. Dependent on the region of Africa from which the slaves were brought
2. Which of the following is not a feature of Liberation Psychology?
   a. Developing a strong sense of independence and separation from one's original culture
   b. Challenging social conditions that foster social injustice
   c. Supporting actions against the exploitation of others
   d. Lobbying for the needs of migrant workers
   e. Interventions that develop individual and collective self-determination
3. Which scholars are associated with providing a critical framework for the amelioration of the psychological effects of racial oppression?
   a. Kardiner and Ovesy
   b. Fanon and Martin-Baro
   c. Markus and Kitayama
   d. Kardiner and Kitayama
   e. Nelson and Prilleltensky
4. Prevention programs are more effective and enhanced when they:
   a. Are comprehensive
   b. Target multiple ecological levels
   c. Utilize combined approaches that facilitate individual and collective enhancement
   d. Reduce risk
   e. All of the above
5. Fill in the blank. ___________ is the concept related to the transition from adolescence to adulthood.
   a. Mentoring
   b. Usiko
   c. Maaf
   d. Rites of passage
   e. Generational transitioning
6. Maat is a:
   a. Philosophical system that incorporates both an expression of resistance and spiritual healing
   b. Form of modern slavery
   c. Racist defence mechanism
   d. African cultural rite of passage
   e. Colonist method for disempowering slaves
7. African-born people living in the United States are:
   a. Largely temporary visitors
   b. The consequence of the Diaspora
   c. Illiterate economic migrants
   d. Well educated and upwardly mobile
   e. Inevitably in need of counseling
8. Colonialism resulted in:
   a. The dysfunctionality of all Black families
   b. The urgent need to offer counseling to all people of African origins
   c. The economic advancement of Black nations
   d. Mutuality of purpose
   e. None of these
9. Neo-colonialism led to:
   a. The psychological empowerment of colonized peoples
   b. The renaissance of traditional cultures
   c. Psychological independence and growth
   d. All of the above
   e. None of these

Answers to the multiple-choice questions are provided at the back of the book

PART 2
CONTEXTS OF COUNSELING

Section Editor
Terri Bakker

7 School Counseling

Elias Mpofu, Jacobus G. Maree, Joseph M. Kasayira, and Carol Noela Van der Westhuizen

OVERVIEW. This chapter focuses on the circumstances under which counseling in schools developed in Africa, then examines research and practices in school counseling with some illustrative examples from countries such as Botswana, Malawi, South Africa, Zambia, and Zimbabwe. In addition, the organizational structures within which counseling services are conceived and delivered at the school level are analyzed. Finally, issues in the development of current school counseling services in sub-Saharan African schools are explored.

LEARNING OBJECTIVES

By the end of the chapter, the reader should be able to:

1. Outline the comparative evolutionary history of research and practice in sub-Saharan African countries.
2. Describe the current practices in school counseling in southern Africa.
3. Discuss the importance of professional, legal, and ethical considerations in the provision of school counseling services.
4. Articulate how the practice of school counseling in sub-Saharan African countries can be enhanced.

INTRODUCTION

As learners mature, they experience a variety of challenges for which they may need counseling. School is the place that learners spend most of their daytime, and therefore is a major influence in the development of learners. School is a community within the wider community, and what happens in school, in part, reflects the character of the community from which learners come. The broader community is always in transition, and presents with a myriad of challenges and opportunities that learners and their families transact, and that influence the quality of school life (Lazarus et al., 2006). Inevitably, the purposes served by school counseling depend on the level of development of the educational system in a particular society so that more developed education systems would have better established school counseling services (Mpofu, Peltzer, Shumba, Serpell, & Mogaji, 2005). The more developed education school counseling services address a greater range of counseling needs in learners with appropriate resources, and in a timely fashion.

Learners in sub-Saharan Africa experience many developmental challenges, including those from evolving and underfunded education systems, widespread poverty, fragile sociopolitical systems that generate ever growing numbers of vulnerable families, and very scarce basic social services (see also Chapters 11, 12, and 20, this volume). For many students, the school is a haven of stability in a sea of deprivation and uncertainty. Civic and multilateral organizations seeking to reach learners in sub-Saharan Africa often find schools the natural place to reach larger numbers of learners, and through the school, the learners' families and community leaders.

The school is a complex structure, both in terms of the wide range of developmental needs among its major customers – the students – and also in regard to the multilayered curricula to which students are exposed. The school is a living and growing entity influenced by the real-world transactions in which it engages with external partners such as families, governmental and civic organizations, and private sector enterprises necessary for it to achieve its mission or goals. It is the hub for the regeneration of communities and nations through its ability to impart and transform culture, and for the development of the human resource base for the economy. In the next section, we consider in greater detail the significance of school and related needs in students for whom in-school counseling is a critical resource.

IMPORTANCE, DEFINITION, AND SCOPE OF KEY TERMS AND CONCEPTS

Students need counseling to make the best they can of the school as a resource for development. As noted previously, in African settings, this need is particularly urgent in view of the underdevelopment of school systems on the continent, the greater vulnerability of families and communities from national and global economic influences, consequences of endemic civil strife, poverty, and poorer health care. Students enroll in schools presenting with vulnerabilities imputed on them by the vulnerabilities from the families and communities from which they come. They bring along to their experience of school the resilience they acquired from grappling with socioeconomic disadvantage, including effects of neglect by families, communities, and national governments. Students need counseling to make sense of their personhood, role as learners, community participation, and potential as future leaders of their communities (Brown & Trusty, 2005; Mpofu, Maree, & Oakland, 2009). School counseling entails the provision of educational, vocational, social, and personal services to enhance their development as learners (Bemak, 2000; Mpofu et al., 2009).

Educational Counseling

Educational counseling involves providing learning support to students to achieve maximally on curriculum goals (Johnson & Johnson, 2003; Mpofu & Nyanungo, 1998). Students may receive counseling in areas in which they have significant strengths and limitations. Counselors may use the results of aptitude or ability tests to counsel students on areas of the curriculum where they have potential to excel. They may counsel students on the basis of results from teacher-made tests and other achievement and diagnostic tests. Based on their learning needs, students may get counseling to best direct their learning efforts. Students may receive counseling to inform choices among subjects in the curriculum important to higher education studies or career goals. In addition educational counseling involves working with students to understand and utilize their individual study orientations to best support their learning efforts (Mpofu & Oakland, 2001; Stroud & Reynolds, 2006; Watkins, Akande, & Mpofu, 1994).

Vocational Counseling

Students in the primary and secondary schools in sub-Saharan Africa often lack knowledge about the formal employment sector, and counselors have a vitally important role in providing education on the various jobs available in the local economy. In-school vocational counseling in sub-Saharan Africa typically involves vocational orientation activities such as lectures about job opportunities and career fairs at the school where students can learn from employers and other exhibitors. Vocational counseling involves educating students on potential career options based on their interests, preferences, and abilities. It includes educating students about the preparation they would need for the various careers they may be interested in pursuing post-school. Vocational counseling activities include training students in job search skills, including resume preparation and interview skills. Research could be of help to counselors to assist them to better understand learners' needs and choice of careers. This need is highlighted in Discussion Box 7.1.

Social Development Counseling

The quality of school life influences how learners develop according to the socioeducational opportunities the school provides. School is a microcosm of society, and students need to learn how to function in the school community, including demonstrating qualities of good citizenship. Social development counseling includes learning support to enable students to know and enact appropriate learner roles in the school setting as a learning community and to enhance their positive self-esteem (Mpofu & Thomas, 2006; Watkins et al., 1996). It includes support to learn and use appropriate social skills (Wentzel, 2003a, 2003b). Life-skills counseling is part of social development counseling, and schools in sub-Saharan Africa teach life skills as a curriculum subject (see also later section on typical issues for counseling).

Personal Development Counseling

Personal development counseling seeks to influence student self-perceptions (Greven, Harlaar, Kovas, Chamorrow-Premuzic, & Plomin, 2009) and students with positive self-perceptions (self-concepts) and higher social skills (social competence) are more likely to succeed in school (Elliot, Malecki, & Demaray, 2001;Wentzel, 2003a, 2003b). Positive self-evaluations predict achievement more than IQ scores (Greven et al., 2009). Self-perceptions by students are lenses by which students appraise their learner roles and self-worth. Sources of self-worth among students influence their personal development in that students may be willing to enact certain learner roles only under conditions or contingencies they perceive to support their self-worth. School counseling is important for supporting positive personal development in students, and in particular, their positive self-perceptions.

Contingencies of self-worth are sources of self-perception that are salient to individuals or the groups to which they belong (Crocker & Wolfe, 2001). These contingencies influence the perceptions they hold about the self in relation to domains of life such as school, peer relations, family, and physical self. Individuals will invest more energy in projecting and protecting self-presentations consistent with their priority sources of self-worth. If students are challenged in an area important to their self-worth, they may need supportive counseling to maintain a positive sense of selfhood and to be perceived by others as competent (Mpofu et al., 2007; Mpofu & Watkins, 1997; Wentzel, 2003a).

Emotional intelligence is an aspect of personal development important for in-school counseling. Emotional intelligence includes four separate although interrelated components: perceiving, using, understanding, and managing emotions (Bar On, Maree, & Elias, 2005). It includes the way in which one succeeds in adapting to one's immediate (and changing) surroundings and coping with

Discussion Box 7.1: Understanding the Reasons Why Young People Choose or Do Not Choose a Career (Maree, 2006)

After extensive research, Maree (2006) concluded that the reasons why young people either choose or do not choose a career are unclear and that our understanding of these reasons needs to improve to prevent policy and planning faults (Cosser & du Toit, 2002; Crouch, 2001). Negative perceptions of the lack of employability, in an ever-shrinking labor market for new employees abound, are spurred on by suggestions of ever-increasing unemployment figures in Africa. The implications of these factors for the labor markets could be disastrous in the long term. The growing number of employees dying or leaving professions because of HIV and AIDS, and career systems clogged with inappropriately or inadequately skilled employees, suggest that the crisis of supply and quality may have severe negative consequences for the African labor market. Creative and bold strategies are essential to facilitate career choice and decision making by learners in Africa. New ways are needed to attract talented learners to fields of study to empower them to become professionals capable of aiding social transformation in Africa. The "chronic mismatch between the output of higher education and the needs of a modernising economy" (*National Plan for Higher Education* (NPHE); Department of Education, 2001, p. 3) and the "shortage of highly trained graduates in fields such as science, engineering, technology and commerce [which] has been detrimental to social and economic development," are areas of particular concern. Maree (2006) supports the assertion that career guidance and counseling of any kind will impact positively on learners' aims to further their studies at the tertiary level (Cosser & du Toit, 2002). Clearly, it is vital to conduct research to help professionals understand learners' idiosyncratic needs and their career choice behavior to preempt the labor crisis looming in Africa.

Questions

1. How much do we really know about learners' reasons for choosing or not choosing a career?
2. In particular, why is it essential to conduct research on learners' career choices in Africa?
3. What is meant by "shifts in learner enrollments at tertiary training institutions"?
4. Discuss some reasons why it has become extremely important to facilitate these shifts.

The preceding few paragraphs lead to the deduction that the time has come to develop a framework for school guidance and counseling that is specifically aimed at addressing the idiosyncratic needs and position of African learners. This need is highlighted in the example described in Discussion Box 7.2.

changes. Particularly, it is salient in collectivist African cultures in which socioemotional ability is critical to effective community participation.

Guidance

Guidance entails the provision and dissemination of consequential information to individuals and groups who may have limited access of resources important for their development or to the fulfilment of their goals (Mpofu, 2006). It differs from counseling in being more directive and educational. Aspects of counseling entail some guidance, although the goal of such guidance is typically to facilitate self-exploration with a view to attaining a higher level of self-knowledge. As discussed subsequently, guidance of students is relatively more established in school in sub-Saharan Africa than counseling.

HISTORY OF RESEARCH AND PRACTICE IN SCHOOL COUNSELING IN SUB-SAHARAN AFRICA

The history of school counseling in the sub-Saharan Africa context is tied to the development of formal schooling in the subregion. Formal schooling in sub-Saharan Africa is one of the heritages from Africa's recent colonial past, and particularly the legacy of European settler occupation. European (settler) colonialism maintained a racially based education system, and a whole series of legislative instruments were put in place to establish and maintain the differential educational rights and privileges for Whites and Blacks (Mpofu et al., 2007; Watson & Fouche, 2007).

The Colonial Period

In colonial Africa, Blacks were both completely denied professional counseling and other psychology-related services, or they were provided with minimal services (see also Chapter 8, this volume). Christian missionaries provided schooling to most African communities and with it Christian or religious counseling. The goal was ministering for spiritual salvation, although Christian counseling provided for personal and social counseling for the practice of Christianity in everyday life. The quality of counseling was heavily influenced by the religious denomination that founded the school and area of emphasis varied somewhat within the same Christian counseling (see also Chapter 10, this volume). Some church schools provided vocational counseling and training, and mostly through the industrial education centers that they instituted at residential mission schools. The counseling was for the most part aimed at training convert or prospective students in vocations that could lend jobs in the formal employment sector or for own enterprises in the village communities. Examples of such trade-oriented vocational training provided by the mission schools included brickwork, carpentry, animal husbandry, and market gardening. Generally, educational counseling was neglected, as there were state-imposed enrollment caps for Black students so that only a few highly motivated and capable students remained in school (Mpofu & Nyanungo, 1998).

National governments in the colonial era delayed their involvement in providing school counseling to Black students, and they perceived basic literacy for menial labor positions in the colonial economy to be the inevitable destiny for schooled Blacks. For instance, although school counseling services were instituted in Rhodesian/Zimbabwean schools in 1971, the then Rhodesian government provided such services only to White, Indian, and Colored students (Mpofu & Nyanungo, 1998; Mntungwana-Hadebe, 1994). It was only during 1981 that the South African government introduced "school guidance" (which included a career education component) as a subject in Black schools, possibly as a "palliative following the Soweto uprisings of 1976" (Akhurst & Mkhize, 2006, p. 142), while "school guidance" had become a compulsory subject in White schools as far back as 1967. In 1984 the Human Sciences Research Council Guidance Working Committee recommended the introduction of school guidance in all schools in South Africa. As part of its institutionalization, school guidance was included in all teacher education programs in South Africa around 1981. A four-year diploma course was introduced in all training institutions (Marais, 1987). On the other hand, in other sub-Saharan African countries such as Botswana, Malawi, Zambia, and Zimbabwe serious efforts to establish full-fledged programs was made after independence.

In Botswana, churches managed schools for some time; later they were run and owned by tribes (*merafe*) and managed by the Tribal School Committees on the strength of the African Education Proclamation No. 26 of 1938 (Ministry of Education, Republic of Botswana, 2008). Similarly, in Zambia, school counseling was nonexistent during the colonial times except insofar as it occurred in traditional settings outside schools.

Although professional school counseling was not institutionalized in many sub-Saharan African countries before independence from European colonialism, some forms of guidance and counseling were instituted in the form of lay counseling and advice given by teachers and elders from the community in line with the African tradition of raising learners. Communities in the sub-Saharan region had their own traditional systems in the provision of adolescence and marriage counseling. Some aspects of the system continue to exist today.

Postcolonial Period

The advent of independence from colonialism was accompanied by efforts to regularize the provision of counseling services in schools. For example, at independence from Britain in 1966, the Botswana government passed the Education Law that ended the Tribal School Committee system so that schools were the direct responsibility of the central government. This legal instrument for the state to provide education enabled policy initiatives toward the institutionalization of school guidance and counseling in Botswana schools. For example, in 1996, the Policy Guidelines on the Implementation of Guidance and Counseling in Botswana were instituted and directed schools to become places for equipping young Batswana with skills to promote lifelong functioning as responsible, self-respecting citizens (Ministry of Education, Department of Curriculum Development and Evaluation, 1996). In Malawi, a career guidance forum was launched through the Ministry of Education and Culture in 1988. The purpose of the forum was to provide a two-way communication between the Ministry of Education and Culture and its education institutions with regard to education and careers in Malawi (Ministry of Education, Malawi, 1988). Further, the Malawi Ministry of Education and Culture distributed to schools a career guidance forum publication that provided teachers and students with information on how best career counseling needs could be addressed. Subsequently, the Ministry of Education and Culture in Malawi introduced career guidance syllabuses for secondary schools (Ministry of Education, Republic of Malawi, 1991). The syllabus was an important first step in introducing formal school counseling in Malawi schools (Maluwa-Banda, 1998). The Zimbabwean government introduced school guidance and counseling to all schools in 1987 (Ministry of Education, Sports & Culture, 1987). The school counseling services has a life-skills orientation and provided only to high school students. The Zambian government introduced school guidance and counseling in 1967, under the auspices of the Ministry of Science, Technology and Vocational Training. Formal psychological assessment started around the time of Independence with the Northern Rhodesia Mental Abilities Survey (McArthur, Irvine, & Brimble, 1964) and the Educational and Occupational Assessment Service within the government's Ministry of Labor and Social Services.

CURRENT PRACTICES IN SCHOOL COUNSELING

In many sub-Saharan African countries, school counseling services are conceived within the Ministry of Education. The services are provided by a unit, division, or a department represented at the Ministry's headquarters. For instance, in Botswana, the guidance and counseling unit is part of the Department of Curriculum Development and Evaluation; in Zambia, School Guidance Services

Case Study 7.1: Schooling in Developmental Perspective: The Case of Tebogo

In 2003, the mathematics teacher of Lebo (pseudonym), a young man who lived in a squatter camp with his unemployed mother and five siblings, contacted the University of Pretoria's Student Counseling Center to inquire about the possibility of having Lebo assessed and counseled regarding the choice of a field of study and a future career. Lebo was subsequently brought to the attention of Prof. Maree and Dr. Van der Westhuizen (both of whom were deeply involved with outreach programs). Lebo (who had until then achieved above average marks throughout his life, despite his depressing surroundings) was assessed by Prof. Maree and decided to study teaching. He was awarded a loan (depending on his academic achievements, part of this loan was to be converted into a bursary). However, it took some time before Lebo began to find his feet in his new environment. During the first number of months at university, Lebo was, for example, assigned a mentor, received classes in life orientation (including classes on how to spend his money wisely, address his lecturers, study, and take part in student activities), and provided the most with basic necessities by Prof. Maree and Dr. Van der Westhuizen. In his own words: "It took me eighteen months to adapt to this completely foreign country before I eventually began to settle in. Very few people understand what a young Black student from a disadvantaged environment is up against when first he arrives at university. I was certainly not prepared at all at school for that. I never received career counseling at school, I was never prepared for what awaited me in a tertiary environment; in fact, virtually everything was totally new and strange and bewildering. If it hadn't been for the support that I received, I would have dropped out after a few weeks." Lebo qualified in 2007 and subsequently decided to continue with postgraduate studies.

Questions

1. What are the most essential messages to school counselors, as well as education authorities that are clear from Lebo's story?
2. In which ways can the strategies employed in the case under discussion be employed, not only in similar contexts, but also on a larger scale?

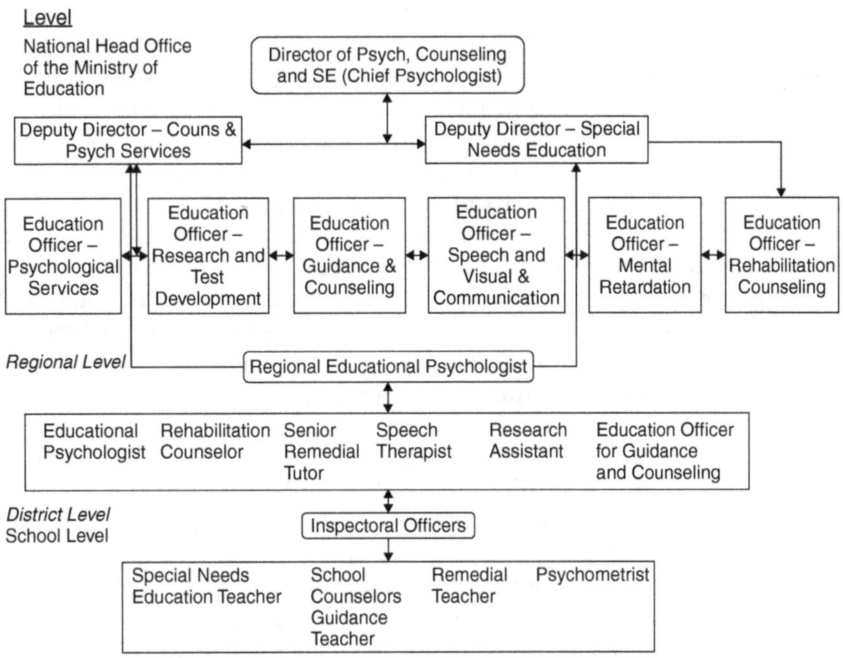

Figure 7.1. Organization chart of psychological services, counseling, and special needs services in an African country.

Unit is responsible for the guidance and counseling program (Kayungwa, personal communication, July, 2009); while in Zimbabwe, guidance and counseling is housed under the school's Psychological Services and Special Needs Education Division (Mpofu, Mutepfa, Chireshe, & Kasayira, 2007). The administrative structure of an ideal school guidance and counseling program in a sub-Saharan country is presented in Figure 7.1.

Questions

1. Describe the possible roles of professionals listed in Figure 7.1 by level.
2. What do you perceive to be the strengths and limitations of the school counseling services structure presented in Figure 7.1?
3. Explain the multidisciplinary character of school counseling as a profession?

In this section we consider the organization of school counseling services in sub-Saharan Africa, typical practices, and the qualifications and experience of personnel who deliver these services. We consider the role of social services allied to school counseling in addressing the needs of students that enhance their school adjustment.

Organizational Structure and Provision of Services

The organizational structure that manages the Guidance and Counseling program at school level varies from country to country. However, typically, the services are provided at the high school level, and by a Guidance and Counseling Committee comprising teachers. For example, in Zimbabwe, the Guidance and Counseling Committee is constituted very much like any other subject department, with a Guidance and Counseling Coordinator who is the equivalent of a head of department for any teaching subject. Working with the Coordinator are teachers responsible for the pastoral care of individual streams of classes (also called Form masters/mistresses). The appointment of a member of the teaching staff to the post of Guidance and Counseling Coordinator at the school is over and above the usual teaching assignment of every teacher (Moeletsi, 2005; Mokopakgosi, 2005). Botswana has more broadly conceived school guidance and counseling services in the sense that they span both primary and secondary school levels (Ministry of Education, 1993, 1994). Each primary school in Botswana is required to have a school guidance and counseling teacher (Ministry of Education, 2000). The duties of the Guidance and Counseling coordinator include:

- In-servicing other members of the staff who are from time to time called upon to offer Guidance and Counseling service to the various classes
- Conducting a needs assessment and drawing up a Guidance and Counseling Program that addresses the needs of the students and other needs as perceived by the staff and community
- Keeping detailed records of learners and setting up Guidance and Counseling resources that can be used by all the staff involved in providing Guidance and Counseling
- Networking with Commerce and Industry and other community resources for inputs into the Guidance and Counseling Program

Like in Zimbabwe, in Malawi, some schools use the committee system. The committee's counseling function is perceived by the school administration to complement the student discipline role. For example, students who breach school rules may receive punishment from the school administration before they receive counseling from the guidance and counseling committee members. Membership to the committee is based on seniority and strong religious inclinations, among other virtues (J. Banda, personal communication, August 26, 2009).

Qualifications of Guidance and Counseling Teachers

The majority of guidance and counseling teachers in sub-Saharan Africa have no relevant training in counseling (Mpofu et al., 2005). The Guidance and Counseling teacher at the school level is appointed as a subject specialist in some areas and then takes on the extra duty of being a guidance teacher. Training for teaching guidance is typically included within the teacher education program, and varies widely across countries in depth and focus. For instance, most life orientation teachers in South Africa have attended only one- to three-day courses on teaching life orientation. One provincial education department staff member is responsible for visiting up to 150 schools in a district to "provide assistance to the [life orientation] teachers to develop learning materials, administer psychometric tests and to provide in-service training" (Kay & Fretwell, 2003, p. 28). Pre-service training of Malawian primary school teachers on Life skills for HIV and AIDS Education includes a few lectures on the following: Basic facts about HIV and AIDS; sexuality and sexual relationships; values and attitudes; and preventing and coping with HIV and AIDS (Malawi Government, MIE and USAID/DFID, 2004). The Zambian and Zimbabwean life-skills teacher preparation curriculum is similar to that for Malawi.

In Zambia, guidance teachers hold relevant qualifications for appointment to their positions. The minimum professional qualifications for appointment to that position are the Diploma in Guidance, Counseling and Placement (DGCP) from the Technical and Vocational Teachers' College (TVTC) or the National In-Service Teachers College (NISTCOL), or a bachelor's degree in guidance and counseling from the Zambia Open University (ZAOU). Guidance teachers are expected to be affiliated with one of the following professional bodies: the National Guidance and Counseling Association of Zambia; the Zambia Counseling Council (ZCC); or Guidance, Counseling and Youth Development for Africa (GCYDA), headquartered in Malawi.

Guidance and counseling is a student development subject and not examined for high school graduation requirements. As a result of the appointment of generalist teachers to teach the learning area, it is not highly regarded by learners (Van Deventer, 2008).Training in guidance and counseling is increasingly widely available in several sub-Saharan countries, making it likely that qualified school counselors will be appointed to such positions.

Typical Services Offered

School guidance and counseling services in sub-Saharan Africa tend to be provided as a school subject rather than a professional service. For instance, students follow a life skills curriculum taught by guidance teachers. The life skills curriculum is timetabled to be taught for one to two hours per week (Flederman, 2008; Van Deventer, 2008). For example, in South Africa the life orientation program subsumes the school guidance and counseling service, and is a compulsory learning area for all students ([Revised] National Curriculum Statement; Flederman, 2008, p. 26). The life orientation curriculum covers student counseling in the areas of personal development, community and environmental health, social development and citizenship, personal development, physical education, and career guidance (Du Toit, Van der Merwe, & Rossouw, 2007). The Malawian secondary school guidance and counseling module includes the following topics: educational guidance; vocational guidance; personal and social guidance; and adolescence counseling (Ministry of Education, Republic of Malawi, 2005).

The guidance lessons are conducted using a wide variety of approaches, some of which are lectures by teachers and guest speakers; debates on topical issues such as gender roles in the modern world; role play for job interviewers and interviewees; group investigations on such topics as the role of the individual in the community; field trips to commercial and industrial sites; and case studies of successful members of various communities that may be inspirational to the students and other people.

Personal–social counseling is offered by the school guidance coordinator and members of the guidance and counseling committee. Many students have experienced the prolonged illness and death of one or both parents, and the consequent needs for emotional support are widely recognized. There is a high level of public awareness of the vulnerability of adolescents to HIV infection through unprotected sexual intercourse. Much of the activity of guidance teachers in high schools appears to be concentrated on preventive health education in this regard, including the distribution of advisory literature and the promotion and support of anti-AIDS student clubs. In many cases these activities benefit from financial sponsorship by programs emanating from outside the school system. In sub-Saharan school settings, there is a tendency for the counselors to prescribe solutions for learners who are often willing to have solutions prescribed for them.

Allied Services

As can be seen in Figure 7.1, school counseling is a multidisciplinary service and intersects the services of school (or educational) psychologists, school counselors, educators, and special education needs personnel. Often, social workers and clinical psychologists may be called upon to provide ancillary services important to comprehensive interventions for student welfare (Mpofu, 2003). We consider the role of school psychologists in supporting the school guidance and counseling services in sub-Saharan Africa settings.

School Psychologists

School or educational psychologists provide psychological services that include conducting individual assessments and offering counseling to learners. According to Mpofu and colleagues (2009), educational psychologists are involved in assessment, diagnosis, and intervention to optimize functioning in the broad context of learning and development. In the realm of psychological assessment, they perform assessments of cognitive, personality, emotional, and neuropsychological functions of people in relation to learning and development in which they have been trained. They identify and diagnose psychopathology in relation to learning and development and identify and diagnose a broad range of barriers to learning and development. Post-assessment, educational psychologists characteristically (1) apply psychological interventions to enhance, promote, and facilitate optimal learning and development; (2) perform a range of therapeutic interventions in relation to learning and development; and (3) advise on policy development and program design, particularly on the development of policy applicable to a variety of sectors and issues.

The extent to which educational psychologists are engaged in these functions varies from country to country. Where the role and functions may be similar, the emphasis per role may be different (see Table 7.1).

Adapted from Mpofu, Peltzer, Shumba, Serpell, & Mogaji (2005).

QUESTIONS

1. Speculate on possible reasons for country differences in role counseling functions for school psychologists.
2. What additional information would you need to better understand the role and function of school psychologists in the six sub-Saharan African countries?

As can be observed from Table 7.1 across countries, educational psychologists carry multilayered functions, with major involvement in the delivery of counseling services.

School psychologists in several sub-Saharan African countries conduct psychological assessment for various educational counseling purposes. Educators, parents, and students in Botswana seek psychological assessment for student counseling in the following areas: aptitude

Research Box 7.1: Traditional Play as a Therapeutic Tool

Kekae-Moletsane, M. (2008) *Masekitlana*: South African traditional play as a therapeutic tool in child psychotherapy. *South African Journal of Psychology*, *38*(2), 367–75.

Background: Research has shown that learners experience their world on an experiential level rather than on a cognitive level. They use play as a medium to express both their feelings and their experiences. Thus, play forms the foundation for learners' more cognitive styles in adulthood.

Objective: The purpose of this study was to exemplify the importance of indigenous knowledge, and, more particularly, the value, effectiveness, and importance of *masekitlana* (a traditional Sesotho game) in administering psychotherapy to learners in severe distress.

Method: A case study was employed. The emphasis was on a traumatized child participant who was referred for psychotherapy because he displayed severe signs of posttraumatic stress disorder (PTSD) after witnessing the murder of his mother and grandmother. The learner refused to respond to the administration of standardized tests, but instead responded positively to *masekitlana* during the process of psychotherapy. Kekae-Moletsane (2008) analyzed and interpreted the learner's drawings, play, behaviors, and reactions during the first five therapy sessions.

Results: The participant showed great improvement after the first five sessions and the majority of PTSD symptoms had in fact disappeared by the end of the fifth session. Seemingly, the learner's fears were resolved to the extent that he started playing with all his toys again. Furthermore, he started talking about his parents and grandmother and remembered things that he used to do with his mother and grandmother. Sad memories were replaced with happy ones and he was transformed into a cheerful, energetic, talkative, and funny young boy.

Conclusions: The research suggests that not only *masekitlana*, but also probably all forms of traditional play may be utilized during psychotherapy with learners to facilitate the healing of miscellaneous forms of pathology. The author concludes by calling for a renewed emphasis on research about African culture and psychology and suggests that an inclusive approach to psychology be accepted in Africa (*id est*, all cultures should be embraced and not one or more to the exclusion of others).

Questions

1. Which traditional forms of intervention can you think of in addition to *masekitlana* that can be applied to resolve psychopathology in learners?
2. What are the implications of this type of intervention (and its success) for school guidance and counseling in an African context?
3. In your opinion, to what extent (and why) does this case study confirm the view that an inclusive approach to the theory and practice of school guidance and counseling presents counselors with the "best" opportunity to resolve the type of pathology described here?

assessment, motivation, individual needs, communication skills, societal influence, socialization, and personality (see Figure 7.2). In some cases they develop intervention programs that could be instituted in ordinary classes as a way of facilitating inclusive education, including for the purpose of placing learners with special educational needs.

QUESTIONS

1. What factors may influence priority assessment needs for school counseling in a country?
2. What use could school counselors make of assessment information in the domains mapped in Figure 7.2 in their practice?

However, the services of school psychologists in many sub-Saharan African countries are often unavailable as a result of the dire shortage of appropriately trained personnel.

LEGAL, PROFESSIONAL, AND ETHICAL ISSUES

In most sub-Saharan African countries, teachers who offer guidance and counseling are not professional counselors. In most cases these teachers are allowed to offer counseling in schools based on their teaching qualifications, which do not necessarily contain any elements of counseling theory or practice. In the absence of a body that oversees the work of the teachers who provide guidance and counseling and that define their professional area, ethical breaches are likely to be prevalent (Foster, Young, & Hermann, 2005; Richards, 2004).

Pending the adoption of legal and professional standards for school counseling, Ministries of Education in the subregion should consider training personnel involved in the use of positive ethics as personal guidelines in the delivery of school counseling services. Positive ethics emphasize practices that enable or empower learners in the areas of functioning important to them (Bush, 2010).

Research Box 7.2: Violence Prevention in Schools

Sathiparsad, R. (2003). Addressing barriers to learning participation: Violence prevention in schools. *Perspectives in Education*, *21*(3), 99–111.

Background: Research has shown that South African schools have become sites of escalating violence for many thousands of learners. This deeply disturbing trend can probably be best described as a barrier to learning, since it denies learners the opportunity to participate fully in society or to realize their potential optimally.

Objective: The purpose of this study was to demonstrate the potential value and efficiency of implementing a conflict resolution program by establishing whether it created consciousness of the benefits of adopting a nonviolent approach to and applying nonviolent strategies to conflict resolution.

Method: A conflict resolution program was implemented, containing elements of both a quantitative and a qualitative research design. The conflict resolution program was developed during phase 1, and in phase 2, facilitators were trained to implement the program. In phase 3, samples were drawn (the program was to be implemented at three racially integrated, coeducational schools). The program was implemented during phase 4 and data were analyzed during phase 5. Pre- and post-test responses to a vignette (conflict scenario) were eventually compared.

Results: A marked post-test decrease in aggressive responses in the face of conflict emerged among participants when compared with pre-test responses. Furthermore, the majority (approximately 54 percent) of participants indicated that they would adopt a problem-solving approach to conflict resolution (post-test) compared with approximately 13 percent pre-test.

Conclusion: The research suggests that the conflict resolution program developed and implemented did indeed create an awareness of the need for and advantages attached to adopting nonviolent responses to conflict. Seemingly, developing and implementing similar conflict resolution programs in (South) Africa on a broader scale (as is done elsewhere in the world) holds much promise. However, sociohistorical factors need to be accounted for before an effective strategy can be developed for all schools. Furthermore, this type of program should ideally become part of the school curriculum, while the focus should be on the transformation of the entire spectrum of education and training services.

Questions

1. To what extent and why can lack of ability to solve conflict be regarded as a barrier to learning?
2. Generally, to what extent can this type of intervention impact positively on conflict resolution and violence prevention in Africa?
3. Discuss some of the caveats to the development and implementation of this type of program in schools in Africa.
4. What are your experiences regarding conflict resolution in schools? How do you feel about the potential of this type of program to facilitate a safer environment in our schools, one that is more conducive to learning than the current environment?

In Research Box 7.2, an educational psychological intervention program to prevent violence in schools is described (Sathiparsad, 2003).

ISSUES OF RESEARCH AND OTHER FORMS OF SCHOLARSHIP

One cross-cutting challenge seems to be the human power that is involved. For instance, even with a long history of powerful professional associations and international networks as in South Africa, there is acute understaffing of school counseling services. The vast majority of the teachers who are in charge of counseling in schools do not have a counseling qualification of any kind. There is great urgency for training more counselors at the correct level of competence in all the countries. Sadly, there is no controlling body to regulate the activities of the various professionals that offer counseling in schools. The regulation of school counseling services would add to the quality of services and also accountability in their delivery. In countries in which school counseling is nonexistent, counselors working in school settings could affiliate with existing allied professional associations to form interest groups that would be the nucleus for growing full-fledged professional associations (Mpofu et al., 2005).

School counseling services in sub-Saharan Africa tend to provide guidance more than they do counseling. The limitation may, in part, be from the shortage of appropriately trained counselors as previously discussed. Professional counselor preparation for school counselors in sub-Saharan Africa should be responsive to the sociocultural

Table 7.1. Roles, functions, and perceived adequacy of training of educational psychologists*

Role	Botswana (n = 14)	Malawi (n = 1)	Nigeria (n = 28)	South Africa (n = 32)	Zambia (n = 3)	Zimbabwe (n = 12)
Consultation						
Academics	Yes (86)	Yes	Yes (84)	Yes (57)	Yes (100)	Yes (67)
Social Behavior	Yes (60)	Yes	Yes (63)	Yes (82)	Yes (67)	Yes (75)
Guidance and Counseling	Yes (53)		Yes (81)	Yes (75)	Yes (67)	Yes (75)
Health-related	No (73)	Yes	No (69)	Yes (79)	No (100)	No (75)
Major Functions and Importance*						
Special education eligibility	No (85)	No	^{1}Yes (72)	^{1}Yes (64)	Yes/No (50)	^{1}Yes (58)
Career counseling	^{3}No (85)	^{3}No	^{2}Yes (59)	No (54)	^{1}Yes (67)	No (66)
Grief Counseling of students	^{2}No (57)	^{2}No	^{4}No (78)	^{2}Yes (68)	$^{2.5}$Yes (67)	No (58)
Preventive health counseling	^{1}Yes (79)	^{1}No	^{4}No (69)	^{3}Yes (68)	$^{2.5}$Yes (67)	^{2}Yes (83)
Report writing	Yes (64)	No	No (66)	Yes (82)	Yes (67)	No (58)
Parenting skills	Yes (79)	No	No (59)	No (53)	Yes/No (50)	^{3}Yes (67)
Perceived Adequacy of Training						
Basic	Inadequate–substantial	Thorough	Thorough	Substantial	Substantial	Thorough
On-the-job	Inadequate–substantial	Substantial	Thorough	Thorough	Substantial	Substantial
In-service	Inadequate–substantial	—	Substantial	Thorough	Substantial	Substantial

*The numbers in parentheses are percentages of participants endorsing (Yes) or not endorsing (No) a particular role or function for school psychologists in their country. Superscripts are ranked importance ratings by function or role.

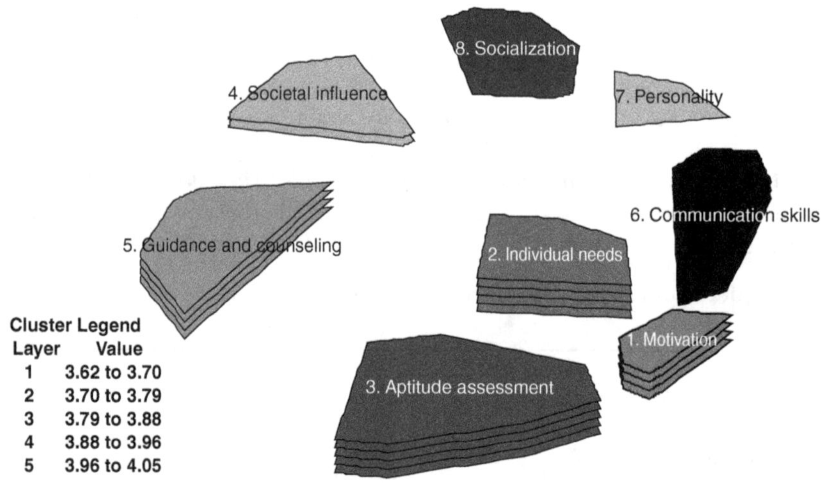

Figure 7.2. Aspects of student counseling needs valued by educators, parents, and students in Botswana schools. Higher stacked clusters portend areas of relative importance compared to others (Mpofu, Maree, & Oakland, 2009).

context of practice to enhance the relevance and appropriateness of the services provided. Appropriate frameworks for the delivery of socioculturally appropriate school counseling services should be developed in consultation with educators, students, parents, and other advocates for students in the community.

The preceding few paragraphs lead to the deduction that the time has come to develop a framework for school guidance and counseling that is specifically aimed at addressing the idiosyncratic needs and positions of African learners. This need is highlighted in the example described in Discussion Box 7.2.

A framework for the delivery of school counseling services in sub-Saharan African school is proposed in Figure 7.1. It is essential to use a demand-driven framework or one that is responsive to the needs of learners in

Discussion Box 7.2: Pointers for Theory, Research, and Practice in Guidance and Counseling (Perry, 2009)

Perry (2009), in a recent article in the *South African Journal for Higher Education*, asserts that guidance and counseling must adjust to a rapidly changing twenty-first century landscape of work, information, and technology, characterized by promise, on the one hand, and uncertainty, on the other. These inequalities are exacerbated by the numerous changes brought about by the information age and the phenomenal growth in and acceptance of the global economy. Perry (2009) emphasizes the fact that school guidance and counseling finds itself in the middle of a paradigm shift in which the important influences of culture and sociopolitical context are highlighted. The author provides the following pointers for theory, research, and practice with secondary school learners by using a "psychology of working" perspective. He highlights the roles of self-determination theory, critical consciousness, and social support as mechanisms for encouraging and stimulating school engagement and preventing school dropout.

The author emphasizes the fact that North American theorists have created their own models of guidance and counseling. Yet, despite the special emphasis and unique language endorsed, theorists agree that guidance and counseling cannot be accurately understood or successfully applied without a sound understanding of how social contexts and systems proffer meaning and purpose. This specific trend has led to an increase in studies that use non-traditional methods (including qualitative and multiple methods), to conduct research on diverse populations and not only on typical White, middle-class learners.

Perry (2009) stresses the fact that the success of future research will depend on its grounding in theoretical principles, its emphasis on clear and measurable goals, basing it on empirical evidence, taking into account culture, as well as bringing together multiple approaches (Hage et al., 2007). An interdisciplinary approach and collaboration with school-linked programs is important, however, and it should be noted that there could be a measure of resistance to such an approach.

Questions

1. Which "paradigm shift that emphasizes the important influences of culture and sociopolitical context" does Perry refer to, and how does this shift affect the theory and practice of guidance and counseling in Africa?
2. Discuss some determining factors in regard to the success of future research in guidance and counseling.

their diversity. Regrettably, in the vast majority of African countries, these services are still available only to those who can afford the services of a private professional school counselor, thereby cementing existing inequalities. As a result, many thousands of learners with vast potential never get the opportunity to realize their potential and contribute to the economies of their respective countries.

The need for training and regular retraining of all persons involved with school counseling (e.g., guidance teachers, officers, and other users and consumers) is a sine qua non. All too often teachers with little or no training in psychology are appointed as, for example, life orientation teachers. Since these colleagues offer an essential and crucially important service (administering, e.g., career counseling to learners), they deserve to be treated with the same amount of respect as other teachers (e.g., mathematics teachers). In addition, training of professionals in the field of school counseling on the ethical use of assessment instruments is imperative, and a Continuing Professional Development (CPD) system should ideally be instituted to ensure that these colleagues become life-long learners in this rapidly evolving field.

Collaboration and cooperation between all stakeholders at all levels is non-negotiable. Collaboration between psychologists registered in various categories – between school psychologists, school counselors, and guidance teachers; between different categories of schools (e.g., private and public), different levels of schooling (primary and secondary) and tertiary training institutions; between different African countries respectively; and between African and non-African countries – is vitally important to facilitate cross-fertilization at the various levels.

It is necessary to train counselors and guidance teachers alike in postmodern paradigms and not only traditional ones. Lessons learned elsewhere should be kept in mind: It is, for instance, necessary to avoid the classical pitfall of over-reliance on a positivist approach. Instead, the global movement toward implementing multiple methods during assessment and guidance (e.g., adopting a qualitative–quantitative approach) needs to be introduced into African school guidance systems as well. In other words, one approach can no longer be overemphasized at the expense of the other.

It seems important to stress the fact that in providing school counseling, a deficit model should to be avoided. The emphasis in testing, assessment, and practice should be on identifying strengths, too, instead of focusing only on weaknesses, pathology, or problems. The global movement toward focusing on solutions instead of problems is an idea whose time has come.

Lastly, research on the issues referred to in this chapter (and others, including but not limited to issues of inclusion, the importance of emotional intelligence training, giftedness, etc.) is important, and counselors; and in particular, guidance teachers need to be trained in the skill of conducting research and disseminating research results. Realization has dawned that these practitioners have access to a gold mine of information that needs to be tapped into and unearthed. Gone are the days when guidance teachers could work in relative isolation, never sharing their experiences with colleagues.

SUMMARY AND CONCLUSIONS

School counseling is an essential service to support students in their development. In African school settings, students experience many challenges to their quality of schooling from deprivations in their families and communities. Most education systems in sub-Saharan Africa are underdeveloped and under-resourced, so that they offer only limited in-school counseling services. Nonetheless, the foundations for comprehensive counseling services are in place in several sub-Saharan African countries from a recognition by national governments of the importance of school counseling to quality of education and the institutionalization of school counseling services in most countries in sub-Saharan Africa.

Prospectively, comprehensive school counseling programs will evolve out of the currently guidance focused services, with more trained professional counselors taking up positions as school counselors. The role of guidance teacher may still be needed to meet the urgent information needs of students, many of whom may be limited in their access of basic knowledge acquisition skills or resources from the effects of poverty and underdevelopment. Guidance teachers could work under the direction and supervision of professional counseling services to be more responsive to students presenting with needs for which counseling would be more appropriate. Socioculturally appropriate school counseling services are possible from taking into account priority needs for counseling by students and their families.

REFERENCES

Akhurst, J., & Mkhize, N. J. (2006). Career education in South Africa. In G. B. Stead & M. B. Watson (Eds.), *Career psychology in the South African context* (pp. 139–53). Pretoria, South Africa: Van Schaik.

Bar-On, R., Maree, J. G., & Elias, M. (2005). (Eds.). *Educating people to be emotionally intelligent*. New York: Praeger.

Bemak, F. (2000). Transforming the role of the counselor to provide leadership in educational reform through collaboration. *Professional School Counseling*, *3*, 323–31.

Brown, D., & Trusty, J. (2005). Designing and leading comprehensive school counseling programs: Promoting student competence and meeting student needs. Belmont, CA: Thomson Brooks/Cole.

Bush, S. (2010). Legal and professional issues. In E. Mpofu & T. Oakland (Eds.), *Assessment in rehabilitation and health* (pp. 22–36). Upper Saddle, NJ: Pearson.

Cosser, M., & du Toit, J. (2002). Factors affecting student choice behaviour in the course of secondary education with particular reference to entry into higher education. Research Report. Pretoria: HSRC.

Crocker, J., & Wolfe, C. T. (2001). Contingencies of self-worth. *Psychological Review*, *108*, 593–623.

Crouch, L. (2001). Turbulence or orderly change? Teacher supply and demand in the age of AIDS. Pretoria: Department of Education.

Department of Education. (2001). National plan for higher education. Pretoria: Department of Education.

du Toit, D., Van der Merwe, N., & Rossouw, J. P. (2007). Return of physical education to the curriculum: Problems and challenges facing schools in South African communities. *African Journal for Physical Health Education, Recreation and Dance (AJPHERD)*, *13*(3), 241–53.

Elliot, S. N., Malecki, C. K., & Demaray, M. K. (2001). New directions in social skills assessment and intervention for elementary and middle school students. *Exceptionality*, *9*, 19–32.

Flederman, P. (2008). Navigational tools for learners, really? What is available, what are the challenges and what should be done? Report undertaken on behalf of SAQA (South African Qualifications Authority). Pretoria: SAQA.

Foster, L. H., Young, J. S., & Hermann, M. (2005). The work activities of professional school counselors: Are the National Standards being addressed? *Professional School Counseling*, *8*, 313–21.

Greven, C. U., Harlaar, N., Kovas, Y., Chamorro-Premuzic, T., & Plomin, R. (2009). More than just IQ: School achievement is predicted by self-perceived abilities – But for genetic rather than environmental reasons. *Current Directions in Psychological Science*, *20*, 753–62.

Hage, S. M., Romano, J. L., Conyne, R. K., Kenny, M., Matthews, C., Schwartz, J. P., & Waldo, M. (2007). Best practice guidelines on prevention practice, research, training, and social advocacy for psychologists. *The Counselling Psychologist*, *35*(4), 493–566.

Johnson, S., & Johnson, C. C. (2003). Results-based guidance: A systems approach to student support programs. *Professional School Counseling*, *6*, 180–4.

Kay, L. L. E., & Fretwell, D. H. (2003). Public policies and career development: A framework for the design of career information, guidance and counselling services in developing countries. Country Report on South Africa, World Bank, April 15.

Kekae-Moletsane, M. (2008). *Masekitlana*: South African traditional play as a therapeutic tool in child psychotherapy. *South African Journal of Psychology*, *38*(2), 367–75.

Lazarus, S., Bojuwoye, O., Chireshe, R., Myambo, K., Akotia, C., Mogaji, A., & Tchombe, T. (2006). Community psychology in Africa: Views from across the continent. *Journal of Psychology in Africa*, *16*(2), 147–60.

Malawi Government, MIE and USAID/DFID. (2004). Life skills for HIV and AIDS Education for teacher training in Malawi: A training manual for use by tutors in the pre-service training of primary school teachers. Malawi: Author.

Maluwa-Banda, D. W. (1998). School counsellors' perceptions of a guidance and counselling programme in Malawi's secondary schools. *British Journal of Guidance and Counselling*, *26*(2),287–95.

Marais, J. L. (1987). Guidance and counselling in the Republic of South Africa: A future perspective. *Proceedings of the Council of Psychologists 45th Annual Convention*, New York, August 22–26.

Maree, J. G. (2006). Current issues in South African career counselling and the availability of teachers in science and technology. *Psychological Reports*, *98*, 151–2.

McArthur, R. S., Irvine, S. H., & Brimble, A. R. (1964). *The Northern Rhodesia Mental Abilities Survey, 1963*. Communication No. 27. Lusaka: Rhodes Livingstone Institute: University of Zambia Press.

Ministry of Education. (1993). *Report of the National Commission on Education*. Gaborone, Botswana: Government Printer.

Ministry of Education. (1994). *The Revised National Policy on Education*. Gaborone: Gaborone, Botswana: Government Printer.

Ministry of Education. (1996). Policy Guide-Lines on the Implementation of Guidance and Counselling in Botswana Education System. Guidance and Counselling Division. Gaborone, Botswana: Author.

Ministry of Education, Department of Curriculum Development and Evaluation. (1996). *The Policy Guidelines on the Implementation of Guidance and Counselling in Botswana's Education System*. Gaborone, Botswana: Author.

Ministry of Education. (2002). Primary School Guidance and Counselling Curriculum Guidelines. Gaborone: Guidance and Counselling Division.

Ministry of Education and Culture, Republic of Malawi. (1991). *Career Guidance Forum*, Issue No. 2, May 1991. Malawi: Author.

Ministry of Education, Republic of Malawi. (2005). Resource material for secondary school management, Module 5: Guidance and counselling. Lilongwe: Author.

Ministry of Education, Sports & Culture. (1987). Director's Circular no. 23. Implementation guidelines for the institutionalization of the guidance and counselling program in all primary and secondary schools. Harare: Ministry of Education, Sport and Culture.

Mntungwana-Hadebe, J. A. (1994). History of special education in Zimbabwe. *Teacher in Zimbabwe Newsletter*, August 31, 7–12.

Moeletsi, B. (2005). An investigation on the implementation of guidance and counselling in Botswana primary schools. Gaborone: University of Botswana.

Mokopakgosi, M. L. (2004). Challenges faced by senior teacher guidance in implementing guidance in primary schools. Gaborone: University of Botswana.

Mpofu, E. (2002). Psychology in Africa: Challenges and prospects. *International Journal of Psychology*, *37*, 179–86.

Mpofu, E. (2003). Conduct disorder: Presentation, treatment options and cultural efficacy in an African setting. *International Journal of Disability, Community and Rehabilitation*, *2*(1), http://www.ijdcr.ca/VOL02_01_CAN/articles/mpofu.shtml.

Mpofu, E., Maree, J. G., & Oakland, T. (2009). *Developing a framework for the use of psychometric tests in Botswana schools*. Gaborone, Botswana: Ministry of Educationn and Skills Development.

Mpofu, E., Mutepfa, M. M., Chireshe, R., & Kasayira, J. M. (2007). School psychology in Zimbabwe. In S. R. Jimerson, T. Oakland, & P. Farrell (Eds.), *The handbook of international school psychology* (pp. 437–52). Thousand Oaks, CA: SAGE Publications.

Mpofu, E., & Nyanungo, K. R. L. (1998). Educational and psychological testing in Zimbabwean schools: Past, present and future. *European Journal of Psychological Assessment,14*, 71–90.

Mpofu, E., & Oakland, T. (2001). Predicting school achievement in African school settings using Bigg's Learning Process Questionnaire. *South African Journal of Psychology*, *31*, 20–8.

Mpofu, E., Peltzer, K., Shumba, A., Serpell, R., & Mogaji, A. (2005). School psychology in sub-Saharan Africa: Results and implications of a six country survey. In C. R. Reynolds & C. Frisby (Eds.), *Comprehensive handbook of multicultural school psychology* (pp. 1128–51). New York,: John Wiley & Sons.

Mpofu, E., & Thomas, K. R. (2006). Classroom racial proportion: Influence on self-concept and social competence in Zimbabwean adolescents. *Journal of Genetic Psychology*, *167*, 93–111.

Mpofu, E., & Watkins, D. (1997). Self-concept and social acceptance in African multiracial schools: A test of the insulation, subjective culture and bicultural competence hypotheses *Cross-Cultural Research*, *31*, 331–55.

Perry, J. C. (2009). Career counselling with secondary school-aged youth: Directions for theory, research, and practice. *South African Journal of Higher Education*, *23*, 482–504.

Sathiparsad, R. (2003). Addressing barriers to learning participation: Violence prevention in schools. *Perspectives in Education*, *21*(3), 99–111.

Stroud, K. C., & Reynolds, C. (2006). *School Motivation and Learning Strategies Inventory (SMALSI)*. Los Angeles, CA: Western Psychological Services.

Van Deventer, K. J. (2008). Perceptions of life orientation teachers regarding the implementation of the learning area in grades 8 and 9: A survey in selected Western Cape high schools. *South African Journal for Research in Sport, Physical Education and Recreation*, *30*(2), 131–46.

Watkins, D., Akande, A., & Mpofu, E. (1994). Student approaches to learning: Some African data. *Ife Psychologia*, *2*,1–18.

Watkins, D., Akande, A., & Mpofu, E. (1996). Assessing self-esteem: An African perspective. *Personality and Individual Differences*, *20*, 163–9.

Wentzel, K. R. (2003a). School adjustment. In W. M. Reynolds & G. E. Miller (Eds.), *Handbook of psychology: Educational Psychology* (Vol. 7, pp. 235–58). New York: John Wiley & Sons.

Wentzel, K. R. (2003b). Sociometric status and adjustment in middle school: A longitudinal study. *Journal of Early Adolescence*, *23*, 5–28.

SELF-CHECK EXERCISES

1. Define school counseling. How is it different from guidance?
2. Outline the comparative evolutionary history of counseling research and practice in sub-Saharan African countries.
3. What counseling needs may students in sub-Saharan Africa present in school settings? To what extent are these needs being addressed?

Case Study 7.2: Child Abuse Counseling Intervention: The Case of Mary

In one urban school in Zimbabwe, a teacher noticed that despite the warm weather, Mary wore her school jersey all the time. The teacher became concerned and asked why. Mary said she never felt hot. This continued into summer and she called Mary to her office and asked her to take off her jersey. Mary started crying as she was taking it off because she had fresh burn marks all over her arms that had stuck to the jersey. The teacher told her that she had to tell the school counselor, the headmaster, and the police, because what Mary was experiencing, was abuse. Mary was afraid, for she thought the perpetrator, her mother, would kill her. The head called the school psychologist and the police. The psychologist introduced herself to Mary and told her that they had to tell a social worker, who would take her to a safe place after listening to her story. She told her that although their conversation would be kept confidential, she had to tell the social worker for her to be able to assist her and her younger brother, who was experiencing the same abuse. Mary disclosed that each time she and her brother did not do household chores well or did anything that infuriated their mother she would switch on the iron and burn their hands, arms, buttocks, and back. They had iron marks all over their backs, hands, and thighs. The mother had marital problems, and seemed to have used the children to vent her frustration. Her husband had moved out to stay with another woman. The children were taken to the children's home for a few days until the social worker had contacted their father. The children underwent several counseling sessions. The psychologist would look away while talking to the children. The mother was said to have a mental problem and had to undergo therapy.

Questions

1. How would you characterize the counseling needs for Mary and other people involved in her situation? What interventions would be possible in each case?
2. What additional information would you need to best plan for counseling Mary? Why would that information be important?

4. What are the main challenges in the implementation of counseling programs in schools in sub-Saharan Africa?
5. Discuss the importance of professional, legal, and ethical considerations in provision of school counseling services.
6. How may the practice of school counseling in sub-Saharan African countries be enhanced?

FIELD-BASED EXPERIENTIAL EXERCISES

1. Interview a secondary school learner to determine counseling needs at schools and how these counseling needs are met by the school and community in which the student lives.
2. Observe primary school learners and secondary school learners interacting anywhere and with anybody. Determine any possible counseling needs. Compare and contrast possible counseling needs for the two groups of students.
3. Interview two secondary school teachers and two primary school teachers to determine some of the counseling needs at schools and how these counseling needs are met by the school and community. Compare and contrast their responses.
4. Discuss with an education official the Ministry of Education's expectations on school guidance and counseling programs in both primary and secondary schools. Evaluate the extent to which the official seems satisfied with the implementation of the program.

MULTIPLE-CHOICE QUESTIONS

1. Learners need in-school counseling to:
   a. Replace that of the ignorant parents at home
   b. Further enhance their development as learners and persons
   c. Learn about far away places
   d. Know what they have been missing from staying at home
   e. Teach others how to live
2. School counselors in sub-Saharan Africa tend to provide more:
   a. Counseling than guidance
   b. Guidance than counseling
   c. Discipline than guidance
   d. Administration than help
   e. Help than is needed

   Refer to Case Study 7.2: Child Abuse Counseling Intervention: The Case of Mary.
3. Mary's mother vented her anger on the learners mainly because:
   a. Their father had left to live with another woman and there was a discipline problem in the home
   b. She could not control her anger and frustration when they did not do their household chores well or made her angry
   c. The learners were reluctant to fulfil household chores since their father had left to live elsewhere
   d. She was afraid the social worker would place the learners in a place of safety

   e. Of her belief that the learners would not tell anyone about the abuse
4. The problem in Mary's house was initially identified as a result of the fact that:
   a. Mary and her brother told the teacher everything
   b. The teacher saw marks on Mary's body in summer when she did not wear a jersey
   c. Mary refused to take off her jersey, even in the warm summer weather
   d. The two learners informed their father that they were being abused by their mother
   e. The teacher found out that Mary's father had left to live with another woman
5. The psychologist referred the learners for further counseling because:
   a. Their mother abused them merely because they neglected their household chores
   b. Their father had left to live with another woman and wanted to them to join him
   c. They no longer wanted to stay with their mother and wanted to join their father
   d. Their father had left them and their mother abused them because of her mental problem
   e. To treat the effects of abuse and also prevent further abuse
6. Counseling services in sub-Saharan Africa tend to focus on:
   a. Life-skills education
   b. Diagnostic assessment
   c. Interagency referrals
   d. Family counseling
   e. HIV counseling
7. Legal and professional services for school guidance and counseling in sub-Saharan Africa are:
   a. Relatively advanced in their development
   b. Nonexistent to elementary in their development
   c. Widely advertised
   d. Accessible to a majority of the citizens
   e. Culturally sensitive
8. School counseling services in sub-Saharan Africa are more likely with further development and growth in the:
   a. Legal system
   b. Tribal affiliations
   c. Education systems
   d. Government expenditure
   e. School admission age for students

Answers to the multiple-choice questions are provided at the back of the book

8 Counseling Students at Tertiary Institutions

Ilse Ruane, Joseph M. Kasayira, and Elizabeth N. Shino

OVERVIEW. This chapter provides information concerning the counseling of students within the context of tertiary institutions, such as universities and other institutions of higher education. The chapter explores the counseling needs of African students or students of African heritage. Practical examples are taken from Zimbabwe, South Africa, and Namibia to illustrate various points. Furthermore, the chapter explores who is available at tertiary institutions to provide counseling to students and whether or not this assistance is suited for their presenting problems.

LEARNING OBJECTIVES

By the end of the chapter, the reader should be able to:

1. Outline the history of research and practice pertaining to provision of counseling services to tertiary level students of African origin.
2. Distinguish between counseling at tertiary and other levels of education.
3. Identify and discuss common problems and challenges faced by African university students in Africa and relevant solutions.
4. Outline the major approaches used to counsel for student diversity at African universities.
5. Evaluate the role of student counselors and other support services in a tertiary learning environment.
6. Describe and justify the competencies of effective student counselors.

INTRODUCTION

In a tertiary education setting, such as a university, there exists a great diversity in sociocultural, political, religious, and racial backgrounds among students and staff. Consequently, students present with a diversity of counseling needs. However, the diversity equips students to respond to an increasingly complex global environment. Diversity also makes it possible for the generation, advancement, and dissemination of knowledge, which is one of the key mission characteristics of university education (see also Chapter 13, this volume). Students enrolled in tertiary institutions are typically in late adolescence and early adulthood. These are important developmental stages, during which students engage formative influences for life-style and career development, in anticipation of becoming productive members of a workforce. Commencing university studies (tertiary level education) is a milestone for many African young adults. Entry into institutions of higher education (i.e., universities, technikons, and colleges) is highly competitive and selective. This atmosphere of competition also brings to the forefront needs for which counseling is necessary.

University students are faced with many challenges, including academic pressure, financial pressure, and social adjustment to the university lifestyle, to name a few. Counseling assists students to navigate difficulties and challenges that they may be experiencing while at university. For example, sharing thoughts and feelings, in the context of a therapeutic relationship, can assist students to feel less isolated, and enable them to understand more clearly what is happening now, and how they would like things to change. Students come for counseling with a broad range of difficulties, for example, examination anxiety, depression, suicidal feelings, mental health problems, past traumas, bereavements, issues concerning relationships, sexuality, family problems, self-harm, and eating disorders (Itsoseng Clinic, 2007; Phala, 2008).

Today, many African universities provide counseling for the students enrolled at their institutions. Although traditional counseling has existed in many African communities before the importation of professional guidance and counseling, compared to other professions, professional psychological services are fairly new (Biswalo, 1996; Ruane, 2006). Professional counseling at African tertiary institutions of higher education is even newer (Kasayira, Chipandambira, Hungwe, & Mupawose, 2007).

According to Bell (1996), only about 4 percent of British students tend to see counselors. Similar results were obtained by Flisher, De Beer, and Bokhorst (2002) at the University of Cape Town in South Africa. Potentially, this small percentage implies that the majority of students do successfully negotiate the complex educational system with other forms of assistance or support than formal counseling. Nonetheless, a large number of students may not access the available services for various reasons, such as lack of services, insufficient knowledge regarding available services, or fear of being labeled as having emotional or psychological problems (Phala, 2008; Ruane, 2006).

IMPORTANCE, DEFINITION, AND SCOPE OF KEY TERMS AND CONCEPTS

The term "university" is used here to refer to institutions of higher education or tertiary level educational institutions. Similarly, "tertiary level students" refers to students at institutions of higher learning, such as universities, technikons, colleges, and other tertiary institutions. In the present chapter, the term "Africans" is used to describe people of African descent. African origin, African heritage, and African ancestry are used interchangeably. Other important terms requiring definition are cultural competence and acculturation. "Cultural competence" refers to the student counselors' ability to engage successfully in cross-cultural counseling. "Acculturation" involves taking on the way of life of the dominant culture. "Student counselor" or "counselor" refers to the professionally trained counselor who provides counseling to tertiary level students. These include professionals such as psychologists and social workers. "Clinic" refers to the counseling setting within which a student receives counseling, and includes counseling clinics and student counseling centers within university settings. "International students" refers to African and foreign students at African universities outside their own countries. The chapter further seeks to provide information concerning the counseling of students within the context of tertiary institutions.

HISTORY OF COUNSELING IN TERTIARY INSTITUTIONS IN AFRICA

The history of counseling, in tertiary education in Southern Africa, specifically in Zimbabwe and South Africa (and Namibia by default), was based on curricula designed on racial lines during the colonial period (Zvobgo, 2007). The curriculum for indigenous Africans that was developed was heavily biased toward practical skills that were just adequate to produce semi-skilled workers to provide a labor force to service the needs of the White community. At the secondary school level, the level of training in vocational schools for Black students was deliberately kept low to limit indigenous African competition with Whites for skilled jobs. Thus, when technical colleges were introduced, during the time when vocational and technical education had become a worldwide trend to meet the demands of industrialization, Africans were excluded from the colleges that offered technical and commercial courses. Africans were by then socialized into regarding any form of education and training that required the use of one's hands as inferior. As a result, indigenous African youth preferred academic programs, despite a shortage of white-collar jobs. Gaidzanwa (2007) observed that as a result of the alienating environment, the minority Black student body experienced pressure to graduate and secure good jobs that would enable them to support their extended families while defending the struggles against racism and class discrimination.

Counseling Services in the Colonial Period

During the colonial period, government-sponsored counseling services were accessed only by White students and others of non-African origin who were regarded as suitable for skilled positions. The school psychological services structure was established so that personal, academic, and career-oriented issues could be addressed for this group of privileged students from primary through tertiary education. Black students typically received counseling from their families, friends, and churches. The counseling from families and friends would focus more on reminding the student of their social responsibility. In terms of career choices, very little career counseling was needed, as the focus was to remind the students that they should pass well in the competitive examinations, so as to access the few jobs available for educated Blacks. Besides their teachings, which emphasized moral uprightness, churches also provided school psychology–related services to a minority of Black students attending schools at church mission stations (Mpofu, Mutepfa, Chireshe, & Kasayira, 2007).

The history of higher education in Namibia dates back to the early 1980s. Before that time, students seeking higher education studied in South Africa, overseas, or in neighboring African countries (Rogerson, 1980). Similarly, professional psychological services in Namibia are relatively new. It is thus likely that counseling of students was provided through other channels within the community, such as the elders, family, teachers, and religious and community leaders. For example, counseling services at the University of Namibia through the Office of the Dean of Students commenced in approximately 1992/3 (Kambaru, 1999), following the establishment of the University of Namibian after independence from South Africa in 1990. The implication is that the availability of formal counseling services to Black students within pre-independence Namibia was limited.

The Postcolonial Period

Postcolonial Africa witnessed a dramatic increase in number of unemployed school leavers. To address the problem, tertiary institutions previously reserved for Whites opened their enrollment to Black students. Several new colleges were also established to absorb the school leavers. The expansion of tertiary education seemed not to focus on industrial training (Mama & Barnes, 2007).

Research Box 8.1: Counseling Provision for Tertiary Level Students

Mapfumo, J. (2008). Freshmen: The counseling they received in high school and the counseling they need in college/university. *THE DYKE: A Journal of Midlands State University*, *3*(1), 57–71.

Objective: Mapfumo (2008) sought to establish whether freshmen had received any counseling in high school. The objective of the study was to compare counseling services expected by tertiary level students and the counseling services they received in high school.

Method: Three hundred and seventy freshmen responded to a questionnaire that solicited information on the existence of counseling in their former high schools, topics covered where counseling had existed, and the areas in which the participants needed counseling as tertiary level students.

Results: Mapfumo reported that 80 percent of the respondents stated that counseling was necessary in institutions in the areas of careers, personal and social matters, stress and anger management, time management, and spiritual matters. The respondents showed less interest in dating, academic issues, adjustment to the new environment, medical counseling, and substance abuse and addiction problems. There were only small differences between the counseling needed by male and female undergraduate students. In general, women have a more pronounced help-seeking behavior than men, with more women in general desiring more help than men (except in the areas of addictions, careers, and time management). Mapfumo (2008) observed that responses by female students seem to suggest that women would make themselves available for counseling whenever they had a need, while men were less likely to seek help with some of their problems. In general, irrespective of sex, tertiary students required the same sort of services, with minor variations between the sexes. This implies that counseling programs should be delivered to all tertiary level students. Mapfumo (2008) advised that counselors may need to make some adjustments in areas of special interests, such as in dating matters, as required by the female students, and anger management, as required by the male students.

Conclusion: Mapfumo concluded that the wide variety of counseling needs expressed by students implied that counselors in tertiary institutions needed a wide variety of skills to carry out their tasks effectively. Where this was not possible, the counselors should call for the assistance of appropriately qualified professionals to render any necessary specialist services.

Questions

1. Identify areas of student counseling needs mentioned above for which a student counselor might have to seek assistance from appropriately qualified personnel.
2. Based on Mapfumo's (2008) study, explain why it is important to have counseling services in all tertiary level institutions.
3. Discuss possible reasons why female students would readily seek counseling more than male students.
4. Examine some gender differences in counseling needs that were identified in Mapfumo's (2008) study.

Resources were also scarce to support quality educational experiences; many students had no formal guidance in their selection of education programs in tertiary institutions. For example, Moyo (2001) conducted a study revealing that a mismatch between university first-year students' expectation and the reality of learning at a university in some areas adversely affected the students' academic performance. Some students enrolled in programs or courses they did not like because of a lack of counseling.

After the attainment of national independence from colonial rule, the right to schooling was extended to all children and school segregation was abolished, while school psychology services were extended to Black students. For instance, in Zimbabwe, a formal policy was adopted to introduce guidance and counseling in secondary schools. Thus, with a large number of modifications, efforts were made to transfer the systems of counseling developed in the colonial period, with diverse student enrollment obtaining in most schools and institutions of higher learning. However, lack of qualified personnel affected the governmental effort to offer psychological services, in particular, counseling services to all students who need the services (Mpofu et al., 2007). Thus, some students begin tertiary level education without having benefited from counseling, despite needing the service. In the next section, we discuss various issues that a student counselor must take into account when counseling students of African origin.

CONSIDERATIONS WHEN COUNSELING STUDENTS OF AFRICAN ANCESTRY

In this section, we consider the influences of linguistic and cultural diversity as well as diversity on campus and international students. We also consider the influence of religion, gender, academic challenges, family expectations, and scarcity of resources.

Linguistic and Cultural Diversity

The counseling needs of tertiary level students of African origin are as diverse as their backgrounds, which differ in terms of geography, religion, language, world view, and culture, among other aspects. Thus, it is difficult to treat students of African ancestry as a single group. A counselor has to consider these differences and treat each student who comes for counseling as a unique individual who shares, with other students of African origin, some heritage of colonial or apartheid education or legacy of slavery. These students share the history of being one of the most disadvantaged groups in terms of educational rights, opportunities, and expectations (Bakker et al., 2000; Bojuwoye, 2006; Mamdani, 1993; Ruane, 2006; Williams, 1986; Zvobgo, 2007). Contemporary tertiary level students of African ancestry consist of a mixture of advantaged and disadvantaged people despite the shared history of being excluded from participating in the mainstream of society. For some disadvantaged students, however, their being a minority group within the university setting in terms of race, ethnicity, language, gender, and physical and learning disabilities exacerbates the situation.

Students typically come from many language groups. For example, Zimbabwe comprises the following major cultural–linguistic communities: Asians, Kalanga, Ndebele, Shangani, Shona, Tonga, Venda, and White languages (Mpofu, Kasayira, Mutepfa, Chireshe, & Maunganidze, 2006), such as English and Afrikaans, whereas in South Africa, the population comprises cosmopolitan communities with 11 official languages that include Sotho, Zulu, Tswana, Venda, Xhosa, English, and Afrikaans. In Namibia, English is the official language and is the medium of instruction at all institutions of higher learning. However, Afrikaans and German are widely spoken, as are numerous indigenous languages such as Oshiwambo, Otjiherero, Nama/Damara, Silozi, Rukwangali, and Tswana. Many of the indigenous languages have distinct dialects.

However, although it cannot be expected of each student counselor to be conversant in the language of each student, it is important for counselors to have an awareness of the diversity of languages among the student population to whom they offer counseling services. It is well known that language influences thought processes and how people articulate their thoughts. For counselors to understand the student's world view, it is important to have an awareness that students express their counseling needs in various ways and might use different concepts or terminologies to express them. For example, a student whose language does not have an equivalent expression for the word "depression" might say "I feel bad" instead of saying "I feel depressed." Similarly, a student's home language influences his/her accent, which might make communication with the counselor and others challenging.

Diversity on Campus and International Students

The faces of many university campuses have changed drastically since their inceptions. Hence, many universities now boast a great diversity. Diversity can refer to a range of variables and aspects such as age, gender, sexual orientation, culture, religion, language, physical and mental ability, racial heritage and ethnicity, national origin, and socioeconomic status. These aspects form part of the multiculturalism of African universities (Ruane, 2008a).

With globalization and many contextual factors, many African universities enroll students from overseas (e.g., exchange students) as well as students from other African countries. Although some students come from neighboring countries, others are from countries much farther away. For example, in recent years, the University of Namibia has enrolled students from Botswana, Angola, South Africa, Ghana, Nigeria, Ethiopia, Democratic Republic of the Congo (DRC), Sudan, Kenya, and Sierra Leone (Shino, 2008). These students from other countries, with a nationality different from that of the host country, are often referred to as international or foreign students. They range from children/spouses/relatives of diplomats to refugees who have been based in refugee camps for years in the host countries. Similarly, some of students are immigrants who have fled poverty or political conflicts in their own countries.

Apart from dealing with other challenges that face university students, international students face a host of other challenges (Chen, 1999), which include sociocultural, environmental, and physiological adjustments. Owing to these difficulties, international students might experience anxiety, a sense of loss, loneliness, helplessness, and depression. Language barriers and communication might be a potential source of distress (Ruane, 2008a). For some students, their home language or language in which they previously received instructions might be different from the language of instruction at university. For example, an international student from DRC might have difficulties with English or Afrikaans, which is used in a number of southern African universities. Because of this, a student might doubt his/her own abilities to learn and might feel incompetent and inferior, confused, and less willing to communicate with others.

International students might also experience educational stressors. These include adjusting to a new educational system, performance expectations, test- or exam-taking anxiety, and adjusting to a new university culture. Many international students also experience culture shock as a result of transition from one culture to another. This culture shock occurs when students find some of their own values incompatible with those of their host culture. At their new host institution, social norms might be different from their own norms. Social isolation and alienation are additional stressors for international students. At the very least, many such students have lost significant social relationships, such as the support of

Case Study 8.1: Andrew

Andrew is a seventeen-year-old bi-racial young man of Colored and Zulu heritage who has just moved to suburban Pretoria, South Africa. He is originally from a multi-ethnic community in Kwa-Zulu Natal. He speaks English and Zulu fluently. He was raised as a Roman Catholic and had, until recently, attended Catholic schools in Kwa-Zulu Natal. He had experienced little or no negative bias from his peers or others in his school there. His family's move to Pretoria was due to his father being transferred by the mine for which he works as a mechanic. The family misses the close extended family in the Kwa-Zulu Natal area, especially the father's mother, who lived next door and helped to raise Andrew and his younger sister. At university, he is ignored by most of the White and Black students on campus. Most of the students are Protestant. Andrew has also been unsuccessful in meeting girls. He is isolated and shows signs of low mood.

Questions

1. What are some of the problems and challenges Andrew experiences?
2. As a university counselor, how would you go about assisting Andrew?
3. In your view, how might a first-year student's adjustment be different from that of a more senior student?
4. Why is it essential for student counselors to address the issue of religion?
5. If you were a student counselor, how would you go about creating awareness about religious tolerance?
6. Critically discuss the issues of cultural differences at universities and the transition between traditional and Western lifestyles. How is this situation exacerbated for Andrew?

parents, former schoolmates, and their friends, and might experience homesickness. In addition, they might have fewer opportunities to establish networks of social support and hence find themselves facing uncertainty, isolation, and loneliness. Financial stressors are a reality and any breakdown or unexpected disturbance in their financial resources (e.g., becoming ill or supporting a parent who had lost a job) threatens a student's educational pursuit and life style. In turn, this threat creates uncertainty and anxiety (Shino, 2008).

Experiences of discrimination and prejudice, among international students in their host countries stemming from ethnic origin, nationality, political background, culture, religion, and language, have been reported. The sources of these prejudices could be other students, faculty, or institutional systems. Such experiences could play a role in causing low self-esteem and self-confidence, and further complicate the adjustment of international students.

Religiosity

Many tertiary students in Africa subscribe to some religion or other (see also Chapter 16, this volume). Religion and spirituality are central aspects of many African students. Although often used interchangeably with spirituality, religion refers to institutional beliefs, practices, and ritual expressions of one's denomination, church, or religious institution (Kelly, 1995). Religions among university students may include, but are not limited to, Christianity, Islam, and Judaism. Religious beliefs are important to many African students; and counselors need to respect and validate them within the counseling process. Closely linked to the issue of religion is that of spirituality. In the traditional African world view, spirituality is paramount. According to a study by Ruane (2006), more traditional African people, including students, define problems requiring psychological intervention in terms of disharmonious social relationships and spiritual encounters, which implies that treatment needs to be more holistic and needs to address a variety of issues (e.g., treatment of an ailment would require the family as a whole actively participating in the healing of the ailment).

Gender

Most tertiary students are at a stage of life where their identity development will be very important to them as young adults. At this stage, they have to find out what it means to be a woman or a man, and some need support to help them to be comfortable with their gender. This is a time when they could develop various relationships including choosing a marriage partner. Student counselors may have to come in to help students become aware of their unique roles in developing positive and lasting relationships. To this end, student counselors need to understand the socially ascribed duties for males and females coming from different cultures. Embedded in the concept of gender role is the power relation between men and women. In this respect, women are traditionally disadvantaged, as some of their ascribed roles keep them in subordinate positions. However, at universities or any other institutions of higher learning, female and male students are generally treated as equals, and this might not be consistent with some cultural expectations. Somerai (2001) argues that the general perception that institutions of higher learning promote gender equity is misplaced, as this is not supported by what female students experience in and outside the institutional environment.Thus, female students need to be empowered so they are able to deal with their doubly disadvantaged circumstances.

Academic Pressures

Unlike in high schools, where most of the academic work is guided by the teacher, tertiary education students find themselves forced to adjust to a new learning environment. At universities, students are expected to make their own decisions about academic issues. This new experience creates pressure for some students. Although this applies to first-year students more than any other academic level, it should be noted that, at any academic level, there are students who let work accumulate until it is too late. Such students need the help of the student counselor in terms of learning and study skills, time management, task management, and examination skills. The student counselor must also take note that some students face academic pressure because of conditions beyond their control, for example, students living with disabilities or health-related conditions. The student counselor should work with the university disability unit, and other stakeholders to make sure that students benefit from all resources and services available to them.

Family Support

Tertiary education students face so much pressure that the support from the student counselor may not be enough. Some of the pressures are better met by the family. Most families would expect a tertiary education student to raise the status of the family and not to embarrass it. As a result, family members would feel obliged to support one of their own members in any way possible to facilitate the students' successful completion of their studies. Family support could come in material form or moral support. Where need be, it is the duty of the student counselor to help the student identify some family members who would provide various types of support when needed.

Resource Needs

The challenges that university students face are exacerbated by the prevailing economic crisis in some African countries. With the increases of student enrollment, most universities have shifted the financial burden of running the institutions back onto the students and hence students are dealing with new kinds of challenges over and above other common stressors that most tertiary level students face, making provision of professional counseling very important.

APPROACHES AND STRATEGIES IN COUNSELING TERTIARY EDUCATION STUDENTS

Three approaches that are deemed to be most contextually relevant are developmental, systemic, and narrative approaches, discussed briefly in the text that follows.

Developmental Approach

Late adolescence and early adulthood can be viewed as a time of great adjustment and often characterized by turmoil. Of particular significance, at this stage of development, are issues of identity including sexual identity and orientation. It thus becomes the task of the counselor to be aware of the developmentally appropriate milestones that students are grappling with at that time.

Students have the difficult task of forming their identities as well as their sexual identity and orientation, that is, their preference for partners of the same or other sex, or both (Sigelman & Rider, 2008). Both identity and sexual identity are vitally important issues requiring resolution. Resolving identity is a process that begins earlier in adolescence and continues throughout adulthood (Sigelman & Rider, 2008), but that is molded largely by experiences that occur during university years. For example, negative feedback from lecturers or friends to a fragile and still forming identity could have dramatic effects on a student and make him or her feel worthless and outcast. Similarly, resolving sexual identity and orientation is a process that peaks during the age at which students are busy with their university studies (Somerai, 2001). According to Sigelman and Rider (2008, p. 364), most students establish their "heterosexual sexual orientation without much soul-searching." However, for those attracted to members of their own sex, the process of accepting their homosexual orientation and establishing positive identity within society's negative attitudes can be a very difficult journey. Furthermore, being aware of the nature of student dating behaviors, sexual behaviors, and consequences such as teenage pregnancies all fall into the realm of necessary developmental knowledge each counselor should possess.

Systems Approach

University students can present to counseling centers with normal developmental issues, such as developing autonomy or establishing identity. However, students must also cope with additional influences that affect their cognitive, social, moral, educational, and psychosocial development occurring at different systemic levels. For example, a students' success socially and their emotional well-being are linked intimately with success in their academic achievement. Thus, students must function within a multilevel system that includes societal rules, family rules and regulations, university practices and policies, and student dynamics. Thus, counselors need to increase their knowledge of systems theory (Becvar & Becvar, 1982, 1996) and enhance their skills in this area. It is imperative that counselors are aware that student clients function within a multileveled system, for example, self, nuclear family, extended family, university, society and greater global economy, etc.

Narrative Approach

As humans, we are narrative by nature (i.e., we live our lives through stories) (Payne, 2000; White, 1995; see also Chapters 2 and 3, this volume). The stories we have about our lives are created through linking certain events together in a particular sequence across a time period, and finding a way of making sense of them (Morgan, 2008). For example, students have stories about themselves, their abilities (actual or perceived), struggles, competencies, relationships, and failures. The way each student develops their story is determined by how they have linked certain events together in a sequence and by the meaning they have attributed to them. There are many stories occurring at the same time and different stories can be told about the same events. Thus, our lives are multi-storied (Morgan, 2008; Payne, 2000; White, 1995). The ways in which we understand our lives are influenced by the broader stories of the cultural context in which we live. For example, a student coming from a rural context will have different stories than a student coming from an urban context and vice versa. Students of African ancestry bring with them many rich stories of their communities, families, religious beliefs, and rituals, all of which a counselor needs to be aware of. According to the narrative approach, this awareness need not necessarily derive from having knowledge of the particular story but from having a willingness and curiosity to investigate the story further.

ISSUES FACED BY AFRICAN STUDENTS AT UNIVERSITY

Counseling at universities is offered by student counselors with various qualifications, including those in psychology, social work, nursing, and sport and recreation. Most of the students requesting counseling approach the various psychology clinics through self-referral. However, in some cases, students, especially those experiencing poor academic performance or needing career counseling, are typically referred by faculty officers and lecturers. Some students might be referred for counseling or assessment by the university bursary committee. We consider next the services involved in tertiary education counseling settings.

The Clinic

Counseling settings within African universities take many forms. Whereas some universities have counseling clinics, at others counseling is offered through counseling centers or offices of counseling services. The most common issues handled by psychology clinics include relationship problems (e.g. friendship and love), academic concerns, family conflicts, career concerns, substance abuse, sexual reproductive health issues, and violence-related issues. Other less common problems attended to are low self-esteem/lack of confidence, stress-related illness, HIV/AIDS, depression, and posttraumatic stress. Some students come to the clinic not with a specific problem but with a general problem of finding difficulties in adjusting to university environment. Student counselors work closely with the student affairs personnel, who work under the dean of students, the medical personnel, and the chaplain. Student counselors achieve more success with voluntary clients than with those referred by university authorities.

Adjustment to the University Environment

Entry into university requires a student to adjust to university life and culture. This adjustment is multifaceted and entails social, environmental, emotional, and educational adaptation. Social adjustment includes many new friends and establishing a network of social support. For many students, it might be the first time leaving home for extended periods of time and hence they are removed from their usual social support systems of friends and family. Similarly, the university environment and new setting might be foreign to them, especially for African students coming from rural areas (Blake, 2006). Hence, they are required to learn to negotiate living in their new environment. The education systems, values, and expectations at the university might be different from what they were accustomed to in high school. Students might experience a sense of loss, loneliness, confusion, and frustration, especially during the initial periods. This initial and continuous adjustment and adaptation to university life plays an essential role in the students' overall adjustment.

Health-related Issues

Substance use, sexual health, and emotional health are a few of the health-related issues for which students may seek counseling. We consider these issues next.

Substance Abuse

Substance abuse is a major problem for many young people (see also Chapter 18, this volume). It includes the abuse and misuse of tobacco, alcohol, and drugs. This is in turn also true at many institutions of higher learning. Contributing factors include socialization, peer pressure, boredom, academic pressure, a desire to experiment, and a lack of recreational activities. It leads to addiction, non-attendance to academic programs, academic failure and dropout, vandalism, conflict, verbal and physical abuse, sexual violence, and crimes. Abuse of substances negatively affect students in their career development, and hence need to be addressed. Adolescents and young adults are more prone to the use of substances owing to peer pressure. Entry to university coincides with a developmental stage wherein the need to be accepted by ones peers is important. Similarly, for many students, it might be the first time being away from home and hence parental supervision is not available (Shino, 2008).

Research Box 8.2: Counseling Needs of Tertiary Level Students

Kasayira, J. M., Musingarabwi, S., Nyanhongo S., Chipandambira K. S., & Sodi, T. (2007). *A survey of the views of college students on academic dishonesty. Journal of Psychology in Africa, 17*(1&2), 123–128; and

Kasayira, J. M. (2008). *Counselling tertiary level students of African origin.* Unpublished manuscript, Midlands State University.

Objective: In a study that was conducted by Kasayira, Musingarabwi, Nyanhongo, Chipandambira, and Sodi (2007), some tertiary level students suggested that professional counseling should be provided to students who engage in love relationships with lecturers for the purpose of getting inappropriate assistance from those lecturers. Kasayira (2008) made a follow-up study to identify counseling needs of tertiary level students.

Method: Interviews were conducted with various people: college students, lecturers, and college principals.

Results: In an interview, some former agricultural college students (personal communication, October 24, 2007), current and former lecturers of a teachers' college (October 30, 2007), and two former principals of teachers' colleges (personal communication, November 6, 2007) identified the following problems that need counseling:

- Drunkenness by male students
- Love relationships, especially between female students and married men
- Balancing academic performance and other aspects of their lives
- Financial management, especially during industrial or field experience attachment where they survive on meager allowances
- STI-, HIV-, and AIDS-related issues
- Unwanted pregnancies
- Sexual and reproductive health issues
- Domestic violence
- Inappropriate relationships with lecturers

Conclusion: There are many problems at a tertiary level requiring the intervention and assistance of counselors.

Questions

1. Discuss the findings of these interviews in relation to the influence of culture on counseling needs of tertiary level students. Are these needs context specific?
2. Discuss the suggestion that students who engage in love relationships with lecturers, in order to pass, should seek counseling assistance.
3. As a student counselor, how will you assist "students who engage in love relationships with lecturers for the purpose of getting inappropriate assistance from the lecturers involved"?
4. What are important considerations that a student counselor should take into account when dealing with each of the nine problems listed above?

Many students with the problem of substance abuse might not be willing to admit their problem and search for counseling. Hence, preventative programs that include psychoeducation on substance abuse could be a good alternative. If the student already has a substance abuse problem, the student counselor could assist him/her in dealing with the problem. This assistance entails making the student aware of the negative impact and effects of his/her behavior, addressing the causes of the abuse, and helping the student find alternative and more productive ways to deal with the causes of the substance abuse.

Sexual Health: HIV/AIDS, STIs, and Pregnancy

Given the prevalence of HIV/AIDS in Africa, it is likely that almost everyone is affected (directly or indirectly) by the HIV epidemic in one way or another. Hence, HIV/AIDS is a challenge for many governments, nongovernmental organizations (NGOs), agencies, and universities. University students are particularly at risk of and susceptible to HIV infection because they are young (today's youth is the HIV/AIDS generation) and ignorant about HIV (Kelly, 2003). According to Poku (2005), a deadly combination of factors such as poverty, gender inequality, low access to reproductive health care, the presence of sexually transmitted infections, and extensive labor migration create an environment for the spread of HIV. HIV infects people of all ages; however, across the continent the infection is concentrated among the socially and economically productive groups ages fifteen to forty-nine years (Poku, 2005).

Thus, university counselors are faced with a great challenge pertaining to HIV/AIDS. Counselors might have to

Discussion Box 8.1: HIV/AIDS Policies at Tertiary Educational Institutions

Kelly (2003) points out that HIV/AIDS is a major challenge for universities in Africa and cannot be ignored. He calls upon university leadership and management committees to commit their full potential and resources in the struggle against HIV/AIDS. This commitment entails establishment of policies, plans, and implementation structures. Many African universities now have HIV/AIDS policies. One such example is the University of Namibia. The University of Namibia's Policy on HIV/AIDS (University of Namibia, n.d.) emphasizes the commitment of the university to address issues pertaining to HIV/AIDS: the rights of student and staff affected and infected by HIV (e.g., right to admission, comprehensive treatment, confidentiality etc.); the integration of HIV/AIDS into teaching and research (e.g., compulsory core curriculum on HIV/AIDS); provision for prevention, care, and support services on campus (including counseling and support); and the implementation and review of the policy.

Questions

1. In your opinion, what are some of the topics that need to be included in the HIV/AIDS policy of a university?
2. Why is it important for universities to address aspects of HIV/AIDS?
3. Should issues pertaining to HIV/AIDS be included in the university curriculum? Provide a rationale for your response.
4. Some universities offer HIV counseling and testing to students and staff. Do you think this is an essential service? Provide a rationale for your response.

counsel students who are infected with HIV, are anxious about the possibility of HIV infection, have a loved one who is infected, have faced a loss of a loved one due to HIV/AIDS, have added responsibilities of taking care of siblings (e.g., in the case of a death of a parent from AIDS), and so forth. The role of the student counselor is complex in this regard. Apart from providing counseling to those already infected or affected, it is important for counselors to play a vital role in the prevention of the spread of HIV for a number of reasons:

- Entry to university coincides with the stage of development at which young people start dating and become sexually active.
- Students might lack knowledge about sexually transmitted infections.
- Students might face peer pressure from other students to engage in sexual activities.
- Students might not have the skills to negotiate safer sex.
- Students might lack information regarding the transmission of HIV.
- Students might hold myths about HIV/AIDS.
- Students might engage in other activities, such as substance abuse, that place them at greater risk for contracting HIV.

Counselors can play a role in educating students about HIV/AIDS. It has, however, been found that education alone does not change behaviors. It thus becomes imperative for student counselors to develop programs that are targeted toward behavior modification.

Emotional Difficulties

Potential sources of students' emotional difficulties are numerous. They might be due to personal problems and conflicts, family problems, peer conflicts, or academic pressure. Emotional problems, such as stress, depression, and suicide ideation and attempts, among others, have been noted among university students. Emotional problems negatively impact students and disrupt their overall well-being. It is therefore important for students' emotional problems to be addressed through counseling. While some of these students might find this flexibility reassuring, others might feel that they have already failed because they have not arrived via the "normal" route. They might feel that they have to prove themselves, and might be overanxious about their academic performance and their right to be at university (Bell, 1996, p. 34).

Residence and Accommodation

With ever-increasing student enrollments at universities across the continent, accommodation for students becomes a challenge. Many universities are able to provide residences for only a limited number of students. At the same time, many students (especially undergraduates) might desire to live on-campus. Living on-campus offers many benefits for students. First, they become part of the campus community and form friendships with other students (e.g., roommates, other students in the dormitories/hostels) (Somerai, 2001), which enhances students' adjustment, sense of self-esteem, and sense of belonging. Second, students residing on campus are closer to facilities, such as lecture halls and libraries, which reduces the cost (in money and time) of traveling to and from campus. Third, living on-campus might foster a sense of security. Many university campuses are relatively safe and have secure/reliable security services; hence crime on many campuses is relatively low, in contrast with the higher crime rates in communities outside of the universities.

Students who rent rooms off campus are faced with numerous crime-related problems (Somerai, 2001) including theft, fear of being physically attacked or raped, and intimidation by older or wealthier members of the community, to name but a few.

Student counseling and accommodation services might thus play a role in assisting students to find off-campus housing that is affordable, safe, and in closer proximity to the university. Many university students come from out of town, and might not be familiar with their new vicinity and environment (Shino, 2008). A potential challenge for counselors is to assist students in adjusting to their environment, choosing the type of accommodation desired (e.g., apartment, student house, commune, rooms), and finding appropriate room-/flat-/housemates.

Students might also encounter difficulties within university accommodation settings. Potential challenges and problems include conflicts between roommates, adherence to rules, and issues such as noise. Typically, these problems are dealt with and resolved through the intervention of housing committee representatives or resident assistants.

Faculty and Academic Challenges

University academic systems challenge students. Academic competency is pivotal to students' successful completion of their studies, and students need to learn the skills that are essential for this success. In the guidelines for structuring student counseling, career and development services, the Society for Student Counseling in Southern Africa (SSCSA, 2001) points out the importance of learning and study skills acquisition. These include aspects such as cognitive skills (e.g., creative writing, brainstorming, problem-solving, critical thinking, decision making), motivation, time management skills, and test- and examination-taking skills.

Lack of academic competencies can contribute to academic failure and make the learning process frustrating to students. Some students enter university with a lack of appropriate/adequate study skills, and might employ the same learning strategies used in high school. Student counseling services can assist students to acquire study skills that are needed for their success at university. Faculty members might also assist students in this regard. However, because of challenges such as large student numbers and high teaching/lecturing volumes for faculty members, lecturers are not always available (or willing) to address issues of study skills.

Sport, Recreation, and Student Associations

For many students, sport and recreation activities assist in dealing with a wide range of challenges that they face at university (see also Chapter 11, this volume). Students may seek assistance from student clubs and associations. These clubs and associations provide a safe haven for students to express their issues and perhaps the opportunity to receive lay counseling from leaders in the clubs and association as well as advice from other members. Coaches, club leaders, and the Student Representative Council normally address issues within this context. In the event that the issues fall outside of the area of lay counseling and advice giving, typically that student would be referred to the university clinic or a more formal counseling center.

Finance and Counseling

In more developed countries, students often obtain sufficient grants/scholarship/funding for their studies, either from governments or other agencies. However, this is not true for many African students. Some African countries (e.g., Botswana) invest heavily into education and hence cater sufficiently for their students. Lack of resources, however, makes it impossible for many African nations.

Owing to this lack of resources, many African students rely on the income of their parents, spouses, or their own incomes if they have been or are employed. In addition, there often are not enough opportunities for students to do casual and/or part-time jobs. For many students, the issue of lack of finance remains an ever-present concern, and poses a threat to the students' security and sense of well-being (Bell, 1996).

Studies that surveyed challenges faced by university students include those done by Chagonda (2001), Ndlovu (2001), and Somerai (2001). Ndlovu (2001) revealed that female students on campus residence who faced financial difficulties dealt with the challenges of resisting seduction by material goods potentially accessible through waged and salaried men off campus. On the other hand, male students on campus faced challenges to their masculinities because of the wealthier men off campus who date the female students they would like to date (Chagonda, 2001). While some female students met economic challenges by exploring relationships with materially comfortable men (Ndlovu, 2001), the male students were forced to channel their effort to studying, financially and politically motivated demonstrations, and politics (Chagonda, 2001). Somerai (2001) argued that, in addition to being ill-treated by landlords and landladies, students residing off campus faced problems pertaining to transport, books, and access to other university facilities. As a way of coping with these difficulties, some students are made "subservient to the whims of landlords, transport providers, fellow students who sometimes take notes for them when they are late for lectures" (Somerai, 2001, p. 7) and in addition, female students may also rely on males whom they date and on whom they sometimes depend for material goods and services. Gaidzanwa (2001) revealed that class issues loomed very large at the university, with most of the distressed men belonging to the working and peasant classes. These are the same classes that are suffering economic hardship nationally. Many of these young men

Case Study 8.2: Tebogo

Tebogo is a second-year university student, currently enrolled for a BCOM law degree. Since commencing her studies two years earlier, she has found herself in a position in which she has doubts as to whether becoming a lawyer is the correct choice for her, owing to issues regarding adjustment and problems within the university residences. Within her family, she had been through a difficult time after suddenly losing her father to illness. As a result, she failed several of her semester tests as she was unable to concentrate or get the necessary amount of studying done. Furthermore, since her father's death she found herself needing to seek financial aid from the university. Recently, she became interested in becoming a doctor. In an attempt to remedy her confusion, she has discussed her uncertainty with her lecturers. After numerous discussions with her lecturers in the law faculty, she is more confused as to whether she is studying for the correct degree and thus wants to stop pursuing the law degree immediately. Thus, she needs further direction.

Questions

1. What are some of the challenges that Tebogo may face at university?
2. Are these challenges unique to Tebogo or do other university students have similar problems?
3. Should Tebogo necessarily stop her studies in law? Provide a rationale for your answer.
4. How would you advise Tebogo to proceed in order to get clarity regarding this issue?
5. If you were her student counselor, how would you go about resolving this problem of financial aid?

demonstrated continuously against dwindling loans and grants to finance their studies, but these demonstrations did not address their growing unemployment, underemployment, and social marginalization on and off campus.

It hence becomes part of the task of the student counselor to assist students in exploring and obtaining financial assistance. Student loans might be available through financial institutions (such as banks) or divisions/ministries of education. Counselors need to provide students such information and assist them to secure such loans. A number of organizations, companies, and NGOs offer scholarships or grants for studies. This implies that student counselors at institutions of higher education need to explore and be aware of various funding possibilities and hence assist students in this regard.

Career Counseling

Some students enter universities knowing what they would like to study. However, some might not have clear goals pertaining to their field of study and career. This uncertainty is possibly due to a number of factors including lack of career guidance at the high school level, lack of self-knowledge, and lack of information or knowledge about various careers. Although students might spend the first academic year taking a variety of courses and hence exploring their likes and dislikes, they eventually have to make a career choice. According to Lamprecht (2002), career choice is undoubtedly one of the most significant decision anyone can make. Studies have also indicated that choosing a career is one of the primary reasons for which students seek counseling at university counseling centers (Carney & Savitz, 1980).

In assisting students to choose a career, it is imperative for a counselor to carry out assessment. Lamprecht (2002) suggests a holistic approach that takes into account the totality of the student, and that includes both qualitative and quantitative assessment. Quantitative assessment includes the use of psychometric assessment instruments, such as questionnaires, whereas the qualitative assessment uses non-testing techniques to gain in-depth insight into the unique profile of the student, such as individual interviews. A comprehensive approach to career counseling enables a student to make an informed decision regarding his/her career.

The aspect of career choice is complicated further by other contextual factors such as sources of funding. For example, a student might have secured a government scholarship that will specifically cover for studies toward adult education that might be considered a priority in the country. However, such a student might desire to study fine arts, which is in line with his/her interest, personality, and values. This student might also face a problem of finding a suitable job in fine arts in his/her country upon completion of his/her studies.

Therefore, the task of career counselors is a complex one. Student counselors need to be well versed in the major career theories, have knowledge of the various career assessment tools and strategies, and possess knowledge of the various contextual factors that influence career choices among African university students. These aspects need to be integrated fully and the students need to be actively involved in this process.

Job-finding Skills

Students enter universities with the aim of completing their studies, gaining relevant skills and knowledge, and finding a job upon completion. Although the knowledge and skills are acquired through various academic courses,

Discussion Box 8.2: Multicultural Competence of Psychologists

According to Tuckwell (2002, p. 61), multiculturalism "is based on a broad, inclusive view of culture, which provides a metaphor for understanding self and others." Thus, the term *multiculturalism* reflects the changing composition of society, especially in urban areas where culturally and racially different communities reside in close proximity. According to Pederson (1994, p. 15), the "multicultural perspective seeks to provide a conceptual framework that recognizes the complex diversity of a plural society, although at the same time it suggests bridges of shared concern that binds culturally different people to one another."

Questions

1. Do universities present a context where multicultural issues may be problematic?
2. What are some of the issues, with regard to multiculturalism, that counselors and psychologists need to be aware of?
3. Is it important for universities to train psychology students in multiculturalism? OR is it important for psychology students to at least be aware of multicultural issues? Provide a rationale for your response.
4. In your opinion, how would multicultural assistance to students differ at African universities as opposed to Westernized universities?

students often are not taught the skills that would enable them to find employment. These include writing curriculum vitaes (CVs), networking, identifying potential employers, applying for jobs, and interviewing skills. Many university counseling centers might be approached by potential employers seeking new graduates.

ISSUES FOR RESEARCH AND OTHERS FORMS OF SCHOLARSHIP

In this section, we address the following issues that impact the delivery and quality of counseling services in African tertiary institutions: counselor training and the scarcity of resources. These are only two of several other significant issues, some of which we addressed in earlier sections of this chapter.

Counselor Training

Given the various challenges that are faced by university students, the role of student counselors is pivotal to the development and psychosocial well-being of students. According to SSCSA (2001), student counselors should be professionally trained as experienced practitioners whose aims should be to provide comprehensive and holistic services to "guide and counsel students with personal, social and academic needs, render career and lifelong learning consultation and development planning, and orchestrate developmental programmes and initiative that support and promote academic and meta-curriculum life on campus" (SSCSA, 2001, p. 10).

Apart from having an awareness of the various problems of students at university, student counselors must have the necessary training and competencies to deal with these challenges. Competencies such as listening skills, general counseling skills, and assessment skills are essential. Therefore, it is essential that counselors are trained professionals, whether possessing a Bachelor's or Master's degree in Psychology, with professional registration with the relevant board/council of the residing country to ensure counselor competence. For example, in South Africa, the relevant professional board would be the Health Professions Council of South Africa to which every registered counselor (whether Bachelor in Psychology or Master in Psychology registration) is a member (Ruane, 2008b). Ruane argued that owing to the ever-increasing diversity of university student populations, counselors also need to have an awareness of student diversity and challenges that result due to diversity. It hence becomes imperative for counselors working with university students to gain multicultural competencies.

Pederson (1994) defined multicultural counseling as a helping relationship in which two or more people (counselor and client/s), with different ways of perceiving their environments, interact. Both the counselor and student being counseled enter the helping relationship with their own values, cultures, world views, expectations, beliefs and attitudes. Effective multicultural counselors have an awareness of their own values and world views and do not impose them on their clients. They take the client's social, cultural, and political contexts into account and tailor their interventions to these world views. Unless counselors are willing to recognize diversity issues, and enter into and understand their client's worlds, they are likely to lose their clients in the helping relationship (see also Chapter 13). According to Ruane (2008a), this is equally applicable to counselors in the African university settings.

In most countries in Africa, counseling trainees are instructed in English, which may result in acculturation. The situation is aggravated by the fact that the trainees are taught Euro-American–centered counseling theories, principles, and practices (Ruane, 2008a). Thus, counselors may develop Western models of conceptualizing and understanding human behavior. As a result, counselors may develop a concept of confidentiality and for that matter therapy and intervention that is different from their clients' (Rukuni, 2007). For instance, for many indigenous Africans confidentiality is between the individual and his/her extended family while counselors who are trained in the Euro-American context consider confidentiality to be between counselor and client. A further example is the fact that indigenous sub-Saharan Africans consider seeking to promote the goals of one's community as one criterion of psychological well-being (Mpofu, 2006), which is in contrast to Western values, norms, and behaviors. In South Africa, large quantities of counselors who received training at tertiary institution are White; thus they do not necessarily possess the necessary culturally appropriate and sensitive skills in dealing with problem originating from an African world view (Ruane, 2008a).

Student counselors have a responsibility in providing counseling and upholding ethical conduct. As in any other counseling settings, ethical principles such as informed consent, confidentiality, what would benefit clients, and not doing harm must be adhered to in student counseling. In the event where university policies are applicable, it is the obligation of the student counselor to explain such policies and procedures to the student receiving counseling. This will allow students to make informed decisions regarding counseling.

Scarcity of Resources

With the exception of some universities, most tertiary institutions do not have counseling as stand-alone services for students. Members of staff who are given the counseling responsibility as an extracurricular activity or as a voluntary service often assist those who need the service. For example, in some teachers' colleges, counseling services are provided by the department of Family, Health and Life Skills (FHLS), whose main task is to provide AIDS education. Members of this department provide counseling to students on a part-time and voluntary basis since they have their own teaching loads to take care of. Other members who provide counseling services to students include the college nurse and hostel wardens. The dean of students and deputy dean of students are at times given the responsibility for providing counseling services on a part-time basis. The head of the department or the dean of student in most cases is the one who provides AIDS education. These members involved are not necessarily qualified counselors, which has ethical implications for all involved (Ruane, 2008a). However, some do hold counseling qualifications, such as Bachelor of Psychology degrees (BPsych) or Master in Psychology degrees (MA), or have attended in-service courses on HIV/AIDS.

SUMMARY AND CONCLUSIONS

The provision of counseling services at institutions of higher learning in African settings is essential. This is influenced by the variety of challenges that students are faced with. These problems and challenges range from adjustment to university life, academic and learning skills, career issues, accommodation, financial problems, emotional problems, substance abuse, HIV/AIDS, student diversity, and presence of international students. To address these issues effectively, counselors must have an awareness of these problems. Furthermore, student counselors must have the necessary competencies to provide effective counseling services. Owing to the ever-increasing diversity on university campuses, student counselors must strive to become effective and culturally sensitive and gain skills that will enable them to be multiculturally competent counselors.

In this chapter we looked at the history of tertiary education in Africa, comparing precolonial and postcolonial education in relation to the provision of counseling services to university students. We explored the challenges brought about by economic crisis by reviewing some studies on challenges faced by tertiary level students. We also explored some counseling service provisions in tertiary institutions. In some tertiary institutions, there are no professional counseling services. The evidence for the need for provision of counseling services in tertiary institution is overwhelming. Where professional counseling services are provided, they can be more beneficial only if clients' cultural–linguistic background is taken into account. Thus, counselors of tertiary level students of African ancestry must study the common characteristic of this group, diverse as it is, and then study the specific cultures of the clients they are likely to serve on day-to-day basis.

REFERENCES

Bakker, T. M., Blokland, L. M., Fouche, J. B., Korf, L., May, M. S., Pauw, A., et al. (2000). Perceptions of psychology students from a historically disadvantaged black South African university of circumstances impacting on their lives. *Journal of Psychology in Africa, 10*(1), 26–48.

Becvar, D. S., & Becvar, R. J. (1982). *Systems theory and family therapy: A primer*. Lanham: University Press of America.

Becvar, D.S., & Becvar, R. J. (1996). *Family therapy: A systemic integration*. Boston: Allyn & Bacon.

Bell, E. (1996). *Counselling in further and higher education*. Buckingham: Open University Press.

Biswalo, P. M. (1996). *Introduction to guidance and counseling in African settings*. Dar es Salaam: Dar es Salaam University Press.

Blake, A. C. (2006). The experience and adjustment problems of Africans at historically black institutions. *College Student Journal, 40*(4), 808–813.

Bojuwoye, O. (2006). Training of professional psychologists for Africa: Community psychology or community work? *Journal of Psychology in Africa, 16*(2), 161–6.

Carney, C. G. & Savitz, C. J. (1980). Student and faculty perception of student needs and the services of a university counseling center: Differences that make a difference. *Journal of Counseling Psychology, 27*, 597–604.

Chagonda, T. (2001). Masculinities and resident male students at the University of Zimbabwe: Gender and Democracy issues". In R. B. Gaidzanwa (Ed.), *Speaking for ourselves: Masculinities and femininities amongst students at the University of Zimbabwe*. Harare: UZ AAP/GSA Ford Foundation.

Chen, C. P. (1999). Common stressors among international college students: Research and counseling implications. *Journal of College Counselling, 2*, 49–65.

Flisher, A. J., De Beer, J. P., & Bokhorst, F. (2002). Characteristics of students receiving counseling services at the University of Cape Town, South Africa. *British Journal of Guidance & Counselling*, http://www.informaworld.com/smpp/title~content=t713406946 ~db=all~tab=issueslist~branches=30 – v3030(3), 299–310.

Gaidzanwa, R. B. (2001). Masculinities and femininities: An introduction. In R. B. Gaidzanwa (Ed.), *Speaking for ourselves: Masculinities and femininities amongst students at the University of Zimbabwe*. Harare: UZ AAP/GSA Ford Foundation.

Gaidzanwa, R. B. (2007). Alienation, gender and institutional culture at the University of Zimbabwe. *Femininities Africa 8: Rethinking Universities, 1,8*, 60–82.

Itsoseng Clinic. (2007). *Itsoseng Clinic statistics*, University of Pretoria, Department of Psychology, Mamelodi Campus.

Kambaru, E. K. (1999). *The counselling needs of students at the University of Namibia*. Unpublished bachelor's dissertation, University of Namibia, Windhoek.

Kasayira, J. M. (2008). *Counselling tertiary level students of African origin*. Unpublished manuscript, Midlands State University.

Kasayira J. M., Chipandambira, K. S., Hungwe, C., & Mupawose, A. (2007). Stressors and coping strategies of state university students in a developing country. *Journal of Psychology in Africa, 17*(1&2), 45–50.

Kasayira, J. M., Musingarabwi, S., Nyanhongo S., Chipandambira K. S., & Sodi, T. (2007). A survey of the views of college students on academic dishonesty. *Journal of Psychology in Africa, 17*(1&2), 123–8.

Kelly, E. W. (1995). *Spirituality and religion in counselling and psychotherapy: Diversity in the theory and practice*. Alexandria, VA: American Counseling Association.

Kelly, M. J. (2003). The significance of HIV/AIDS for universities in Africa. *JHEA/RESA, 1*(1), 1–23.

Lamprecht, J. C. (2002). Career assessment skills. In K. Maree & L. Ebersohn (Eds.), *Life skills and career counseling*. Sandown: Heinemann.

Mama, A., & Barnes, T. (2007). Editorial: Rethinking Universities 1. Femininities *Africa 8: Rethinking Universities, 1*(8), 1–7.

Mamdani, M. (1993). University crisis and reform: A reflection on the African experience. *Review of African Political Economy, 58*, 7–49.

Mapfumo, J. (2008). Freshmen: The counselling they received in high school and the counselling they need in college/university. *THE DYKE: A Journal of Midlands State University, 3* (1), 57–71.

Morgan, A. (2008). What is narrative therapy? Retrieved August 2008 from www.dulwichcentre.au/alicearticle.html.

Moyo, H. J. (2001). First year student's expectations versus the reality of learning at the University. *International Journal of Open and Distance Learning, 1*, 95–107.

Mpofu, E. (2006). *Theories and techniques for counsellors applied to African settings*. Harare: College Press.

Mpofu, E., Kasayira, J. M., Mutepfa, M., Chireshe, R., & Maunganidze, L. (2006). Inclusive education in Zimbabwe. In P. Engelbretcht & L. Green (Eds.), *Responding to the challenges of inclusive education in southern Africa*. Pretoria, South Africa: Van Schaik Publishers.

Mpofu, E., Mutepfa, M. M., Chireshe, R., & Kasayira, J. M. (2007). School psychology in Zimbabwe. In S. R. Jimerson, T. Oakland, & P. Farrell (Eds.), *The handbook of International school psychology*. Thousand Oaks, CA: SAGE Publications.

Ndlovu, S. (2001). Feminities amongst resident female students at the University of Zimbabwe. In R. B. Gaidzanwa (ed.). *Speaking for ourselves: Masculinities and Feminities amongst students at the University of Zimbabwe*. Harare: UZ AAP/GSA Ford Foundation.

Payne, M. (2000). An overview of narrative therapy. In M. Payne *Narrative therapy: An introduction for counsellors* (pp. 6–17). Thousand Oaks, CA: SAGE Publications.

Pederson, P. B. (1994). A *handbook of developing multicultural awareness*. Alexandria, VA: American Counseling Association

Phala, A.V. (2008). *Service delivery at Itsoseng psychology clinic: A programme evaluation*. Unpublished master's dissertation, University of Pretoria, Mamelodi Campus.

Poku, N. K. (2005). *AIDS in Africa: How the poor are dying*. Cambridge, UK: Polity Press.

Rogerson, C. M. (1980). A future "University of Namibia"? The role of the United Nations Institute for Namibia. *The Journal of Modern African Studies, 18*(4), 675–83.

Ruane, I. (2006). Challenging the frontiers of community psychology: A South African experience. *Journal of Psychology in Africa, 2*, 283–92.

Ruane, I. (2008a). Obstacles in the utilisation of mental health resources in a South African township community. Paper presented at the 5th African Conference in Psychotherapy, Polokwane, South Africa.

Ruane, I. (2008b). *Counselling tertiary level students of African origin*. Unpublished manuscript, University of Pretoria.

Rukuni, M. (2007). *Counsellor training and multicultural counselling in Zimbabwe: Relationship with multicultural counselling competencies*. Unpublished manuscript, Zimbabwe Open University.

Shino, E. (2008). *Counselling tertiary level students of African origin*. Unpublished manuscript, University of Namibia, Namibia.

Sigelman, C. K., & Rider, E. A. (2008). *Life-span human development*. Canada: Wadsworth Cengage Learning.

Somerai, P. (2001). Female non-resident students: Femininities under stress?. In R. B. Gaidzanwa (Ed.), *Speaking for ourselves: Masculinities and femininities amongst students at the University of Zimbabwe*. Harare: UZ AAP/GSA Ford Foundation.

SSCSA (May 2001). *The role of student counseling, career and development services in higher education: Guidelines for structuring and developing student counseling, career and development services*. Potchestroom, South Africa.

Tuckwell, G. (2002) *Racial identity, white counsellors and therapists*. Buckingham, Philadelphia: Open University Press.

University of Namibia (n.d.). University of Namibia Policy on HIV/AIDS. Retrieved October 21, 2008 from www.unam.na/student%20life/aids/draft-policy.pdf

White, M. (1995). The narrative approach to therapy. In M. White (Ed.), *Re-authoring lives* (pp. 11–40). Adelaide, South Australia: Dulwhich Centre Publications.

Williams, J. (1986). *American racism*. In M.W. Macht & J. K. Quam (Eds.), *Social work: An introduction*. Columbus: Merrill.

Zvobgo, R. J. (2007). *Contextualising the curriculum: The Zimbabwe experience*. Harare: College Press.

SELF-CHECK EXERCISES

1. Outline the problems and challenges experienced by university students.
2. In your view, how might a first-year student's adjustment be different from that of a more senior student?

3. Why is it essential for student counselors to address the issue of HIV/AIDS?
4. If you were a student counselor, how would you go about creating awareness about HIV/AIDS at your university?
5. In what ways are international students' and non-international students' problems different?
6. Consider the transition from secondary to tertiary education. How do students negotiate and adjust to their new environment?
7. Critically discuss the issues of cultural differences at universities and the transition between traditional and Western lifestyles.
8. A student comes to see the student counselor due to financial problems. How would the counselor go about assisting the student?
9. Should lecturers act as counselors in universities where no other counseling services are available?

FIELD-BASED EXPERIENTIAL EXERCISES

1. Visit the student counseling services at your university and write two pages about the importance of student counseling. More specifically, your write-up must include a brief outline of the history of counseling services as your university, the type of counseling provided, the service providers, and the benefits of student counseling.
2. Visit the psychology and social work departments at your university and interview at least one lecturer in each department. Specifically, ask them about whether or not they provide counseling to students. What type of counseling do they provide, if at all? What are the pros and cons of providing counseling to their students?
3. Interview a high school student to determine some of the expectations that high school students have about the tertiary level educational experience.
4. Design and administer a questionnaire to students so as to identify types of academic problems they could be facing. Cluster the problems into two groups: of those due to conditions within the person (e.g. disability or laziness) and those due to external factors (e.g. lack of reading materials). Identify the problems you think you can help with on your own and then go ahead and help; refer those you can not handle to appropriate personnel or service providers.
5. List all the counseling-related services that are available to students at your institution, both at the institution and in the community near the institution. Interview some students to find how much they know about the services available to them and whether they are accessing the services.
6. Contact the student counselor at your university and interview him/her about skills that are required to be an effective student counselor.

MULTIPLE-CHOICE QUESTIONS

In this exercise, for some questions there may be more than one answer; however, you are required to choose the best possible answer according to the chapter.

1. Select the exception:
   a. African student
   b. African ancestry
   c. African origin
   d. African heritage
   e. African descent
2. The following is the closest to one of the key missions of university education:
   a. Provide career to young adults
   b. Provide a milestone for young adults
   c. Provide education for young adults
   d. Accommodate young adults of diverse backgrounds
   e. Create and disseminate knowledge to young adults
3. In the present chapter, the following theoretical approaches are recommended for counseling students of African heritage at tertiary institutions:
   a. Behavioral, cognitive, and psychoanalytic
   b. Cognitive, humanistic, and psychoanalytic
   c. Developmental, narrative, and systemic
   d. Cognitive, behavioral, developmental, and systemic
   e. Humanistic, psychoanalytic, and systemic
4. Fill in the blanks. An African student's confidentiality is between _______, while a Euro-American–oriented trained counselor's confidentiality is between_______.
   a. client and counselor; counselor and client
   b. counselor and client; client and extended family
   c. client and extended family; counselor and client
   d. counselor and extended family; client and extended family
   e. client and extended family; counselor and extended family
5. The following is true for both advantaged and disadvantaged contemporary university students of African ancestry:
   a. Being excluded from the mainstream society
   b. Having some heritage of colonial education
   c. Having some heritage of apartheid education
   d. Having a legacy of slavery
   e. All of the above
6. Which of the following is the least desirable termination of the counseling process?
   a. When the counseling goal has been accomplished
   b. When the counselor chose to terminate counseling
   c. When the presenting problem has been addressed
   d. When the student chose to terminate counseling
   e. None of the above
7. All of the following are correct about aspects of multiculturalism except:
   a. Social status
   b. Refugee status

c. Mental status
d. Citizenship status
e. Economic status

8. Fill in the blanks. The role of student counselors is to______ as competencies of effective student counselors is to______.
   a. consultation; career counseling
   b. counseling; consultation
   c. career counseling; personal guidance
   d. consultation; listening
   e. assessment; counseling
9. The following is a challenge likely to affect an international student more than local students:
   a. Environmental adjustments
   b. Test- or exam-taking anxiety
   c. Loneliness
   d. Financial stressors
   e. Performance expectations
10. Which statement is out of place?
   a. Informed concern
   b. Confidentiality
   c. Informed decision
   d. Not doing harm
   e. Client benefit

Answers to the multiple-choice questions are provided at the back of the book

9 Family Therapy within the African Context

Vinitha Jithoo and Terri Bakker

OVERVIEW. Family relationships play a pivotal role in the mental and physical well-being of individuals and hence require a healthy balance of connection as well as individuation. The historical, social, and therapeutic foundations of family counseling have emerged from research and practice based in the Euro-American context, and thus extrapolating these models to other contexts, such as the African one, may omit the importance of the unique interactions families have with major environmental systems. In this chapter, we consider the social and psychological factors that differentiate clients of African ancestry; the history, research, and practice of family counseling; the utility of traditional therapeutic modalities; and current practices, legal and professional issues, research on counseling, within the African context.

LEARNING OBJECTIVES

By the end of the chapter, the reader should be able to:

1. Define the social and psychological factors that differentiate families of African ancestry from European and American families.
2. Understand the first- and second-order cybernetic techniques used in the counseling of families.
3. Discuss the importance of an ethically based practice.
4. Appreciate the operational difficulties inherent in using the nuclear family as the foundational basis for the conceptualization of family therapy.
5. Understand the impact of globalization on family well-being.
6. Evaluate prospective areas of research that would advance our understanding of the family dynamics within an African context.

INTRODUCTION

Africa is rich in its diversity of cultures, religions, and linguistic preferences. It has a multilayered legacy from several and recurrent forced geographic and cultural migrations or displacement as a direct consequence of colonialism, apartheid, racism, and social and economic marginalization of the indigenous population. The emotional ethos of these collectivist cultures shares a legacy of conflict and violence, loss and grief, and many unrealized dreams that form an integral part of their shared identity. Families are at the centre of the cultural regeneration of Africa. They need support in that role, and counseling is one of several resources available to African families in their development.

IMPORTANCE, DEFINITION, AND SCOPE OF KEY TERMS AND CONCEPTS

Family therapy has been structured in ways that support the dominant value system and keep invisible organizing principles of people's lives, including culture, class, race, and sexual orientation (McGoldrick, 1998). For instance, there is a tendency to focus on the nuclear family and underplay the importance of the community and the context for the family experience. Usually, contemporary Western family therapies do not include cultural variables, and its principles are also presumed to be universally valid. Ironically, default, scholarly engagement, within the African context, has prepared family therapy practitioners to function more efficiently within the American context. In many societies, the formal education system is essentially chauvinistic, patriarchal, racist, and sexist, which arose from research based on dominant White groups in America and other Western countries. As a result, families whose norms and values differ tend to be labeled and pathologized (as deficient or dysfunctional). The traditional framework of family therapy associated with people like Bowen, Minuchin, Ackerman, Bateson, the Milan group, Haley, and others defined "family" as an intact, middle-class, heterosexual, White family organized with the man as the head of the household and the women as the primary caretaker of all family relationships. The theoretical basis focused on members interacting as systemic units, and family relationships were understood in terms of complementarity, homeostasis, feedback loops, enmeshment–engagement, and overfunctioning–underfunctioning. There was no acknowledgment of the influence of unequal power.

Euro-Americocentric family therapy frameworks may be inappropriate for use in African settings. Within an African context, family therapy is influenced by its indigenous heritage. This framework may not fit neatly into the Western traditional theoretical constructs used to understand families at different phases in the life cycle. According to Ancis (2004), culturally responsive approaches incorporate the individual client or clients' biography, style, social network, and specific techniques and strategies appropriate to the client's culture, customs, and life habits. Hence, discourses around family conflict and discord may defy theoretical explanations and require a qualitative analysis of issues. Nwoye (2000) argues that modern African therapy incorporates sociological dimensions that either were ignored or unrecognized by Western therapists.

HISTORY OF RESEARCH AND PRACTICE OF FAMILY COUNSELING

Indigenous African family counseling has existed in Africa for millennia. Traditional African families were hierarchically structured with parents and grandparents in executive positions (Nwoye, 2006a). Children and younger people were regarded as on a journey to responsible adulthood. Essentially, indigenous family counseling was preventive and psychoeducational. The goal was to minimize or prevent disordered development. When there was conflict in a family, uncles and aunts or other extended family mediators intervened. For example, a mediating team of elders would serve as mediators in marriage or family conflict (Nwoye, 2001). According to Nwoye (2004), interventions were moral and didactic. However, because of the nuclearization and fragmentation of the modern African family, the old structures are being dismantled. People now turn more and more to counselors, psychotherapists, psychiatrists, social workers, and members of the clergy when family relationships are disturbed. Many of these practitioners are educated or trained in Western contexts and influenced by international trends in family therapy and counseling.

The idea of family therapy and counseling as a distinct therapeutic modality first entered Western mental health services during the 1950s when systems thinking was introduced to the field (Becvar & Becvar, 2000). The family came to be viewed as a system, with the individual members mutually influencing each other so as to maintain the family as a whole. Counselors started viewing problems as arising from the system the individual was part of (interpersonal) rather than from internal problems that developed from within the individual (intrapersonal). The focus in treatment shifted from individual pathology to family relationships. Later this focus was extended to thinking about problems within not only the extended family but also the larger social and cultural context.

During the 1960s and 1970s, a number of South African mental health professionals became interested in family therapy, which later developed into the establishment of the South African Institute (later Association) of Family Therapy (SAAMFT) in 1981. These mental health workers were attracted to the emphasis on family relationships and viewing problems as part of a greater family and community context. They felt that these ideas were familiar in the African context and better fitted with local realities. Subsequently, SAAMFT organized a number of international conferences where therapists from all over the world could share ideas and showcase their work. This conference resulted in an exchange of ideas in that African counselors could learn about family therapy while adapting its principles to the African context. In Zimbabwe, an organization called CONNECT and a Zimbabwe Institute of Systems Therapy were established soon after SAAMFT (Mason & Shuda, 1999). In this way, the Euro-American domination was challenged, while new counseling options were developed to fit with African realities. Since then, African therapists, such as Nwoye (2004), have continued to contribute new ways of working in Africa, while staying in touch with overseas colleagues. However, there are few formal family therapy organizations situated within Africa. Most family counselors work from universities, schools, colleges, churches, and social service agencies and were trained overseas (Nwoye, 2004).

Research in Family Therapy

The international family therapy movement has produced a large number of professional organizations and training institutes, resulting in an extensive literature and a great number of research studies in especially the United States. For example, the Journal Family Process has been in existence for forty-seven years. However, research on family counseling with African people and in African countries is limited. Although there has been a movement toward more cultural (Krause, 2002), gender (Hare-Mustin, 1994), and social sensitivity and inclusivity (McGoldrick, Giordano, & Pearce,1996) as well as social justice (Aldorondo, 2007), few studies have originated from Africa by Africans themselves. However, there are a few notable exceptions, such as Boyd-Franklin's (1989) book on Afro-American families in therapy.

One of the most influential international research journals *Family Process*, recently, regretted that in the forty-six years of its existence, it has not published a single article with first authors from the Middle East, Asian countries outside Japan, and Africa (Imber-Black, 2008). A number of articles published elsewhere have opened the way for serious engagement with African concerns in family counseling (e.g., Bakker & Snyders, 1999; Mason, Rubenstein, & Shuda, 1992; Nwoye, 2001, 2004; Wilson, 1982). There is a recent movement, in the counseling field as a whole, to develop indigenous psychological practice (Kim & Berry, 1993; Nwoye, 2000) and integrate traditional healing practices into psychotherapy and counseling (Moodley & West, 2005).

The Scope of the Need

Today, counseling, and especially formal family counseling, services are still few and far between in African countries, so that these services have been described as

Discussion Box 9.1: Personal Reflections

Divide the class in groups of four to five people. Have each person write down a story remembered from his or her own family of origin. Discuss the following:

- How have their family of origin stories shaped their lives?
- How do these stories impact their relationships with others?
- How do these stories affect how they feel about their family of origin?

"underdeveloped" and "suffering from retarded growth" (Nwoye, 2004, pp. 143, 146). The underdevelopment of African formal services for family counseling tends to mirror other aspects of underdevelopment in African countries, such as economic underdevelopment. A number of counselors do offer these services and have developed locally appropriate approaches to family counseling that fit well with traditional understandings of family counseling (Nwoye, 2004). There is a great need for social services addressing family problems and linking individual problems to family contexts in a culturally appropriate way in African societies. Currently, the traditional extended African family is fragmented and has moved toward nuclearization, so that senior family members are not approached for counseling any more (Nwoye, 2004). More and more Africans are approaching formal health and social services for assistance with problems in living. African people have a rich tradition in family counseling practices. The challenge for the counselors of the future would be to integrate this tradition so as to appropriately address current problems of both rural and more urbanized, globalized people of African descent.

FUNDAMENTAL CONCEPTS AND APPROACHES TO FAMILY COUNSELING

Individual models of counseling tend to put the individual's inner life at the center of the counseling process while family counselors are more interested in the recurring patterns of interactions between individuals in families. It is assumed that the way the family functions – its rules, structure, forms of communication, and the meanings, understandings, and assumptions of the family about its world and itself – all impact on the well-being of family members (Goldenberg & Goldenberg, 2000). Family counselors are interested in the meanings and stories or narratives that families have created, and the way such meanings and stories may unfold during counseling so that family members can improve their well-being and move forward constructively in their lives.

The family is a social system; it does not exist in isolation. All families are subject to gender, cultural, ethnic, and social class influences. The history of each family is interwoven with the history of a community or communities. Providing an overview of families with African ancestry is very difficult because of diversity, not only in race and ethnicity, but also in social, geographical, and cultural backgrounds. Darling (2005) suggests that these varied family dimensions can influence perceptions and reactions to age, family composition, family characteristics, gender roles, family interests, health issues, economic conditions, education, and religion.

Changing Definition of the Family

There are multiple ways of constructing a definition of what constitutes the family: family of origin, family of procreation, family of commitment or affiliation. There is no consensus as to what constitutes a family. Hence, adopting a broad definition that encompasses a social construction that is overinclusive and nonexclusionary is beneficial. Darling (2005) suggests that it may be meaningful to view the family as a bonded unit of interacting and interdependent individuals who have some common goals, resources, and values, and who may share living space – at least for some part of their life cycles. Roopnarine and Gielen (2005) assert that families are not static entities, but "composed," "decomposed," and "recomposed," with the traditional family serving as a life-phase transition to the other family arrangements.

The existence of multiple families form challenges to the traditional family theory which was formulated on the notion of marriage as the basic building block to family formation, monogamy, and two-parent heterosexual unions. Family therapists need to enable their clients to transcend these limited conceptualizations of family constellation and widen the net to include all significant relationships (e.g., siblings, grandparents, housekeepers, nannies, etcetera).

The lengthening of grandparental life course has resulted in grandparents either assisting their adult children in the rearing of their offspring, or assuming total responsibility for providing the necessary care and socialization to their grandchildren (Burton, Dilworth-Anderson, & Merriwether-deVries, 1995). The HIV and AIDS pandemic in sub-Saharan Africa has resulted in the early death of many parents, leaving a large population of children orphaned. Grandparents have become the primary caregivers of their grandchildren. Thus, "family therapists are poised to play a critical role in strengthening existing familial bonds, understanding transgenerational phenomena and easing reactivity to life-cycle demands for monumental coping" (Brown-Standridge & Floyd, 2000, p. 185). Initially, grandparents may assist by co-parenting and upon the death of their children, take on all the childrearing responsibilities. The duration of this arrangement may vary from short term to long term.

Family counselors are especially sensitive to the unique cultural and historical *context* of clients. For example, economic hardship may influence the structure of a family in that it may force a parent into migrant labor. The HIV and AIDS pandemic may impact family structure, leading to child-headed households. Political oppression may have family members incarcerated. Even "positive" developments such as economic advancement may impact the family in that members may move to an affluent suburb and lose contact with extended family members in rural areas. Family counselors need to explore family members' interpretation of the effects of such events in their lives. Regardless of family arrangements, the ability to execute different family roles, in these diverse cultural systems amidst political, social, and economic transitions globally, will determine the stability of societies and their ability to raise children who are more likely to develop multiple cultural identities (Arnett, 2002).

Culture

Culture refers not only to customs, values, family patterns, and religious beliefs, but also to the social and political forces that have shaped family life over time (Almeida, Woods, Messineo, & Font, 1998). Cultural norms prescribe certain behaviors and norms for men and women, young and old, "ill" and "healthy"; these dimensions and associated socio-identities may also be considered cultural constructs (Ancis, 2004). Culture plays a major role in the various dimensions of the therapeutic process, namely the etiology of the distress, the symptom picture and diagnosis, the coping strategies, as well as the modality of treatment sought. According to Ancis (2004), complaints of distress are often expressed through culture-specific idioms. Alarcon and Foulks (1995) assert that self-concept and self-image are influenced by cultural factors, such as childrearing practices, intrafamily roles, and social expectations. This influence sometimes leads to diagnostic challenges.

Family therapists need to transform their definitions and diagnostic impressions to achieve cultural competence. McGoldrick (1998, p. 8) asserts that "cultural competence" requires us to go beyond the dominant values and explore the complexity of culture and cultural identity – not without values and judgments about what is adaptive, healthy, or "normal," but without accepting unquestioningly our society's definitions of these culturally determined categories.

In collectivist cultures, such as those that exist in Africa, the family rather than the individual is prized and valued. The individual is seen as a product of the generations of his or her family. Frequently, collectivism is reinforced and perpetuated through ancestor worship, family rituals, funeral rites, mythologies, and festivity celebrations. The individual is expected to have clearly defined roles and positions based on age, gender, and social class. These bonds are characterized by a strong sense of family commitment, obligation, and mutual responsibility. A strong sense of interdependence and loyalty and respect to the community at large also exists.

Families of African descent vary hugely along most variables such as language, gender roles, and kinship structures. Traditionally, most Africans grow up in extended kinship networks, and communal values predominated over individualism. Families have clear structures of authority and childhood, and gender roles are clearly defined. Within tribes and extended families, specific people were designated to assume leadership and decision-making roles and offer advice on a range of issues. A specific protocol existed regarding the handling of important family matters. Before globalization and migration, family discord was mediated by members of the extended family. According to Nwoye (2004), the aim of indigenous family therapy in Africa was preventative or psychoeducational to prevent disordered development in children.

The need for family therapy grew in response to the dissolution of old structures and the emergence of a new family constellation that was influenced by factors such as globalization, the impact of HIV/AIDS, political unrest, urbanization, or scarcity in resources (Creighton & Omari, 2000). The changing sociodemographics of families have significantly altered the psychosocial resources and adaptive mechanisms of families. Family support and the unifying bonds that the extended family provided previously have begun to erode owing to the pursuit of autonomy by individuals and mobility of family members who no longer live in close proximity to each other. In fact, some children grow up not knowing their family members. The changing value system has made it easier to get divorced without being stigmatized. Divorce is seen as providing an escape from a dysfunctional relationship and a second opportunity for happiness.

Other cultural factors to consider may be the expectations of clients that the counselor would take a directive position, in line with traditional healers or advice from senior family members. Strictly, gender roles and hierarchies may be defined, with strong expectations of the father or senior man being a spokesperson for women and younger family members. Last, but not least, spiritual dimensions prominently may feature and should be respected, addressed, or referred to an appropriate healer, whether traditional or connected to a religious institution.

Often cultural misunderstanding and communication difficulties prevent African people from accessing appropriate services. Understanding and contextualizing the lives of people of African descent is a prerequisite to being a family therapist. This prerequisite may entail some self-exploration and analysis on the part of the family therapist. Burton, Winn, and Clark (2004, p. 406) suggest that this process involves an "exploration of the therapist's

Discussion Box 9.2: Sources of Bias

Divide the class into groups of four or five people. Discuss the importance of counselor-awareness of diversity issues and the impact these issues have on the counseling process. Students must identify current issues that contribute to cultural bias.

own racial, economic, gender, and political histories, tensions and resolution of these tensions in relation to their clients' racial, gender, economic, and political histories." Culturally competent family therapy requires the therapist to attend to culture-bound characteristics of the family's thinking and behavior throughout the therapeutic process (Ariel, 1999).

Gender

In the African context, family structure has been premised on the patriarchal system, which advocates rigid gender identities, thereby maintaining male dominance. Men and women are reared with different role expectations, communication patterns, experiences, goals, problem-solving techniques, and opportunities. Later, such gender dichotomy and differential family experiences may lay the foundation for future conflict in family relationships.

According to the systems perspective, participants in any family interaction, including sexual abuse and violence, exert reciprocal influence on each other's behavior, thereby sharing the patterns of circular causality that serve both to stabilize the family and maintain the problematic behavior (Bloch & Harari, 1996). The General Systems Theory has been widely criticized by feminist theorists for discrediting the power imbalance and for asserting that women and men are equal participants in problem interactions. Feminist philosophy has been used as the conceptual basis to vehemently challenge the impact of gender on the process of family therapy. Although feminism is many things – a social movement, an epistemology, a political stance, an approach to therapy – at its heart, it is a moral enterprise, a naming of what is unjust and a call to redress inequity (Doherty, 2001, p. 152). Hence, feminist family therapy has focused on the client's context, especially the patriarchal structure and traditional forms of authority which are considered damaging to women. Harris, Moret, Gale, and Kampmeyer (2001) suggest that when therapists fail to consider gender, they are implicitly ignoring the power differentials that exist between women and men in a patriarchal society as well as implicitly accepting definitions of women and men that are determined by the dominant discourse. Doherty (2001) asserts that feminism's stance was not just a clinical appeal to more effective ways to help women be healthier, but also a profoundly moral appeal for therapists to redress inequities that women experience in private and public spheres. Family therapists need to reconstruct gender in the process of therapy to help families build relationships based on social justice and human rights rather than male dominance.

Poverty and Economic Marginalization

Economic trends indicate that more and more families are struggling to survive financially. Poverty-stricken families may be found in a wide spectrum of cultural and racial groups and reside in urban as well as rural settings. Economic class determines access to resources such as housing, health care, jobs, and education.

The major source of stress for poor families is not only to cope with maintaining family cohesion and individual well-being, but to simultaneously cope with the challenges of poverty and meeting basic needs for survival. It is not uncommon for families in poverty to face limited access to basic resources, confront a host of personal and familial stressors, conceptualize life as an endless series of crises, and require multiple forms of social service (Ziemba, 2001, p. 214). While mental health services could potentially enhance the quality of family and interpersonal functioning, they often are difficult to access, largely because of scarcity of resources and difficulty accessing community-based mental health centers. Barriers to the client-therapist relationship include perceived disrespect by the client or therapist and client perception that the treatment is irrelevant. These difficulties may arise from social class difference, and in some cases, stigmatization of the client by care providers. Rarely is client oriented care integrated by multiple service providers. In formal clinical training, the neglect of poverty and social class issues has led to a professional culture that shares stereotypical beliefs about families in poverty (Schnitzer as cited in Ziemba, 2001).

APPROACHES TO FAMILY COUNSELING

During the early days of family therapy, the role of the therapist was to study the family system from a relatively objective position as an outsider, and to make interventions to change the family's functioning. This position is called a *"first-order cybernetics"* (Becvar & Becvar, 2000). (*Cybernetics* refers to the study of the way information flows through a system through feedback loops.) For example, the therapist would intervene to change the family's communication patterns, structure, or ways of problem solving. This position would imply that the counselor has some model for understanding what kinds of family behaviors are healthier than others. This carries dangers in that the values of the therapist may be different from those of the family, especially if the family is from a different cultural background. Considering that most theories about the family were developed in Western contexts, one may conclude that these theories may not be applicable to all people from African and other cultural backgrounds.

Recently, there has been a move toward *"second-order cybernetics,"* which assumes that the counselor cannot remain outside the system but becomes part of the observing system and a participant in constructing the reality being observed. This view of the role of the therapist/counselor corresponds to the influential theories of social constructionism and narrative therapy. The counselor would be interested in co-creating new realities or narratives with family members, rather than making interventions from the outside. The counselor cannot assume that he or she knows which is the "best" way for the family to be, or that there is an objective "truth" about a family. This approach thus lends itself to a more respectful way of working with people who may be different from middle-class Western clients who form the majority of clients described in the family literature.

Both these positions are reflected in the following major approaches to family therapy (Becvar & Becvar, 2000; Goldenberg & Goldenberg, 2000).

First-order Approaches

Our discussion identifies mostly Western approaches, and is mindful of the lack of evidence for relevance and effectiveness in African settings. We mention these in passing.

Psychodynamic

Nathan Ackerman, a pioneer of family therapy, initiated this approach, which attempts to integrate psychoanalytic and systems thinking. A fundamental goal of this work is for family members to support each others' needs for attachment, individuation, and personal growth.

Experiential

The counselor uses the therapeutic process to facilitate the family's natural growth and fulfillment of family members' potentials. Carl Whitaker and Virginia Satir are therapists who developed this approach.

Structural

This approach was initiated by Salvador Minuchin. The counselor would understand the structure of the family in terms of roles, coalitions between members, boundaries, wholeness, subsystems, and organization. It is assumed that a family becomes dysfunctional if the structure and organization prevent it from effectively dealing with changes from within and without the system. The counselor attempts to change dysfunctional family functioning through active intervention.

Communication and strategic approaches

Communication theories developed at the Mental Research Institute by theorists such as Bateson, Jackson, and Watzlawick heavily influenced family therapy. Human problems are viewed as interactional and situational. Strategic family therapists use these theories to understand the way families manage change, and to actively intervene so that therapeutic change can take place. The work of Jay Haley and Cloe Madanes falls into this school. The therapist is directive, carefully plans tactics, and may use paradoxical interventions such as prescribing a symptom.

Behavioral/cognitive

Therapists such as Gerald Patterson married behaviorism with family therapy. Traditional behavioral and cognitive therapy techniques are applied in a family context. Counselors may, for example, do behavioral parent training to improve parenting skills in families.

DIFFERENT MODALITIES OF FAMILY THERAPY

It is important to note that family therapy may take many forms and does not necessarily imply one therapist in a room with one nuclear family. Different variations are possible; for example, only one individual may meet with the counselor, who works from a family system perspective. Couples, family units, and subsystems may be seen together. Couples or families could meet together with other couples or families in groups. In addition, family networking focuses on the larger systems surrounding a family and may involve multiple therapists meeting with whole communities at a time. What all these different modalities have in common is the idea of treating individual behavior within a family and social context.

Second-order and Postmodern Approaches

The Milan systemic approach

The first therapists to initiate a second-order approach to therapy worked in Milan, Italy and included Luigi Boscolo and Gianfranco Cecchin. The most outstanding feature of their work was recognition that the therapist is part and parcel of what is being observed and cannot have an objective view of the family and what is in their best interest. This paved the way for the postmodern approaches to develop.

Counselors with a *postmodern* outlook argue that preconceived ideas of what constitutes a functional family are in the eyes of the beholder and thus influenced by the background of the beholder. The culture, ethnicity, gender, sexual orientation, and economic class will inevitably influence judgments. No counselor can be objective or unbiased. Postmodern counselors tend rather to take a "not-knowing" stance (Anderson & Goolishian, 1988) and work together with families to examine belief systems and different realities.

Case Study 9.1: Multigenerational Family Dynamics

Mrs Mkize married at the age of nineteen years because she was pregnant. Her parents initially disliked Mr. Mkize because he was irresponsible, "lazy," drank too much, and had a bad temper. After their marriage, they lived in Mr. Mkize's family home. They had two children: Musa (eighteen years) and Thabile (fourteen years). Mr. Mkize has a poor employment record and worked erratically. Shortly after Thabile was born, Mrs. Mkize was forced to work in order to support the family. Mr. Mkize spent most of his time at the local shabeen and frequently came home intoxicated and became verbally and physically abusive toward his wife. Mrs. Mkize suspected that her husband was having an extramarital affair; but he denied it. Mrs. Mhize urged her mother-in-law to stop her son's behavior; but she asked Mrs. Mkize to be tolerant and interpreted her son's violent outbursts as a sign of affection. She (the mother-in-law) suggested that it was acceptable for Zulu men to have multiple partners and confessed that her late husband was no exception. The Mhize family was referred for family therapy after Musa was treated for stab wounds that he sustained while protecting his mother.

Questions

1. Describe the family dynamics.
2. Describe the mutual influences of each generation on each other.
3. Comment on gender roles and division of labor and the power dynamics.
4. What part did the extended family play?
5. How have religion and cultural values shaped their lives and that of the family?
6. What therapeutic modality would be most effective in assisting this family?
7. What challenges would you anticipate as a counselor?

Social constructionist approaches

Social constructionist therapists do not view reality as something objective out there, but as something that is socially constructed in conversation with others (Freedman & Combs, 1996). The implication is that counseling becomes a conversation wherein the counselor, together with clients, co-constructs realities. Language and meaning become central to the therapeutic process. Stories, interpretations, meanings, values, and beliefs are held up for discussion and their implications for the lives of clients are evaluated. These principles may be applied in different ways. One example is the "collaborative language systems approach" of Harlene Anderson and Harry Goolishian (1988). They assume that problems are "stories that people have agreed to tell themselves" and therapy becomes a process wherein the therapist and client are conversational partners who together engage in a shared inquiry unique to each relationship. The problem exists in language and is " dis-solved" in language. There is a dedication to developing consensual meaning through dialogue (Bird, 2004). This extends beyond work with families. Strictly speaking, social constructionist and narrative therapies are not family therapy models, as they may involve work with individuals or various groupings of people depending on the specific client, the problem, and the situation. However, many practitioners working from this perspective were trained in family therapy and share some of the vocabulary and ways of thinking of family therapists.

Narrative approaches

Michael White and David Epston pioneered this approach in New Zealand. They believed that our sense of reality is maintained through stories. These stories shape and constitute our lives; and they are informed by cultural narratives specifying the dominant view of how one "should" be in a specific context. Some of these "truths," perpetuated by the dominant culture (including psychological theories of health and pathology), may be constraining and oppressive. Narrative therapy allows clients to reexamine the stories of their lives and choose alternative stories that are more in line with their values. This approach especially is sensitive to the oppressive effects of racist, sexist, and class beliefs and aims to expose these. The counselor collaborates with people to construct self-narratives that are in line with their preferred values, beliefs, and spirituality.

RELEVANCE OF EXTANT FAMILY THERAPY MODELS TO THE AFRICAN CONTEXT

There is no one "African family" (Boyd-Franklin, 1989). One may add that there is no one "African family counselor." Counselors working in African contexts may use ideas from any school of family therapy effectively, provided they remain sensitive to and respectful of the fact that their clients (and more importantly, they themselves) may not fit the model as it is portrayed in most Western-based textbooks. All therapeutic models carry cultural and ideological power and may influence our values of "healthy" functioning. These values are not universal. Family therapy has been accused of being oppressive, elitist, neo-colonial, and irrelevant to African contexts. For example, Bulhan (1993) accuses family therapists of imposing Euro-American values on clients in developing countries such as in Africa. However, most family counseling models have moved away from the rigid

Research Box 9.1: Children, Play, and HIV/AIDS in Family Counseling

Erasmus, E. (2004). *Play in psychotherapy with HIV/AIDS-affected children and families*. Unpublished MA (Counseling Psychology) dissertation, University of Pretoria.

Background: During her formal training as a counseling psychologist, Elrika Erasmus (2004) volunteered at a support group for HIV/AIDS affected people at a government hospital, and it struck her how few children attended these sessions. She wondered if only adults affected by HIV/AIDS needed therapy and support. She wondered if the seriousness of the subject did not make therapy a closed space, which excluded children. If we included playfulness in counseling, could this open up the therapeutic space for children? This idea led to her research question:

Research Question: Can counseling and psychotherapeutic interventions be introduced in a playful manner to families and children affected by HIV/AIDS?

Method: A qualitative, narrative research stance was adopted. Working from an ecosystemic world view, the researcher undertook an investigation into the possibilities of working with HIV/AIDS–affected children and families in South Africa in a playful manner in family counseling. Through a process of co-creating and reflecting, the narratives of four therapists were used to describe their experiences of playfulness and psychotherapy with HIV/AIDS–affected persons. These narratives were presented against a background of a research literature discussion of HIV/AIDS and play in therapy.

Results: The following were themes emerging from the narratives: Few psychotherapists had experience of working with children together with families with regards to HIV/AIDS. Reasons for this included that they felt they were not adequately trained. Some noticed that parents are sometimes overprotecting their HIV-positive children and not allowing them to continue to develop and grow. Counseling with HIV/AIDS–affected children and families was often hampered by a lack of basic resources and poverty sometimes prevented children from receiving psychological assistance. In general, the stigma surrounding HIV/AIDS and sex contributed to a reluctance to use assistance. Counselors had different interpretations of playfulness in therapy but felt that children and adults responded positively to more playfulness if introduced in a culture-sensitive way. One therapist used guided imagery to deal with the more difficult parts of the disease. Counselors found that a positive attitude and social contact helped HIV/AIDS–infected people to survive longer and continue to live a fuller life. It was, however, easy for counselors to fall prey to the stigmas surrounding their HIV/AIDS–affected clients, and they felt this detracted from their ability to be playful and helpful with their clients. However, all these psychotherapists believed in their clients' abilities to excel and grow despite or perhaps, because of, the presence of HIV/AIDS in their lives.

Conclusions: Playful psychotherapeutic interventions with HIV/AIDS–affected children and families could be possible, given four criteria. First, the basic resource requirements including food, clothing, and transport of the children and family members must be in place before emotional needs can be adequately addressed. Second, children should be allowed in the therapeutic space with the rest of the family, but in a culture-sensitive way. Third, psychotherapists should be trained to make psychotherapy more child friendly. Lastly, these therapists should be willing to engage in a playful manner with their clients, and not fall prey to the stigma of HIV/AIDS.

Questions

1. Do you agree that children have a place in family counseling? If so, how would you include them in sessions?
2. If parents feel it is inappropriate to have children present when talking to the counselor about HIV/AIDS, how could the counselor ensure that the children's needs are also attended to?
3. Imagine you are having a counseling session with three siblings younger than thirteen years, from an HIV/AIDS–affected family. How would you assist them in a sensitive manner to express their feelings and experiences? (Remember there are other ways of communicating besides words!)

individualism of mainstream counseling approaches and fit well with the holistic world view underlying traditional African values (Bakker & Snyders, 1999). In addition, social constructionist and narrative approaches have an explicit liberatory and social justice agenda that allows for a wide variety of local beliefs and practices to enter the field. The Care Counselors of Malawi (1996) have used narrative counseling principles in community gatherings, in a number of villages in Malawi, to initiate conversations about HIV and AIDS, combining this with drama and song in the local language. Nwoye (2006 b) illustrates how Western and African cultural and therapeutic practices may be integrated in a narrative approach to child and family therapy with an African family.

LEGISLATIVE AND PROFESSIONAL ISSUES

Professional Issues

The family therapy field has always crossed disciplinary and professional boundaries. Prominent family therapists

Discussion Box 9.3: Ethical Issues

In small groups, reflect on how you would overcome the following ethical issues identified by Goldenberg and Goldenberg (2000):

- To whom and for whom does the counselor have primary responsibility? The identified patient? The entire family? Or only the members of the family who attend sessions?
- Is the primary goal to increase family harmony or the growth of individual members?
- How should family secrets be handled? What if a spouse reveals an extramarital affair in a private conversation with the counselor?
- Should the counselor agree to have individual sessions with one family member while the family as a whole attends family sessions?
- Should the contents of this session be confidential or not?

have emerged from psychiatry, social work, clinical and counseling psychology, school counseling, and other settings. In the United States and Europe, family therapy has developed a separate professional identity with professional associations, training institutes, and specialized diploma and degree programs leading to licensing or certification as family therapists (Becvar & Becvar, 2000). Professional practice is regulated by specialist regulating bodies. However, such specialization and regulation does not yet exist in Africa, where practitioners work in universities, schools and colleges, and social and health services, and local training in working with families is often limited and introductory. Each professional is regulated by the professional body. In addition, clients may not be aware of what to expect from "family counseling," which has ethical implications for informed consent.

The ethical issues that are unique to family counseling are not always clearly addressed by ethical guidelines that have been developed with individual clients in mind, as is standard in most professions. Guidelines for family therapy exist, however, and are essential to the practice of family counseling. For example, Gladding, Remley, and Huber (2001) have done a detailed analysis of the ethical, legal, and professional issues specific to the practice of marriage and family therapy. Professional associations provide ethical guidelines to practitioners, such as the Code of Ethics published by the American Association for Marriage and Family Therapy (1998).

However, according to Becvar and Becvar (2000), even these guidelines do not address some of the more subtle ethical issues faced by counselors who work from postmodern and social constructionist assumptions. For example, in many cultures and for a long time in history, child and wife abuse was publicly sanctioned and part of a proud family tradition. It was (and still is) believed that good parents would beat their children. Today this practice is defined as a social ill and a sign of dysfunctional family life. Are we acting ethically if we "label" a family as having a problem who previously believed that they were acting in a proud family and cultural tradition? How does one respect cultural differences and the family's values while promoting social justice? Snyman and Fasser (2004) conclude that, although all professionals should adhere to the prescribed ethical standards set by professional bodies, such rules are not enough. Currently, there is an added responsibility of continuous self-monitoring by questioning the ethical implications of each step in therapy. Counselors should also take responsibility for their actions and continually check with clients how the process impacts on them. Finally, it is imperative that all training programs should integrate ethical issues in all aspects of training.

Comparisons with Practices in Other African Settings

The traditional African world view is holistic, communalistic, and anthropocentric. Humans form part of a kinship network that includes spiritual beings and the ancestors. In African societies herbalists, priests, and diviners are specialists in dealing with personal and interpersonal problems. Healing is ritualistic and communal and the source of healing is attributed to the ancestors. Such a view contrasts with that of the counselor, who is believed to be the facilitator of change. Family counseling approaches also do not always include spiritual and physical dimensions. However, a systems view is aligned to the holistic understanding of humans found in traditional African healing (Bakker & Mokwena, 1999; Bojuwayo, 2005).

Nwoye (2004) refers to the traditional African practice of family counseling, which involved senior family members such as aunts or uncles advising families in difficult situations. This practice was largely educational and preventative. However, it is threatened by changes in family lifestyles and structures. However, this cultural conception is sympathetic to the idea of family counseling.

Through consulting traditional healers, many Africans are familiar with the healing rituals in Africanist churches. These faith healers work holistically and may involve family members in healing rituals (Bakker & Snyders, 1999). Similarly, Islamic traditional healers emphasize the role of spirituality, intellect, and religion-based practices and treat the body and mind as one. They view human beings as in continual interaction with their bio-psycho-social, religious, and cultural environment – a

Research Box 9.2: Culturally Sensitive Family Therapy

Pakes, J. & Roy-Chowdhury, S. (2007). Culturally sensitive therapy? Examining the practice of cross-cultural family therapy. *Journal of Family Therapy, 29*, 267–83.

Objective: The article was drawn from a research project that examined cross-cultural family therapy sessions to ascertain what constituted culturally sensitive practice. This research examined cultural assumptions held by therapists that become enacted in therapy.

Method: A discourse analytic approach was used to explore the principal themes and cultural assumptions that informed the therapeutic process. Three sessions of psychotherapy were analyzed. The participants were two families of Sudanese origin, and two therapists who hailed from different ethnic backgrounds to the family.

Findings: The study found that stereotyping and the assumption of homogeneity may cause disrespect, and has the tendency to devalue the uniqueness that exists within ethnocultural groupings. Values connected to "individualistic" cultures should not be generalized to "collectivistic" cultures, for example, open and direct communication was encouraged by the therapists, but in Sudanese culture this is inappropriate; hence, a third party acts as a mediator. In addition, discourse based on binary oppositions (either/or) encourages dichotomous thinking and false distinctions. In the therapeutic context, these binary oppositions negatively impact the way freedom of choice and decision making unfold.

Conclusions: This study highlights the importance of awareness of cultural diversity and self-reflexivity in cross-cultural work. Adopting a therapeutic stance that is able to deconstruct assumptions and artificial dichotomies may have a higher empathic and therapeutic value. Hence, a balance between "knowing" and "not knowing" enhances the cultural sensitivity of therapists. Culture is often seen as an "add on" in therapy and becomes a central metaphor.

Questions

1. What is the value of conducting discourse research in cross-cultural family therapy?
2. How can we become reflexive as therapists in relation to "culture"?
3. Explain what is meant by "doxic."
4. What did Krause mean by adopting a "not-knowing" stance?
5. How are power imbalances managed in culturally sensitive work?

view very close to systems theory. Farooqi (2004) believes that it is possible to integrate Islamic views of mental health and healing with Western methods, and advises counselors to be aware of and respectful of Islamic cultural traditions.

To summarize, family counseling models may come closer to culturally familiar ways of dealing with human problems for people of African descent than individual models of counseling. Family therapy, like traditional and religious healing practices, follows a holistic approach, focusing on relationships within the family and community context. Such an approach may be familiar to many African families. Counselors should be aware of differences between various forms of helping and healing (e.g., the emphasis on the spiritual) and ensure that they are respectful of clients' expectations. Many African people make use of various forms of healing simultaneously. A working and referral relationship or even partnership with other healers may facilitate the work of the family counselor in certain settings (January & Sodi, 2006; Simwaka, Peltzer, & Maluwa-Banda, 2007). Culturally sensitive variations need to be improvised. For example, inviting a senior family member like an advisory aunt to a family session may bridge the gap between a culturally familiar and respected ritual, and the relative strangeness of a formal counseling relationship.

ISSUES FOR RESEARCH AND OTHER FORMS OF SCHOLARSHIP

Although the field of family therapy has become increasingly mindful of the universalistic concerns about human rights and the welfare of children, insufficient attention has been paid to family life within the African context. Family theory and research, from an African perspective, is in a developmental phase, and hence the need to explore the African psyche, within a transitional context encompassing both the modern and indigenous. Thus, family therapy research has to learn how culture and context influence not only clients but also clinicians and the therapeutic process. Attending to the following issues may assist family therapists in both critical scholarship and practice:

- Studying the caregiving practices and strategies for socializing girls and boys, parent–child arrangements, allocation of resources, division of labor, and other aspects of family life would improve our understanding of broad definitions of family life.
- Our views and actions about power, gender, and human interaction/communication need to be continuously critiqued and updated.
- The influences of race and culture in supervision and training need to be addressed. There is a need for

research exploring the relationships between culturally different supervisors and supervisees.

SUMMARY AND CONCLUSIONS

Family therapists play a pivotal role in society, and such a privilege should be associated with advocacy and responsibility. Thus, it is their responsibility to engage critically with theoretical paradigms that collude with the status quo of power, privilege, and oppression and seek out an integrative framework that could bring integrity to the therapeutic process. Ideally, families should be approached from a multifaceted perspective that considers: (1) what constitutes a family in different cultures; (2) how parental roles and responsibilities are defined and carried out; (3) how sociocultural beliefs, gender roles, religion, and spirituality influence the structure and organization of the family system; (4) how such structures influence the social and cognitive experiences of children; and (5) the impact of globalization. In the African context, the task of family therapists would be to integrate culture-specific theories and interventions into contemporary Western approaches, reconfigure traditional Euro-American centric models, and/or implement novel strategies in assisting families.

REFERENCES

Alarcon, R. D., & Foulks, E. F. (1995). Personality disorders and culture: Contemporary clinical views (Part A). *Cultural Diversity and Mental Health*, *1*, 3–7.

Aldorondo, E. (Ed.) (2007). *Advancing social justice through clinical practice*. Mahwah, NJ: Lawrence Erlbaum Associates.

American Association for Marriage and Family Therapy (1998). *AAMFT code of ethics*. Washington, DC: Author.

Ancis, J. R. (Ed.) (2004). *Culturally responsive interventions*. New York: Brunner- Routledge.

Anderson, H., & Goolishian, H. (1988). Human systems as linguistic systems: Preliminary and evolving ideas about the implications for clinical theory. *Family Process*, *27*, 157–63.

Ariel, S. (1999). *Culturally competent family therapy: A general model*. Westport, CT: Praeger.

Arnett, J. J. (2002). The psychology of globalization. *American Psychologist*, *57*, 774–83.

Bakker, T. M., & Mokwena, M. L. E. (1999). African and Western perspectives compared. In P. Avis, A. Pauw, & I. Van der Spuy (Eds.), *Psychological perspectives: An Introductory workbook* (pp. 215–26). Cape Town: Pearson Education South Africa.

Bakker, T. M., & Snyders, F. J. A. (1999). The (hi)stories we live by: Power/knowledge and family therapy in Africa. *Contemporary Family Therapy*, *21*(2), 133–54.

Becvar, D. S., & Becvar, R. J. (2000). *Family Therapy: A systemic integration* (4th ed.). Boston: Allyn and Bacon.

Bird, J. (2004). *Talk that sings: Therapy in a new linguistic key*. Auckland, NZ: Edge Press.

Bloch, S. & Harari, E. (1996).Working with the family: The role of values. *American Journal of Psychotherapy*, *50(3)*, 274–84.

Bojuwoye, O. (2005). Traditional healing practices in Southern Africa. In R. Moodley & W. West (Eds.), *Integrating traditional healing practices into counseling and psychotherapy* (pp. 61–72). Thousand Oaks, CA: SAGE Publications.

Boyd-Franklin, N. (1989). *Black families in therapy: A multisystems approach*. New York: Guilford Press.

Brown-Stanridge, M. D., & Floyd, C. W. (2000). Healing bittersweet legacies: Revisiting contextual family therapy for grandparents raising grandchildren in crisis. *Journal of Marital and Family Therapy*, *26*(2), 185–97.

Bulhan, H. A. (1993). Family therapy and oppression: A critique and proposal. In L. J. Nicholas (Ed.), *Psychology and oppression: Critiques and proposals* (pp. 167–89). Johannesburg: Skotaville.

Burton, L. M., Dilworth- Anderson, P., & Merriwether-deVries, C. (1995). Context and surrogate parenting among contemporary grandparents. *Marriage and Family Review*, *20*, 349–66.

Burton, L. M., Winn, D. M., & Clark, S. L. (2004). Working with African American clients: considering the 'homeplace' in marriage and family practices. *Journal of Marital and Family Therapy*, *30*(4), 397–410.

Care Counsellors of Malawi (1996). Pang'ono pang'ono ndi mtolo – little by little we make a bundle: The work of the CARE counsellors of Malawi. *Dulwich Centre Newsletter*, *3*, 2–24.

Creighton, C., & Omari, C. K. (Eds.) (2000). *Gender, family and work in Tanzania*. Aldershot: Ashgate.

Darling, C. A. (2005). Families in a diverse culture. *Journal of Family and Consumer Sciences*, *97*(1), 8–13.

Doherty, W. J. (2001). Feminism, moral consultation and training. In T. S. Zimmerman (Ed.), *Integrating gender and culture in family therapy training* (pp. 151–56). New York: Hawthorne Press.

Farooqi, Y. N. (2004). Understanding Islamic perspective of mental health and psychotherapy. *Journal of Psychology in Africa*, *16*(1), 101–12.

Freedman, J., & Combs, G. (1996). *Narrative therapy: The social construction of preferred realities*. New York: Norton.

Gladding, S. T., Remley, T. P., & Huber, C. H. (2001). *Ethical, legal and professional issues in the practice of marriage and family therapy* (3rd ed.). Upper Saddle River, NJ: Merrill Prentice-Hall.

Goldenberg, I., & Goldenberg, H. (2000). *Family therapy: An overview* (5th ed.). Belmont, CA: Wadsworth/Brooks/Cole.

Hare-Mustin, R. T. (1994). Discourses in the mirrored room: A postmodern analysis of family therapy. *Family Process*, *33*, 19–35.

Harris, T., Moret, L. B., Gale, J., & Kampmeyer, K. L. (2001). Therapists's gender assumptions and how assumptions influence therapy. In T. S. Zimmerman (Ed.), *Integrating gender and culture in family therapy training* (pp. 33–60). New York: Hawthorne Press.

Imber-Black, E. (2008). Editorial: Making family process truly international. Retrieved January 28, 2008 from http:/www.familyprocess.org/current_issue.asp?

January, J., & Sodi, T. (2006). The practices of Apostolic faith healers in mental health care in Zimbabwe. *Journal of Psychology in Africa*, *16*(2), 315–20.

Kim, U., & Berry, J. W. (Eds.) (1993). *Indigenous psychologies: Research and experience in cultural context*. Thousand Oaks, CA: SAGE Publications.

Krause, I. (2002). *Culture and system in family therapy*. London: Karnac.

Mason, J., Rubenstein, J., & Shuda, S. (Eds.) (1992). *From diversity to healing*. Durban: South African Institute of Marital and Family Therapy.

Mason, J., & Shuda, S. (1999). The history of family therapy in South Africa. *Contemporary Family Therapy*, *21*(2), 133–54.

McGoldrick, M. (1998). Belonging and liberation: Finding a place called "home." In M. McGoldrick (Ed.), *Re-visioning family therapy: Race, culture and gender in clinical practice* (pp. 215–28). New York: Guilford Press.

McGoldrick, M., Giordano, J., & Pearce, J. K. (1996). *Ethnicity and family therapy* (2nd ed.). New York: Guilford Press.

Moodley, R., & West, W. (Eds.) (2005). *Integrating traditional healing practices into counselling and psychotherapy*. Thousand Oaks, CA: SAGE Publications.

Nwoye, A. (2000). Building on the indigenous: Theory and method of marriage therapy in contemporary Eastern and Western Africa. *Journal of Family Therapy*, *22*, 347–59.

Nwoye, A. (2001). History of family therapy: The African perspective. *Journal of Family Therapy*, *12*(4), 61–77.

Nwoye, A. (2004). The shattered microcosm: Imperatives for improved family therapy in Africa in the 21st century. *Contemporary Family Therapy*, *26*(2), 143–64.

Nwoye, A. (2006a). A narrative approach to child and family therapy in Africa. *Contemporary Family Therapy*, *28*(1), 1–23.

Nwoye, A. (2006b). Theory and method of marriage therapy in contemporary Africa. *Contemporary Family Therapy*, *28*, 437–57.

Pakes, J., & Roy-Chowdhury, S. (2007). Culturally sensitive therapy? Examining the practice of cross-cultural family therapy. *Journal of Family Therapy*, *29*, 267–83.

Roopnarine, J. L., & Gielen, U. P. (Eds.) (2005). *Families in global perspectives*. Boston: Pearson.

Simwaka, A., Peltzer, K., & Maluwa-Banda, D. (2007). Indigenous healing practices in Malawi. *Journal of Psychology in Africa*, *17*(1), 155–62.

Snyman, S., & Fasser, R. (2004). Thoughts on ethics, psychotherapy and postmodernism. *South African Journal of Psychology*, *34*(1), 72–83.

Wilson, N. R. (1982). Family therapy in Kenya. *Journal of Family Therapy*, *4*(2), 165–76.

Ziemba, S. J. (2001). Therapy with families in poverty: Application of feminist family principles. In T. S. Zimmerman (Ed.), *Integrating gender and culture in family therapy training* (pp. 205–38). New York: Hawthorne Press.

Zimmerman, T. S. (Ed.) (2001). *Integrating gender and culture in family therapy training*. New York: Hawthorne Press.

USEFUL WEBSITES

http://www.abacon.com/familytherapy/index.html
http://www.aamft.org/
http://www.familyprocess.org/

SELF-CHECK EXERCISES

1. Define family in the African context.
2. What is the difference between individual models of counseling and family models of counseling?
3. What contextual factors impact on the families' psychosocial functioning?
4. How can family therapists minimize cultural value conflicts and develop a strong therapeutic alliance with clients?
5. Should contemporary family therapy approaches be replaced by culture-specific approaches?
6. How can family therapy approaches be adapted to meet the needs of clients from African ancestry?

FIELD-BASED EXPERIENTIAL EXERCISES

Divide the class into groups. Each group will research one ethnic cultural grouping and learn about their "typical" customs, beliefs, values, traditions, childrearing practices, division of labor, gender roles, health beliefs, systems of healing, experiences with oppression, and so forth.

- Allow each group to discuss their findings.
- Allow students who represent members of the discussed cultural group to relate their own personal experiences of their culture and how it fits, or does not fit, with what the group reported.
- Highlight the differences and discuss within-group differences, to help students understand that not all representatives of a group will ascribe to what is typical for the group as a whole.
- Discuss the role stereotyping plays and how harmful those consequences are to the counseling process and relationship.

MULTIPLE-CHOICE QUESTIONS

1. When was family therapy and counseling introduced to the mental health services?
   a. During the 1800s
   b. During the 1950s
   c. During the 1980s
   d. After 2000
2. The traditional framework of family therapy is associated with the following people:
   a. Freud, Adler, and Jung
   b. Watson, Bandura, and Pavlov
   c. Bowen, Minuchin, Ackerman, and Bateson
   d. Michael White
3. According to McGoldrick (1998), traditional family therapy has been structured in ways that failed to take into account:
   a. The patriarchal structure of the family
   b. The matriarchal structure of the family
   c. Culture, class, race, and sexual orientation
   d. All of the above
4. Fill in the blank. According to Nwoye (2000), African-based family counseling takes into consideration ________________ dimensions that are unrecognized by Western-based therapies.
   a. sociological
   b. anthropological
   c. biomedical
   d. neurological
5. Feminist family therapy focuses on:
   a. Shifting the locus of power to women
   b. Achieving equilibrium

c. The patriarchal structure and traditional forms of authority considered harmful to women
d. Respecting the father as the head of the family

6. In which postmodern approach to family therapy is objective "reality" unimportant and language and meaning of central importance to the therapeutic process?
a. Social constructionist approach
b. Structural approach
c. Experiential approach
d. Strategic approach

7. The therapist's stance in theories that are clustered into first-order cybernetics is:
a. To study the family from a relatively objective position as an outsider
b. To engage with the family as a participant in constructing reality
c. To study the whole therapeutic system including the therapist
d. None of the above

Answers to the multiple-choice questions are provided at the back of the book

10 Pastoral Care and Counseling

Daniël Johannes Louw

OVERVIEW. This chapter focuses on the the unique contribution of pastoral care and counseling to processes of healing. The dimension of healing is connected to existential realities that reflect real-life issues. The emphasis is on the healing of life in order to connect to African spiritualities and its interconnectedness to spiritual forces believed to determine the destiny of everyday life. A systems approach, taking into consideration processes of interculturalization, appears best suited to African settings.

LEARNING OBJECTIVES

By the end of the chapter, the reader should be able to:

- Explain the unique contribution of pastoral care and counseling to processes of healing within a holistic approach to pastoral therapy.
- Describe the interplay between culture and the spiritual realm of life.
- Propose a pastoral assessment/diagnosis in terms of life issues that are a threat to spiritual health.
- Outline the basic features of African spiritualities.
- Relate basic counseling skills to the demands coming from African spiritualities on counseling procedures.
- Critique different anthropological models from a pastoral anthropological perspective.

INTRODUCTION

Any theory of counseling people in Africa, even a definition of care and counseling, should deal with an African world view, philosophy, and spirituality. The concept "Africa" is complex and does not denote a homogeneous group (Long, 2000). Rather, Africa is a philosophical concept, describing the complexity and diversity of different cultural, local, and contextual settings as related to a state of being and mind. Africa is also a "spiritual category." It is an inclusive category describing the "spirit" of people living in Africa. Africa functions as a hermeneutical paradigm indicating a unique approach to life that differs from the analytical approach emanating from Western secular thinking and Hellenism. *Hellenism* refers to the rationalistic and positivistic approach to life that is an attempt to explain all life issues in terms of the rational categories of the human mind. Waruta and Kinoti (2000) referred to the spiritual dimension of care with African communities. Let us consider some of the terms associated with this understanding of an African world view.

IMPORTANCE, DEFINITION, AND SCOPE OF KEY TERMS AND CONCEPTS

First, we explain the concept of hermeneutical understanding. Next, we briefly define the comstruct of pastoral care and counseling.

A *hermeneutical understanding* is an understanding wherein one assesses meaning within a systemic network of dynamic relationships. It is not an analytical approach wherein one begins by separating the entities from their context and thereafter starts to reason in terms of a cause-and-effect approach. For example, the value of a human being should not be assessed in terms of individuality, but in terms of one's place wihin a relational system of interconnectedness. Hermeneutics represents a qualitative approach and is an attempt to understand texts or phenomena, including people, within contexts. It probes into the meaning dimension of texts (intentionality) as well as of human behavior.

Pastoral is derived from the Latin term *pascere*, which means to feed and to care for the flock. These terms underline the fact that human crises have a spiritual dimension and cannot be fully overcome until the spiritual yearnings of the human being have been met. Pastoral care and counseling falls within the field of *theology*, the science that deals with the care of human souls (*cura animarum*). It operates within the realm of *spirituality*, that is, life as related to the awareness of a transcendent dimension. The term *soul* (Hebrew: *nĕfĕsj*/quality of human life; Greek: *kardia*/heart, or *noes*/mind) refers to the qualilty of human life as embedded in the network of human relationships and determined by the presence of God. It represents life as directed to the ultimate dimension of human existence. The soul, as a spiritual entity, is engaged in the existential, human quest for meaning. Also, the soul connected to *ethos*. An appreciation of soul is based on an understanding of the importance of virtues, norms, values, and the moral dimension of our humanity.

Discussion Box 10.1: African Spirituality

The notion of African spirituality is not clear. The concept "Africa" refers to a vast continent, to geography or demographic issues. It encompasses different local settings and represents different cultures. Because of democratization and liberalization, the concept is associated with different political issues and ideologies.

Africa represents different spiritualities. It is actually impossible to reduce the cultural and spiritual diversity to one model. Even the attempt to use *Ubuntu*-philosophy, as a cultural and spiritual schema of interpretation, stirs many critical and scientific questions.

Questions

1. What is the necessity for an African approach to epistemology and can one use the concept "African epistemology"?
2. Discuss the implications of a philosophical approach to a pastoral hermeneutics to gain clarity on the notion of African spiritualities.
3. What is the impact of an "African" approach to counseling on theoretical paradigms for pastoral counseling? How does it influence theory formation in pastoral care?

The African pastoral theologian Emmanual Lartey (1997) referred to the now traditional definition of *pastoral care* as the helping act performed by representative Christian persons, directed toward the healing, sustaining, guiding, and reconciling of troubled persons, whose troubles arise in the context of ultimate meanings and concerns. Pastoral care fulfills psychospiritual functions: the functions of nurturing, liberating, and empowering. It is a normative science in that it does not prescribe using the Bible as a handbook or manual for life. It deals with people's existential struggles from a spiritual perspective. In such a model, the comfort and will of God play a fundamental role. Pastoral care, with its emphasis on relational spirituality, is evident in various aspects of the lives of Africans. Pastoral care in an African context is practiced within the context of certain traditions. These are now described.

TRADITIONS INFORMING PASTORAL CARE AND COUNSELING IN AN AFRICAN CONTEXT

Christian traditions, African traditions, and Biblical counseling are recognized.

Christian Traditions

Within the Christian tradition, soul care is exercised from the perspective of salvation. It deals with the comfort of God as enfleshed in the cross and resurrection of Christ, and exhibited by the inhabitational presence of the Spirit of God in human bodies. Thus, spiritual care is about the ensoulment of the human body and the embodiment of the human soul. With such an anthropological understanding of the human soul, my preference is for a systemic and relational understanding of the soul rather than a substantial understanding (i.e., soul as a thing). Such a conceptual framework is closer to the understanding of our being human within most African spiritualities. Although it is difficult to generalize, there exists a general tendency to see the core of our human existence as an interrelated network of connections and communalities (see the ubuntu paradigm; see also Chapters 1 and 4, this volume) influenced by and related to life forces/spiritual entities. Ethics, values, norms, and morality, are integrated within the Christian tradition of comfort and consolation.

African Traditions

Traditional healers are at the forefront of spirituality and health in many African communities (see also Chapters 1 and 4, this volume). Three main types of traditional healers exist in South Africa (Hemshorn de Sánches, 2003, p. 72): the *isangoma* (diviner), the *izinyanga* (doctors), and the *umthandazi* (prophet healers) (Oosthuizen, 1992; see also Chapter 1, this volume). The question at stake is: How could they be incorporated in pastoral care and counseling? The important point to understand is that the traditional healers provide a safe space for the sick or traumatized person.

Counseling African people is to counsel life. In Africa, epistemology is embedded in the wisdom of systemic relationships as expressed through the interconnectedness and communality of life (Oguejiofor, 2003, pp. xiv–xv). *Epistemology* refers to theory formation, in science, pertaining to the question of how to gain knowledge from an entity or phenomenon. It is the theory regarding processes of knowing and the sources for valid knowledge. It operates with the questions: What is the source of knowledge; and where do I get my knowledge from? How do I know? One can describe counseling within the African context as wisdom counseling. *Wisdom counseling* refers to the moment in counseling wherein the counselee needs to make a true discernment pertaining to what really counts

Case Study 10.1: Nomsa X

Nomsa X is a woman in a small village. Because she has been living positively with HIV for more than three years, she has experienced a great deal of rejection from her community. They talked about her and referred to her as the woman with the "sickness." The stigmatization of being labeled a "patient" caused emotional pain. Because of a lack of intimacy, she suffered from anxiety and a fear of rejection.

She visited a medical doctor in the city who identified her pain as depression. Medication was prescribed. However, back in the village the emotional pain and burden became too "heavy" for her to carry. She decided to visit a divine healer (who was a Christian) in a nearby village.

When she returned, she was a totally new person. She smiled and started to reach out to other people in her neighborhood. One day her eighteen-year-old daughter asked her: "Mother what happened because you have changed a lot?" She smiled and said: "I left my burden with Him. I don't need to carry it myself. I am not alone anymore."

What happened and changed?

Questions

1. Apply a narrative explanation to the case of Nomsa.
2. What aspects of her spiritual healing could have supported her recovery?

Discussion Box 10.2: Perspectives on Pastoral Care

Pastoral care is actually a concept that emanates from the Christian tradition and a Western understanding of life and humanity. A Western approach to counseling procedures has been influenced heavily by counseling procedures coming from psychology. Approaches are often very analytical. Counseling procedures are affected by listening skills. Within the practical setting of counseling, the Rogerian technique has established itself as the ABC of counseling, thus the importance of an empathetic approach.

Thus, one must consider how to translate counseling skills into a practice of care that deals with an African approach to life issues. The interculturalization of care and counseling has become a vital issue.

Questions

1. What is meant by the interculturalization of care and counseling? Discuss the notion of empathy and its relatedness to the concept of "interpathy" within the African traditions.
2. Narrative therapy in psychology evolved from philosophical processes of globalization and postmodernization. In this therapy, the client is the expert and; a new story has to be created. In this process, exisiting paradigms and rational concepts should be deconstructed. How does such an understanding of narrative therapy fit into the African tradition to tell stories and to interpret life with the aid of symbols and metaphors?

in life. It deals with the human quest for meaning, with questions about the significance of life. Norms, values, and virtues play a decisive role in wisdom counseling.

This emphasis on wisdom can be linked to what is called *Biblical counseling* in the Christian tradition of pastoral care. "Pastoral counselors work with a biblically informed wisdom framework and perspective" (Schipani, 2003, p. 81). This framework corresponds with the pastoral counselor's confessional affirmation concerning Scripture. In light of this framework, Schipani (2003, p. 81) concluded that pastoral counselors, like teachers and ministers, give due consideration to the teachings, narratives, poetry, prophecy, and other biblical materials, as these expressions of the written Word illuminate and address their counselees' existential challenges and struggles. In this regard, pastoral counselors give special attention to a unique hermeneutical counseling process with the goal of wise discernment, wise decision making, and wise living.

Psychological Foundations

From a psychological perspective, the field of pastoral counseling focuses on the application of spiritual content and processes to the alleviation of human distress. The following primary functions of the pastor are brought into play: spiritual direction, prayer, administration of the sacraments, pastoral guidance, and interpretation of Scripture (Miller & Jackson, 1995). Clinebell (1996) regarded pastoral care and counseling as having moved from a person- and client-centered model to a relationship-centered model. He also described the overarching goal of all pastoral care and counseling (and of all of ministry) as to liberate, empower, and nurture wholeness centered in Spirit.

Table 10.1. Stages in pastoral care and counseling

	Phase 1	Phase 2	Phase 3	Phase 4
Patient person	Self-insight Self-understanding	Self-integration Acceptance of situation	Active involvement Action/program designs for living	Trust in God Appropriateness of God-images
Pastor's skill	Listen Empathy Interpathy Interpretation Understanding	Knowledge of theodicy Summary of facts Information Story analysis Liturgical acts	Assistance in formulating objectives/goals Facilitation Motivation	Organic use of scripture Prayer Serving the sacraments
Objective	Building trust Relationship Communicating Understanding and sensitivity	Building perspective Generating hope Vision Insight	Cooperation Purposeful Behavior Reaching out to systemic interaction	Growth in faith Maturity in faith Imparting meaning Receiving meaning
Core component	Emotion and affection Love Cultural system	Content Thought Will Pastoral style and attitude	Actions Support network Family and friends	Faith God's promises Cultural/ religious values and norms
Summary	FEEL	THINK/WILL	DO	BELIEVE/TRUST

The normative dimension does not imply that pastoral counseling is directive in the sense of prescriptive advice counseling. In this regard, an interdisciplinary approach is imperative. For instance, Miller and Jackson (1995) advocated for the integration of psychology and religion. Taylor (1991) referred to four phases of counseling: clarification, formulation, intervention, and termination, and added to these the important dimension of theological assessment.

The Central Role of Theological Assessment in Pastoral Care and Counseling

With regard to forming a pastoral assessment, Louw (1998, pp. 321–45) emphasizes the role of God-images. Fundamental to a theological assessment is helping people to differentiate between appropriate God-images (images that can help people to hope and find meaning in life) and inappropriate God-images (images that contribute to anxiety, false guilt, despair, helplessness, self-rejection, and destructive anger and hatred).

Louw (1998, pp. 349–65) developed a four-phase model of counseling, based on the three-stage model of Egan (1990). The four-phase model is illustrated in Table 10.1.

Application to People of African Ancestry

To apply pastoral care to counseling people of African ancestry, a *systems approach* to counseling is paramount. In a systems model, one works with the interconnectedness of relationships and one's position within the network of relationships rather than with individuality and personality (see also the Chapter 8, this volume). According to Friedman (1985), systems thinking focuses less on content and more on the process that governs the data. Additionally, it focuses less on the cause-and-effect connections that link bits of information and more on the principles of organization that give data meaning. "The components do not function according to their "nature" but according to their position in the network" (p. 15).

Within an African setting, the notion of interculturality and counseling across cultures becomes extremely important. For instance, Augsburger (1986) underlined the importance of the counseling skill of *interpathy* in cross-cultural care as follows:

> Interpathy is an intentional cognitive envisioning and affective experiencing of another's thoughts and feelings, even though the thoughts rise from another process of knowing, the values grow from another frame of moral reasoning, and the feelings spring from another basis of assumptions. (p. 29)

Pastoral care and counseling is about "thinking with" and bracketing one's own beliefs to enable understanding the spiritual other.

HISTORY OF RESEARCH AND PRACTICE IN PASTORAL CARE AND COUNSELING IN AFRICA

An accurate account of the history of research in pastoral care, within an African context, is still to be achieved. Most written historical accounts have strong Western influences. For instance, on the one hand, there is a Western emphasis on psychotherapy and personality theories, processes of representation of the vestiges of colonialization, and church missionary influences (see also Chapters 6 and 7, this volume). On the other hand, there is the oral tradition in Africa, embedded within African spirituality and an African view on life, scholarship on which is emerging.

Research Box 10.1: Restoring the Sick

Berinyuu, A. A. (1988). *Pastoral care to the sick in Africa. An approach to transcultural pastoral theology*. Frankfurt am Main: Verlag Peter Lang.

Objective: The study is an attempt to probe into the realm of African spirituality and to research the mechanism in which traditional African healers (diviners) can contribute to health and welfare. It also investigated the possible interplay between a Western and African understanding of health and healing. The contextual and cultural setting was Ghana. The guiding question was: What is the appropriate pastoral approach for Ghananian with its long history of both indigenous African and Christian traditions?

Method: Participants included traditional healers. Qualitative approaches were used for both the data analysis and interpretation.

Results: Participants believed that health is not merely about the absence of bacteria, germs, or diseases, but that good health also includes positive human relationships.

Conclusion: Ghananians hold a relational view of spirituality and health.

Questions

1. What is meant by healing within a Western concept; and how can it be linked to an African traditional understanding?
2. Discuss any strengths and limitations of the health perspective held by the Ghananians. Explain your selection of perceived strengths and limitations.

Table 10.2. Life dimensions of existential healing

Existential issues		Life needs being needs: courage to be		Christian spiritual healing/therapy
Anxiety: experience of loss/ rejection	⟶	Intimacy: affirmation and self-actualization	⟵	Grace: unconditional love role of God-images
Guilt/shame	⟶	Freedom/deliverance	⟵	Forgiveness/reconciliation
Despair/doubt	⟶	Anticipation: meaning	⟵	Eschatological realm of hope/salvation
Helplessness/vulnerability	⟶	Support system	⟵	Fellowship & service/*koinonia*/*diakonia*
Frustration/anger (Disappointment and frustration; structural issues: poverty/unemployment/violence/crime)	⟶	Life fulfillment/ direction/ transformation	⟵	Gratitude and joy/*promissio* therapy/ethics (*Promissio* refers to the fulfilled promises of God as expressed in the Biblical text)

The history of pastoral care in the Christian tradition is linked to the classic formulation of *cura animarum*: care of the human souls (McNeill, 1951). According to Oden (1987, p. 187), care of souls means the care of the inner life of persons. God is the chief carer of souls. Therefore, history is intrinsically linked to the Biblical image of the shepherd (Mills, 1990). Proposing a shepherding perspective, Hiltner (1958) referred to the solicitous concern expressed within the religious community for persons in trouble or distress.

Within the Christian tradition, the historical development of pastoral care can be divided into five broad approaches: the (1) *kerygmatic approach*, in the reformed tradition, with the emphasis on sin, confession, and proclamation; (2) *sacramental approach*, in the Roman Catholic tradition, with the emphasis on the sacrament of confession and the liturgy of intercession; (3) emphasis is on deliverance and exorcism within more *charismatic* approaches; (4) the influence of Western psychology; and (5) bipolar model, which emphasizes the interplay between the spiritual dimension of care (the human quest for meaning) and the human/personal/existential dimension of care (need-satisfaction and the empirical aspect).

This interplay is portayed in Table 10.2.

In terms of history and theory formation for counseling people in an African setting, it is important to link care and counseling to the processes of liberation and empowerment of people (*the justice and freedom paradigm*). The emphasis in the African context is less on individual counseling, as understood by many person-centered theories in Western psychology, and more on social, political, and public healing.

In an African epistemology, daily life events and the interrelatedness of people should be seen as ingredients for a holistic and integrated understanding of healing. Life describes a dynamic network of systemic relationships.

For Africans, life is an integral whole of cosmic and social events (Berinyuu, 1988). For this reason, broken ties and relationships must be restored in order to heal. In this regard, role fulfilment is more important than personal self-actualization (although one can self-actualize in role function). Role is in itself a therapeutic principle for the healing of life (Kahiga, 2005a; Twesigye, 1996).

Therefore, the African paradigm regarding history is about life and human events, guided by the principle of *Ubuntu* (Mandela, 2005; Pobee, 1992; Van Binsbergen, 2003; see also Chapter 1, this volume). Life never stands on its own and is embedded in the dialectics between life events and death. "Life is a thesis and death is its antithesis. Life is to embrace and death is to depart and to isolate. The synthesis between life and death is becoming" (Kahiga, 2005 b, p. 190). Many Africans perceive human life as an infinite becoming or progression, and each human person ought to be an agent of this traditional cultural reality.

Rather than to try to describe the history of counseling African people, it will be more appropriate to pose the question: How is counseling related to the the notion of culture? In different cultural settings, the history of counseling in Africa will be different. For instance, Bate (1995) advocated for the connection between inculturation and healing. His basic argument was that an analysis of culture is the key to understanding the sickness-healing process. Bellagamba (1987) referred to inculturation as the attempt to create a spirituality that is rooted in the basic experience of life.

PASTORAL INTERVENTION AND DIAGNOSIS WITHIN THE DIMENSION OF SPIRITUALITY

Because a human is a societal being within the totality of transcendental and religious powers, the spiritual dimension should play a decisive role in counseling procedures and well-being. The roles of community, ancestors, God-image, and immanency in African settings are discussed next.

Community

According to Skhakhane (1995), the community is the core of African spirituality. By "community" is meant not only the living, but also the ancestors.

> African Spirituality consists of an intimate relationship of people with their ancestors; a relationship initiates and governs their activity in life in such a way that they relate to all other beings in a manner that guarantees harmony and peace. (p. 112)

"Community" also includes the state of the whole family. Ackermann (1993) and Mtetwa (1996) referred to this state as the priority of community: the extended family. Within the extended family, role assignment and the quest for humanity are of the utmost importance. According to Bellagamba (1987, p. 107), "a spirituality which does not incorporate all people, their events, their richness, their hopes and concerns, cannot speak to Africans who are fundamentally communal and relational."

Bosch (1974) was of the view that "African spirituality is structured, not along the lines of a pyramid, but a circle – community and communality as the centre of religious life" (p. 40). African spirituality places emphasis on communal procedures that incorporate the community, the extended family, as well as an understanding of God as related to life and daily events (Bujo, 1992, p. 18). "For most African peoples, God is present in everyday life because he is just and he punishes sin" (Long, 2000, p. 23). Therefore, people are dependent on God and need to keep good relations with God. African spirituality is connected to an integral and holistic understanding of life (Kretzschmar, 1996, pp. 63–75). This perspective should be included in any pastoral intervention and diagnosis.

Ancestors

In an African setting, pastoral diagnosis is a diagnosis of the spiritual realm and the interplay between the supreme being, the realm of the ancestors, and the quality of life relationships. The ancestors are part of daily life events and believed to be reckoned with in life decisions. The ancestral spirits are believed to continue to play a vital role in the lives of their descendants, often acting with benevolence, protecting and guiding those in whom they continue to live, and mediating their request to the deity or more powerful spirits. For instance, Setiloane (1989) linked the interaction of one's "Seriti" (vital forces) with those of other people in the community, as an integral part of African spirituality. Even after death, the vital participation of the deceased is believed to be experienced in the community in general and in the home and clan circle in particular.

God-image and Divinity

A pastoral assessment and diagnosis should also include an assessment of the appropriateness of God-images and their role in life events. God-images refer to the conceptualization of experiences as related to a transcendent being (God). A God-image represents a very specific perspective and understanding of God and is often expressed in metaphors and symbols. Divinity refers to a transcendent being as well as to the ultimate realm of the beyond. In this regard, the concept of divinity is important. Gehman (1989) conceived divinity to be a dynamic concept that related to "vitalism" as a force that moves and rules humanity and determines their fate in the world. Setiloane (1989) considered this vitalism to be present in everything. Similarly, Frank (1999) observed that tradition-led Africans believed the divine Spirit to penetrate everything and everywhere. Tradition-led Africans believe things exist because they participate in

Discussion Box 10.3: Shame Culture

Because of African spirituality, a pastoral assessment of well-being and healing cannot be separated from the complexity of guilt and shame experiences. It can be argued that in rural and semirural communities, the predominant African world view cannot be separated from a culture of shame. According to the research done by Wiher (2003), a shame culture is dominated by a shame-oriented conscience, which is linked mainly to honor and status. Harmony and acceptance imply honor and lead to a good conscience. A bad conscience arises when one has not met the expectations and norms of the group. When one is discovered, one loses status and honor and can become totally marginalized.

Questions

1. How could one's position and status within the network of relationships play a decisive role in healing?
2. How may changed perceptions facilitate the physical process of healing?

God (Nwachuku, 1994). Setiloane (1989) concluded from the Sotho-Tswana word for God (*Modimo*) that God was never conceived as a "person" but as something intangible, invincible, a natural phenomenon able to penetrate and percolate into things. Likewise, Bujo (1992), Kriel (1989), and Tempels (1969) considered that indigenous Africans associated divine power with a vital force for living, which reflected a cultural preference for power-charged objects.

Immanency

Immanency is the understanding that the divine element is part of everyday life and can be presented by cosmic entites and events (such as in the African belief in the indwelling presence of spirits and life forces within the realm of relationships). On the one hand, the traditional African understanding is that God is omnipresent and intervenes in life events. On the other, Africans also view God as supreme, and therefore too remote to enter into close relationships with people. Therefore, Africans hold a complex view of God in perceiving that "God is immanent in his actions" and also "distant and unknowable in his person, what all men and women can do is passively accept his will" (Long, 2000, p. 25).

Tradition-led Africans perceive God as the "Great Ancestor." Ancestors are revered because of their influential position within the system of spiritual powers. Therefore, the divine is expressed symbolically in stories, which link the divine to the realm of ancestors (Bujo, 1992; Kabasélé, 1991; Pobee, 1979). It seems that African religion is both communal and anthropocentric. It is communal in the sense that religion is experienced within the realm of social relationships and the networking of daily life events. Anthropocentry refers to the central position and role of human beings within daily life events. African religion is athropocentric because it focuses predominantly on the well-being of human beings

Christian theologians in their pastoral care with tradition-led Africans attempt to link the mystery of Christ to brotherhood and ancestorship. Christ is projected as the Brother-Ancestor (Nyamiti, 1984, p. 23) or the "proto-ancestor" (i.e., the unique ancestor who is the source of life and the highest model of ancestorship" (Nyamiti, 1984, p. 7). The role of the pastor is of the utmost importance within the African context.

In a certain sense the pastor assumes the role of the "prophet healer." Augsburger (1986, p. 13) advocates what he calls the pastoral counselor as an intercultural person. The counselor needs the basic skill of *interpathy* besides the general skill of empathetic listening and reflective understanding.

HEALTH AND ILLNESS IN AN AFRICAN CONTEXT

Concerning the notions of health and illness in an African context, research has pointed out that health should be assessed as a communal concern (see also Chapters 1 and 4, this volume). Tradition-led Africans believe health means the correct relationship to one's environment. Illness means that the societal order, equilibrium, and harmony are disrupted and destabilized. Thus, illness actually is a sociological phenomenon: the interests of the family, clan, or society are affected. Illness is also a religious concept (Saayman & Kriel, 1992). If the spiritual chain of protection has been damaged and this gives rise to the anger of the ancestors and spiritual powers, which harm or wreak evil upon the person and community. It is within this context that the actions and power of the so-called witchdoctor or *isangoma* figure must be understood and further researched. In this regard, it is important to take the magic dimension of the health–sickness continuum within an African context into consideration.

Illness implies suspicion; thus, together with the patient, one must search for deeper underlying factors. With this suspicion the diagnosis and rituals of the prophet healer/diviner could be of assistance because "by definition, a diviner is a person who discloses the causes of misfortune and death" (Berinyuu, 1988, p. 37). However, tradition-led Africans recognize illness from biological or animate organisms that they believe to be enabled by the spiritual world.

Well-being and Communality

The African understanding of themselves within roles and societal relationships can be linked to the therapeutic principle in the fellowship of believers, namely mutual care (*koinonia*). The impact of culture, a holistic approach to healing is imperative. Culture implies that healing does not circle around an individual but is concerned with a group, the family, or neighbors from the community. The healing process is a communal task (Hemshorn de Sánches, 2003, p. 72).

In the African cultural life view, the healing process leads toward three aims (which should further be researched):

- Bringing the disturbed relation back to its good order. This might be achieved by conversations with all the parties concerned in the house. It also includes calming the rage of the ancestors by respective sacrifices.
- Cleansing of the polluting subject. "For this are applied methods of interior and exterior cleansing such as bathing, inhaling, emetics (ukuphalaza) and enemas (ukuchatha)" (Ngubane, as cited by Hemshorn de Sánches, 2003, p. 72).
- Restoring the balance of power in relationships. The African primal world can be conceived of as a universe of distributed power. To heal the disease, the healer must redress the imbalance of power, either by decreasing the evil power or countering it with healing power.

Long (2000, p. 123) mentions the following strategies to achieve this:

1. Remove the source of the evil power.
2. Confront and overwhelm the evil power.
3. Appease the powers that are causing the suffering.
4. Manage the powers to protect from attack.

In counseling African clients, an individual approach must be supplemented by group counseling. Group counseling should include the family (Gehman, 1989, pp. 50–1), the social group, and other important figures in the community. However, as noted in Chapter 1, the active ingredients that result in treatment success or cure based on this world view are yet to be fully researched.

STRATEGIES AND TECHNIQUES IN PASTORAL CARE AND COUNSELING IN TRADITION-LED AFRICAN SETTINGS

Without any doubt, the dimension of spirit possession in an African approach cannot be ignored. Health problems are often attributed to the work of spirits, usually in the service of a declared or undeclared enemy.

Spirit Possession, Exorcism, and Deliverance

In the African world view, there are legions of spirits who inhabit the "the world between" and intersect everyday life. According to Long (2000, p. 31), the spirits may act on their own accord, perhaps punishing a person for tearing the web of relationship by breaking a taboo, or they may be summoned and sent to do harm by a living enemy. Even a neglected ancestral, who desires attention or wishes to preserve tradition, may also possess someone and cause illness in the person or signficant others. Also it is possible that a witchcraft spirit may possess a person with diabolical consequences. Witches are seen as the enemies of life. "In Xhosa culture *umona* signifies the quintessence of witchcraft, the personification of evil. The person who has umona has turned his back on the community and is seeking gain at another's expense" (Long, 2000, p. 96). In this regard diviners and sorcerers are seen as powerful figures that can manipulate the spirits, either by discovering a reason or by countering their strategy of power through different rituals.

In an African approach to pastoral care, the notion of balance and peace are extremely important. Liturgy as well as rituals can play an important role to help restore balance and create integration. According to Kiriswa (2002, pp. 23–4), "psychological illnesses are either treated by ritual purifications, exorcisms or sacrifices."

Touching

Another question is whether the healing touch of a sick person should be introduced in pastoral, healing practices. Touch and embraces communicate connectedness. Touch also communicates the sharing of life. Here the laying of the hands can play a significant role in the display of God's blessing (Acts 8, pp. 14–7). The touch also communicates full identification with that person's suffering in order to bring about full restoration (Long, 2000, p. 112).

Use of Metaphors, Symbol, and Language

Another critical area for research is the language of the pastoral caregiver A pastoral caregiver should be an interpretor of language, metaphors, and symbols in an African context. To be human means to speak and to speak is to be both divine and human (Twesigye, 1996). Therefore, a human is embedded in an oral society and part of a collective story. Both verbal and nonverbal or symbolic languages are essential mediums for humanization. Authentic humanity or *Ubuntu* is expressed through nonverbal and effective symbolic language of works, ritual, attitudes, and behavior. Thus, the contention is that explicit deeds and actions (unintentional and intentional) speak louder than words alone.

Externalizing

The notion of externalization can be linked to the African view in that the problem is often not within. Therefore, the person in him/herself is not the problem but the problem is the issue as it impacts on human behavior and responses.

Narrative Therapy or Storytelling

Because of the importance of language and the oral tradition in African spirituality, pastoral care typically incorporates the technique of storytelling (see also Chapter 2, this volume).The drama of life and death is embedded in a spiritual realm where stories, symbols, and metaphors play a decisive role in the process of healing. Storytelling is very influential when it comes to the question of attitudinal change and cognitive restructuring. The technique of storytelling can be most helpful to build new perspectives and change in schemata of interpretation.

Pedagogical and Directive Counseling

The intention behind education and the pedagogical dimension in pastoral care is to prepare people for life.

> A pedagogical method (pedagogical counselling) was mainly employed not only as a preventive measure but also as a process of socialization and maturation. It was done in view of preventing future problems and helping a person to grow into a responsible adult. (Kiriswa, 2002, p. 27)

Pastoral care seeks to liaise with cultural leaders in the community to cooperate in terms of *initiation ceremonies* or rites of passage, using stories, proverbs, riddles, and other appropriate means to develop an indirect and preventive approach in care (Kiriswa, 2002). Through the community and their stories, younger people are introduced to morals and core life issues. The role of elders is important in the African community.

ISSUES FOR RESEARCH AND OTHER FORMS OF SCHOLARSHIP

One of the most critical areas to be researched is the understanding of the human being within an African context. The pastoral caregiver must have a clear understanding of this construct to be effective and credible. How one assesses a human being is determined by one's theory on the essence of our beingness.

Dynamism of Being Human

The African understanding of the human is a dynamic approach. "An African concept of a human person (Motho-Umunto), as evidenced in daily contact and traffic, is that of a dynamo" (Setiloane, 1989, p. 13). As previously discussed, an African traditional conception of being views the potential in human beings as an energy or force, which is immanent in all things. Berinyuu (1988, p. 10), for example, referred to an Akan tribe (Nigeria) who have their own unique view of the person. According to Akan, "The ntroro spirit is the energy which links him/her to the ancestral lineage." The human spirit is not regarded as an identifiable self, but as a personal consciousness of powers, which are associated with the concept of "destiny." This destiny can be modified, so that one can adapt within circumstances and within a social context. These concepts need to be operationalized in the practice of pastoral care and counseling with many Africans.

Intervention, Cause, and Purpose

Counseling in an African setting should take the mystic dimension of life into account, together with the deterministic cause–effect of African thinking. For example, as Kiriswa (2002) and Nyirongo (1997) observed, many traditional African communities still believe that illness or sickness never occurs on its own but has a fundamental spiritual causation. There are no clear or established procedures as yet for pastoral care providers, in the modern sector, to counsel at various levels of physical and spiritual causation.

Offerings may be delivered as compensation for wrongdoing. Because the bringing of an offering and compensation play such an important role in regaining balance in human relationships, pastoral care must make a special effort to follow up the Christian concept of the vicarious grace of Christ's offering which brings about restoration in relationships. It may be challenging to link these practices in settings where Christ was perceived as other than a divine Big Brother.

Because of the very vulnerable position of women in tradition-led African culture, an important issue to be addressed is the role of spirituality within a patriarchal cultural system. Spirituality as a healing force in women is recognized in many African cultures. Studies need to examine how gender role expectations influence the types of pastoral care African women receive in their communities.

SUMMARY AND CONCLUSIONS

Pastoral care deals with the spiritual realm of our being human and how this spiritual dimension (soul) is related to existential, relational, and life issues. In the Christian tradition, the healing dimension is related to the notion of salvation and peace (*sjalom*). Within an African setting, pastoral care should incorporate the notion of interculturality and deal with the spiritual assessment of life in terms of African spirituality. As argued in this chapter, pastoral counseling must be interdisciplinary – connected to psychology and psychotherapeutic skills such as empathetic listening. Another important theory is systems thinking, as proposed in many family counseling models. Another important model is narrative therapy with its emphasis on storytelling.

The African lifestyle is in itself a therapeutic system of counseling. The so-called authoritarian missionary pattern, in which the Western model is regarded as superior and the African model as inferior, must be guarded against. If the African world view is not adopted, pastoral care may be perceived by many as too aloof to address their needs (Taylor, 1983).

Pastoral care occurs within a systemic framework, so that counseling is part and parcel of the interconnectedness of a communal understanding of human relationships. Counseling is a relational and systemic issue, not a professsional technique to be taught as a skill. To counsel is a mode of life, in terms of how you deal with the other within a system of a family (extended family) or tribe/community, hence the argument for a holistic–cultural and systems approach.

REFERENCES

Ackermann, E. (1993). *Cry beloved Africa! A continent needs help*. Munich, Kinshasa: African University Studies.

Augsburger, D. W. (1986). *Pastoral counseling across cultures*. Philadelphia: Westminister.

Bate, S. C. (1995). *Inculturation and healing. Coping-healing in South African Christianity*. Pietermaritzburg: Cluster Publications.

Bellagamba, A. (1987). New attitudes towards spirituality. In A. Shorter (Ed.), *Towards African Christian maturity* (pp. 95–109). Kampala: St Paul.

Berinyuu, A. (1988). *Pastoral care to the sick in Africa. An Approach to transcultural pastoral theology*. Frankfurt: Peter Lang.

Bosch, D. J. (1974). *Het evangelie in Afrikaans gewaad*. Kampen: Kok.

Bujo, B. (1992). *African theology in its social context*. Faith and Cultural Series. New York: Maryknoll.

Clinebell, H. J. (1996). *Basic types of pastoral counseling*. Nashville, TN: Abingdon Press.

Egan, G. (1990). *The skilled helper. A systematic approach to helping*. Pacific Grove, CA: Brooks/Cole.

Eybers, H. H. (1991). *Pastoral care to Black South Africans*. Atlanta, GA: Scholars.

Frank, M. E. (1999). *African notions of sickness and death in pastoral care to the dying*. Unpublished Masters dissertation, University of Stellenbosch.

Friedman, E. H. (1985). *Generation to generation. Family process in church and synagogue*. New York: Guilford Press.

Gehman, R. J. (1989). *African traditional religion in Biblical perspective*. Kijabe: Kesho Publications.

Hemshorn de Sánches, B. (2003). Violence, trauma and ways of healing in the context of transformative South Africa: A gender perspective on the dynamic and integrative potential of "Healing" in African religion. *Journal for the Study of Religion, 16*(1), 65–81.

Hiltner, S. (1958). *Preface to pastoral theology*. Nashville: Abingdon.

Kabasélé, F. (1991). Christ as ancestor and elder brother. In R. J. Schreiter (Ed.), *Faces of Jesus in Africa*. New York: Orbis Books.

Kahiga, J. K. (2005a). Epistemology and praxis in African cultural context. *African Ecclesial Review, 47*(3), 184–98.

Kahiga, J. (2005b). Homosexuality: An antithesis to life. Homosexuality and the African culture. *African Ecclesial Review, 46*(4), 380–7.

Kiriswa, B. (2002). *Pastoral care in Africa: An integrated model*. Eldoret: AMCEA Gaba Publications.

Kretzschmar, L. (1996). A holistic spirituality. A prerequisite for the reconstruction of South Africa. *Journal of Theology for Southern Africa, 95*, 63–75.

Kriel, A. (1989). *Roots of African thought: Sources of power – a pilot study*. Pretoria: University of South Africa.

Lartey, E. M. (1997). *In living colour. An intercultural approach to pastoral care and counselling*. London: Cassell.

Long, W. M. (2000). *Health, healing and God's kingdom. New pathways to Christian health ministry in Africa*. Carlisle: Regnum Books.

Louw, D. J. (1998). *A pastoral hermeneutics of care and encounter. A theological design for a basic theory, anthropology, method and therapy*. Cape Town: Lux Verbi.

Mandela, N. (2005). *In the words of Nelson Mandela*. London: Penguin Books.

McNeill, J. T. (1951). *A history of the cure of souls*. New York: Harper & Row.

Miller, W. R., & Jackson, K. A. (1995). *Practical psychology for pastors*. Englewood Cliffs, NJ: Prentice-Hall.

Mills, O. (1990). Pastoral care (history, traditions, and definitions). In R. J. Hunter (Ed.), *Dictionary of pastoral care and counseling* (pp. 836–44). Nashville: Abingdon Press.

Mtetwa, S. (1996). African spirituality in the context of modernity. *Bulletin for Contextual Theology in Southern Africa & Africa, 3*(2), 21–5.

Nyamiti, C. (1984). *Christ as our ancestor: Christology from an African perspective*. Gweru: Mambo Press.

Nyirongo, L. (1997). The Gods of Africa or the Gods of the Bible? The snares of African traditional religion in Biblical perspective. Series F2: Brochure of the Institute for Reformational Studies. Potchefstroom: PU vir CHO.

Oden, T. C. (1987). *Pastoral theology: Essentials of ministry*. San Francisco: Harper & Row.

Oguejiofor, J. O. (2003). Introduction. Philosophy and the question of good governance in Africa. In J. O. Oguejiofor (Ed.), *Philosophy, democracy and responsible governance in Africa* (pp. i–xv). Münster: Litt Verlag.

Oosthuizen, G. C. (1992). Diviner-prophet parallels in the African independent and traditional churches and traditional religion. In G. C. Oosthuizen & J. Hexam (Eds.),*Empirical studies of African independent/indigenous churches* (pp. 163–94). Lewiston: E. Melden Press.

Pobee, J. S. (1979). *Toward an African theology*. Nashville: Abingdon Press.

Pobee, J. S. (Ed.) (1992a). *Exploring Afro-Christology*. Frankfurt: Peter Lang.

Pobee, J. S. (1992b). In search of Christology in Africa: Some considerations for today. In J. S. Pobee (Ed.), *Exploring Afro-Christology*. Frankfurt: Peter Lang.

Schipani, D. S. (2003). *The way of wisdom in pastoral counseling*. Elkhardt: Institute of Menonite Studies.

Shorter, A. (1985). *Jesus and the witchdoctor*. Maryknoll, New York: Orbis Books.

Skhakhane, J. 1995. African spirituality. In M. Makobane, B. Sithole, & M. Shiya (Eds.), *The church and African culture*. Germiston, South Africa: Lumko.

Taylor, C. W. (1991). *The skilled pastor. Counseling as the practice of theology*. Minneapolis: Fortress Press.

Taylor, H. (1983). *Tend my sheep. Applied theology* 2. TEF Study Guide 19. London: SPCK.

Tempels, P. (1969). *Bantu philosophy*. Paris: Présence africaine.

Twesigye, E. K. (1996). *African religion, philosophy, and Christianity in Logos-Christ. Common ground revisited.* New York: Peter Lang.

Van Binsbergen, W. (2003). *Intercultural encounters. African and anthropological lessons towards a philosophy of interculturality.* Münster: Lit Verlag

Waruta, D. W., & Kinoti, H. W. (2000). *Pastoral care in African Christianity.* Nairobi: Acton Publishers.

Wiher, H. (2003). *Shame and guilt. A key to cross-cultural ministry.* Mission Academics (Vol. 10). Bonn: Verlag für Kultur und Wissenschaft.

SELF-CHECK EXERCISES

1. What is the difference between pastoral counseling and the other disciplines within the field of care and healing?
2. Within a pastoral anthroplogy, what is meant by the human soul? Should one differentiate between the soul and the body?
3. Is there a difference between African spiritualities and their understanding of life issues and an existential interpretation of life?
4. How does wisdom counseling fits into an African epistemology and understanding of the cosmos (cosmology)?

FIELD-BASED EXPERIENTIAL EXERCISES

1. Interview elderly people in a local village and ask them to tell and share their life stories. Take field notes and identify specific metaphors and symbols being used to "paint the picture of life."
2. Read some of the works of African philosophers (e.g., Kenneth Kaunda) and try to describe an African approach to life issues.
3. Observe a divine healer and take note of his/her practices and approaches.

MULTIPLE-CHOICE QUESTIONS

1. A pastoral caregiver should listen to:
   a. Sins
   b. Personality traits
   c. Positions within the network of relationships
   d. Role functions within a community
2. The human soul is:
   a. A "thing" within a human being
   b. A description of the quality of life
   c. A reference to meaning and life goals
   d. An indication of a human being's commitments and convictions.
3. In African epistemology, "Africa" refers to:
   a. Context
   b. Philosophy of life
   c. Culture and tradition
   d. Political issues and ideolgies
4. An African interpretation of counseling includes:
   a. Wisdom counseling
   b. Storytelling
   c. Intervention strategies
   d. Exorcism
5. Counseling, as related to life issues, should deal with:
   a. Touching and bodily expressions
   b. Rituals and dancing
   c. Pedagogical issues
   d. Interpathy
6. A systems approach to counseling refers mainly to:
   a. The individual
   b. Personality
   c. Character and traits
   d. Position within networks of relationships.
7. A pastoral diagnosis implies:
   a. A medical model
   b. Classification of people
   c. Assessment of personality
   d. Assessment of the appropriateness of God-images
8. Anthropology within an African context deals fundamentally with:
   a. Dynamic life forces
   b. Energy of life
   c. Personhood
   d. Psychoanalytical issues
9. Health within African spirituality is concerned with:
   a. Behavioral changes
   b. Personal introspection
   c. Human relationships
   d. Communal issues
10. Traditional healers are:
    a. A threat to pastoral processes of healing
    b. Unacceptable within a Christian approach to healing
    c. Should be rejected as paganism
    d. Fulfill an important role within a holistic approach to health and healing

Answers to the multiple-choice questions are provided at the back of the book

11 African Refugees: Challenges and Prospects of Resettlement Programs

Clemente Abrokwaa, Mary Shilalukey Ngoma, Edward Shizha, and Elias Mpofu

OVERVIEW. Since independence in the 1950s and 1960s, postcolonial African societies have been characterized by civil wars and ethnic conflicts. Many Africans had hoped that independence from European colonial rule would usher in a period of peace and prosperity in all areas of life for the entire population. However, this anticipation has rather been usurped by several unending civil wars and ethnic conflicts that have not only claimed millions of lives but have also produced – and continue to produce – streams of desperate refugees fleeing across national borders in search of security and protection. Many of these victims have been women and children. This chapter examines the history of the African refugee problem; the major theories on the subject; national, regional, and international initiatives on African refugees; current practices of refugee hosting inside and outside the continent; legal issues; cultural and diversity concerns; and issues for research on African refugees.

LEARNING OBJECTIVES

By the end of the chapter, the reader should be able to:

1. Define *a refugee* based on the UN definition of the term.
2. Outline the historical causes of the refugee problem in Africa.
3. Identify, describe, and evaluate the major theoretical paradigms on refugees.
4. Outline the legal rights, as well as the major problems facing African refugees both inside and outside Africa.
5. Discuss peace-building strategies in efforts to end the African refugee problem.

INTRODUCTION

Wars and conflicts, of any kind, form an integral part of human existence; hence both national and international communities continue to search for global peace and security. Conflicts and wars result in needless loss of lives and typically displace millions of people from their homes, ancestral lands, and countries of birth, forcing them to seek protection and security elsewhere. Usually, these survivors endure physical and psychological trauma as they flee for their lives. Women and children are the most vulnerable and may lose their entire families from the conflicts and displacements. The plight of these survivors continues in the host countries where they are involuntarily resettled in that the survivors may experience significant human indignities, including deprivation of basic health and socioeconomic necessities. The constant fear and uncertainties of repatriation, and the cultural pressures of their host countries, add to their burdens. We consider definitions and term for refugees and related terms to clarify the subsequent discussion.

IMPORTANCE, DEFINITION, AND SCOPE OF KEY TERMS AND CONCEPTS

Several definitions of refugee have been proposed (e.g., New York Protocol, 1967; UN Convention, 1951). The UN *Convention Relating to the Status of Refugees* of July 28, 1951 and *The New York Protocol* of 1967 define a refugee as

> any person who, based on well-founded fear of being persecuted for reasons of race, religion, nationality, membership of a particular social group or political opinion, resides outside the country of his or her nationality and is unable, or owing to such fear, is unwilling to avail himself/herself of the protection of that country.
>
> (UNHCR, 1951 Convention, Article 1; The New York Protocol, 1967, unhcr.org).

A *refugee*, therefore, is any person who has been "recognized as a refugee and granted asylum or protection," within the definition of Article 1 of the UN Convention of 1951 as amended by The New York Protocol of 1967.

Recent research has broadened this definition to include the role of economic, environmental, and other factors as major contributors to the creation of refugees. For example, Wood (1994) provided an encompassing definition of refugees that included political instability, persecution and war, life-threatening economic decline, and ecological crisis and religious conflicts. The survivors of these conditions are forced to cross national and international borders in search of protection, assistance, and safety, and the security that they cannot get in their own country (Veney, 2007). The refugee problem cannot be fully defined using a single disciplinary approach. Instead, it requires a multidisciplinary approach that includes economics, sociology, psychology, health, counseling, anthropology, law, political science, history, and geography (Ngoma & Mudenda, 2001; Veney, 2007). This chapter employs the UN definition of refugee stated in the preceding text.

HISTORY OF AFRICAN REFUGEES

Africa is one of the world's richest continents in natural resources today, and yet it has the largest concentration of refugees both within and outside of its borders (Brooks & Yassin, 1970; Kibreab, 1985; Zolberg et al., 1989). The refugee problem facing African governments and their societies is not a new one but dates back to the forced migrations on the continent beginning, especially with the Atlantic slave trade in the fifteenth century through the colonial period of the late nineteenth and mid-twentieth centuries (Veney, 2007). The African refugee problem has increased dramatically as a result of the liberation wars of the 1950s and 1960s, and in particular, in the post-independence era due to ethnic and civil wars. For instance, Africa's total number of refugees at the end of 2003 was 2.9 million, excluding refugees in North Africa (UNHCR, 2004c). During the liberation wars, large populations were displaced from their communities and relocated to "safer free zones" within the country. Some others sought asylum and refuge in neighboring countries, while others found sanctuary in North America and Europe. These refugees, however, were in smaller numbers compared to the new waves of refugees in the post-independence period, victims of political persecution and repression, human rights abuse, and ethnic and civil wars. For example, in 1960 the total African refugee population was 300,000 but had increased to 5 million by 1989 (USCR, 1990). In 1994 alone, the total number of refugees was 7 million, representing 43 percent of the total world refugee population in that year (UNHCR,). These increases were generated by civil wars in the Sudan, Burundi, Democratic Republic of the Congo (DRC), Somalia, Ethiopia, Eritrea and Libya; the genocide in Rwanda; and the collapse of the rule of law in Zimbabwe under the Mugabe dictatorship.

Refugee Hosting and Exporting Countries

According to the United Nations High Commissioner for Refugees (UNHCR), some African countries have repeatedly received and hosted refugees at great expense to their own citizens. Given the preexisting socioeconomic conditions in those countries, others have actually become perennial exporters of refugees into neighboring countries and outside the continent. The sub-Saharan countries that have historically been receiving and hosting refugees have included Botswana, Mozambique, Zambia, Tanzania, Kenya, Uganda, Zimbabwe, Ghana, Nigeria, Uganda, South Africa, and Guinea, while the exporting countries have included Somalia, Sudan, Eritrea, DRC, Burundi, Angola, Uganda, and Zimbabwe. For example, in 2001 there were 400,000 Angolan refugees in Zambia and the DRC; 520,000 Burundian refugees in Tanzania; 275,000 DRC refugees in Angola, Congo-Brazzaville, Tanzania, and Zambia; 325,000 Eritrean refugees in Sudan; 210,000 Liberian refugees in Côte d'Ivoire, Ghana, Guinea, and Sierra Leone; and 150,000 Sierra Leonean refugees in Guinea and Liberia (Mahmoud, 2005).

In the Horn of Africa, the Great Lakes Region, and Southern Africa (particularly Zimbabwe), deterioration in the economic and political situation has led to a massive exodus of people fleeing political repression and war. Despite a reported decrease in the overall number of conflicts and those displaced across international borders by UNHCR, recent refugee movements from lower-profile ethnic clashes still persist. These include both new emergencies, such as in Côte d'Ivoire and the Central African Republic, and more protracted ones, including those in Burundi, the DRC, Somalia, and Sudan (UNHCR, 2006). In addition, there has been a large number of refugees produced by domestic xenophobia such as in South Africa, as well as from the abuse or persecution of citizens who are members of opposition parties such as in Zimbabwe. These people seek refuge with their extended family members in other parts of the city or country, or in churches or in police camps within their vicinity, to escape from maltreatment or even death. Despite the fact that the plight of these people does not make the headlines of the world news, it must be acknowledged that they face conditions similar to those of any other refugee groups.

NATIONAL, REGIONAL, AND INTERNATIONAL INITIATIVES ON AFRICAN REFUGEES

At the global level the UN is mandated, through its agency the UNHCR, to assist refugees worldwide, including African refugees, in terms of protection and security, providing shelter and food, and repatriation and resettlement of refugees. At the regional level, the African Union (AU), the Economic Community of West African States (ECOWAS), and the Southern African Development Committee (SADC) work directly with the UNHCR and both local and international nongovernmental organizations (NGOs) to assist refugees and internally displaced persons on the continent. This assistance has been evident during the Liberian and Sierra Leonean civil wars, in Sudan, Rwanda, Eritrea, Ethiopia Somalia, the DRC, Togo, the Ivory Coast, and currently in Darfur. These regional institutions are guided by the Agreements contained in the 1951 UN *Convention* and *The New York Protocol* stated earlier.

Post-September 11, 2001 World Trade Center Tragedy and Refugee Policy Changes in North America and Europe

Until the late 1990s, and especially since the World Trade Center tragedy of September 11, 2001 in the United States, most African and Western nations had been

Discussion Box 11.1: Refugee-producing Countries and Asylum Countries

The table reports the main origins of African refugees and host countries, January 2005

Origin of refugees	Main countries of asylum	Number of refugees*
Sudan	Chad	225,000
	Uganda	215,000
	Ethiopia	91,000
	Kenya	68,000
	Democratic Republic of the Congo	45,000
Burundi	United Republic of Tanzania	444,000
	Democratic Republic of the Congo	19,000
	Rwanda	4,700
	South Africa	2,100
	Canada	1,900
Republic Democratic Republic	United Republic of Tanzania	153,000
	Zambia	66,000
	Congo	59,000
	Burundi	48,000
	Rwanda	45,000
Somalia	Kenya	154,000
	Yemen	64,000
	United Kingdom	37,000
	United States	31,000
	Djibouti	17,000
Liberia	Guinea	127,000
	Côte d'Ivoire	70,000
	Sierra Leone	65,000
	Ghana	41,000
	United States	20,000

*This table includes UNHCR estimates for refugees in industrialized countries on the basis of recent resettlement arrivals and recognition of asylum seekers. Source: UNHCR (2006).

Questions

1. Discuss the major implications of African refugees resettled in Canada, Britain, and the United States as indicated in the table.
2. Do you think that your country should continue to receive and resettle African refugees under the UN Convention Agreement? What is your view on the opinion that Western countries should opt out of the agreements since there seems to be no end in sight for African wars that create refugees?
3. What suggestions do you have for the African Union regarding African refugees?

willingly accepting African refugees from Sudan, the DRC, Mozambique, Angola, Algeria, Libya, and many other areas on the continent. For instance, in 2000 the U.S. government resettled 3,600 Sudanese refugees in American cities. In Europe and North America, as well as in Australia, the same "compassionate" attitude prevailed toward African refugees. However, since 2001 the United States and Canada, European countries such as Great Britain and France, and Australia have begun to tighten their border controls and immigration laws to restrict entry to African refugees (CCR, 2005; Odhiambo-Abuya, 2007).

Initiatives by the international community to address the root causes of the African refugee problem have included working with regional bodies (such as the Southern African Development Coordinating Conference (SADCC) or the continental body, the African Union (AU) to improve governance issues. The regional blocks are still to deliver substantive interventions to curtail the African refugee problem. Several of the leaderships of the same organizations are major instigators of the refugee problem through political repression, corrupt practices, and other human rights abuses.

Effects of National Refugee Policy Changes

Some Western countries, including the United States, have since September 2001 made their refugee status application and selection process too time-consuming

Discussion Box 11.2: Canadian Council for Refugees' Campaign for Refugees Asylum

Hundreds, perhaps thousands, of people have been living in Canada for years in legal limbo, unable to return to their home country because of insecurity there – a danger explicitly recognized by the Canadian government – and unable to get on with their lives in Canada because they are denied permanent residence. They are from Afghanistan, Burundi, Democratic Republic of the Congo, Haiti, Iraq, Liberia, Rwanda, and Zimbabwe, the countries on which the government has imposed a moratorium on removals. They were denied refugee status, under a determination process that has been the subject of considerable criticism and with no right of appeal. However, the Canadian government, to its credit, has recognized that they should not be forced back to these countries because of the situation of generalized risk faced by the entire civilian population. Therefore, the citizens of these countries are protected from immediate removal, but they remain in Canada in a state of limbo that can continue for years, or even decades, without any prospect of resolution. In this situation, they are not allowed to reunite with their family members, even spouses and children, or to pursue their education; they are ineligible for federal child tax benefits, even if they work and pay the same taxes as Canadians, and they have very limited job prospects.

Source: Canadian Council for Refugees (CCR, 2005, p. i)

Questions

1. State your opinion on the Canadian government's policy refusing refugee status to some African refugees in the country.
2. How does this policy violate the UN *Convention* and the *Protocol* Agreements?
3. Do you think that these refugees should be denied employment opportunities, access to Canadian education, and child tax benefits even if they pay their share of the country's taxes?
4. Suggest ways of resolving this issue.

and difficult for refugees to apply. The U.S. application, for example, requires refugees to provide "proof of life in immediate danger, proof of being a former employee of the US government, proof of immediate relatives in the US, or to be considered as a special humanitarian concern to the government" (USCR, 2002). Since September 2001, refugee resettlement in Western countries has become more difficult, particularly for African refugees, because of the assumption that the new refugees could serve as a threat to national security (Trans Africa Forum, 2002). In 2001, the United States admitted 18,979 refugees from Africa, but this number dropped to only 2,548 in 2002 and increased to 10,717 in 2003. Similarly, in 2002, out of the total number of 84,130 African refugees who applied for refugee status to Britain, only 8,270 (10 percent) were accepted (McConnachie, 2005). Several African refugees in North America and Europe are now living in a state of limbo, uncertain when their host governments will grant them the leave to stay permanently (CCR, 2005; Hughes & Liebaut, 1998; Spitzer, 2006; UNHCR, 2002). The trend of border tightening against African refugees in Western countries will continue into the foreseeable future due to the political, social, and economic concerns of the governments and citizens of these countries.

THEORIES ON REFUGEES

Two theories can be identified: the push and pull migration factors and the coercive migration theory. We consider these next.

The Push and Pull Migration Factors

The extant literature on refugees posits three main theories on the subject: the voluntary, involuntary, and the coercive migration models. The voluntary migration theory focuses on the "push and pull" factors dictated by the rational choices of migrants, and based primarily on wage differentials between countries (Faist, 1997; Heisler, 2000; Massey, Arango, Hugo, Kovaouci, & Pelligrino, 1993; Portes, 1985). Higher economic incentives elsewhere are capable of pulling migrants into that economy, while the depressing economic conditions at home rather push migrants to flee such conditions for a better life elsewhere. Conversely, the involuntary migration theory contends that migrants leave their own countries of origin, or cross international borders based on their own accord.

The Coercive Migration Theory

This theory identifies two types of refugees: the reactive fate groups and the purpose groups (Kuntz, 1981). According to Kuntz, the reactive fate groups are those who flee their countries with no plans on how they will return, as in the case of civil and ethnic war victims or victims of an environmental disaster, such as a volcanic eruption or flooding caused by a tsunami or dams. The purpose groups, on the other hand, are those who leave their countries of origin to organize resistance for eventual return, using the host country as asylum. This model was greatly used by freedom fighters during the colonial period and by the anti-Apartheid groups, including the African National Congress (ANC; Nyaba, 2007). These theoretical suppositions on the African refugee problem are rooted in the historical legacies of the African continent and its peoples.

A closer examination of the two theories indicates that both are similar in their examination of the causes underlying the production of refugees. For example, in the case of Africa, the growing harsh economic conditions engendered both by local and world economic events, as currently occurring with the global economy, generally tend to "push and pull" desperate citizens seeking better lifestyles out of their local or country's economies into others. Concerned Africans living in war-torn countries are equally "pushed and pulled" out of their countries or communities into more stable political environments of other countries or areas where they are assured of the safety of their lives. In the case of sub-Saharan Africa in particular, it is appropriate to conclude that the Coercive Theory better explains the subregion's refugee problem than the Voluntary or the "Push and Pull" Theory.

CURRENT REFUGEE HOSTING PRACTICES

The Role of the UNHCR

The current practice of hosting refugees inside and outside Africa is based on the injunctions outlined in the *UN Convention Relating to the Status of Refugees of 1951* and *The New York Protocol of 1967* discussed earlier (unhcr.org). However, these international laws or agreements are subject to local or national interpretation. The current practice identifies the UNHCR as the lead UN agency in matters of global refugee protection, assistance, and welfare. However, it contracts its work to local nongovernmental organizations (NGOs) and international nongovernmental organizations (INGOs) for administrative and operational purposes. The World Food Program (WFP) is the primary international agency responsible for delivering food to refugees for their survival. The UNHCR provides leadership and assists refugee-hosting governments to acquire resources for use by refugees. For instance, refugees fleeing their country arrive in the host country of asylum often sick, malnourished, and wounded from war and conflict, highly traumatized psychologically from the acute exposure to the sight of death and destruction, particularly with children. Thus, they need immediate assistance including food, shelter, clean water, medicine, clothes, security, and counseling (Ngoma, Mudenda, & Ngoma, 2001).

Location of refugee settlements is determined by physical feasibility in that refugees are likely to be provided services in border areas next to their countries of origin. Many refugees are exhausted, hungry, and sick from the usually long and difficult sojourn from their homes of origin. Their plight would be worsened if the host country deliberated to settle them in distant locations from their entry points. Furthermore, many countries hosting refugees do not have the resources to provide settlements away from the border areas for external refugees.

Refugee Hosting

On the issue of hosting refugees, a Zambian study conducted by Mary Ngoma and Choolwe Mudenda (2001) found that the Zambian Ministry of Home Affairs and Ministry of Health collaborated strongly with the UNHCR and several other agencies, such as Medicins san Frontier, Red Cross, African Humanitarian Aid, Jesuit Refugee Service, Care International, Lutheran World Federation, Mennonite Central Committee, World Vision International, Young Men's Christian Association Refugee Project, and the Zambia Red Cross, as well as smaller local NGOs such as "HODI" that provided information and interdisciplinary support to refugees living in Zambia. In Ghana the UNHCR works directly with the Ministry of Interior and local NGOs and INGOs. This practice is similar in other countries across Africa including Kenya, Tanzania, South Africa, Egypt, Guinea, Uganda, and Ethiopia. This administrative setup provides a practical basis for the *modus operandi* of the host governments and their responsible ministerial agencies and the UNHCR, in their efforts both at providing for the needs of refugees as well as sharing refugees' concerns with all other collaborating agencies. Former liberation movement leaders turned oppressors generate millions of refugees escaping political repression and economic malaise.

Location of Refugee Camps in Host African Countries

Concerning the welfare of refugees and refugee camp administration and supervision in Africa, host countries are obliged to care for the safety and well-being of their citizens, first and foremost. Thus, the majority of refugee-hosting African nations tend to locate their refugee centers in more remote and rural parts of their countries. According to Ngoma and Mudenda (2001), the Zambian camps and settlements of their study were set up toward the border areas of Northern, North-Western, and the Western Provinces of the country. Similarly, in Kenya the Kakuma, refugee camp hosting refugees from Sudan, Ethiopia, Rwanda, and the DRC. The refugee camp is located sixty miles north of Nairobi in a desert area lacking direct contact with the Kenyan society and the nearest communities in the area. Also, this situation was true of the Liberian refugee camp in Ghana and those of Tanzania.

Changing Refugee Hosting Practices

The practice of hosting refugees in remote rural areas has not always been the policy of these welcoming governments. For instance, during the period 1960–1990s, both Tanzania and Kenya were credited for having open and generous asylum policies toward refugees (Veney, 2007). These policies allowed refugees access to free medical services, free education, social services, and permission to travel around the country freely; and the refugees were not forced into camps. However, since the early 1990s, several host countries across Africa, including Kenya and Tanzania, have introduced new oppressive and containment policies instituting forced encampment restricting refugee mobility, employment outside the camps, education, and general participation in the host country's economy. These countries have used their military to force refugees into the camps (Rutinwa, 1999; Veney, 2007).

Factors Affecting Refugee Hosting Policies

The changes in the policies of the hosting of refugees across Africa have been the consequence of three major factors: introduction of the World Bank/IMF's Structural Adjustment program (SAP), effects of democratization, and protracted regional political instability (Veney, 2007). The World Bank and the IMF's Structural Adjustment policies introduced in the early 1980s not only removed the central government from the African economy by privatizing almost all public services, but adversely affected the economies of African countries, causing higher inflation and worsening the poverty conditions of the people (Engberg-Pedersen, Gibbon, Raikes, & Udsholt, 1996; Mkandawire & Solido, 1998). The SAP policies forced both host and conflict countries to grapple with a decline in living standards of their people, residents living in areas that hosted refugees faced new challenges as refugees competed with them for scarce resources, fragile infrastructure collapse, and the emergence of new economic dynamics resulting from the presence of refugees. Furthermore, African nations faced issues of environmental problems, mounting foreign debts, less land for agriculture, and less employment opportunities for their populations.

In addition to the economic plight, the emergence of democratization across the African continent, particularly in the 1990s, also brought in its wake the spirit of ethnocentrism. Local residents perceived refugees as intruders and foreigners illegally invading ethnic lands and communities and using their scarce resources, causing resentment and hatred against the latter despite their already deplorable conditions. Protracted political conflicts as have been occurring in the Horn of Africa and in the Great Lakes regions have continued to force host countries such as Kenya, Tanzania, Uganda, Zambia, and South Africa to literally become "tired" of the continued influx of refugees into their countries, as they see no end in sight of the wars producing these streams of refugees.

Local Attitudes toward Refugees

In their Zambian study, Ngoma and Mudenda (2001) reported that the local leaders interviewed in Zambia's provincial capitals confessed that despite their genuine concern for the plight of the refugees, they felt that the refugees destabilized the status quo, in all sectors of the local lifestyle. These areas included health and disease, land and agriculture, water, cross-cultural conflict as men and women competed for marriage, economic activities, language of communication, food and nutrition, education, and other social services. The researchers found that hosting border town communities, although sympathetic toward the refugees, similarly expressed fatigue at the refugees' nonstop dependence on their meager resources. In some cases the local communities expressed anger and hostility based on the perception that services such as roads, clinics, and food rations were better in the refugee settlements and camps, than for local communities. Similarly, in 2007 conflict broke out between the Darfur refugees in Accra, Ghana and the local residents who charged that the refugees were "overstepping their bounds" by "impregnating their women " (ghanaweb.com, July13, 2007). Many of these reasons were given for the xenophobic attacks on refugees and immigrants by local residents in South Africa. The attacks, which were directed at Zimbabwean, Malawian, Somali, Mozambican, and Nigerian immigrants occurred in May 2008 in South Africa and left more than sixty people dead. More than 35,000 foreign nationals – mostly Zimbabweans and Mozambicans – fled the country or were displaced inside South Africa. The United Nations Children's Fund (UNICEF) reported that more than 600 of the displaced people in Gauteng (a province in South Africa) were children and women.

Refugees and Economic Participation

Refugees are almost strictly barred from joining the mainstream economy to compete for the limited jobs with the local residents or citizens of the host country, despite the fact that this policy violates the UN *Convention* Agreement on refugee status in host countries. Refugees flee their countries with almost nothing except their lives, thus making life in the camps economically harsh for them, particularly for women with children as well as unaccompanied children. During times of shortages of food and medical care and high unemployment in the host economy, tensions arise, adversely affecting the relationship between refugees and communities close to the camps. However, it needs to be mentioned that the services provided for the refugees by the UNHCR and other NGOs, in turn, benefit the host country and their immediate communities close to the camps in terms of the construction of accessible roads, clinics, food supply, medical care, water supply in the form of boreholes, and improvement of general infrastructure, particularly in education.

Women and Children Refugees

While earlier research on refugees focused mainly on the victims as a whole, recent research rather identifies not only the different types of refugees and their needs

Discussion Box 11.3: Phasing of Refugees' Statuses in Conflict Africa

The descriptions below refer to the various stages of refugees in a refugee camp.

1. The Acute Phase Refugee (New Arrival)

The "new arrival" tends to be culturally and ethnically different from his/her hosts. In the process of "flight and flee," the new arrival may not have had time to collect essential items, visit the granary for food, or buy essential supplies. Running from a bullet or "panga" (large knife used by rural dwellers as a hunting or agricultural tool) is in itself a terrifying and stressful situation. It is a question of life and death and happens with little thought. For women and young girls, there is the added danger of rape or sexual abuse, with consequences of unwanted pregnancy and sexually transmitted infection, in addition to fending off hunger, wild animals, mosquitoes, bad weather, and bugs. Although just grateful to be alive, most refugees during this phase are dogged by poverty worse than they experience in their home environment. They are destabilized, frightened, and unsettled for a period of up to two years. They live in temporary or makeshift shelters, such as canvas tents or grass shelters. They may be maimed or suffer from acute diseases such as dysentery, respiratory infections, and others. They live in a confined area and are answerable to gatekeepers as they come and go.

2. The Intermediate Phase Refugee

Ranging from two to five years, this time frame is when refugees settle into the new environment. There will be issues of adjustment to the culture, the food, the environment, and lifestyle. During this adjustment period, issues of mental health often arise. These issues are linked to the realization of material and human loss. Where children have died, surviving parents wish to replace these children. Where a partner is lost, remarriage is an option.

Where the food is different, the breadwinner will try by all means to forage for food similar to the usual diet. The diet tends to be cassava and fish over the maize mealie-meal and beans provided by the UNHCR and other collaborating agencies. Male members of the family would cycle or walk great distances to source or exchange the beans and mealie-meal for cassava. They would go to other points for food handouts and have double or more portions to resell or barter.

Focus group discussions with the male refugees showed that after the acute phase and arrival, during which they felt useful, setting up structures to live in and fetching for firewood and water, they now had too much time on their hands and often did not know what to do with themselves. With no alternative for occupation for most men, this often leads to increased sexual and reproductive activity or mental health problems such as depression and feelings of inadequacy, leading sometimes to outbursts of anger, confusion, and suicidal tendencies. Women appeared to adapt better as they transition to house keeping and keep busy all day. They may have fears of the enemy within the camp environment.

Children have limited access to school and spent more time around adults. Some young adolescents confessed to being sexually abused by older or married men. Others felt obliged to agree to these advances given that men are considered dominant. There seems no future for most inhabitants of settlements at this stage, short of repatriation and recovering their original lifestyle.

3. The Settled or Long Stay Refugee

In this case refugees have lived in the host country for thirty years or more. Some children are now adults and do not have experience of their parents' original home. Shelter is as for any rural population, with water, sanitation, and access to health facilities, and for most refugees, no electricity. Population dynamics are evident during the long stay interaction. There are less physical barriers and restrictions. A small number, fewer than 1 percent, may live in urban settings and become integrated into the local communities. Repatriation may be an option, but becomes less likely during this phase.

Questions

1. What are your suggestions for the UNHCR and local governments concerning the needs of the "new arrivals" into the refugee camps?
2. Briefly summarize the condition and needs of each of the three phases of refugees in your own words.
3. Suggest some adaptation strategies for the "new arrival."
4. Why do you think that the search for specific cultural foods, as indicated by the Intermediate refugee phase, is important at this phase of the refugee's life in the camp?
5. What suggestions do you have to relieve boredom on the part of the male refugees at the Intermediate stage?
6. Do you support refugee education on sexually transmitted diseases and unwanted pregnancies, or do you think that their safety and basic needs should gain more attention?
7. Would you consider Settled refugees still refugees or grant them citizenship in the host country?

Case Study 11.1: Children Refugees and Trauma: The Case of John Jok from Sudan

At the Kakuma Camp in Kenya, all the refugees from the Democratic Republic of the Congo, Rwanda, Ethiopia, and Somalia were required to visit the only clinic in the Camp once each month. One day, I went to the clinic with about fourteen other boys to see the doctor. Actually, we didn't know what to tell the doctor; but we were all having nightmares from the war, and I could see my father being shot and dying in front of my mother every time I went to bed. The government soldiers began to rape the women of my village and my mother pushed us boys into the bush to hide. It was horrible what we saw; we still remember it in our sleep. Also, some of the boys had become quite ill from the journey, due to the fact that we saw some of our friends being eaten by lions and crocodiles as we tried to cross the river into Ethiopia. It was horrible. One particular boy had lost all his family; and he was about seven years old. He sat in front of me at the clinic; and he began to fall asleep. When his turn came to see the doctor; he didn't get up. I thought he was asleep so I shook him to wake him up ... he was dead. I still see that boy in the line at the clinic in my dreams – after ten years! It has affected our minds.

Questions

1. Suggest effective ways of treating refugee children experiencing problems associated with psychological trauma.
2. What suggestion do you have for the UNHCR concerning children refugees and psychological trauma?

in terms of length of stay in refugee camps, but more so, emphasizes on gender and age (Forbes, 2004; Human Rights Watch, 2000; Ngoma et al., 2001; Veney, 2007). A greater emphasis is now placed on the needs of women refugees and children, particularly unaccompanied children. Refugees everywhere go through both physical and psychological traumatic experiences that could last a lifetime. For instance, an interview with a group of the so-called "Lost Boys" from Sudan resettled in Philadelphia revealed that some of them were still having nightmares about the war and the many deaths they witnessed – even after ten years (Abrokwaa, 2007).

Case Studies

The cases described below are hypothetical and the names used are not those of real persons. Any similarity to the names or case histories of particular individuals is purely coincidental.

Similarly, Ngoma and Mudenda's Zambian study observed that children refugees often pose a particular challenge in that they may become separated from their parents and other adults they know. They may be sexually abused or they may need food more frequently, and may be abused to work for adults. More importantly, they may need greater medical care than the adults (Arie, Bjornstad, Clacherty, Kistner, & Mazibuko, 2007; Toole & Foster, 1989; Toole, Nieburg, & Waldman, 1988). In the Sierra Leonean and Liberian wars, children were not only recruited to fight for both government and rebel forces – they were also subjected to torture and psychological trauma and were made to commit heinous acts beyond the capabilities of children (Stepakoff et al., 2006). These experiences remain with them throughout their lives. Women refugees need more assistance than their male counterparts becausee they are prone to rape, sexual harassment, unwanted sexual advances, unplanned pregnancy, domestic violence and sexism in the camps, and general sanitation requirements for their health (Africa Watch, 1993; Hackett, 1996; Omaar & de Waal, 1993; Schafer, 2002).

The Zambian study cited earlier identified three main types of refugees: the Acute Phase Refugee, the Intermediate Phase Refugee, and the Settled or Long Stay Refugee, applicable to all other refugees across the continent.

CULTURAL AND DIVERSITY ISSUES

African refugees resettled in non-African countries – particularly Europe and North America – are greatly affected not only by their limited numbers but also their absence from the social, economic, and political activities that promote both diversity and integration into their host countries. According to Haines and Mortland (2001), the adjustment of African refugees to North American life can be understood largely in terms of the interplay between social convergence with the mainstream and cultural distance from it. Most African refugees, especially those who do not communicate in English or the official language of the host country, there is a mixture of the two but with greater social and cultural distance from the members of the host nation. Thus, cultural distance becomes a barrier to cultural integration in the host society, restricting access to enriched social contact between refugees and the mainstream population (Goodman, 2004; Ogbu, 1995).

Refugee Integration into Host Society

Cultural *integration* concerns how refugees relate and adjust to their host community's local values, norms, and behavioral patterns, as well as the host society's reactions to aspects of the cultural practices and customs of refugees. However, *complete integration* does not always occur on many levels of the society; hence the

Case Study 11.2: Refugees in Zambia and Child Molestation

In trying to ease the pain of a thirteen-year-old refugee girl from an urban setting, a Zambian family invited her to live with them for a short time. She was reasonably relaxed with the daughter, who was slightly younger than she was. She would, however, look troubled and tensed up whenever the father of the home appeared or spoke. She relaxed totally with the mother and even laughed whenever she found something funny.

One day, shortly after her visit of three weeks, she began to sing while in the bath and looked decidedly happier. She would soon be going back to her home country and reunited with her family. She opened up and began to talk more openly. Her uncle, who should have been her protector, had sexually molested her younger sister during the flight. She, being larger in build, was able to fight him off and run away. Her younger sister, however, could not. She now had HIV infection.

(Ngoma & Mudenda, 2001)

Questions

1. In what ways do you think children refugees could be better protected from sexual molestation in the refugee camps?
2. How do you think the host country's laws should punish the men who molest children refugees in the camps? Do you think that the UN should create an international law on sexual molestation against children in refugee camps? If yes, what type of punishment do you suggest?
3. Suggest counseling strategies for refugee children who have been sexually molested in refugee camps, as well as for refugee women who have been raped.

Research Box 11.1: Rights and Protections for Children

Meeting the rights and protection needs of refugee children: An independent evaluation of the impact of UNHCR's activities. UNHCR (2002). Geneva: Author.

Objective: To strengthen UNHCR's operational effectiveness to fulfill its mandate on behalf of refugees and other displaced persons, particularly children.

Method: The study used field missions, focus groups, and a confidential field questionnaire. Extensive interviews were held with more than sixty UNHCR staff members in Geneva, and also its Senior Regional Advisors on Refugee Children.

Results: The study uncovered general confusion at all levels – headquarters, regional, and local – about what child protection meant or what the policy priority on refugee children entailed. This confusion was due to lack of understanding of child rights as the framework for child protection; lack of situational analysis; and insufficient integration with community services and the Agency's work with community networks.

Conclusion: Accountability for child protection should be clarified at all levels. Resources need to be increased.

Question

1. Comment on the UNHCR's current definition of Refugee Children's Rights. Suggest ways of improving the definition to assist the Agency in protecting refugee children more effectively.

two communities remain differentiated, so that there is no singular "host society" to which the refugees could be integrated (Beiser, 1999). Bloch (2006) contends that whereas integration in one way or another always happens, it is not necessarily to the mainstream society. Similarly, Samovar and Porter (1991) equally argue that despite the appreciation of the contributions of refugees to the Canadian racial and cultural diversity, African refugees continue to remain socially isolated because of their race and culture. The refugees can equally well be integrated into their various ethnic enclaves, into a specific social class, or into client status in the social welfare system (Berry, 1997; Kamali, 1997;).

Resettlement Problems Facing Refugees and Host Residents

Some members of the host society misinterpret the behavioral actions and cultural practices of African refugees due to a lack of adequate background knowledge of the history and culture of the newcomers into their communities. Thus, whether they are in Europe, North America, or in neighboring African countries, African refugees become potential targets of discrimination based on their language and cultural and religious practices (Beiser, 1999) – and sometimes due to their skin color as well. For instance, in an interview conducted with the "Lost Boys"

Case Study 11.3: Refugee Resettlement and Cultural Orientation: The Case of John Deng

In Sudan we had no knowledge of homosexuality where men "married" had slept with other men, while women slept with other women. The refugee agency in Philadelphia put us into various American homes and I was put into a house with two men. It never crossed my mind that the two men were having a sexual relationship! How? Why? Well, one day I returned from school and found the two of them kissing in the kitchen. I was shocked! I could not believe it! I asked them: Why are you two behaving this way? One guy asked me: which way? I responded: Why are you two men kissing each other? Shouldn't you be kissing a woman? Well, they laughed and they explained to me that in America men can get married to men and women could marry other women. I told them not in Sudan! They told me this country was not Sudan. From then on, I saw them many times in the kitchen and they would open their bedroom so I could see them there as well. You know, it's hard to get it out of your mind, I tell you, since it was new to me. Perhaps they should tell us about it before they bring us here – to prepare us for this society.

Questions

1. Design a cultural orientation curriculum to include topics that you think would be important for African refugees to know, before arriving for resettlement in your country or city.
2. Do you agree or disagree that African refugees should not be resettled in the homes of homosexuals? Give your reasons.

studying at Penn State University in 2007, almost all the sixteen "Lost Boys" interviewed confirmed experiencing some form of racial discrimination in Philadelphia, where they had been resettled from the Kakuma camp in Kenya in 2002 by the U.S. government (Abrokwaa, 2007). For example, they stated that because of their "very dark skin" some American commuters – both Black and White – would not even sit beside them on public buses, while some preachers at the bus stops preached *only* to them about "sin and evil," of the "dark forces of Satan and his children," as they completely ignored the rest of the commuters in the bus line. In addition, they confirmed that some of them, unknowingly, were resettled in the homes of gays and lesbians – a cultural practice with which they were completely unfamiliar.

Effects of Cultural Differences between Refugees and Host Communities

Given their status as refugees and the cultural differences that exist between African refugees and the mainstream North American and European population, the former are more likely to experience an identity crisis. In their daily interactions with the mainstream society, they "receive messages" that communicate to them the impression or feeling that they "do not belong." Thus, without social recognition and acceptance, African refugees may experience isolation and loneliness and the stress of "rejection" and discrimination that act as barriers to integration (Din-Dziethham, Nembhard, Collins, & Davis, 2004; Finch & Vega, 2003). In Canada, social isolation is prevalent among the Sudanese, Somali, Congolese, Sierra Leonean, and Eritrean refugees whose cultures are perceived as vastly different from the mainstream Anglo-Saxon and French-Canadian cultures. Most African refugees, strong communal identity, solidarity, sharing, reciprocity, trust, support, and religion played central roles in their lives at pre-migration (Goodman, 2004). Therefore, the loss of this community identity and the sense of belonging created the pressure of feeling different in their host country, requiring them to rebuild their disrupted social networks (Golding & Baezconde-Garbanati, 1990; Hagan, 1998; Simich, Mawani, Wu, & Noor, 2004).

LEGAL ISSUES

International Law on Refugees

Refugees around the world, including African refugees, are governed under two major international legal instruments: *The UN Convention Relating to the Status of Refugees* of 1951, and *The New York Protocol* of 1967. These two form the most comprehensive instruments governing the legal status of refugees adopted to date at the international level (un.org/millennium/law/v-14.htm). They constitute the minimum humanitarian standards for the treatment of refugees, strengthen international cooperation and solidarity on behalf of refugees, and depoliticize the act of granting asylum (unhcr.org). The *Convention* contains both time and geographical limitations (the latter being optional). The purpose of the *Protocol* was to remove such limitations. Thus, the *Protocol* is an independent, though integrally related, international treaty thereby underlining the universality of the two fundamental instruments concerning refugees.

The UN Convention (1951) and The New York Protocol (1967)

Contracting Parties to the *Convention* and the *Protocol* undertake to protect refugees according to the terms outlined therein, namely:

a. The *Convention* provides the definition of a refugee.
b. It stipulates when a person ceases to be a refugee and excludes from refugee status persons who have

Research Box 11.2: Acculturation in Refugee Status

DeWitt, Pearson, J., Wolf, K., Tyma, A., & Kahl, D. (2008). *At Home Among Strangers: The Acculturation Process of Female African Refugees in the upper Midwest of the United States*. Allacademic.com.

Objective: The study investigated the problems facing female African refugees as they transitioned to life in the United States. The research was conducted among the female African refugees in Fargo, North Dakota.

Method: The study employed the Action Research method to ascertain some of the major transitional problems facing female African refugees in the community.

Results: Existence of a lack of a centralized network to offer female refugees required assistance. Female African refugees faced constant racism in the workplace and sometimes in the community by being ignored completely by local residents. Reversal of domestic roles occurred: Husbands had abandoned their traditional role of providing for the family, with women now having to work double jobs to take care of the family, and the men not helping.

Conclusion: The development of a Fargo governmental and organizational-based program designed to aid in the continued success of the female African refugees in Fargo is needed.

Questions

1. Write a paragraph justifying the importance of this research.
2. Discuss the following: Should African refugees hold onto their traditional cultural norms or adopt their host country's cultural practices concerning the family?

committed crimes against peace, war crimes, crimes against humanity, and serious crimes committed outside the country of refuge.

The two legal instruments identify the rights and obligations of refugees stating that refugees should:

c. Not be expelled or returned to territory where their life or freedom would be threatened on the basis of their race, religion, nationality, or membership in a particular social group or political opinion.
d. Not be penalized for having entered or being illegally in the country where they seek asylum
e. Not be expelled except in exceptional circumstances to protect national security and public order.
f. Be obliged to conform to the laws and regulations of the country in which they find themselves, including measures taken to maintain public order.
g. Not be discriminated against based on race, religion, or country of origin (unhcr.org).

The *Convention* grants refugees access to the courts and the justice systems, as well as the educational provisions and scholarships. Also, access is granted to travel freely both within and outside their new countries of residence, when the situation permits, and does not infringe upon the national security of the host nation. All Contracting Member States agree to cooperate with the Office of the UNHCR in its efforts to protect and provide for refugees. This agreement is recognized by all African states, as evident in the 1969 OAU Convention on African Refugees (OAU Convention on Refugees, 1969, Article VIII), and also in the current Constitutions of the African Union, ECOWAS and SADC on refugees. However, as stated earlier these laws are subject to local and national interpretation based on the conditions prevailing in the host country.

ISSUES TO BE RESOLVED BY RESEARCH AND OTHER FORMS OF SCHOLARSHIP

The preceding discussion on African refugees indicates that while national and international literature exists on European and other refugees, there is paucity of literature and published research on African refugees, with the only available information being the few compiled by local African governments, UNHCR, and other supporting agencies. The health reports of refugees can be accessed only through local health management teams, such as Provincial Hospitals and District Health Centers. In addition to the physical instability of refugee life, the Zambian Case study indicated that psychosocial, and gender and children's issues are of utmost importance requiring immediate attention at all phases of the lives of African refugees.

The many problems facing refugees are to be fully addressed by research. Counseling services must be established to address the mental health of refugees, particularly children, including tackling issues of domestic violence, rapes, and child molestation. Counselors are needed to assist refugees in handling the stresses from fear, discrimination and social rejection, and depression. Familiar social networks need to be set up to assist African refugees resettled in Western countries to enable them to cope with these conditions. Cultural integration and multiculturalism should be made integral parts of the cultural fabric of the host societies (Beiser & Hou, 2006; Simich et al., 2004; Spitzer, 2006).

Peace-building strategies must be strongly pursued in Africa to stem the relentless creation of the waves of refugees on the continent and eliminate the indignities and unnecessary hardships placed on innocent women and children.

SUMMARY AND CONCLUSION

African refugees are protected under the statutes of the *UN Convention Relating to the Status of Refugees of 1951*, implemented and supervised by the UNHCR. Officially, refugees are recognized by the United Nations as persons or groups requiring economic, social, and political assistance. The main organization of the United Nations mandated to protect refugees worldwide, including African refugees, is the UNHCR, which is assisted by the WFP, and UNICEF at the international level. At the regional and national levels, the UNHCR works directly with African governments through the African Union, the ECOWAS, and SADC in the areas of refugee protection, removal and resettlement, feeding, and shelter. Currently greater emphasis is placed on protecting women and girls from male abuse, rape, and other forms of sexual maltreatment in refugee camps. Similarly, emphasis is being placed on caring for unaccompanied children.

Research has shown that both the physical and the psychological well-being of refugees are equally important to be addressed as health needs. The necessity for cultural integration strategies to assist refugees to adapt and embrace their new societies is greatly needed, particularly those resettled in Western countries. Increasingly, the United Nations is recognizing the need to educate refugee children in the camps to assist in the rebuilding of their communities upon their return. Strategies for lasting peace on the African continent are needed to alleviate the hardships and discomforts endured by refugees.

REFERENCES

Abrokwaa, C. (2007). African conflicts and refugees: The resettlement experiences of the "Lost Boys from Sudan" in the US. Unpublished manuscript.

Africa Watch. (1993). Seeking refuge, finding terror. *Africa Watch, 5*(13). New York: Human Rights Watch.

Arie, K., Bjornstad, C., Clacherty, G., Kistner, J., & Mazibuko, M. (2007). *Children on the move: Protecting unaccompanied migrant children in South Africa and the region*. A report by Save the Children, UK.

Beiser, M. (1999). *Strangers at the gate: A 10-year study of refugee settlement in Canada*. Toronto: University of Toronto Press.

Beiser, M. N. M., & Hou, F. (2006). Ethnic identity, resettlement stress and depressive affect among Southeast Asian refugees in Canada. *Social Science & Medicine, 63*(1), 137.

Berry, J. W. (1997). Immigration, acculturation and adaption. *Applied Psychology: An International Review, 46*(1), 5–68.

Bloch, A. (2006). Emigration from Zimbabwe: Migrant perspectives. *Social Policy & Administration, 40*(1), 67–87.

Brooks, H. C., & Yassin El-Ayouty. (1970). *Refugees south of the Sahara: An African dilemma*. Westport, CT: Negro University Press.

Canadian Council for Refugees (CCR). (2005). *Lives on hold: Nationals of Moratoria countries living in limbo*. Montreal: Canadian Council for Refugees.

DeWitt, L., Pearson, J., Wolf, K., Tyma, A., & Kahl, D. (2008). At home among strangers: The acculturation process of female African refugees in the upper Midwest. Retrieved on September 21, 2007 from Allacademic.com.

Din-Dzietham, R., Nembhard, W., Collins, R., & Davis, S. (2004). Perceived stress following race-based discrimination at work is associated with hypertension in African Americans. The Metro Atlanta Heart Disease Study, 1999–2001. *Social Science & Medicine, 58*, 449–61.

Engberg-Pedersen, P., Gibbon, P., Raikes, P., & Udsholt, L. (Eds.). (1996). *Limits of adjustment in Africa*. Copenhagen: Center for Development Research.

Faist, T. (1997). The criminal meso-level. In Hammer, T., et al. (Eds.), *International Migration Immobility & Development*. New York: Berg Publications.

Finch, B. K., & Vega, W. A. (2003). Acculturation stress, social support, and self-rated health among Latinos in California. *Journal of Immigrant Health, 5*, 109–17.

Forbes, M. S. (2004). *Refugee women*. Lanham, MD: Lexington Books

Golding, J., & Baezconde-Garbanati, L. (1990). Ethnicity, culture and social resources. *Journal of Community Psychology, 18*(3), 465–86.

Goodman, J. H. (2004). Coping with trauma and hardship among unaccompanied refugee youths from Sudan. *Qualitative Health Research, 14*(9), 1177–96.

Hackett, P. (1996). *Pray God and keep walking: Stories of women refugees*. Jefferson, NC: McFarland.

Hagan, J. (1998). Social networks, gender and immigrant settlement: Resource and constraint. *American Sociological Review, 63*(1), 55–67.

Haines, D. W., & Mortland, C. A. (Eds.). (2001). *Manifest destinies: Americanizing immigrants and internationalizing Americans*. Westport, CT: Praeger.

Heisler, B. S. (2000). The sociology of immigration: From assimilation to segmented integration, from the American experience to the global arena. In C. B. Brettell & J. F. Hollifield (Eds.), *Migration theory: Talking across disciplines*. New York: Routledge.

Hughes, J., & Liebaut, F. (Eds.).(1998). *Detention of asylum seekers in Europe: Analysis and perspectives*. The Hague: Kluwer Law International.

Human Rights Watch. (2000). *Seeking protection: Addressing sexual and domestic violence in Tanzania's refugee camps*. New York: Author.

Kamali, M. (1997). *Distorted integration: Clientization of immigrants in Sweden*. Uppsala, Uppsala Multiethnic Papers No. 41/ Centre for Multiethnic Research, Uppsala University.

Kibreab, G. (1985). *African refugees: Reflections on the African refugee problem*. Trenton, NJ: Africa World Press.

Kunz, E. F. (1981). Exile and resettlement refugee theory. *International Migration Review, 15*(1), 42–51.

Mahmoud, A. I. (2005). *Somalia between state collapse and national reconciliation: A study in conflict resolution in Africa*. Cairo: Al-Ahram center for Political and Strategic Studies.

Massey, D. S., Arango, J., Hugo, G., Kovaouci, A., Pelligrino, A., & Taylor, J. E. (1993). Theories of international migration: A review and appraisal. *Population and Development Review, 19*, 431–66.

McConnachie, A. (2005). Asylum policy for Great Britain: Restoring integrity. *Sovereignty*. http://www.sovereignty.org.uk/features/articles/immig3.html

Mkandawire, T., & Solido, C. S. (1998). *Our continent, our future: African perspectives on structural adjustment*. Trenton, NJ: Africa World Press

Ngoma, M. S., & Mudenda, C. (2001). *Appraisal report of refugee human rights in Zambia*. The Inter-African Network for Human Rights and Development.

Ngoma, M. S., Mudenda C., & Ngoma, J. (2001). *The health situation of refugees, women and children in Zambia: Lessons from the complex emergency influx of 2001*. (Unpublished manuscript).

Nyaba, P. A. (2007). *What is African liberation?* African File, Pambazuka News 336 http://www.africafiles.org/article.asp?ID=16965

Odhiambo-Abuya, E. (2007). Reinforcing refugee protection in the wake of the War Against Terror. *Boston College International and Comparative Law Review*, *XXX* (3), 277–330.

Ogbu, J. U. (1995). Understanding cultural diversity and learning. In J. A. Banks & C. A. M. Banks (Eds.), *Handbook of research on multicultural education* (pp. 582–93). New York: Macmillan.

Omar, R., & de Waal, A. (1993). *The nightmare continues: Abuses against Somali refugees in Kenya*. London: African Rights.

Organization of African Unity. (1969). *Convention governing the specific aspects of refugee problems in Africa*. Addis Ababa: Refugee Convention.

Portes, A. (1985). Urbanization, migration and models of development in Latin America. In Walton, J. (Ed.), *Capital and labor in the urbanized world*. London: SAGE Publications.

Rutinwa, B. (1999). The end of asylum? The changing nature of refugee policies in Africa. *New issues in refugee research*. Working Paper no. 5. Refugee Studies Program, Oxford University. http://www.unhcr.ch/ref-world/pub/wpapers

Samovar, L. A., & Porter, R. E. (1991). *Communication between cultures*. Belmont, CA: Wadsworth.

Schafer, L. H. (2002). True survivors: East African refugee women. *Africa Today*, *49*(2), 29–48

Simich, L., Mawani, F., Wu, F., & Noor, A. (2004). *Meanings of social support, coping, and help-seeking strategies among immigrants and refugees in Toronto*. Toronto: CERIS Working Paper No. 31.

Spitzer, D. L. (2006). The impact of policy on Somali refugee women in Canada. *Refuge*, *23*(2), 42–49.

Stepakoff, S., Hubbard, J., Katoh, M., Falk, E., Jean- Baptiste, M., Potiphar, N., & Omagawa, Y. (2006). Trauma healing in refugee camps in Guinea: A psychosocial program for Liberian and Sierra Leonean survivors of torture and war. *American Psychologist*, *61*(8), 921–32.

Toole, M. J., & Foster, S. (1989). *Famines: The public health consequences of disasters*. Atlanta: Centers for Disease Control and Prevention.

Toole, M. J., Nieburg, P., & Waldman, R. J. (1988). Associations between inadequate rations, under-nutrition prevalence, and mortality in refugee camps. *Tropical Paediatrics*, *218*–22.

Trans Africa Forum. (2002). Refugees: Post WWII to Post 9–11. Trans Africa Forum Issue Brief. June http://www.transafrica-forum.org/reports/refugees_issuebruef0602.pdf

UNHCR. (2002). Branch Office in Canada. *Comments on the Proposed Immigration and Refugee Protection Regulation*. Ottawa: Submission to the House of Commons Standing Committee on Citizenship and Immigration.

UNHCR. (2004a). *Refugees by numbers* (pp. 9 and 14).

UNHCR. (2004b, June 15). 2003 Global refugee trends: Overview of refugee populations, new arrivals, durable solutions, asylum-seekers, and other persons of concern to UNHCR. Geneva: Author. http://www.unhcr.ch.statistics

UNHCR. (2006). *The state of the world's refugees 2006. Human displacement in the new millennium*. Oxford: Oxford University Press.

UNHCR. (2008). Meeting the rights and protection needs of refugee children: An independent evaluation of the impact of UNHCR's activities. Geneva: Author.

United Nations. (1951). *Convention relating to the status of refugees adopted on 28 July 1951 by the United Nations Conference of Plenipotentiaries on the Status of Refugees and Stateless Persons convened under General Assembly Resolution 429 (V) of 14 December 1950*.Geneva: Author.

United Nations.(1967). *The New York protocol on refugees*. Geneva:Author.

U.S. Committee for Refugees (USCR). (1989). *World refugee survey* 1988 (p. 46). New York: American Council for Nationalities Service.

U.S. Committee for Refugees (USCR). (1990). *World refugee survey* 1989 (p. 31). New York: American Council for Nationalities Service.

U.S. Committee for Refugees (USCR). (2002). *World refugee survey* 2002 (p. 81).New York: Immigration and Refugee Services of America.

Veney, C. (2007). *Forced migration in Eastern Africa*. New York: Palgrave.

Wood, B. (1994). Forced migration: Local conflicts and international dilemmas. *Annals of the Association of American Geographers*, *84*(4), 607–34.

Zolberg, A. R., Aguayo, S., & Sulurke, A. (1989). *Escape from violence: Conflict and refugee crisis in the developing world*. New York: Oxford University Press.

USEFUL WEBSITES

http://www.amnestyinternational.org
http://www.allafrica.com
http://www.refuge.com
http://www.unhcr.ch.refworld
http://www.refinternational.org
http://www.refugees.org
http://www.hrw.org
http://www.reliefweb.int
http://www.unhcr.org
http://www.crisisweb.org
http://www.lchr.org
http://www.au.org

KEY REFERENCES ON REFUGEES

Forbes, M. S. (2004). *Refugee women*. Lanham, MD: Lexington Books

Hackett, P. (1996). *Pray God and keep walking: Stories of women refugees*. Jefferson, NC: McFarland

Kibreab, G. (1985). *African refugees: Reflections on the African refugee problem*. Trenton, NJ: Africa World Press

Kunz, E. F. (1981). Exile and resettlement refugee theory. *International Migration Review*, *15*(1), 42–51.

Rutinwa, B. (1999). The end of asylum? The changing nature of refugee policies in Africa. *New issues in refugee research*. Working Paper no. 5. Refugee Studies Program, Oxford University. http://www.unhcr.ch/ref-world/pub/wpapers

UNHCR. (2008). Meeting the rights and protection needs of refugee children. Geneva: Author.

UNHCR.2006. *The state of the world's refugees 2006. Human displacement in the new millennium*. Oxford: Oxford University Press.

UNHCR.(2004). *Refugees by numbers* (pp. 9 and 14).

UNHCR.. (2004c, June 15). 2003 global refugee trends: Overview of refugee populations. New arrivals, durable solutions, asylum-seekers, and other persons of concern to UNHCR. June 15. Geneva: Author. http://www.unhcr.ch.statistics

Veney, C. (2007). *Forced migration in eastern Africa*. New York: Palgrave.

Wood, B. (1994). Forced migration: Local conflicts and international dilemmas. *Annals of the Association of American Geographers*, *84*(4), 607–34.

Zolberg, A. R., Aguayo, S., & Sulurke, A. (1989). *Escape from violence: Conflict and refugee crisis in the developing world*. New York: Oxford University Press.

SELF-CHECK EXERCISES

1. Define *a refugee* as contained in the *UN Convention Relating to the Status of Refugees of 1951* and *The New York Protocol* of 1967:
2. Identify the major factors that contribute to the creation of refugees in Africa.
3. Why is the African refugee problem incapable of being defined using a single disciplinary approach?
4. Identify five African countries plagued by civil war since independence.
5. Briefly explain the three main refugee theories in your own words.
6. What three factors have contributed to the changing refugee hosting policies in Africa today? Why have the refugee hosting policies changed in Western societies, particularly in North America and Europe?
7. Explain briefly why most African governments tend to locate refugee camps in remote rural areas of their countries.
8. State some of the major problems facing women and children in African refugee camps.
9. Outline some of the major problems faced by refugees resettled in Western countries.

FIELD-BASED EXPERIENTIAL EXERCISES

1. Interview a refugee to discover why he/she fled his/her country, and the dangers he or she faced in the process.
2. Interview a refugee concerning life in the refugee camp, in terms of:
   a. Safety
   b. Shelter
   c. Food
   d. Education
   e. Health
   f. Counseling
3. Interview women refugees on issues pertaining to rape, sexual assault, unwanted pregnancy, and domestic violence in the refugee camps.
4. Design and conduct a community research survey on the hosting of refugees and its economic, social, and cultural effects on local residents.
5. Discuss the topics of cultural differences and multiculturalism with your class members.
6. Invite a refugee to speak to your class or community regarding his/her experiences as a refugee both in Africa and in the West.
7. Interview a refugee on the dangers and hardships created by African civil wars to refugees, particularly women and children.

MULTIPLE-CHOICE QUESTIONS

1. The *UN Convention* and *The New York Protocol* define a refugee as any person:
   a. Staying at a refugee camp
   b. Engaged in conflict or war
   c. Who has been recognized as a refugee and granted asylum or protection
   d. Who works for the UNHCR
2. The African refugee problem cannot be defined using just one disciplinary approach because:
   a. It is not the best approach
   b. It is not based on law
   c. It is narrow
   d. It is multidisciplinary
3. The main international institution mandated to protect and provide assistance for refugees around the world is:
   a. The World Bank
   b. The UNHCR
   c. Amnesty International
   d. The International Refugee Association
4. Cultural Integration means:
   a. Cultural differences
   b. Complete integration of cultures
   c. Ability of refugees to speak their host country's language
   d. How refugees relate and adjust to their host community's local values and norms
5. African refugees in North America are more likely to experience identity crisis because of:
   a. Their status as refugees and the cultural differences that exist between African refugees and the North American population
   b. The language barriers existing between the two groups
   c. The reluctance of African refugees to embrace the North American culture
   d. The refugee policies of North American governments

Answers to the multiple-choice questions are provided at the back of the book

12 Counseling Orphans and Vulnerable Children in Africa

Gertie Pretorius, Brandon Morgan, Magen Mhaka-Mutepfa,
Mary Shilalukey Ngoma, and Thokozile Mayekiso

OVERVIEW. Africa has the greatest proportion of orphans globally, with the HIV and AIDS pandemic one of the foremost reasons for this situation (UNAIDS/UNICEF/USAID, 2004). Despite the high numbers of orphans and other vulnerable children on the continent, state and federal governments repeatedly consider these children a last priority in social service provision. Furthermore, many services addressed toward these children attend to their basic needs and seldom address their emotional well-being. In this chapter, the psychological experiences of orphans and other vulnerable children are explored and counseling techniques that can be applied to this population group discussed. Examples of current programs in Africa are also presented.

LEARNING OBJECTIVES

By the end of the chapter, the reader should be able to:

1. Outline the challenges of defining orphans and vulnerable children (OVCs) in an African context.
2. Explain the importance of providing counseling to OVCs, especially within the framework of children's rights.
3. Evaluate the role of HIV and AIDS in the psychosocial experiences and well-being of OVCs.
4. Discuss appropriate counseling supports for OVCs.
5. Describe areas requiring further research in the counseling of OVCs.

INTRODUCTION

Statistics paint a poignant picture of the landscape of OVCs in Africa. According to the *Children on the Brink Report* (UNAIDS/UNICEF/USAID, 2004), in 2003, approximately 43 million orphans resided in sub-Saharan Africa. Of these children, roughly 11 million have become orphans as a result of the HIV and AIDS pandemic (UNAIDS, 2008). These statistics suggest that the majority of orphans – after Asia, which has approximately 87 million orphans – reside in Africa (Altman, 1994; UNAIDS/UNICEF/USAID, 2004). The situation of OVCs in Africa has reached a critical level, especially as fueled by the HIV and AIDS pandemic (UNAIDS/UNICEF/USAID, 2004; UNAIDS/WHO, 2006, 2007; UNICEF, 1998), incessant civil strife and wars that have come to define Africa in recent decades (Laband, 2007; Sendabo, 2004), and child neglect and abuse by national or state governments (Joint Learning Initiative on Children and HIV/AIDS [JLIC], 2009).

The increasing numbers of orphans are alarming for health care professionals, government agencies, and local communities, as OVCs tend to experience many psychosocial challenges that impact their development and well-being. These challenges include stigmatization and discrimination, illegal labor practices, malnutrition, health problems, poverty, physical and sexual abuse, and a lack of educational opportunities (Smart, 2003; Subbarao & Coury, 2004; UNAIDS/UNICEF/USAID, 2004). A variety of other factors, such as grief, exploitation, and excessive responsibilities at home may further erode the well-being and quality of life of OVCs (FOST, 2002; Shilalukey Ngoma & Chanda, 2002; UNAIDS, 2002, 2006).

IMPORTANCE, DEFINITION, AND SCOPE OF KEY TERMS AND CONCEPTS

The key terms used throughout this chapter are child, orphan, vulnerable child, and family, and are defined in the following subsections.

Child

The definition of a child is challenging in Africa, as it varies between countries (Smart, 2003). According to Smart (2003, p. 3), most African countries define a child as a boy or girl "up to the age of 18 years." This definition applies to Namibia and South Africa, with these countries defining a child as any person who is younger than the age of eighteen years (Children's Act of South Africa, 2005; Children's Status Act of Namibia, 2006; Children's Status Bill of Namibia, 2005). However, exceptions to this definition do exist (Smart, 2003). For example, in Zimbabwe, the Children's Act of Zimbabwe (2002) defines a child as any person younger than the age of sixteen years.

Another challenge in defining a child is that there are many indigenous definitions of childhood that are not captured by policy documents (Mutepfa-Mhaka et al., 2008). For example, in some cultures in Zimbabwe, a person is no longer considered a child when he or she is able to complete household chores without supervision. Some religious groups may marry off girls at the age of thirteen years, and thus do not observe the legal definition of child (Apostolic Sect Members, personal communication, October 3, 2008).

Orphan

The term *orphan* is problematic as "its meaning varies among cultures and is potentially stigmatizing" (Levine, Foster, & Williamson, 2005, p. 3). The definition used to describe OVCs is an important consideration, as these definitions impact the decisions made about OVCs (Levine et al., 2005; Skinner et al., 2004). For example, "it can result in the inappropriate categorisation and labelling of children, and it may generate conflicts over resources and priorities at community and household levels" (Levine et al., 2005, p. 3). There is also no absolute definition of an orphan, as these definitions are a function of social roles and therefore vary between cultures (Barnett & Whiteside, 2006).

A frequently cited definition of an orphan is a child younger than the age of fifteen years who has lost a mother, father, or both parents due to death (UNAIDS/UNICEF/USAID, 2002). An orphan can be further defined as either a maternal, paternal, or double orphan (UNAIDS/UNICEF/USAID, 2004). According to the *Children on the Brink Report* (UNAIDS/UNCIEF/USAID, 2004), a double orphan is any child who has lost both a mother and father, whereas a maternal orphan and a paternal orphan is defined as the loss of a mother or father respectively, due to death. Various other definitions of OVCs exist. Smart (2003) provides an overview of definitions of orphans from several countries in Africa; the reader is referred to this document for a delineation of these definitions.

Vulnerable Child

As with the definition of orphan, the concept of vulnerability remains elusive and difficult to define, as no single definition adequately captures what constitutes a vulnerable child (Skinner et al., 2004). Generally, a vulnerable child is any child who has limited access to his or her basic needs. Thus, a child may be vulnerable but not an orphan. For example, a child may reside with his or her parent(s), yet still have access to his or her basic rights denied (Dawes, van der Merwe, & Brandt, 2007; Skinner et al., 2004). According to Subbarao and Coury (2004), definitions of vulnerable children are usually broad and include many children. In addition, definitions used by the community are often different from those of external agencies (Skinner et al., 2004).

The *Children on the Brink Report* (UNAIDS/UNICEF/USAID, 2004, p. 6) defines a vulnerable child as a child "whose survival, well-being, or development is threatened by HIV and AIDS." It would, however, be erroneous to consider only children affected by HIV and AIDS as vulnerable, as various other children are vulnerable. Local and community definitions of a vulnerable child include children who are terminally ill, children who have living conditions in which their parent(s) has(ve) limited opportunities for obtaining an income, or a child who is abused (Bambisanani, 2001 cited in Smart, 2003). Vulnerable children also include children who are disabled, destitute, or have poor hygiene; street children; children in conflict; neglected children; and children with a parent(s) in prison[1] (Skinner et al., 2004; Smart, 2003).

Skinner et al. (2004, pp. 16–17) conducted a research report to create a working definition of OVCs. Following the research report, Skinner et al. (2004) center their definition of OVCs on three core areas: *material problems*, *emotional problems*, and *social problems*. Material problems include lack of access to money, shelter, and food. Emotional problems include inadequate care, support, and love. Social problems consist of lack of role models to follow, a supportive peer group, and guidance in difficult situations.

Family

The idea of family in African culture is often different from that in Western countries. For example, in the Zulu culture of South Africa the family consists of the *Umndeni* and the *Imideni*. The Umndeni includes the nuclear family and can also include the extended family members. The Imideni, however, is a family that consists of all the people in a community – who are not necessarily related. Foster (2000) mentions that marriage in Africa is not a partnership of two individuals, but rather a connecting of two families, highlighting the importance of family in these cultures.

Many OVCs in Africa are cared for by the extended family (Ngalazu Phiri & Tolfree, 2005). The extended family is broad and includes uncles, aunts, grandparents, and other relatives. Although the sense of duty and responsibility of the extended family to provide support to OVCs was historically without limit, a variety of factors have weakened extended families' capacities to care for orphans (Foster, 2000; Foster, Makufa, Drew, & Kralovec, 1997; Foster & Williamson, 2000; Plan Finland, 2005; UNICEF, 2001; van Dyk, 2005a). The extended family may be a beneficial and positive experience for OVCs; however, some OVCs who reside with the extended family are subject to abuse and exploitation (FOST, 2000, Foster & Williamson, 2000; Mahati et al., 2006; Shilalukey Ngoma & Chanda, 2002; Tsheko, 2007; UNAIDS, 2006).

HISTORY OF PRACTICE IN COUNSELING OVCS

This section briefly considers the history and evolution of important OVC-related events. The focus here is on

[1] This list is not exhaustive, as many other definitions of vulnerable children exist. The reader is referred to Smart (2003) for an overview of these definitions in the African context.

Discussion Box 12.1: The Extended Family as a Source of Support

The following case study demonstrates the complexities of OVCs residing with extended family members.

A ten-year-old boy comes to counseling because he is being abused by an uncle. His mother has recently died from a stroke and his father is in prison. The boy moved in with his aunt and uncle after his mother's death, but the uncle is convinced that his mother died due to AIDS. He also repeatedly mocks the boy and reminds him that his mother and father are worthless. The boy's aunt, concerned for his well-being and worried about his aggressive behavior at school, decided that counseling is necessary. The aunt is clearly very caring toward the boy, and provides him with all the resources she has at her disposal.

Questions

1. How might the extended family be both an asset and a cost to orphan children?
2. What counseling interventions would be helpful to the child described in this case study? Explain your choices.

the global strategies and goals as set out by the United Nations.[2] Research on the psychological experiences of OVCs is then presented, setting the stage for a discussion on current practices addressing OVCs and intervention techniques that can be applied to OVCs.

Within the last two decades, various important events occurred that had direct implications for OVCs. Foremost, among these events, is the Convention on the Rights of the Child (CRC), which was promulgated by the United Nations in 1990 (van Dyk, 2005a). The CRC has become important in assisting orphans and other vulnerable children in realizing an environment that is both safe and supportive (Gruskin & Tarantola, 2005; Richter, Mangold, & Pather, 2006), and many countries are signatories of this convention (Gruskin & Tarantola, 2005).

Following the promulgation of the CRC, several notable events between1994 to 2000 occurred. A workshop was held in Zambia on providing support to children and families who are affected by HIV and AIDS. At this workshop, factors related to children's well-being were debated. Several years later a UN General Discussion was held on *Children Living in a World with AIDS*. This committee highlighted the importance of following the CRC and focusing interventions for children based on these rights. In 1998, a conference was held in South Africa in which several countries committed themselves to establishing OVC task teams (Smart, 2003).

In 2000, the *Millennium Summit* was held, in which many countries agreed to implement strategies to create a safer world and end poverty by the year 2015 (UNAIDS, 2008). After this event, enhanced coordination and greater efforts were established to enhance the well-being of OVCs. A UN Special Session in 2002 resulted in the *World Fit for Children Declaration*. In the same year, numerous countries in Africa committed themselves to establishing task teams and creating a plan of action in responding to the OVC crisis (UNAIDS, 2008).

The African Leadership Consultation also followed, which focused on developing priorities for responding to the OVC crisis (Smart, 2003). In 2004, the *Framework for the Protection, Care and Support of Orphans and Vulnerable Children Living in a World with HIV and AIDS* (UNICEF, 2004) was published. This framework promoted an effective response from a variety of stakeholders in addressing the problem of OVCs and HIV and AIDS. The *Children on the Brink Report: 2004* (UNAIDS/UNICEF/UNAIDS, 2004) was also published in which orphan estimates and intervention strategies were discussed.

More recently, the *Joint Learning Initiative on Children and HIV/AIDS* report explored areas of addressing responses to children's needs and provided recommendations for these responses (JLIC, 2009). In 2006, several countries committed themselves to providing access to prevention programs, treatment, and support for people impacted with HIV and AIDS (UNAIDS, 2009). The recently published *Outcome Framework for 2009–2011* highlights eight priority areas in which a greater response to the HIV and AIDS pandemic is needed. These priority areas envisaged to assist in achieving the Millennium Development Goal outcomes (UNAIDS, 2009).

THE PSYCHOLOGICAL EXPERIENCES OF OVCS

Research has demonstrated that orphans tend to have higher levels of psychological distress than non-orphans (Musisi, Kinyanda, Nakasujja, & Nakigudde, 2007). In this section, the psychological experiences of OVCs are succinctly discussed before presenting current practices used in addressing the needs of OVCs in Africa.

Depression and Internalizing Behaviors

Various studies have indicated that orphans tend to experience higher levels of depression than non-orphans. According to Straker (1986), OVCs are likely to experience a sense of helplessness because of a perceived lack of control over aspects of their lives, a sense of meaninglessness and emptiness, a loss of self-esteem, emotional blunting, and feelings of isolation and alienation. The traumatic stress that OVCs experience may also result in these

[2] The history of events discussed here is in no way exhaustive.

Research Box 12.1: Living on the Street

Tudorić-Ghemo, A. (2005). Life on the street and the mental health of street children – A developmental perspective. Unpublished master's thesis, University of Johannesburg, Johannesburg, South Africa.

Objective: The study explored the mental health of street children and how street life affects healthy personality development.

Method: Participants were twenty-one Black street children (ages thirteen to eighteen years) living in a street youth shelter in the East Rand of Johannesburg, South Africa. The children took the Draw-a-Person projective personality test.

Results: The results suggest that healthy development in these street children was compromised, indicated by an absence of autonomy, dependency, security, and the need for achievement. These street children also appeared to be arrested at their first level of development.

Conclusion: Children living on the street all have unique experiences. Healthy personality development in these children is not based solely on their street or home experiences. Street children's behavior should not be pathologized, but rather seen in context.

Questions

1. What were the strengths and limitations of the study instrument?
2. Explain the findings of the study in terms of children's adaptation to street life.
3. What interventions would work with children living on the street?

children experiencing anxiety, depression, withdrawal, psychosomatic complaints, sleep disturbance, irritability, and excessive aggression (Straker, 1986).

Cluver, Gardner, and Operario (2007), sampling children from South Africa, found that orphans who lost a parent to HIV and AIDS were more prone to depression and suicidal ideation than other orphans. Musisi et al. (2007) also found that orphan participants from Uganda tended to have significant levels of emotional and behavioral problems. In their sample, depression, anxiety and suicidal ideation were common (Musisi et al., 2007). Similar findings were demonstrated by Atwine, Cantor-Graae, and Bajunirwe (2005), who found that orphans who had lost a parent or both parents to an AIDS-related illness tended to have higher levels of anxiety, depression, and anger. Makame, Ani, and Grantham-McGregor (2002), sampling orphans from Tanzania, found that their sample experienced more internalizing problems than non-orphans.

Externalizing Behaviors

Orphans are likely to experience various externalizing behaviors. Cluver and Gardner (2006), sampling children from South Africa, found that orphans who lost a parent to an AIDS-related illness were more likely to experience higher levels of posttraumatic stress disorder (PTSD) symptoms; this may be due to the traumatic nature of their parent's death. Cluver et al. (2007) found that orphans are likely to experience peer and conduct problems. Similarly, Olley (2006) found that street children in Nigeria are vulnerable to antisocial and conduct problems, including substance abuse, oppositional behavior, and violent behavior.

Many children in Africa are impacted by war (Bayer, Klasen, & Adam, 2007; Onyut et al., 2005). Although not all orphans become child soldiers, the increasing amount of orphans in Africa is adding to the abundance of child soldiers used in war (Barnett & Whiteside, 2006). Within the Great Lake districts of Africa, many children have been drawn into war, either as child soldiers or as victims. Child soldiers, many of whom are younger than the age of fourteen, often witness extreme forms of violence and torture against other people. During war, sexual assault is also common, placing female children at risk of rape and sexual mutilation, and consequently HIV and AIDS (Craddock, 2004; Laband, 2007; McKay, 2005; Mills, Singh, Nelson, & Nachega, 2006). Children who witness shootings, beatings, death, and sexual abuse are, in turn, at particular risk for experiencing PTSD symptomatology (Bayer et al., 2007; Kohrt et al., 2008; Summerfield, 2000).

Although many OVCs experience psychological issues, it is important to consider arguments against labeling these children as exhibiting pathological behavior. Research Box 12.1 presents evidence that not all OVCs may necessarily be experiencing psychological distress.

CURRENT PRACTICES WITH OVCS

In Africa, there are gaps in the offering of culturally acceptable psychosocial supports to adults and children (van Dyk, 2005a; Essex et al., 2002). These gaps in provision are an area of concern, as OVCs are faced with many issues that require a multidisciplinary approach to resolve. These issues include limited supervision and care, inadequate medical and psychological care, poverty, exploitation, stunted growth, hunger, limited education, abuse, forced or early marriage, stigma, inadequate housing, limited life skills, and child labor practices (Foster, 2004; Levine et al., 2005; Smart, 1999). The desperation of OVCs may also make them more vulnerable to exploitation and abuse than non-orphans, which increases their susceptibility to HIV infection (Foster, 2004; Foster & Williamson, 2000; Mahati et al., 2006; Oleke, Blystad, Rekdal, & Moland, 2007; Tsheko, 2007).

In Africa, various strategies are used to address the well-being of OVCs, mostly by civic society or nongovernmental organizations (NGOs). The *Framework for the Protection, Care and Support of Orphans and Vulnerable Children Living in a World with HIV and AIDS* (UNICEF, 2004) promotes the use of five key strategies in intervention: (1) strengthening of the family and/or extended family's capacity to cope with the increasing amount of orphans; (2) strengthening and mobilizing of community-based responses; (3) ensuring that access to essential services are available; (4) the creation of legal protection through laws and policies, and the development of essential services for vulnerable children; and (5) raising awareness, and creation of environments that support children (UNAIDS/UNICEF/USAID, 2002, 2004; UNICEF, 2004). Each of these five areas is briefly discussed and examples of current programs addressing these presented.[3]

Strengthening of the Family or Extended Family's Capacity to Cope with the Increasing Number of Orphans

The family is a child's first source of support in life. Thus, when a child loses a parent(s), it is preferable to keep the surviving children together under the care of a surviving parent or extended family members. However, these families require support, such as financial, agricultural, and psychological support. These needs provide opportunities for areas of intervention to assist families in coping. Examples of programs that can be used include support groups, peer support, group counseling, and individual counseling. Other important areas that can be addressed include providing assistance to the caregivers on child development, assisting parents in succession planning, and providing life skills training for families, where needed (UNICEF, 2004).

The Nelson Mandela Children's Trust Fund (NMCF) provides many programs that address the aforementioned. One such program is the *Alternative Models of Care* program, which explores appropriate care for vulnerable children and explores different forms of support that can be provided. Social and financial support is also provided to orphans and child-headed homes (http://www.nelsonmandelachildrensfund.com).

Another program, in South Africa that aims to facilitate the living environments of OVCs, is the New Africa Foundation, which acts as a financial bridge between companies and social projects. In turn, the New African Foundation supports workers at the grass-roots level by ensuring that they receive funds from the corporate sector. Examples of beneficiaries include the Polokego Shelter for Abused Women and Children and the Mohlangeni Informal Settlement project (http://www.newafricafoundation.com).

The Firelight Foundation also provides financial resources to organizations in the greater sub-Saharan region. This organization provides grants to organizations that work with OVCs and that have gained the trust of the community in which they function. The supported organizations provide essential services such as assisting children to remain in school and supporting youth clubs, home-based care programs, and psychosocial support centers. This foundation therefore assists children in remaining in family-based care (http://www.firelightfoundation.org; Firelight Foundation, 2008).

Strengthening and Mobilizing of Community-based Responses

The community is important in African culture. Therefore, local leaders and community members should be included in any intervention, as well as in providing support to OVCs. Communities can be mobilized to prevent abuse and exploitation of OVCs and also provide support-based responses, such as food gardens, child care services, and home visits (UNICEF, 2004). According to the NMCF (http://www.nelsonmandelachildrensfund.com), the head of the community must first be addressed before any intervention is conducted and also receive education on important aspects impacting on OVCs.

In Rwanda, initiatives by local NGOs are available for children in child-headed households. Examples of assistance provided include vocational training, financial assistance, and implementation of income generating activities. The aim of these initiatives is to improve children's well-being and to cover basic expenses that they accrue (MacLellan, 2005). Mutepfa-Mhaka et al. (2008) write that the Zambian government has implemented similar initiatives, providing skills that will enable children to improve their own well-being. Organizations that are involved include Aid to the Child Orphan in Zambia (ACOZ) and the Bauleni Street Kids Project and Community School (Mutepfa-Mhaka et al., 2008).

Ensuring that OVCs Have Access to Essential Services

OVCs face a host of psychosocial needs. However, they are often denied access to essential services and assistance.

[3] Programs presented serve as examples; the authors do not include these programs in order to promote them. Each of the programs mentioned cannot be confined to any of the five areas as done in the text, as the services they provide mostly overlap across the five areas.

Discussion Box 12.2: Legislation Contradictions in South Africa

Legislation may act as a buffer toward adequately defining OVCs in Africa. However, another concern is that legislation may be contradictory, creating confusion and ethical dilemmas for health professionals. One such example is presented in the context of South Africa.

In South Africa, the Choice on Termination of Pregnancy Act states that a person younger than 18 years of age may undergo an abortion without parental consent. However, the Bill of Rights states that every person has the right to life, creating a dilemma in relation to abortion. The Child Care Act states that a child who is fourteen years old can consent to his or her own medical treatment, and a person older than the age of eighteen years may consent to an operation. Thus, a child who is fourteen years or older is able to give consent for an HIV test and to be treated for sexually transmitted diseases. A child must be sixteen years old to give consent to sexual activity. Furthermore, any sexual intercourse with a child younger than sixteen years of age is considered statutory rape by South African law. Thus, there is a dilemma, as a child may give consent to an abortion before the age of sixteen years, but may be involved in sexual activity only when sixteen years or older.

Questions

1. How do policy and legal definitions of OVC differ from local and community definitions?
2. How might these differences in definitions impact on intervention programs aimed at OVC?

Assistance can be provided in keeping OVCs in school and ensuring that they receive a good education (http://www.nelsonmandelachildrensfund.com). Other support that can be provided includes supplying meals to OVCs, addressing health and nutritional needs, providing essential health services, offering legal assistance, and ensuring that OVCs and their families have safe drinking water (UNICEF, 2004).

The Harriet Shezi Clinic at Baragwanath Hospital in South Africa is one of the largest clinics providing support to HIV- and AIDS-affected children in Africa. There are various programs that address these children in a holistic manner. On one spectrum, medical assistance and antiretroviral treatment are provided. Other programs, however, address the psychosocial functioning of the children and include support groups, holiday programs for the children, school outreach programs, parenting workshops, and individual counseling (http://www.witsecho.org.za). Appropriate referrals within the hospital are also possible.

Creation of Legal Protection through Laws and Policies, and the Development of Essential Services for Vulnerable Children

Governments have a responsibility toward caring for OVCs and must therefore provide them with assistance. This can be done through national polices and strategies to care for OVCs, and providing resources to address OVCs needs. Programs should be implemented and well monitored by governments. Policy issues that can be addressed include child abuse, exploitation, HIV and AIDS, and provision of recreational facilities (http://www.nelsonmandelachildrensfund.com; UNICEF, 2004).

Various governmental policies to support vulnerable children exist. In South Africa, the Department of Social Development's *National Action Plan for Orphans and Other Children Made Vulnerable by HIV and AIDS South Africa 2006–2008* identifies strategic priorities in the care of OVCs. These priorities include strengthening of families to protect OVCs and mobilizing community-based responses (Department of Social Development, 2005). Similar protection mechanisms are enshrined in the Constitution and legislation of Uganda (Mutepfa-Mhaka et al., 2008).

Raising Awareness and Creation of Environments That Support Children

Orphans who have lost a parent to an AIDS-related illness often face discrimination and stigmatization from their peers and the community. Undue discrimination against OVCs must be addressed, and a supportive environment for these OVCs created. Public figures can be used to address the HIV and AIDS pandemic, and leaders must speak on behalf of OVCs. Raising awareness is therefore a form of social mobilization that ensures the protection of OVCs (UNICEF, 2004).

The Firelight Foundation assists in this process. The foundation aims to engage in advocacy for their grass-roots level organizations, allowing for enhanced community- and family-based care. They make use of outreach programs, publications, and joint campaigns as part of their advocacy efforts (http://www.firelightfoundation.org; Firelight Foundation, 2008).

The Farm Orphan Support Trust (FOST) is an example of a program that aims to reduce the deleterious impact of HIV and AIDS on children in farming communities in Zimbabwe. The main goal of this program is to provide a supportive and nurturing environment for the children and to increase the capacity of farm worker communities in responding to the growing number of orphans. Programs presented by FOST include community awareness raising and advocacy, psychosocial support, home-based care, and feeding programs (Hadziucheri, Chiwandire, Makawara, & Walker, 2006).

STRATEGIES FOR COUNSELING OVCS

OVCs require both psychosocial and emotional support to address their well-being. Material support alone is inadequate in alleviating the needs of these children (Atwine et al., 2005). In this section, strategies that can be used by counselors and other professionals to address the emotional needs of OVCs are presented.

According to Deacon and Stephney (2007), various factors need to be taken into consideration when providing counseling to OVCs: (1) the child's living environment including access to food, education, and health care; (2) if HIV and AIDS related, whether the child is infected, the level of symptoms evident in the ill caregiver or child, the child's thoughts about the situation, and emotional distress; (3) characteristics of the child such as gender, age, and personality attributes; (4) support available to the child such as the level of psychosocial support; and (5) stigma and discrimination.

Memory Box Technique

A strategy that has become popular in the counseling of children and their families in the context of HIV and AIDS is the *memory box*. This technique may be especially useful in bereavement counseling. The memory box allows people to record their life stories for their children, hereby leaving behind important information on the family history, culture, and beliefs. It also captures the journey through HIV and AIDS. The memory box contains a variety of materials and memorabilia, including stories, books, letters, photos, drawings, words, and pictures (Baumann & Germann, 2005; Frohlich, 2005; Kanabus, n.d.; van Dyk, 2005a).

The memory box technique makes use of facilitated workshops and group work, or may be done individually. This technique can assist with the process of bereavement, and may prevent the experience of complicated grieving experiences in children after the loss of a parent(s) (Baumann & Germann, 2005; Frohlich, 2005; van Dyk, 2005a). The memory box also empowers parents, in that it enables them to communicate with their child, and facilitates future planning with their child. The child is provided with an opportunity to discuss his/her parent(s), illness. The memory box also provides information on HIV and AIDS, potentially enabling the child to withstand stigma and discrimination (Baumann & Germann, 2005).

The Three-stage Approach

An intervention model described by Pynoos and Eth (1986) may be useful in providing counseling to OVC. This model adopts a three-stage approach: *open (exploration)*, *trauma (support)*, and *closure*. This model makes use of projective drawings and storytelling techniques to encourage the discussion of the actual traumatic situation as well as the aftermath and consequences of the experience on the child.

In the opening phase (stage 1), expressive representation such as art and drawings are used by the counselor rather than making a direct inquiry, because such methods are considered to be less threatening. The counselor encourages the child to "draw whatever you would like – but something you can tell." Elaboration and extension of the story is then encouraged by making use of questions, such as "what happens next?" Through this technique, the traumatic events experienced by the child are projectively represented.

The second stage (trauma support) includes a two-pronged approach, and involves (1) reliving the experience and (2) coping with the experience. The counselor attempts to provide safety and comfort for the child as he or she is provided with an opportunity to work through the traumatic experiences. Emphasis is placed on the child's sensory response to the experience. Further questions may promote the discussion of specific details of the trauma that have special meaning for the child. The child is then given an opportunity to reverse the sense of helplessness by formulating a plan of action. It is important that cognitive reappraisals be examined to counteract self-blame and offset the guilt of personal responsibility for the child's circumstances. Concerns about the future are also explored with the child.

The closing stage of the model (stage 3) provides the child with an opportunity to reflect back on the counseling process.

Teddy Bear Therapy

Teddy Bear Therapy (TBT), as developed by Charl Vorster, is a promising intervention in the counseling of children. TBT is based on the General Systems Theory, viewing the child in the context of the family system and hierarchy of subsystems in the family, and is a form of directive child play therapy (Vorster, 2008). TBT is rooted in Gardner's (1971) Mutual Story Telling Technique. However, unlike Gardner's (1971) technique that promotes the child as inferior to the therapist, TBT promotes an equal relationship between the child and therapist. In this way, the TBT approach empowers the child to deal with his or her difficulties, and also provides a corrective emotional experience (Baloyi, 2006; Novello & Vorster, 1999; Vorster, 2008). An important component in the decision to make use of TBT is the "child's ability to create a fantasy world with the therapist" (Vorster, 2008, p. 1). Thus, this technique is suited for children ages between three and ten years (Vorster, 2008).

TBT makes use of a story technique with the child, in which an animal – usually a teddy bear – creates an additional relationship in the system with the child. This

Research Box 12.2: Play Therapy

Baloyi, L. (2006). Teddy Bear Therapy: An application. *Child Abuse Research in South Africa*, 7(2), 17–25.

Objective: The objective of the study was to examine the application of Teddy Bear Therapy (TBT) as a psychotherapeutic intervention with South African children. The therapy was provided by the author over three sessions.

Method: Participants were two siblings (ages three and five) who experienced a car hijacking and a five-year-old boy who had persistent encopresis. The case-study approach was used and data were collected using interviews and clinical observations.

Results: The participants had lower levels of symptoms of trauma after the intervention. Subsequent follow-up sessions several months later confirmed the beneficial effects of TBT as a therapeutic technique for children.

Conclusion: TBT is effective in treating children with trauma in South Africa.

Questions

1. Why would TBT work with Black South African children with trauma?
2. What alternative therapy could work with children with trauma in the African context?

animal is given a problem similar to that of the child, and the child becomes a helper, assisting the animal with the problem (Vorster, 2008). Vorster (2008, p. 3) states that "[h]ow the therapist defines the relationship between him or herself and the client, as well as the manner in which the story is introduced, should always honour the complimentary role definition between child and teddy bear. Everything the therapist does must be in line with this definition of the relationship."

In TBT, it is important to first have a session with the parent(s) or caregiver(s), to obtain a detailed developmental history of the child. This developmental history allows for an indication of the child's capabilities. The aim of TBT is to find an optimal solution to the child's difficulties, and identify coping strategies that are realistic, tangible and appropriate, taking the child's developmental phase into account. The TBT technique is effective with a variety of children's difficulties, including fears and phobias, behavior problems at school, withdrawn behavior, adaptation to a physical disability, grief, depression, rejection by friends, physical and sexual abuse, and parental divorce, among others (Vorster, 2008).

An important element of the TBT technique is that the therapist has a great deal of responsibility, including a strong ethical responsibility toward the child. Thus, despite the simplicity of this technique, supervision, guidance, and adequate training are suggested before TBT is used (Baloyi & Vorster, 2000b cited in Baloyi, 2006; Vorster, 2008). Research Box 12.2 presents an application of TBT for counseling children experiencing trauma. This research suggests that TBT may be useful for a variety of factors pertinent to the experiences of OVCs.

Support Groups

Support groups may be beneficial for OVCs. There is evidence that support groups can assist in reducing symptoms of anxiety, depression, and anger in orphans (Kumakech, Cantor-Graae, Maling, & Bajunirwe, 2009). Support groups, made up of people with similar experiences, assist in addressing problems by sharing experiences and feelings. Support groups can consist of individual one-on-one counseling or participation in larger groups where pertinent topics are presented. Research has found that peer support groups can assist in providing participants with a sense of hope and relationship. These groups may also assist in providing support and acceptance and reducing the negative impact of stigmatization of people infected with HIV (Funck-Brentano et al., 2005; Harris & Larsen, 2007).

Therefore, support groups become a place where OVCs are able to discuss pertinent topics that are a reality in their lives. A variety of techniques can be used in support groups, including drama, poetry, singing, art, storytelling, and debate (Avert, 2008a, 2008b; Harris & Larsen, 2007; Hughes-d'Aeth, 2002; Mutepfa, 2004; Mutepfa et al., 2008). From the experience of one of the authors, support groups allow a safe environment in which pertinent topics can be openly discussed. In turn, this open discussion allows children to discuss their hidden concerns and raise questions.

A Developmental Approach

The *Children on the Brink Report* (UNAIDS/UNICEF/USAID, 2004) proposes a developmental approach to the allocation of resources and the provision of interventions to OVCs at the levels of infancy and early childhood, middle childhood, and adolescence.

During infancy and early childhood, physical proximity to a caregiver and emotional care are important. The death of a parent during this stage will have enormous implications for the developing child. Interventions should thus target the need for proximity and emotional care, and caregivers should receive training on caring for children in this age group. During middle childhood, school attendance and access to loving family care are of

Case Study 12.1: Bereavement Counseling in the African Culture

The following case study provides a culturally contextualized therapy of a young boy in South Africa.

A six-year-old boy was referred for counseling after the death of his mother from an AIDS-related illness. The boy's grandmother became his caregiver; and she told the boy that his mother had gone to heaven. One day, after the boy inquired about his mother, the grandmother said that his mother now lives on a cloud. On a cloudless day the boy would be sad, as he could no longer see his mother. Making use of art therapy, the boy was able to move from bereavement to acceptance. The art therapy was delivered by the first author and was provided over several sessions on a one-to-one basis.

Questions

1. How appropriate was the intervention for the child? Give reasons for your answer.
2. What other interventions may have been appropriate from the child? Explain your answer.

paramount importance. At this age, the child may have a clearer understanding of the finality of death and fear any further abandonment and loss. These children may also regress to earlier forms of behavior (UNAIDS/UNICEF/USAID, 2004).

Adolescence is a period during which many developmental changes occur, including the formation of an identity (Erikson, 1973). The adolescent may experience a variety of emotions with increased intensity, including depression, hopelessness, and anger. OVCs, in this age group, may be at risk of forced sexual activity, unwanted pregnancies, and commercial sex work, necessitating interventions at this level of risk (UNAIDS/UNICEF/USAID, 2004).

The developmental approach proposed by UNAIDS, UNICEF, and USAID (2004) can be used in the context of bereavement counseling. Research has demonstrated that OVCs experience bereavement (Cluver & Gardner, 2007), thus necessitating counseling at this level. The factors surrounding an AIDS-related death may be traumatic for the child, and the grief experienced by children may not always be obvious to adults. Rather, children are likely to express the grief through their behaviors, thoughts, feelings, or physical symptoms (Bauman & Germann, 2005; Cluver & Gardner, 2006; Lewis, 1999; Makame et al., 2002). When counseling children, it is thus important to consider their developmental stage. To obtain a better understanding of bereavement counseling in children, readers are referred to Baumann and Germann (2005); Kanabus, (n.d.; accessed from Avert.org), Kenyon (2001); Lewis (1999), Silverman (2000), van Dyk (2005b); and Webb (2005). Also, various other sources can be consulted.

ISSUES TO BE RESOLVED THROUGH RESEARCH AND SCHOLARSHIP

Much research is still required in the area of emotional care of OVCs. In this section, the authors highlight several of these. Although this chapter explores several possible intervention methods, it is important to note that there is limited research on intervention techniques used with OVCs and on the efficacy of these interventions. This scarcity of research is especially true in the case of girl OVCs, as they are frequently exposed to greater levels of vulnerability than their male counterparts (Subbarao & Coury, 2004).

The developmental approach, discussed in the previous section, and the implication for bereavement counseling, is an important area of future research. Mdleleni-Bookholane (2003) argues that the way in which children conceptualize death is determined by sociocultural practices of a given time and space in history, and these should be taken into account in the counseling of OVCs (Mberi & Makore-Rukuni, 2001; Mdleleni-Bookholane, 2003) However, research into African children's conceptualization of death is lacking, with no published material on this topic from Africa (Mdleleni-Bookholane, 2003).

An important consideration to take into account in counseling OVCs is child development in the African context. Most developmental theories are born from a Western framework. However, theories of child development should recognize socioeconomic and political changes that influence cultural values and the child's development (Ramokgopa, 2001). Ramokgopa (2001) conducted a study on the developmental stages of African children in South Africa by comparing child development in Africa to that of Erikson's theory (Erikson 1973). Ramokgopa (2001) found that African children do experience the same developmental stages as Western children do; however, the developmental changes are different from those proposed by Erikson.

Child development in Africa appears to be more holistic in nature, with developmental stage changes marked by readiness to move to the next stage rather than by age, and are often marked by ceremonies and rituals. Thus, Ramokgopa (2001) recommends that psychotherapeutic techniques applied to children in Africa should acknowledge cultural beliefs and the diversity of the people, as well as traditional African methods of solving problems that could be incorporated into the therapy. However, further research into child development in Africa and African-born theories of child development are required (Ramokgopa, 2001).

SUMMARY AND CONCLUSION

In Africa, many orphans and vulnerable children have negative experiences, including limited access to education, abuse, neglect, forced labor, sexual activity, and destitution. These children may also experience psychological problems such as depression and posttraumatic stress disorder. For these reasons, cultural and context-related counseling is required in Africa to provide effective interventions to orphans and other vulnerable children. Several of the many approaches used in the counseling of these children are discussed in this chapter. Unfortunately, studies in the unique African context are sporadic and limited, and much research is still needed in the context of counseling orphans and other vulnerable children in Africa.

REFERENCES

Altman, L. K. (1994, 21 February). In major finding, drug curbs HIV infection in newborns. *New York Times*.

Atwine, B., Cantor-Graae, E., & Bajunirwe, F. (2005). Psychological distress among AIDS orphans in rural Uganda. *Social Science & Medicine*, *61*, 555–64.

Avert. (2008a). Why HIV/AIDS education? Retrieved October 21, 2008 from http://www.avert.org/aidseducation.htm.

Avert. (2008b). HIV AIDS education and young people. Retrieved October 21, 2008 from http://www.avert.org/aidsyoun.htm.

Baloyi, L. (2006). Teddy Bear Therapy: An application. *Child Abuse Research in South Africa*, (2), 17–25.

Barnett, T., & Whiteside, A. (2006). *AIDS in the twenty-first century. Disease and globalization* (2nd ed.). New York: Palgrave-Macmillan.

Baumann, L. J., & Germann, S. (2005). Psychosocial impact of the HIV/AIDS epidemic on children and youth. In G. Foster, C. Levine, & J. Williamson (Eds.). *A generation at risk. The global impact of HIV/AIDS on orphans and vulnerable children* (pp. 93–133). New York: Cambridge University Press.

Bayer, C. P., Klasen, F., & Adam, H. (2007). Association of trauma and PTSD symptoms with openness to reconciliation and feelings of revenge among former Ugandan and Congolese child soldiers. *Journal of the American Medical Association*, *29*(5), 555–9.

Children's Act of South Africa. (2005). *Government Gazette*. (No. 28944).

Children's Act of Zimbabwe [Chapter 5:06]. (2002). Government of Zimbabwe.

Children's Status Act of Namibia (2006). *Government Gazette*. Government of Namibia.

Children's Status Bill of Namibia. (2005). *Government Gazette* (No. 3761).

Cluver, L., & Gardner, F. (2006). The psychological well-being of children orphaned by AIDS in Cape Town, South Africa. *Annals of General Psychiatry*, *5*, 8.

Cluver, L., & Gardner, F. (2007). Risk and protective factors for psychological well-being of children orphaned by AIDS in Cape Town: A qualitative study of children and caregivers' perspectives. *AIDS Care*, *19*(3), 318–25.

Cluver, L., Gardner, F., & Operario, D. (2007). Psychological distress amongst AIDS-orphaned children in urban South Africa. *Journal of Child Psychology and Psychiatry*, *4*(8), 755–63.

Craddock, S. (2004). Introduction. Beyond epidemiology: Locating AIDS in Africa. In E. Kalipeni, S. Craddock, J. R. Oppong, & J. Ghosh (Eds.), *HIV & AIDS in Africa: Beyond epidemiology* (pp. 1–10). Malden, MA: Blackwell Scientific.

Dawes, R. B., van der Merwe, A., & Brandt, R. (2007). A monitoring dilemma: Orphans and children made vulnerable by HIV/AIDS. In A. Dawes, R. Bray, & A. van der Merwe. (Eds.). *Monitoring child well-being. A South African rights-based approach* (pp. 359–69). Cape Town: HSRC Press.

Deacon, H., & Stephney, I. (2007). *HIV/AIDS, stigma and children: A literature review*. Cape Town: HSRC Press.

Department of Social Development. (2005). Policy framework for orphans and other children made vulnerable by HIV and AIDS South Africa. Briefing paper by the Department of Social Development to the Joint Monitoring Committee. Retrieved February 14, 2008 from http://sabinet.co.za.

Erikson, E. H. (1973). *Childhood and society*. Middlesex: Penguin Books.

Essex, M., Mboup, S., Kanki, P. J., Marlink, R. G., & Tlou, S. D. (Eds.). (2002). *AIDS in Africa*. New York: Kluwer Academic/ Plenum Press.

Firelight Foundation. (2008). Annual report 2007. Retrieved June 1, 2009 from http://www.firelightfoundation.org/annual-reports.php.

FOST. (2000). *The farm orphan support trust annual report 1999*. Harare.

FOST. (2002). *The farm orphan support annual report 2001*. Harare.

Foster, G. (2000). The capacity of the extended family safety net for orphans in Africa. *Psychology, Health and Medicine*, *5*, 55–62.

Foster, G. (2004). Safety nets for children affected by HIV/AIDS in Southern Africa. In R. Pharoah (Ed.), A generation at risk? HIV/AIDS, vulnerable children and security in Southern Africa. Retrieved April 6, 2009 from http://www.iss.co.za/pubs/Monographs/No109/Chap4.htm

Foster, G., Makufa, C., Drew, R., & Kralovec, E. (1997). Factors leading to the establishment of child-headed households: The case of Zimbabwe. *Health Transition Review*, *7*, 155–68.

Foster, G., & Williamson, J. (2000). A review of current literature on the impact of HIV/AIDS on children in Africa. *AIDS*, *14*, s275–84.

Frohlich, J. (2005). The impact of AIDS on the community. In S. S. Karim & Q. A. Karim (Eds.), *HIV/AIDS in South Africa* (pp. 351–70). Cape Town: Cambridge University Press.

Funck-Brentano, I., Dalban, C., Verber, F., Quartier, P., Hefez, S., Costagliola, D., & Blanche, S. (2005). Evaluation of a peer support group therapy for HIV-infected adolescents. *AIDS*, *19*(14), 1501–8.

Gardner, R. A. (1971). *Therapeutic communication with children: The mutual story telling technique*. New York: Science House.

Gruskin, S., & Tarantola, D. J. M. (2005). Human rights and children affected by HIV/AIDS. In G. Foster, C. Levine, & J. Williamson (Eds.), *A generation at risk. The global impact of HIV/AIDS on orphans and vulnerable children* (pp. 134–58). New York: Cambridge University Press.

Hadziucheri, M., Chiwandire, R., Makawara, T., & Walker, L. (2006). Zimbabwe country profile. In K. Izumi (Ed.), *Reclaiming our lives. HIV and AIDS, women's land and property rights and livelihoods in Southern and East Africa – narratives and responses*. Cape Town: HSRC Press.

Harris, G. E., & Larsen, D. (2007). HIV peer counseling and the development of hope: Perspectives from peer counselors and peer counseling recipients. *AIDS Patient Care and STDs*, *21*(11), 843–59.

Hughes-d ' Aeth, A. (2002). Evaluation of HIV/AIDS peer education projects in Zambia. *Evaluation and Program Planning*, *25*, 397–407.

Joint Learning Initiative on Children and HIV/AIDS (JLIC). (2009). Home truths. Facing the factors on children, AIDS, and poverty. Retrieved June 1, 2009 from www.jlica.org/protected/pdf-feb09/Final%20JLICA%20Report-final.pdf.

Kanabus, A. (n.d.). Am I going to die? Living with a progressive disease. Retrieved May 1, 2008 from http://www.advert.org.

Kenyon, B. (2001). Current research in children's conceptions of death: A critical review. *Journal of Death and Dying*, *43*(1), 69–91.

Kohrt, B. A., Jordans, M. J. D., Tol, W. A., Speckman, R. A., Maharjan, S. M., Worthman, C. M., & Komproe, I. H. (2008). Comparison of mental health between former child soldiers and children never conscripted by armed groups in Nepal. *JAMA*, *300*(6), 691–702.

Kumakech, E., Cantor-Graae, E., Maling, S., & Bajunirwe, F. (2009). Peer-group support intervention improves the psychosocial well-being of AIDS orphans: Cluster randomized trial. *Social Science & Medicine*, *68*, 1038–43.

Laband, J. (2007). Introduction: African civilians in wartime. In J. Laband (Ed.), *Daily lives of civilians in wartime Africa* (pp. 1–16). South Africa: University of KwaZulu-Natal Press.

Levine, C., Foster, G., & Williamson, J. (2005). Introduction: HIV/AIDS and its long-term impact on children. In G. Foster, C. Levine, & J. Williamson (Eds.), *A generation at risk. The global impact of HIV/AIDS on orphans and vulnerable children* (pp. 1–10). New York: Cambridge University Press.

Lewis, S. (1999). *An adult's guide to childhood trauma. Understanding traumatised children in South Africa*. Cape Town: David Phillip Publishers.

MacLellan, M. (2005). *Child headed households: Dilemmas of definition and livelihood rights*. Paper presented at the 4th World Congress on Family Law and Children's Rights: Cape Town: South Africa.

Mahati, S. T., Chandiwana, B., Munyati, S., Chitiyo, G., Mashange, W., Chibatamoto, P., & Mupambireyi, P. F. (2006). *A qualitative assessment of orphans and vulnerable children in two Zimbabwean districts*. Cape Town: HSRC Press.

Makame, V., Ani, C., & Grantham-McGregor, S. (2002). Psychological well-being of orphans in Dar El Salaam, Tanzania. *Acta Paediatrica*, *91*, 459–65.

Mberi, E., & Makore- Rukuni, M. N. (2001). *Counselling of special populations*. Harare: Zimbabwe Open University.

McKay, S. (2005). Girls as "weapons of terror" in Northern Uganda and Sierra Leonean rebel fighting forces. *Studies in Conflict & Terrorism*, *28*, 385–97.

Mdleleni-Bookholane, T. N. (2003). *The development of an understanding of the concept of death by Black African learners in a rural area*. Unpublished doctoral dissertation, Rand Afrikaans University, Johannesburg, South Africa.

Mills, E. J., Singh, S., Nelson, B. D., & Nachega, J. B. (2006). The impact of conflict on HIV/AIDS in sub-Saharan Africa. *International Journal of STD & AIDS*, *17*, 713–17.

Musisi, S., Kinyanda, E., Nakasujja, N., & Nakigudde, J. (2007). A comparison of the behavioral and emotional disorders of primary school-going orphans and non-orphans in Uganda. *African Health Sciences*, *7*(4), 202–13.

Mutepfa, M. (2004). *Guidance and counseling programs in Zimbabwean schools*. Harare: Ministry of Education, Sport and Culture.

Mutepfa-Mhaka, M., Phasha, N., Mpofu, E., Tchombe, T., Mwamwenda, T., Kizzito, S., & Jere-Folotiya, J. (2008). Child-headed households in sub-Saharan Africa. In T. Maundeni, L. L. Levers & G. Jacques (Ed.). Changing family systems: A global perspective (pp. 328–61). Gaborone, Botswana: Bay Publishing.

Ngalazu Phiri, S., & Tolfree, D. (2005). Family- and community-based care for children affected by HIV/AIDS: Strengthening the front line response. In G. Foster, C. Levine, & J. Williamson (Eds.), *A generation at risk. The global impact of HIV/AIDS on orphans and vulnerable children* (pp. 11–36). New York: Cambridge University Press.

Novello, A., & Vorster, C. (1999). Stories metaphors and rumours: Psychotherapy in a children's home. *The Social Work Practitioner-Researcher*, *11*(3), 148.

Oleke, C., Blystad, A., Rekdal, O. B., & Moland, K. M. (2007). Experiences of orphan care in Amach, Uganda: Assessing policy implications. *Journal of Social Aspects of HIV/AIDS*, *4* (1), 532–43.

Olley, B. O. (2006). Social and health behaviors in youth of the streets of Ibadan, Nigeria. *Child Abuse & Neglect*, *30*, 271–82.

Onyut, L. P., Neuner, F., Schauer, E., Ertl, V., Odenwald, M., Schauer, M., & Elbert, T. (2005). Narrative exposure therapy as a treatment for child war survivors with posttraumatic stress disorder: Two case reports and a pilot study in an African refugee settlement. *Biomed Central Psychiatry*, *5*(7). Retrieved June 1, 2009 from http://www.biomedcentral.com/1471-244x/5/7/

Plan Finland. (2005). *Helping AIDS orphans in child headed households in Uganda. From relief intervention to supporting centred community coping strategies*. Geneva: UN High Commissioner for Human Rights.

Pynoos, R., & Eth, S. (1986). Witness to violence: The child interview. *Journal of American Psychiatry*, *25*, 306–19.

Ramokgopa, I. M. (2001). *Developmental stages of an African child and their psychological implications: A comparative study*. Unpublished doctoral dissertation, Rand Afrikaans University, Johannesburg, South Africa.

Richter, L., Mangold, J., & Pather, R. (2006). Family and community intervention for children affected by AIDS. Retrieved February 4, 2008 from www.hsrcpublishers.ac.za

Sendabo, T. (2004). *Child soldiers. Rehabilitation and social reintegration in Liberia*. Sweden: Life & Peace Institute.

Shilalukey Ngoma, M., & Chanda, M. (2002). *A situation analysis of adolescent reproductive health in Zambia*. Adolescent and Reproductive Health Unit Directorate of Research and Public Health, Central Board and Ministry of Health, UNICEF.

Silvermann, P. R. (2000). *Never too young to know: Death in children's lives*. New York: Oxford University Press.

Skinner, D., Tsheko, N., Mtero-Munyati, S., Segwabe, M., Chibatamoto, P., Mfecane, S., Chandiwana, B., Nkomo, N., Tlou, S., & Chitiyo, G. (2004). *Defining orphaned and vulnerable children*. Cape Town: HSRC Press.

Smart, R. (1999). *Children living with HIV and AIDS in South Africa*. Pretoria, South Africa: Save the Children Fund.

Smart, R. (2003). Policies for orphans and vulnerable children: A framework for moving ahead. Retrieved February 10, 2008 from http://www.policyproject.com

Straker, G. (1986). The sanctuaries treatment team: The continuous traumatic stress syndrome – the single therapeutic interview. *Psychology in Society*, *8*, 48–78.

Subbarao, K., & Coury, D. (2004). *Reaching out to Africa's orphans: A framework for public action*. Washington, DC: The World Bank.

Summerfield, D. (2000). Childhood, war, refugeedom and 'trauma': Three core questions for mental heath professionals. *Transcultural Psychiatry*, *37*(3), 417–35.

Tsheko, G. N. (Ed.). (2007). *Qualitative research report on orphans and vulnerable children in Palapye, Botswana*. Cape Town: HSRC Press

Tudorić-Ghemo, A. (2005). *Life on the street and the mental health of street children – A developmental perspective*. Unpublished master's thesis, University of Johannesburg, Johannesburg, South Africa.

UNAIDS. (2002). Background paper on children affected by AIDS in Zimbabwe. Retrieved April 6, 2009 from www.harare.unesco.org/hivaids/webfiles/Electronic%20Versions/ChildrenAffectedbyAIDS.doc.

UNAIDS. (2006). *Report on the global AIDS epidemic: A UNAIDS 10th anniversary special edition executive summary*. Geneva: UNAIDS.

UNAIDS. (2008). *2008 report on the global AIDS epidemic*. Geneva: UNAIDS.

UNAIDS. (2009). Joint action for results. UNAIDS outcome framework 2009–2011. Retrieved June 1, 2009 from http://data.unaids.org/pub/BaseDocument/2009/JC1713_Joint_Action_en.pdf.

UNAIDS/UNICEF/USAID. (2002). Children on the brink 2002. A joint report on orphan estimates and programme strategies. Retrieved February 25, 2008 from http:// data.unaids.org/Topics/Young-People/childrenonthebrink_en.pdf

UNAIDS/UNICEF/USAID. (2004). Children on the brink 2004: A joint report of new orphan estimates and a framework for action. Retrieved February 25, 2008 from http://data.unaids.org/Publications/External-Documents/unicef_childrenonthebrink2004_en.pdf

UNAIDS/WHO. (2006). Report on the global AIDS epidemic. Retrieved May 1, 2008 from http://www.unaids.org/en/KnowledgeCentre/HIVData/GlobalReport/Default.asp.

UNAIDS/WHO. (2007). AIDS epidemic update. Retrieved February 25, 2008 from http://www.unaids.org/en/KnowledgeCentre/HIVData/EpiUpdate/EpiUpdArchive/2007/

UNICEF. (1998). Report of an assessment of stimulating orphan programming for families and children affected by HIV/AIDS in Botswana. Developing a supportive environment for exploration. New York: Author.

UNICEF. (2001). A study on street children in Zimbabwe. Retrieved January 20, 2008 from www.unicef.org./evaldatabase/index_14428.html

UNICEF. (2004). The framework for the protection, care and support of orphans and vulnerable children living in a world with HIV and AIDS. Retrieved June 1, 2008 from www.unicef.org/aids/files/Framework_English.pdf.

van Dyk, A. C. (2005a). *HIVAIDS care and counselling: A multidisciplinary approach*. Cape Town: Pearson Education South Africa.

van Dyk, P. (2005b). Bereavement and spiritual counselling. In *HIVAIDS care and counselling: A multidisciplinary approach* (pp. 236–56). Cape Town: Pearson Education South Africa.

Vorster, C. (2008). *Teddy Bear Therapy: Step by step*. Unpublished Manuscript.

Webb, N. B. (Ed.). (2005). *Helping bereaved children: A handbook for practitioners*. New York: Guilford Press.

USEFUL WEBSITES

http://www.avert.org
http://www.avert.org/yngindx.htm
http://www.thebody.com
http://www.hsrcpress.ac.za
http://www.cdc.gov/hiv/
http://www.who.int/hiv/en/
http://www.unaids.org/en/
http://www.unicef.org/
http://www.soulcity.org.za/
http://www.kidshealth.org/
http://www.lovelife.org.za/
http://www.globalhealth.org
http://www.africaaction.org
http://www.aidsinfo.nih.gov
http://www.savethechildren.org

SELF-CHECK EXERCISES

1. Describe some of the psychological experiences of OVCs in Africa.
2. Define OVCs in the African context and provide reasons for including or excluding certain groups of children in your definition.
3. What factors should be taken into account when counseling OVCs?
4. Describe any two counseling approaches that can be used with OVCs, and explain how the African cultural context may impact these counseling techniques.
5. How might a human rights approach to counseling protect the well-being of OVCs?
6. Why do you think an HIV- and AIDS-related death may be traumatic for the child?
7. How might stigmatization and discrimination due to HIV and AIDS impact OVCs?
8. What areas in Africa are under-researched in counseling OVC?

FIELD-BASED EXPERIENTIAL EXERCISES

1. Create a program to provide intervention to OVCs. Describe what activities you would include and the rationale behind the inclusion of these activities. Provide a timetable and working plan of how the program would be run (who are the presenters, how long is the program, who are the participants, what are the topics, etc.). Discuss your program with local community-based projects and NGOs, and decide how your program may be improved (strengths and weaknesses) or implemented.
2. Request an interview with a local NGO or community-based organization and discuss the services that they provide to OVCs. Consider how these services are able to address the needs of OVCs and what other services could be provided. Compare the services provided by these organizations to those discussed in this chapter.
3. Create a list of definitions of orphan and vulnerable child from community members and from available

academic resources (such as the Internet). Explore common themes that occur in these definitions. From these themes create a working definition of OVCs in your community.

MULTIPLE-CHOICE QUESTIONS

1. The term *orphan* is problematic because:
   a. The meaning of orphan varies across countries, and may also cause the child to experience stigmatization.
   b. All orphans are defined in the same way, causing many children to not be recognized as orphans.
   c. In Africa, all children are defined as younger than the age of fourteen years, which excludes children above this age from the definition of *orphan*.
   d. The term orphanhood is not problematic.
2. Which of the following statements is NOT part of the five strategies that can be implemented to provide care for orphans and other vulnerable children as proposed by the *Framework for the protection, care and support of orphans and vulnerable children living in a world with HIV and AIDS?*
   a. The strengthening of the family's or extended family's capacity to cope with the increasing number of orphans
   b. The creation of schools that all orphans must attend in order to receive proper counseling and intervention services without the community interfering
   c. Strengthening and mobilizing community-based responses
   d. The extension of child protection services
3. Orphans should always move in with the extended family because:
   a. The extended family loves all orphans and provides them with good care.
   b. The extended family will ensure that the orphan attends school.
   c. The orphan will help the extended family with finances by working, allowing the orphan to learn important life skills.
   d. The extended family as a resource has weakened considerably due to the HIV/AIDS pandemic, and many orphans also have negative experiences with the extended family; thus, it is not always a solution for the orphan to move in with the extended family.
4. School attendance is important for orphans because:
   a. They can play soccer instead of learning, allowing them to make friends.
   b. It gives them something to do in the morning and afternoon.
   c. It keeps them from wandering the streets, causing trouble.
   d. Educators may be able to provide assistance to orphans, and education is the basic right of the child.
5. Which of the following statements is true?
   a. A crucial intervention for orphans is providing them with work so that they can earn an income.
   b. Orphans are vulnerable to exploitation and abuse.
   c. The community always protects orphans from exploitation and abuse.
   d. In Africa it is legal for children to work as prostitutes, but the community discourages girls from doing this.
6. Orphans always experience the following psychopathology:
   a. Depression
   b. Suicide
   c. Not all orphans experience psychopathology.
   d. Orphans do not experience any psychopathology.
7. Which of the following statements is true?
   a. Child development is universal, so all theories of child development should be considered when creating interventions for orphans and other vulnerable children.
   b. The most important developmental stage in which to provide counseling is adolescence, because all adolescents are sexually active and at an increased risk of acquiring HIV.
   c. Erikson's theory can be used with children in Africa, because all children in all cultures in Africa go through the same developmental stages as proposed by Erikson.
   d. Culture is important in children's development in Africa.
8. The three-stage approach suggested by Pynoos and Eth is:
   a. Exploration, trauma support, closure
   b. Trauma support, closure, exploration
   c. Exploration, closure, follow-up
   d. Intake, trauma support, follow-up
9. Teddy Bear Therapy is effective with:
   a. Divorce
   b. Depression
   c. Abuse
   d. All of the above
10. Which issues should be resolved through further research and scholarship?
    a. Child development in Africa
    b. Exploration of the transmission of HIV and AIDS between mother and child
    c. Statistical data analysis on trends in HIV and AIDS infections in Africa
    d. All of the above
11. The care of orphans and other vulnerable children is:
    a. The government's responsibility
    b. The extended family's responsibility
    c. The responsibility of orphanages and NGOs
    d. Everyone's responsibility

Answers to the multiple-choice questions are provided at the back of the book

13 Diversity Counseling with African Americans

Debra A. Harley and Kim L. Stansbury

OVERVIEW. As a group, African Americans are heterogeneous with a multiplicity of racial compositions largely comprising involuntary immigrants to the United States from Africa, the Caribbean, Latin America, and Europe (Mpofu, 2005). Understanding the diversity that exists within the African American population, their position as one of the historical racial minority groups in the United States, and their unique cultural orientation and values are prerequisites to understanding the emotional consequences of race in the counseling process. This chapter presents an introspection of therapeutic counseling for people of African descent with a focus on African Americans. The multicultural movement in counseling began approximately forty years ago, and gained momentum from observations that clients from minority groups received unequal and poor counseling services (Patterson, 1996). During the past two decades, the counseling literature has increasingly included multicultural counseling. This inclusion, however, has been in part perfunctory, and too infrequently resiliency and strengths-based foci have not been included (Harley & Dillard, 2005). The multicultural movement shaping the United States needs to take place at two levels. On the first level, the United States is coming to recognize, learn about, and appreciate the cultural diversity within the country and among racial, ethnic, and cultural groups that make up its population. On the second level, the United States also needs a global perspective that recognizes and is open to other cultures in other countries (Leong & Blustein, 2000; Monk, Winslade, & Sinclair, 2008).

LEARNING OBJECTIVES

By the end of the chapter, the reader should be able to:

1. Demonstrate an understanding of the culturally appropriate counseling interventions for people of African descent.
2. Illustrate how race, *positionalities*, and culture influence the counseling process.
3. Identify barriers in counseling.
4. Critique advantages and disadvantages of traditional and multicultural counseling approaches.
5. Discuss multicultural counseling from a social justice perspective.
6. Evaluate international movements in counseling for diverse populations.

INTRODUCTION

In a global and international society, racism and oppression have a long history, and are ingrained in the social, cultural, legal, and professional fabric of the United States. Counselors, psychologists, social workers, and other helping professionals, as part of society, have been greatly affected, either consciously or unconsciously, by racism and, through them, the field of counseling in general (Lee, Blando, Mizelle, & Orozco, 2007). Thus, many people of African descent resist counseling and are suspicious of service providers, question assurance of confidentiality, and are mindful of historical hostilities (e.g., discrimination, mistreatment, stereotyping). Cultural mistrust can impact decisions and activities in many ways and frequently result in people of African descent having a lower level of satisfaction with counseling, lower self-disclosure in a counseling situation, and lower positive attitudes toward the seeking of help for mental and emotional concerns (Atkinson, 2004). Whaley (2001) referred to cultural mistrust among African Americans toward White therapists as a "healthy cultural paranoia" because the therapists belong to a group who have been less than hospitable and deserving of mistrust. In fact, the major barriers in counseling for people of African descent include (1) a lack of availability and access to culturally appropriate services, (2) a history of oppression, (3) socioeconomic status (SES), (4) cultural suspicions, and (5) the language or terminology of counseling (Gielen, Draguns, & Fish, 2008; Helms & Cook, 1999; Lee, 1997; Sue & Sue, 2008).

The well-being of people of African descent is linked to the historical, social, and ecological circumstances they encounter. Any discussion of African Americans and African descendants' progress requires an examination of health disparities and risk factors within this group. In the United Kingdom, African Americans and people of African descent are disproportionately represented among those with high blood pressure, cancer, cardiovascular disease, HIV/AIDS, infant mortality, substance abuse, diabetes, various physical disabilities, and homicide rates (Black Health Care, 1999/2000; Centers for Disease Control and Prevention [CDC] 2004, 2008; Net Wellness, 2007; Department of Health and Human Services, 2010) across the life span. In many ways, being Black is a health risk (Williams & Johnson, 2002). African Americans receive less than adequate care and referral to specialists regardless of their SES and insurance status (Fiscella, 2006; Smedley, Stith, & Nelson, 2003; Williams & Johnson, 2002). In mental health care, African Americans are less likely than their White counterparts to receive antidepressants for depression and less likely to receive the newer selective serotonin reuptake inhibitor medications (Blazer, Hybels, Somonsick, & Hanlon, 2000; Melfi, Croghan, Hanna, & Robinson, 2000). In 2002, the U.S. Surgeon General examined mental health care issues among minorities and reported that (1) only one African American in three who needs mental health care receives it, and terminates treatment earlier than White Americans; (2) African Americans are more apt to receive treatment through primary care than specialist services, and as a result, they are over-represented in emergency departments and psychiatric hospitals; (3) errors in diagnosis are made for certain disorders (e.g., schizophrenia and mood disorders) more often for African Americans than for White Americans; and (4) African Americans are also found to metabolize antidepressants more slowly than White Americans and may experience serious side effects from inappropriate dosages (Satcher, 2002).

IMPORTANCE, DEFINITION, AND SCOPE OF KEY TERMS AND CONCEPTS

In its early stages, multicultural counseling focused exclusively on race and ethnicity. More recently, the counseling profession has expanded the definition of cultural diversity to include gender, sexual orientation, age, religion, socioeconomic status/class, geographical location, parental status, marital status, educational background, work experiences, and disability (Chao, 2008; Harley, Feist-Price, & Alston, 1996; Robinson-Wood, 2009). However, many argue that race still remains the most pressing and difficult of all diversity issues to address in health care, counseling, education, and policy development because race is a reminder of the flaws rooted in historic inequities, institutional law, and longstanding cultural stereotypes (Harley, 2008; West, 1993). Proponents of multiculturalism, who believe that the study of ethnic differences affects the counseling relationship, are concerned that the influence of racism will be ignored or diluted if other cultural differences are also included (Anderson & Carter, 2003; Jackson, 1995). It is the taint of the slave health deficit and health scandals like the Tuskegee Syphilis Study that affect the health care choices of both Blacks and their service providers, which is tied to racist, classist, and paternalist medical conduct (Williams & Johnson, 2002). Watkins and Terrell (1988) found that many people of African descent who scored high on the Cultural Mistrust Inventory expected less from counseling regardless of the race of the counselor. Client mistrust correlates positively with client self-disclosure and premature termination. Discussion Box 13.1 further discusses the impact of interpersonal trust in the client–counselor multicultural relationship with clients of African descent.

Just as the context of multiculturalism has changed and expanded, so too has terminology. The terminology of multiculturalism has been transformed and renamed and identified as diversity and inclusion; more recently, the concept of social justice has emerged as an overarching term for multiculturalism and diversity (Alston, Harley, & Middleton, 2006; Harley, Alston, & Turner-Whittaker, 2008). Diversity can be defined as (1) a concept that encompasses acceptance and respect; (2) understanding that each individual is unique, and recognizing individual differences; (3) differences along the dimensions of race, ethnicity, gender, sexual orientation, socioeconomic status, age, physical abilities, religious beliefs, political beliefs, or other ideologies; (4) the exploration of differences in a safe, positive, and nurturing environment; (5) understanding each other and moving beyond simple tolerance to embracing and celebrating the rich dimensions of diversity contained within each individual (http://gladstone.uoregon.edu/~asumca/diversityinit/definition.html). In addition, diversity is a set of conscious practices that involve:

1. Understanding and appreciating interdependence of humanity, cultures, and the natural environment.
2. Practicing mutual respect for qualities and experiences that are different from our own.
3. Understanding that diversity includes not only ways of being but also ways of knowing.
4. Recognizing that personal, cultural, and institutionalized discrimination creates and sustains privileges for some while creating and sustaining disadvantages for other.
5. Building alliances across differences so that we can work together to eradicate all forms of discrimination (www.las.iastate.edu/diversity/definition.shtml).

The practice of multiculturalism/diversity/social justice acknowledges that the definition of diversity and categories of differences are not always fixed but also can be fluid, that individuals have the right to self-identification, people are multidimensional, and no one culture is intrinsically superior to another (Bryan, 2007). The fluidity of diversity becomes even more evident through globalization and internationalization.

Traditional counseling and therapy are based exclusively on European and North American culture (Atkinson, 2004; Parham, 2001; Smith, 2004). The aim of multiculturalism/diversity/social justice in counseling is to understand

Discussion Box 13.1: Interpersonal Mistrust in a Client–Counselor Multicultural Relationship

Research suggests that both African American and White counselors have to contend with mistrust of clients of African descent, with high levels of mistrust related to superficial exploration of counseling issues and potential early termination. Clients tend to show lower levels of mistrust and to provide a greater number of disclosing statements to African American counselors, whereas high levels of mistrust are associated with a lesser number of disclosing statements to White counselors. However, clients are more willing to self-refer and to disclose more intimately when the counselor responds with racial content than are clients who are exposed to universal content (Thompson, Worthington, & Atkinson, 1994). Because of this level of mistrust, African American psychologists propose an *emic* approach to counseling. The *emic* perspective refers to ideas, behaviors, items, and concepts that are culture specific and reflects an individual's world view (Vontress, Johnson, & Epp, 1999).

Vontress et al. (1999) suggest that "counselors need two pairs of spectacles through which to view the experience of their culturally diverse clients: an *emic* pair that allows the counselor to empathize with the client's specific cultural worldview and an *etic* pair that allows the counselor to understand what his or her own cultural worldview is and what demands it makes on those who must adapt to it" (p. 21). The latter is more difficult to achieve because people's awareness of their own culture is unconscious, and ironically, more accessible to those outside of the culture who have not been immersed in it. For counselors to work effectively with clients of African descent, they should learn as much as possible about the client's culture. This learning process can occur through reading, research, active interaction, or interviewing the client.

Questions

1. Explain how the *emic* perspective utilizes the significance of the Black experience as a positive or growth-promoting aspect of the psyche of people of African descent.
2. How can the *emic* approach affect the credibility of counselors?
3. How can counselors balance *emic* and *etic* perspectives when working with clients of African descent?
4. Which perspective should counselors use in diagnosing issues that are presented by clients of African descent? Why?

difference; to foster unity through mutual enrichment in interpersonal relationships, organizations, and societies; and to benefit from differences, especially when power differences and social equity are also addressed (Smith, 2004). At its most basic level, "practicing multiculturalism involves challenging assumptions, valuing others, and being genuine in all interactions" (Smith, p. 11). To work effectively with clients, counselors should have specific multicultural competencies: attitudes and beliefs (awareness), knowledge, and skills (Arredondo et al., 1996) that recognize the client's context (i.e., race, gender, age, sexual orientation, and so forth) (Sue, Arredondo, & McDavis, 1992). *Attitudes and beliefs* refer to the mindset of counselors about ethnic and racial minority clients, as well as counselors' responsibility to (1) check their biases and stereotypes, (2) develop a positive orientation toward multicultural perspectives, and (3) recognize ways in which personal biases and values can affect cross-cultural counseling relationships. *Knowledge* refers to the understanding counselors have of their own world view, their specific knowledge of cultural groups, and their understanding of sociopolitical influences on cross-cultural relationships. *Skills* refer to the specific abilities that are necessary to work with racial and ethnic minorities (Sue et al., 1992). Discussion Box 13.2 includes a broad constellation of components of counselors' multicultural competencies.

RESEARCH AND PRACTICE IN COUNSELING PEOPLE OF AFRICAN ANCESTRY

A considerable amount of the multicultural counseling research has identified the need for counselors to become culturally competent to address the needs of a diverse society appropriately (Arredondo et al., 1996; Robinson-Wood, 2009). According to Coleman and Wampold (2003), "more than 450 approaches to counseling and psychotherapy have been identified" (p. 229). Pack-Brown and Fleming (2004) indicated that, whereas traditional psychology and psychotherapy have expanded their interventions in recent years to emphasize and utilize client diversity, group approaches have been slower to incorporate psychological, emotional, and spiritual factors related to an African American perspective. Overwhelmingly, ethnic minority populations have been neglected by evidence-based practices (EBPs) and treatment (Roysicar, 2009). According to Sue and Zane (2006), the issue is not one of research design and methodology, but of a need for more ethnic research to be conducted, especially into culturally competent interventions. In fact, Sue and Zane emphasized EBPs have not been very helpful in reducing disparities or improving effectiveness for minorities primarily for three reasons:

1. Little research has been conducted on EBPs with clients from ethnic minority groups.

Discussion Box 13.2: Constellation of Multicultural Competencies

The broad constellation of multicultural competencies includes the following chief components:

- Having a good self-awareness of the attitudes or world view into which the counselor has been socialized
- Recognizing and being sensitive to the client's world view and attitudes
- Having knowledge of the cultural groups with which one works
- Understanding effects of racial identity, acculturation, ethnic identity, minority stress, and coping with minority status on the individual
- Understanding the impact of sociopolitical influences on minority persons
- Possessing proficiencies to work with culturally different groups
- Having the ability to be culturally responsive and to translate mainstream interventions into culturally consistent strategies, understanding, skills, and interactional proficiency (Roysircar, 2003; Toporek, 2003)

As a standard, multicultural competence in counseling is an indication that counselors should both appreciate other cultural groups and be able to work with them effectively. In fact, the ultimate goal of counselors should be cultural proficiency (Castro, 1998). Cultural proficiency refers to "an ideal state that involves high mastery, a commitment to excellence in working with minority populations, and a proactive attitude in designing and implementing strategies with a particular cultural group" (Ridley & Kleiner, 2003, p. 8).

Strength-based and empowerment-oriented approaches to counseling and service delivery are recommended as effective ways to work with clients of African descent. Too often, African Americans attributes and behaviors are misinterpreted as problems when in essence they are strengths.

Questions

1. What are the advantages of counselor self-awareness in working with clients of African descent?
2. Why should a counselor have an understanding of his or her own cultural group?
3. In what ways are you culturally competent?

2. A need exists to broaden the current definition of evidence.
3. Research that tests if existing interventions are effective is limiting (p. 330).

Sue and Zane's observation about the lack of EBPs is consistent with earlier reports by the U.S. Surgeon General (2001) and the President's New Freedom Commission (2003) reports about the acute gap between research and practice for racial and ethnic minorities. Others argue that the dilemma we face is the recognition that cultural factors have not been well integrated into traditional models of treatment, and we have not developed models of culturally relevant treatments that have empirical support as to what those treatments should include or when to use those treatments (Coleman & Wampold, 2003).

Given the paucity of ethnic treatment outcome research, one may question (1) how we can be sure that disparities in treatment actually exist and (2) if treatment effectiveness and efficacy have not been demonstrated empirically with these populations, whether we should refrain from using empirically supported treatments (ESTs) when they have not been studied in ethnic populations. Sue and Zane (2006) offer several answers to these questions. First, the preponderance of research of varying degrees of rigor has pointed to service disparities. Second, the assumption of generality of treatment outcomes is hardly "good science" where assumptions should not be made; rather, they must be tested (p. 332). Freeman and Logan (2004) list ten common errors made in research studies on mental health of African Americans, the most common of which is using a dominant lens and ignoring cultural factors to assess people of African descent. This type of violation in research calls increased attention to the demands of science that generality be convincingly demonstrated in some manner. In addition, being aware of how racism continues to appear in the mental health service delivery system is important, especially because dealing with racism is a constant in the lives of people of African descent (Gibson & Denby, 2007). Discussion Box 13.3 lists eight areas in mental health that are influenced by racism.

Most researchers continue to assume that findings obtained from one population can be generalized to other populations (Sue, 1999). Sue refers to this bias-based approach as the selective enforcement of scientific principles. That is, substantial attention is given to the problems of internal validity in research, but relatively little attention to external validity (i.e., generalizability). For racial and ethnic minorities, whose characteristic responses to illness, stress, or dysfunction may be different from the dominant culture, selective enforcement is likely to yield negative outcomes (e.g., mismatch between client goals and counselor goals). These groups are likely to be labeled as abnormal and viewed as deficient (McGoldrick & Giordano, 1996).

Discussion Box 13.3: Areas in Mental Health Influenced by Racism

African Americans continue to face racism in the delivery of counseling and mental health service delivery. The forms of racism are overt and covert, intentional and unintentional, and implicit and explicit. Rollock and Gordon (2000, pp. 7–8) identified eight areas in which racism influences service delivery:

1. The identification and interpretation of deviance and distress
2. Definitions of psychological symptoms including the causes and cures
3. Explanation of the etiology of mental disorder and deficiency
4. Mental health evaluations that are designed to showcase the needs of disadvantaged groups
5. Mental health service delivery lacking providers who are culturally similar to clients
6. Racism that affects the institutional structure, leading to design of programs without the economically disadvantaged in mind
7. Under-representation of diverse populations in research projects
8. Training in mental health services that ignores social context and oppressed populations

Racism is multidimensional in that there are different types of racism, including but not limited to: (1) spatial (e.g., racially and economically segregated areas), (2) institutional (e.g., activities that are designed to protect the advantages of dominant groups or maintain or widen the unequal position of a subordinate group, such as apartheid in South Africa or Jim Crow laws in the United States), (3) internalized (e.g., when people of color see themselves through the eyes of the dominant culture and apply to themselves the negative stereotypes or apply socialized effects of institutions that devalue their presence or contributions), (4) individualized (e.g., when people grow up with a sense of White racial superiority), (5) historical (e.g., based on lineage and common descent), (6) scientific (e.g., characterized with certain physical traits and a hierarchy), and (7) new racism (e.g., not based on any biological notion or assumption of inferiority or superiority, but on new expressions such as immigrant and cultural values) (Hick, 1998–2000; http://www.archchicago.org/departments/racial_justice/workshop). In addition, racism can manifest in different ways, for example, as apartheid, colonialism, Eurocentrism, White privilege, and genocide.

Questions

1. List examples of how the counseling or mental health service delivery system may unintentionally promote racism.
2. As a counselor, how can you change the adverse effects of racism in counseling and mental health service delivery?
3. Identify examples in which racism in counseling can occur in relation to the different types of racism.

Coleman and Wampold (2003) maintained that three approaches to identifying and developing psychological interventions are applicable to diverse groups: (1) generalizability across various populations, (2) culturally specific treatments, and (3) ecological perspectives on clinical practice. The core assumptions of these three approaches and their usefulness for multicultural counseling are described in Table 13.1.

Norcross (2003) suggested that EBPs in counseling must include three essential elements: the therapist/counselor, the therapy/counseling relationship, and the client's nondiagnostic characteristics. In addition, cultural competency depends on contextual factors such as client characteristics, therapist/counselor characteristics, the type of intervention or treatment, and the treatment setting. Likewise, according to the transcendent model, Coleman and Wampold (2003) identified the multiple levels in which culture affects the counseling process. The contextual framework for counseling interventions includes the client, presenting challenge, the client's world, the clinician's world, and ecological systems.

Counseling approaches often pass on to clients the blame when counseling or intervention proves to be ineffective. Subsequently, African Americans are denied access to appropriate cultural interventions. Too often, there is a lack of critical reflection about the interests and inequalities at work in the counselor–client relationship.

DIVERSITY COUNSELING PROCEDURES WITH PEOPLE OF AFRICAN ANCESTRY

The general goal of counseling should be to assist African Americans in the most culturally sensitive and appropriate manner possible. The process of emancipation of the mental health of people of African descent requires intervention, which takes into account the historical and contemporary experiences that haunt the mind and spirit of people of African descent (Logan, 2007). These haunts include, but are not limited to, slavery and plantation life, segregation and discrimination, assimulation and acculturation, and poverty and racism. Treatment that is culture specific has certain characteristics and assumptions

Table 13.1. Approaches to identifying and developing psychological interventions with diverse groups

A. Examine Generalizability Across Various Populations

The generalizability strategy has been recommended as a vital means in multicultural counseling to determine which treatments work best for various racial, ethnic, cultural, and other nonmajority groups. There are several assumptions:

1. The anticipated interaction between the treatment and the characteristics of people assumes that specific ingredients of the treatment work better with one type of individual than another (Coleman & Wampold, 2003, p. 230).

   The problem with this assumption is that it ignores the overwhelming evidence that the specific ingredients of treatment per se do not create the beneficial outcomes of counseling (Wampold, 2001).
2. Therapists are unimportant to the outcome relative to the importance of differences among treatments (Coleman & Wampold, 2003, p. 230).

   The problem with this assumption is that the evidence indicates that much more of the variability in outcomes in treatments is due to differences among treatments; moreover, ignoring therapist effects leads to an overestimate of the true effects due to treatments (Wampold, 2001).
3. Persons can be classified on constructs relevant to their response to treatment (Coleman & Wampold, 2003, p. 230).

   The problem with this assumption is that stratifying, by the relevant constructs (socioeconomic status, generational status, racial identity, degree of acculturation, country of origin, gender), is literally impossible. In the research design, a related problem is present because the grouping variable related to the type of person cannot be randomly assigned (Heppner, Kivlighan, & Wampold, 1999).

B. Culturally Specific Treatments

Culturally specific treatments that are created as modified standard treatments or novel treatments designed for various racial, ethnic, or cultural groups have several assumptions:

1. The variability within African Americans is less important than the differences between African Americans and other racial and ethnic groups.
2. Racial or ethnic group designation is isomorphic with or more important than other personal characteristics such as SES, gender, attitudes, and values.
3. Race and ethnicity are salient constructs that determine how therapy should be designed and delivered (Coleman & Wampold, 2003, p. 232).

C. Ecological Perspectives on Clinical Practice

The ecological perspective has several assumptions that are useful in developing a contextual model of psychological intervention:

1. Reducing our understanding of human behavior, particularly behavior that results from interpersonal interaction, to the linear relationship between proximal factors provides an insufficient explanation of how that behavior is organized within the complex interactions between an individual and his or her immediate (e.g., family, community, and peers), and general (e.g., society, institutions, and heritage) environment.
2. Core human processes involving issues related to such factors as affect, cognitive development, or perception are shared by people across contexts, but to understand how these processes are organized within an individual's life, one has to understand how the individual has made sense of his or her context and used that understanding to develop a repertoire of behavior that can effectively manage the demands of the context in which he or she lives.
3. Change in one part of the ecosystem will lead to changes in other parts of the system (Coleman & Wampold, 2003, pp. 234–5).

Questions

1. What can you conclude about treatment generalizability across populations?
2. What are the advantages and disadvantages to culturally specific treatments?
3. What are the implications of the ecological perspective for clinical practice?

(Coleman & Wampold, 2003). Table 13.2 identifies what it is that culture-specific treatments do.

Identity Counseling

Elements of approaches to counseling and therapy that have been found to be most effective with African Americans are racial identity, trust building, family therapy, group work, gender sensitivity, and the assessment of spiritual and religious content in therapy (see also Chapter 5, this volume; Smith, 2004). Exploration of racial identity allows African Americans to look at how internalized oppression and the coping methods for dealing with racism influence identity development (Helms & Cook, 1999). Building trust with this population requires the counselor to consider several issues. First, the counselor needs to explore the client's fears and concerns about counseling, to respectfully challenge client's misperceptions about the treatment process, and to educate him or her about the counseling process and the counselor's roles and responsibilities. Second, the counselor must possess some knowledge about African

Table 13.2. Function of culture-specific treatments

Culture-specific treatments do the following:

1. Respect and use the culture's definitions of psychological and sociological distress.
2. Respect the culture's assumptions about personal control and responsibility.
3. Use the culture's dominant modes of interaction.
4. Align with the culture's world view.
5. Emphasize developing constructive relationships with other cultural group members.
6. Recognize and address the exogenous as well as endogenous sources of behavior.
7. Emphasize the development of a positive cultural identity as a core strategy for coping with psychological and sociological distress.

Adapted from Coleman & Wampold (2003).

American culture and sensitivity to cultural differences and their impact on the counseling process. In addition, the counselor should carefully examine and clarify clients' expectations and culturally influenced values, and explore differences that may exist between themselves and their clients in these areas. Finally, the counselor should use relevant self-disclosure to increase clients' comfort level (Smith, 2004). Building trust is important to any counseling relationship; however, establishing trust with African American clients is critical because often they will want concrete solutions and may view the counselor as an expert.

Family Counseling

In utilizing family therapy approaches, the counselor must work to understand the client's definition of family, its structure, and its function (see also Chapter 8, this volume; Smith, 2004). For example, genograms are useful in mapping family members and their relationships to one another, major events in their lives, and geographic locations. In addition, the community genogram is a practical strategy for counseling people of African descent because culture, communities, families, groups, and individuals are all interconnected. The African proverb, "It takes a village to raise a child" underlies the community genogram (Ivey, D'Andrea, Ivey, & Simek-Morgan, 2002). The role of extended kinship (blood and non-blood relatives) among African Americans is equally important in both the clinical assessment and counseling process, especially because of nontraditional configurations (Brown-Wright & Fernander, 2005; Smith, 2004). Many African American families may benefit from time-specific therapy approaches that are problem focused or multigenerational in nature. Other effective approaches, in working with families of African descent, include structural, Bowen, and strategic family therapy theories (Boyd-Franklin, 1987). Lee (1995) found psychoeducation to be especially effective with single-parent African American women.

Mental Health

Denby (2007) offers a culturally responsive, three-pronged framework for structuring mental health services for African Americans: a historical perspective, a theoretical and conceptual framework, and intervention strategies. This proposed framework includes six major components: (1) cultural specificity, (2) strengths and empowerment orientation, (3) solution-focused intervention, (4) localized and indigenous regulations, (5) socioeconomic responsiveness, and (6) evidence-based cultural models. First, culturally specific programs must be predicated on the needs, characteristics, and values of African American individuals and families. Second, because of the historical relationship that African Americans have had with traditional service structures, skills inherent in the strengths perspective (e.g., validation and acceptance) are of even greater importance. Third, African Americans respond better to practical means of alleviating areas of need; thus, solution-focused interventions are needed. Fourth, given the limited autonomy and ownership that African Americans have in the shaping of societal structure, it is imperative that they share in the development of alternative mental health programming. Fifth, economic hardships prevent some African Americans from seeking needed mental health services; therefore, they need programming that is not contingent solely upon government funding patterns and whose eligibility criteria are not determined by those patterns. Finally, research is needed to examine the efficacy of mental health treatment models that purport to be culturally specific and training and development of staff so that evidence-based models can be delivered with high fidelity (pp. 27–8).

According to Smith (2004), "group work can be extremely effective for African Americans" (p. 159). People of African descent have a strong orientation to interdependence, community, and collectivistic tendencies (Atkinson, 2004; Lee et al., 2007; Sue & Sue, 2008). Examples of collectivism, among people of African descent, include the seven principles of nguzo saba, which can be incorporated into the counseling process in a more Afrocentric approach (Robinson & Howard-Hamilton, 1994). The seven principles are *umoja* (unity), *kujichagulia* (self-determination), *ujima* (collaborative work and responsibility), *ujamaa* (cooperative economics), *nia* (purpose), *kuumba* (creativity), and *imani* (faith) (Riley, 1995); illustrated throughout African and African American literature, music, art, poetry, and linguistic expressions. Effective group counseling can incorporate each of these aspects along with a focus on issues and resolutions that have clear boundaries and expectations, especially since most African Americans tend to present practical rather than personal problems (Brown-Wright & Fernander, 2005; Helms & Cook, 1999; Smith, 2004).

Case Study 13.1: The Case of Joe Jackson

Joe Jackson is a seventy-six-year-old African American who grew up in the rural South. He worked all of his life as a farmer. His wife and son observed that he is experiencing sleeplessness, loss of appetite, fatigue, and is talking to himself. His wife reported that Mr. Jackson wakes up at night stating that he hears voices and someone calling his name. The son indicated that he has noticed his father looking under the house for someone and calling out names.

Family members came together to talk about how to help Mr. Jackson. They called upon their minister to intervene. The minister and several deacons from the church came and prayed for him and laid healing hands on him. The minister concluded that Mr. Jackson had lost his spiritual center and was distracted by the devil. Consequently, the minister told the family to pray for Mr. Jackson three times a day and to give him holy oil. The minister also suggested that Mr. Jackson should be hospitalized.

Questions

1. What issues should the counselor consider in conducting a cultural assessment with Mr. Jackson and his family?
2. Explain the minister's intervention from a traditionalist or spiritual African American perspective.
3. What health care beliefs in the family would support the minister's intervention and proposed treatment?

Gender Sensitivity

Gender-sensitive practice (e.g., feminist theory) is especially useful for people of African descent. Of particular use, the major tenets of feminist therapy are psychoeducational liberation and personal validation (Smith, 2004). The counselor is able to work with clients to understand the social and historical facts concerning sexism, racism, and discrimination, as well as the impact of these facts on cultural conditioning and racial identity development. In addition, the feminist approach respects individual differences and takes into consideration the intersection of gender and other forms of diversity such as religion and spirituality (Smith, 2004), class, sexuality, and other *positionalities* (Robinson-Wood, 2009; Sue & Sue, 2008).

Spirituality and Religiosity

Many African Americans tend to use their spirituality and religion as sources of support, particularly during difficult times (see also Chapter 11, this volume). Counselors working with this population need to be comfortable incorporating these variables into counseling (Smith, 2004). "To many African Americans the road to mental health and the prevention of mental illness lie in the health *potentialities* of their spiritual life" (Sue, 2006, p. 219). The Black church (used to refer collectively to the many denominations of faith observed by African Americans) has always offered a sense of community, personal and psychological support, coping strategies, role models, and a sense of collective achievement (James & Johnson, 1996). The Black church provides a strong sense of peoplehood and kinship bond (Harley, 2005a; Sue, 2006). Although churches are racially integrated, most African Americans maintain membership in predominately Black churches. African Americans belong to many religious affiliations, including Baptists, African Methodists, Jehovah's Witness, Church of God in Christ, Seventh Day Adventists, Pentecostal churches, numerous Islamic sects, Presbyterians, Lutherans, Episcopalians, Roman Catholics, and Jews (Hines & Boyd-Franklin, 1996). "Today the Black church continues to function as an institution that affects the psychological health of African Americans" (Harley, 2005a, p. 191). The Black church is a strength-based approach that reinforces the psyche of African Americans. According to Harley (2005a), the Black church is an alternative approach that could assist with providing mental health interventions for people of African descent. The church serves numerous functions (e.g., religious, social economic, political) for members of the African American community. Case Study 13.1 presents a case study of working with an elderly African American client.

Language

For African Americans, nonverbal language may play an important role in the counseling relationship. Understanding nonverbal language and its meaning is as critical to the counseling process as overt, verbal communication (Baruth & Manning, 1999). Body language may convey one message, whereas verbal expression may convey another. For example, during counseling, African American males may be very direct, acting overly confident and unconcerned. This directness might be a defense mechanism, which limits disclosure or willingness to discuss difficult topics. Counselors working with people of African descent can benefit from an understanding of certain expressions associated with the population (Barth & Manning, 1999). "Studies in the field of linguistics and sociolinguistics support the fact that language conveys a wealth of information other than the primary content of the message; the cue of background, place of origin, group membership, status in the group, and the relationship to the speaker can all be determined" (Sue, 2006, p. 185). In addition, Sue (2006) suggests that the listener (client) uses this sociolinguistic information to formulate opinions about the speaker and to interpret the message. Styles of communication among most African Americans are often high-key, animated, heated, interpersonal, and confrontational. When looking at African Americans' communication style, along a continuum of the overt activity dimension (the pacing/intensity) of nonverbal communication, the characteristics are (1) speak with affect; (2) direct eye contact (prolonged) when speaking, but less when listening; (3) interrupt (turn taking) when possible; (4) quicker responding; and (5) affective, emotional, and interpersonal (Sue, 2006). Consideration of how this style affects a therapist's or counselor's perception and ability to work with people of African descent is crucial to the counseling process (Atkinson, 2004; Sue, 2006).

The response of African American (and all) clients also must be considered through the lens of six cultural phenomena (Envision Incorporated, 1994):

1. *Communication* refers not only to style but also to word usage and meaning. African Americans have a "code" for communication in which a word has one meaning in a certain context and another in a different context. Inflection of the voice also provides contextual meaning to words.
2. *Spatial needs* are the physical proximity to another person. Spatial preference among Africans varies widely depending on generational differences and acculturation or assimilation rates.
3. *Environmental control* is the individual's perception of his or her ability to manipulate situations to determine outcome. In 1966, Rotter formulated the concepts of internal and external control to explain human behavior. *Internal control* (IC) refers to people's beliefs that reinforcements are contingent on their own actions and that they can shape their own fate. *External control* (EC) refers to people's beliefs that reinforcing events occur independently of their actions and that the future is determined more by chance and luck. Many African Americans tend to have an external locus of control (Harley, 2005b). It is important to remember that locus of control falls along a continuum.
4. *Time orientation* identifies one's orientation either as past (hold onto old values), present (in the here-and-now, without linking outcomes to the future or past), or future (use the present to achieve future goals). African Americans tend to be present oriented (Ho, 1987; Sue, 2006).
5. *Social organization* refers to how culture defines and shapes the person's behaviors and beliefs. African Americans value efforts that promote cooperation and efforts that facilitate group survival (Parham & Parham, 1997).
6. *Biological variation* involves the influence of race and ethnicity and the susceptibility of people to certain conditions and diseases. Although African Americans do not show a propensity for any particular type of mental illness, they do so for certain physical illness (e.g., hypertension, diabetes) (Harley, 2005b). However, African Americans are increasingly recognizing mental health disorders and the ways in which they are manifested among the group (e.g., incarceration, sexual or physical abuse, suicide).

Failure to consider clients' behavior practices and cultural phenomena frequently lead to the assumption that everyone will respond to treatment in the same way, thus prompting stereotyping.

Relationship Factors

One of the most important issues in counseling is trust, especially with African American clients (Lee et al., 2007). Many African Americans follow the path of utilizing family members, the church, and community to assist them with problems, especially psychological ones. This practice is commonly known as "not letting outsiders in your business" (outsiders referring to professionals). For African American women, "kitchen psychology" is commonly practiced, in which they gather with other Black women to tell their story and seek advice (hooks, 1993). Often by the time a decision is made to seek professional help, African American clients may feel desperate and at the end of their rope. When the client enters counseling, he or she may exhibit a great amount of anger and, this anger may be directed at the counselor as part of a social system (something beyond simple transference) that has historically proven inhospitable and deserving of mistrust (Lee et al., 2007). In responding to the client's anger, the counselor should make the client feel more comfortable, use appropriate self-disclosure, and/or let the client vent and help him or her to process the anger through validation. Case Study 13.2 presents a case of responding to surface anger expressed by an African American female client.

CRITICAL RESEARCH ISSUES

For at least two decades, researchers in the United States have increasingly provided incisive critiques on the inadequacies and inequities of counseling approaches for African Americans and other racial minority groups. These various critiques expose the ways in which counseling privileges those who are White, male, heterosexual, Christian, non-disabled, and economically advantaged, while deprivileging those who are female, of racial minority backgrounds, have disabilities, and are poor. Of these categories, people of African descent are disproportionately represented.

Case Study 13.2: The Case of Mary Johnson

Mary is a thirty-six-year-old African American female who was referred to counseling for anger issues. She was cited for disturbing the peace in several public incidents. After her last incident, Mary was court ordered into counseling or to serve six months in jail for throwing items at a store clerk. Mary opted for counseling. She walked into the office of her twenty-six-year-old White female counselor, at which time, she said to the counselor, "I've had enough of dealing with people like you."

Questions

1. Identify several ways in which the counselor should respond to Mary.
2. What are some issues that should be addressed to determine Mary's response pattern?
3. How should the differences in Mary and the counselor's age, race, and cultural background be addressed?

Research Box 13.1: Bi-cultural Competencies

Diemer, M. A. (2007). Two worlds: African American men's negotiation of predominately White educational and occupational worlds. *Journal of Multicultural Counseling and Development*, *35*, 2–14.

Objective: To examine the perspectives and competencies of African American men who negotiate two worlds and suggest that bicultural competence may facilitate participation in the opportunity structure while maintaining identification with one's racial group.

Method: Qualitative interviews were conducted. The researcher served as the instrument because of historical misrepresentation of African Americans in social science literature, and as a European American male to be attentive to this history and to attempt to remain self-reflective regarding potential biases and assumptions in the research process.

Results: Data analysis resulted in one category (two worlds: experiences and motivation) and four subcategories (barriers in the White world, barriers in the Black world, bicultural balance, bicultural skills).

Conclusion: The present study indicates that the capacity to negotiate two worlds reflects one source that may facilitate the career development and full participation of African American men in predominantly White opportunity structures, while they continue to retain an identification with their culture of origin.

Questions

1. How can bicultural competencies help African Americans develop adjustment and coping strategies?
2. How is it possible to retain a healthy identity and maintain positive attitudes toward both cultures?
3. In what ways did the researcher position himself to address the *emic* perspective of participants?

One of the most critical research issues is an examination of practices that avoid overpathologizing and underpathologizing African Americans and those of African descent. According to Sue and Sue (2008), the mandate is for African Americans to monitor their behavior carefully and not expose themselves to the point that their psychological well-being might be threatened. Monk et al. (2008) argue that multiculturalism in the United States is struggling more than in some other places, yet African Americans must continuously negotiate between two cultures. Diemer (2007) examines how African American men negotiated predominately White educational and occupational worlds. See Research Box 13.1.

Lee et al. (2007, pp. 6–8) raised several issues and controversies that required further research:

1. *Is multiculturalism an exclusive or an inclusive concept?* The issue is whether multiculturalism should exclusively involve the study of ethnic differences as they affect the counseling process, especially since other cultural minorities experience discrimination based on permanent aspects of themselves that cannot be changed.
2. *Do the same basic counseling principles and techniques apply to everyone regardless of cultural background?* The controversy is between taking an "etic" or "emic" perspective. That is, the controversy is between using the universal elements of counseling that all cultural groups are assumed to share versus the indigenous characteristics of each cultural group that may have an impact on the counseling process.
3. *Should we be adapting traditional counseling to meet the needs of nontraditional clients or examining nontraditional counseling to enlighten traditional approaches?* Given that traditional counseling is developed from a Eurocentic perspective for use with persons of

Research Box 13.2: Counselor Cultural Capital

Zhang, N., & Burkard, A. W. (2008). Client and counselor discussions of racial and ethnic differences in counseling: An exploratory investigation. *Journal of Multicultural Counseling and Development, 36,* 77–87.

Objective: The study surveyed clients to examine the effect of counselor discussion of racial and ethnic differences in counseling.

Method: Survey packets were distributed to volunteer clients seeking help from counselors who were racially or ethnically different. The study was conducted at a counseling center at a midwestern university and two community mental health agencies in the midwestern part of the United States.

Results: Analysis revealed that White counselors who discussed racial and ethnic differences with their clients of color were rated as more credible and as having stronger working alliances than those who did not discuss such differences.

Conclusion: The initial findings suggest that in order for White counselors to increase the perception of clients of color regarding counselors' credibility and to build a strong working alliance, these counselors may need to at least acknowledge and perhaps discuss the issue of racial and ethnic differences between themselves and their clients of color during counseling.

Questions

1. Why did clients of color give White counselors more credibility if they discussed racial and ethnic differences?
2. Why did White clients not value discussion of these differences as much as clients of color?
3. What were the implications of gender in these discussions?

a European cultural background, professionals now agree that it is important to modify traditional counseling techniques to fit persons of various cultural backgrounds. More research is needed because of the myriad of counseling techniques and specific cultural groups, and the indigenous helping traditions within a specific cultural group.

Zhanf and Burkard (2008) conducted a study of client and counselor discussions of racial and ethnic differences in counseling as an exploratory investigation. The findings from their study may have important implications for cross-cultural counseling and future research on process issues in cross-cultural counseling. See Research Box 13.2.

With the graying of America, the African American community is undergoing a demographic shift. Elders who once played such a central role in guiding the affairs of the community and family now have a diminishing presence (Monk et al., 2008). With increasing stressors and decreasing economic resources, there is a greater possibility that older African Americans, in need of service, are likely to have fewer psychological and social resources for coping (Middleton, 2005). With this population, multicultural counseling must look to expand collaboration across disciplines (e.g., social work, gerontology, health care), especially with evidence-based practice (Roysircar, 2009).

Counseling African Americans and others of African descent is a process in which counselors must be prepared to alter their frame of reference and increase their awareness, knowledge, and skill levels. African Americans bring shared values of group membership and individual life experiences. A one-model-fits-all approach is inappropriate and disregards intracultural differences. Counselors must be able to avoid stereotyping and generalizations in counseling.

CULTURAL, LEGISLATIVE, AND PROFESSIONAL ISSUES

Throughout the counseling and human services profession, practitioners are guided by a code of conduct that regulates their ethical behavior. The African Counseling Association (AfCA), American Counseling Association (ACA), American Psychological Association (APA), Commission of Rehabilitation Counselor Certification (CRCC), and the National Association of Social Work (NASW) each have a Code of Ethics that includes specific requirements that practitioners will (1) respect the dignity and worth of the person; (2) promote social justice and social change; (3) empower people who are marginalized, oppressed, and vulnerable; and (4) communicate information in ways that are both developmentally and culturally appropriate.

As a profession, counselors must undertake efforts to ensure the following goals are achieved:

1. Recruitment of culturally diverse counselors.
2. Provision of pre-service and in-service training in practices that better address the characteristics of culturally diverse clients.
3. Implementation of culturally appropriate assessment procedures (Bullock, 1999).
4. Promotion of social justice and social change with and on behalf of clients (National Association of Social Workers, 2009).

Table 13.3. Sampling of African counseling community

- Amani Counseling Training Centre – Nairobi, Kenya
- Amani Trust – Harare, Zimbabwe
- Botswana Counseling Association
- Childline – Zimbabwe
- Connet-Zimbabwe
- Counseling Institute of South Africa
- Island Line – Zimbabwe
- Kara Counseling and Training trust – Zambia
- Kenya Counselling Association-Kenya
- Life Line – Southern Africa
- Regional AIDS Training Network – Kenya
- The Samaritans – Zimbabwe
- The Centre, AIDS Counseling – Harare, Zimbabwe
- Torture/Violence Treatment Centres
- Transactional Analysis Training – South Africa

5. Training and supervision of counselors to ensure that they are helping clients make transitions across the life span.

One of the major professional issues confronting multicultural counseling is how to remove barriers, real and perceived, and attitudinal and structural to increase cross-cultural counseling. Nonetheless, the counseling profession is growing in many Africanist settings (see Table 13.3) and prospects for increasingly responsive services are encouraging in the years ahead.

RELATED DISCIPLINES INFLUENCING COUNSELING ASPECTS

By nature, multicultural counseling is multi- and interdisciplinary. Many disciplines (counseling psychology, family studies, gender studies, gerontology, medical anthropology, political science, psychology, rehabilitation counseling, religion, social work, sociology) contribute to the philosophical, contextual, and practical assumptions of multicultural counseling. The multiple dimensions of human existence require that both theorists and practitioners understand the sociopolitical forces that globally define diversification (Sue, 2006). In counseling and other human service fields, the common connection is working with people.

Culturally specific counseling approaches take into account the mind, body, and spirit. Each of these areas is present in other disciplines as well. For example, knowledge of anatomy helps one to understand the interplay among the cognitive, physical, and emotional realms. To be an effective counselor, one must gain knowledge in the medical and psychosocial aspects of lived experiences and behavior.

GLOBAL COMPARISON OF COUNSELING ASPECTS

The Afrocentric world view proposes that the African American experience in the United States continues African history, beliefs, values, customs, and culture. The Afrocentric or African world view is holistic, interdependent, and oriented toward collective survival (Ivey et al., 2002). In the Afrocentric worldview, an individual is validated in terms of others (family, community). Although there are many different approaches to healing, which are grounded in different African cultural and religious traditions, they all share a strong sense of the interconnectedness of body, mind, and spirit. According to Cheatham (1990, p. 375), "unlike the Western philosophic system, the African tradition has no heavy emphasis on the individual … Nobles (1975) writes that there is a sense of corporate responsibility and collective destiny as epitomized in the traditional African self-concept: 'I am because we are; and because we are, I am'." Even with transplantation to the United States, for many African Americans, the philosophic linkages with Africa were retained (Cheatham, 1990). Many African Americans continue to practice and sustain the indigenous cultural belief system of Africa (see Chapter 1, this volume). According to Harley (2005b), inclusion of indigenous practices in diagnostic considerations offers the advantage of examining cultural influences in behavior.

The Afrocentric world view is closely related to other cultures. For example, descendants of families of southern Italian, Chinese, Japanese, Puerto Rican, and Mexican origin have a life orientation closer to the Afrocentric world view than to the European–North American world view (Ivey et al., 2002). In counseling, one must be mindful that each individual is likely to have some mixture of cultural frames of reference. Some healing traditions draw on traditional African religions from the Ifa region. Others are based in Christian churches with an African orientation such as the Aladura International Church in the United Kingdom. Still, others draw from Islamic tradition. The East London NHS Foundation Trust emphasizes that there is a growing appreciation that having access to many of the various healing approaches can benefit clients facing a life crisis or major health problem (www.africanhealingforwellbeing.org).

Monk et al. (2008) affirm that the United States is seemingly unaware of what is happening in other parts of the world in creating a multicultural social vision for counseling. Canada, New Zealand, Britain, and France have surpassed the United States in incorporating multiculturalism into the fabric of its political and social life. However, it must be acknowledged that the United States made history in 2008 with the election of the first President of African descent, Barack Obama. Generational difference must also be considered within the goal and international arena. In the United States, African American children are growing up in vastly different communities from their parents. According to Monk et al. (2008), different cultural practices are forever competing and colliding with one another. The impact of mass media and the Internet, both the exporting and importing of images of those classified as "other," is changing the face of globalization as well. Counseling strategies and approaches from around the world can be downloaded from the World Wide Web.

In 2003, a proposal was developed to internationalize counseling psychology in the United States (Takooshian, 2003). The focus was on ways to best achieve this. Other notable initiatives include counseling psychology prevention efforts in Guatemala, the International Counseling Psychology Conference, and Lao Hmong Shamanic healing ceremonials for opium addicts. Sima and West (2005) in Tanzania have initiated a dialogue between modern counselors and traditional healers to share information and remove mistrust on both sides so as to facilitate cooperation and coordination of therapeutic efforts. The objectives of AfCA are to (1) establish a network of counselors and counselor educators with an interest in counseling in Africa; (2) develop counseling theory and practice that is appropriate for the African context; (3) form working relationships with counseling organizations both in and outside of Africa; (4) disseminate information on counseling, counselor education, and counselor supervision; and (5) recognize the achievement of African counselors. The African counseling community consists of a collection of counseling and counseling training centers (see Table 13.3).

THE NEED FOR FUTURE RESEARCH

For a long time, African Americans have not been the focus of research studies that considered their issues from a cultural perspective. A need exists for research to be conducted by educators and researchers of African descent on people of African descent utilizing various research methodologies. Unlike quantitative research, qualitative research and single-subject methods offer information beyond statistical significance.

Several issues and questions that have been raised throughout the course of this chapter need further investigation. Numerous areas of research remain to be addressed:

1. Studies are needed on specific populations of African descent, including the elderly, lesbians and gays, and biracial individuals who self-identify as African American to determine their counseling needs, and effective approaches to intervention.
2. Studies to determine effective cross-training of counselors in multicultural counseling.
3. Longitudinal studies of the sociocultural effects of the intersection of identities (race, gender, socioeconomic status, sexual orientation) on the response to counseling of people of African descent.
4. Research that focuses on African Americans in rural areas.

SUMMARY AND CONCLUSION

Multiculturalism is a fact of life. Likewise, racism and discrimination are as well. The continuation of inequity of people of African descent is not to be condoned in counseling. The consequences of traditional counseling approaches are not identical for all groups, but the effects of inequality are made worse by the intersection of race, a history of slavery, and legal discrimination against African Americans. Discrimination impedes the psychosocial and cultural development of people of African descent. Nevertheless, African Americans have shown resilience and perseverance in spite of centuries of discrimination.

African American clients who view problems residing in *positionalities* may see the constructs surrounding the traditional approaches to counseling counterproductive to their well-being. Although the infusion of multicultural counseling into traditional counseling had not been a central focus in the field of counseling in the past, the historic barriers to integration seen to be slowly dissolving. As researchers and counselors acknowledge that what is culturally relevant to the client is prerequisite to producing successful counseling outcomes, the process of inclusiveness will become solidified in the profession.

REFERENCES

Alston, R. J., Harley, D. A., & Middleton, R. (2006). The role of rehabilitation in achieving social justice for minorities with disabilities. *Journal of Vocational Rehabilitation*, *24*, 129–36.

Anerson, J., & Carter, R. W. (2003). *Diversity perspectives for social work practice*.Boston: Allyn & Bacon.

Arredondo, P. Toporek, R., Brown, S. P., Jones, J., Locke, D. C., Sanchez, J., & Stadler, H. (1996). Operationalization of the multicultural counseling competencies.*Journal of Multicultural Counseling and Development*, *24*, 42–78.

Atkinson, D. R. (2004). *Counseling American minorities* (6th ed.). Boston: McGraw Hill.

Baruth, L. G., & Manning, M. L. (1999). *Multicultural counseling and psychotherapy: A lifespan perspective* (2nd ed.). Upper Saddle River, NJ: Merrill.

Blazer, D. G., Hybels, C. F., Somonsick, E. M., & Hanlon, J. T. (2000). Marked differences in antidepressant use by race in an elderly community sample: 1986–1996. *American Journal of Psychiatry*, *157*, 1089–94.

Boyd-Franklin, N. (1987). The contribution of family therapy models to the treatment of black families. *Psychotherapy*, *24*, 621–9.

Brown-Wright, L., & Fernander, A. (2005). The African American family. In D. A. Harley & J. M. Dillard (Eds.), *Contemporary mental health issues among African Americans* (pp. 19–34). Alexandria, VA: American Counseling Association.

Bryan, W. V. (2007). *Multicultural aspects of disabilities: A guide to understanding and assisting minorities in the rehabilitation process* (2nd ed.). Springfield, IL: Charles C Thomas.

Bullock, L. (1999). *A historical chronology of the CCBD*. Reston, VA: CCBD Mini-Library Series.

Castro, F. G. (1998). Cultural competence training in clinical psychology: Assessment, clinical intervention, and research. In

C. D. Belar (Ed.), *Comprehensive clinical psychology: Vol. 10. Sociocultural and individual differences* (pp. 127–40). Oxford, UK: Pergamon/Elsevier Science.

Centers for Disease Control and Prevention (CDC). (2004). Health, United States: Table 30, 53, *67*. Hyattsville, MD: U.S. Department of Health and Human Services, National Center for Health Statistics. Retrieved January 9, 2009 from http://www.cdc.gov/nchs/data/hus

Centers for Disease Control and Prevention (CDC). (2008). Comprehensive cancer control program. Retrieved January 17, 2009 from www.cdc.gov/Features?CancerHealthDisparities

Chao, R. C. L. (2008). *Multicultural competencies in counseling: A statistical exploration*. La Vergne, TN: Lightning Source.

Coleman, H. L. K., & Wampold, B. E. (2003). Challenges to the development of culturally relevant, empirically supported treatment. In D. B. Pope-Davis, H. L.K. Coleman, W. M. Liu & R. L. Toporek (Eds.), *Handbook of multicultural competence in counseling & psychology* (pp. 227–46). Thousand Oaks, CA: SAGE Publications.

Denby, R. W. (2007). A conceptual and theoretical framework for understanding African-American mental health. In S. M. L. Logan, R. W. Denby & P. A. Gibson (Eds.), *Mental health care in the African-American community* (pp. 15–37). New York: Haworth Press.

Diemer, M. A. (2007). Two worlds: African American men's negotiation of predominately White educational and occupational worlds. *Journal of Multicultural Counseling and Development*, *35*, 2–14.

Envision Incorporated. (Producer) (1994). *Cultural diversity in healthcare: A different point of view* [Video]. (Available from Envision Incorporated, 1201 16th Avenue South, Nashville, TN 37212).

Fiscella, K. (2006). Multicultural medicine and health disparities. *JAMA*, *295*, 2302–3.

Freeman, E. M., & Logan, S. L. (2004). Common heritage and diversity among Black families and communities: An Africentric research paradigm. In E. M. Freeman & S. M. Logan (Eds.), *Reconceptualizing strengths and common heritage of Black families: Practice, research, and policy issues* (pp. 237–65). Springfield, IL: Charles C Thomas.

Gibson, P. A., & Denby, R. W. (2007). African-American mental health: A historical perspective. In S. M. L. Logan, R. W. Denbt & P. A. Gibson (Eds.), *Mental health care in the African-American community* (pp. 3–14). New York: Haworth Press.

Gielen, U. P., Draguns, J. G., & Fish, J. M. (2008). *Principles of multicultural counseling and therapy*. New York: Routledge.

Harley, D. A. (2005a). The Black church: A strength-based approach in mental health. In D. A. Harley & J. M. Dillard (Eds.), *Contemporary mental health issues among African Americans* (pp. 191–203). Alexandria, VA: American Counseling Association.

Harley, D. A. (2005b). African Americans and indigenous counseling. In D. A. Harley & J. M. Dillard (Eds.), *Contemporary mental health issues among African Americans* (pp. 293–306). Alexandria, VA: American Counseling Association.

Harley, D. A. (2008). Maids of academe: African American women faculty at predominately white institutions. *Journal of African American Studies*, *12*, 19–36.

Harley, D. A., Alston, R. J., & Turner-Whittaker, T. (2008). Social justice and cultural diversity. *Rehabilitation Education*, *22*, 237–48.

Harley, D. A., & Dillard, J. M. (Eds.). (2005). *Contemporary mental health issues among African Americans*. Alexandria, VA: American Counseling Association.

Harley, D. A., Feist- Price, S. M., & Alston, R. J. (1996). Cultural diversity and ethics: Expanding the definition to be inclusive. *Rehabilitation Education*, *10*, 201–10.

Helms, J. E., & Cook, D. A. (1999). *Using race and culture in counseling and psychotherapy: Theory and process*. Boston: Allyn & Bacon.

Heppner, P. P., Kivlighan, D. M., Jr., & Wampold, B. E. (1999). *Research design in counseling* (2nd ed.). Belmont, CA: Brooks/Cole.

Hick, S. (1998–2000). Four types of racism. Retrieved April 29, 2009 from http://www.socialpolicy.ca/52100/m17/m17-t2.stm

Hines, P. M., & Boyd- Franklin, N. (1996). African Americans families. In M. McGoldrick, J. Giordano & J. K. Pearce (Eds.), *Ethnicity and family therapy* (2nd ed., pp. 66–84). New York: Guilford Press.

Ho, M. K. (1987). *Family therapy with ethnic minorities*. Newbury Park, CA: SAGE Publications.

hooks, B. (1993). *Sisters of the Yam: Black women and self-recovery*. Boston: South End Press.

Ivey, A. E., D ' Andrea, M., Ivey, M. B., & Simek-Morgan, L. (2002). *Theories of counseling and psychotherapy: A multicultural perspective* (5th ed.). Boston: Allyn & Bacon

Jackson, M. L. (1995). The demise of multiculturalism in America and the counseling profession. *Counseling Today*, *37*, 30–1.

James, W. H., & Johnson, S. L. (1996). *Doin' drugs: Patterns of African American addiction*. Austin: University of Texas Press.

Lee, C. C. (1995). Empowering the African American family: New perspectives on single parenthood. *The Family Digest*, *8*, 1, 3, 11.

Lee, C. C. (1997). *Multicultural issues in counseling: New approaches to diversity* (2nd ed.). Alexandria, VA: American Counseling Association.

Lee, W. M. L., Blando, J. A., Mizelle, N. D., & Orozco, G. L. (2007). *Introduction to multicultural counseling for helping professionals* (2nd ed.). New York: Routledge.

Leong, F. T. L., & Blustein, D. L. (2000). Toward a global vision of counseling psychology. *The Counseling Psychologist*, *28*, 5–9.

Logan, M. L. (2007). Mental health interventions and the Black community. In M.L. Logan, R. W. Denby & P.A. Gibson (Eds), *Mental health care in the African American community* (pp. 39–55). New York: Haworth Press.

McGoldrick, M., & Giordano, J. (1996). Overview: Ethnicity and family therapy. In M. McGoldrick, J, Giordano & J. K. Pearce (Eds.), *Ethnicity and family therapy* (pp. 1–27). New York: Guilford Press.

Melfi, C. A., Croghan, T. W., Hanna, M. P., & Robinson, R. L. (2000). Racial variation in antidepressant treatment in a Medicaid population. *Journal of Clinical Psychiatry*, *61*, 16–21.

Monk, G., Winsslade, J., & Sinclair, S. (2008). *New horizons in multicultural counseling*. Los Angeles: SAGE Publications.

Mpofu, E. (2005). Selective interventions in counseling African Americans with disabilities. In D. A. Harley & J. M. Dillard (Eds.), *Contemporary mental health issues among African Americans* (pp. 237–53). Alexandria VA: American Counseling Association.

National Association of Social Workers. (2009). *Code of Ethics*. Washington, DC: Author.

Norcross, J. C. (2003). Empirically supported psychotherapy relationships. *International Clinical Psychologist*, *6*, 10.

Pack-Brown, S. P., & Fleming, A. (2004). An Afrocentric approach to counseling groups with African Americans. In J. L. DeLucia-Waack, D. Gerrity, C. R. Kalodner, & M. R. Riva (Eds.), *Handbook of group counseling and psychotherapy* (pp. 183–99). Thousand Oaks, CA: SAGE Publications

Parham, T. (2001). Afterword: Beyond intolerance: Bridging the gap between imposition and acceptance. In J. G. Ponterotto, J. M. Casas, L. A. Suzuki & C. M. Alexander (Eds.), *Handbook of multicultural counseling* (2nd ed.). Thousand Oaks, CA: SAGE Publications.

Parham, T. A., & Parham, W. D. (1997). *Therapeutic approaches with African American populations*. Newbury Park, CA: SAGE Publications.

President's New Freedom Commission on Mental Health. (2003). Achieving the promise: Transforming mental health care in America. Report of the President's New Freedom Commission on mental Health. Rockville, MD: Author.

Ridley, C. R., & Kleiner, A. J. (2003). Multicultural counseling competence: History, themes, and issues. In D. B. Pope-Davis, H. L. K. Coleman, W. M. Liu & R. L. Toporek (Eds.), *Handbook of multicultural competencies in counseling & psychology* (pp. 3–20). Thousand Oaks, CA: SAGE Publications.

Riley, D. W. (1995). *The complete concept of Kwanzaa: Celebrating our cultura harvest*. New York: HarperCollins.

Robinson, T. L., & Howard-Hamilton, M. (1994). An Afrocentric paradigm: Foundation for a healthy self-image and healthy interpersonal relationships. *Journal of Mental Health Counseling, 16*, 327–39.

Robinson-Wood, T. L. (2009). *The convergence of race, ethnicity, and gender: Multiple identities in counseling* (3rd ed.). Upper Saddle River, NJ: Pearson.

Rollock, D., & Gordon, E. W. (2000). Racism and mental health into the 21st century: Perspectives and parameters. *American Journal of Orthopsychiatry, 70*, 5–135.

Rotter, J. (1966). Generalized expectancies for internal versus external control reinforcement. *Psychological Monographs, 80*, 1–28.

Roysircar, G. (2003). Counselor awareness of own assumptions, values, and biases. In G. Roysircar, P. Arredondo, J. N. Fuertes, J. G. Ponterotto, & R. L. Toporek (Eds.), *Multicultural counseling competencies 2003: Association for Multicultural Counseling and Development* (pp. 17–38). Alexandria, VA: Association for Multicultural Counseling and Development.

Roysircar, G. (2009). Evidence-based practice and its implications for culturally sensitive treatment. *Journal of Multicultural Counseling and Development, 37*, 66–82.

Satcher, D. (2002). Mental health, culture, and ethnicity. Retrieved February 8, 2009 from http://www.healthyplace.com/communities/depression/minorities3.asp

Sima, R. G., & West, W. (2005). Sharing healing secrets. Counselors and traditional healers in conversation. In R. Moodley & W. West (Eds.), *Integrating traditional practices into counseling and psychotherapy* (pp. 316–25). Thousand Oaks, CA: SAGE Publications.

Smedley, B. D., Stith, A. Y., & Nelson, A. R. (Eds.). (2003). *Unequal treatment: Confronting racial and ethnic disparities in health care*. Washington, DC: The National Academies Press.

Smith, T. B. (2004). *Practicing multiculturalism: Affirming diversity in counseling and psychology*. Boston: Pearson.

Sue, D. W. (2006). *Multicultural social work practice*. Hoboken, NJ: John Wiley & Sons.

Sue, S. (1999). Science, ethnicity, and bias. Where have we gone wrong? *American Psychologist, 54*, 1070–7.

Sue, D. W., Arredondo, P., & McDavis, R. J. (1992). Multicultural counseling competencies and standards: A call to the profession. *Journal of Counseling and Development, 70*, 477–86.

Sue, D. W., & Sue, D. (2008). *Counseling the culturally diverse: Theory and practice* (5th ed.). Hoboken, NJ: John Wiley & Sons.

Sue, S., & Zane, N. (2006). Ethnic minority populations have been neglected by evidence-based practices. In J. C. Norcross, L. E. Beutler, & R. F. Levant (Eds.), *Evidence-based practices in mental health: Debate and dialogue on the fundamental questions* (pp. 329–37). Washington, DC: American Psychological Association.

Takooshian, H. (2003). Counseling psychology's wide new horizons. *The Counseling Psychologist, 31*, 420–6.

Thompson, C. E., Worthington, R., & Atkinson, D. R. (1994). Therapist content, orientation, therapist race, and Black women's cultural mistrust and self-disclosure. *Journal of Counseling Psychology, 41*, 155–61.

Toporek, R. L. (2003). Couselor awareness of client's worldview. In G. Roysircar, P. Arredondo, J. N. Fuertes. J. G. Ponterroto & R. L. Toporek (Eds.), *Multicultural counseling competencies 2003: Association for Multicultural Counseling and Development* (pp. 39–50). Alexandria, VA: Association for Multicultural Counseling and Development.

U.S. Department of Health and Human Services. (2010). *Data 2010: The healthy people 2010 database*. Hyattsville, MD: U.S. Department of Health and Human Services, CDC, National Center for Health Statistics: 2004. Available at http://wonder.cdc.gov/data2010/focus.htm.

U.S. Surgeon General. (2001). Mental health: Culture, race, and ethnicity – A supplement to mental health: A report of the Surgeon General. Rockville, MD: U.S. Department of Health and Human Services.

Vontress, C. E., Johnson, J. A., & Epp. L. R. (1999). *Cross-cultural counseling: A case book*. Alexandria, VA: American Counseling Association.

Wampold, B. E. (2001). Contextualizing psychotherapy as a healing practice: Culture, history, and methods. *Applied and Preventive Psychology, 10*, 69–86.

Watkins, C. E., & Terrel, F. (1988). Mistrust level and its effects on counseling expectations in Black-White therapist relationships: An analogue study. *Journal of Counseling Psychology, 35*, 194–7.

West, C. (1993). *Race matters*. New York: Vintage Books

Whaley, A. L. (2001). Cultural mistrust: An important psychological construct for diagnosis and treatment of African Americans. *Professional Psychology: Research and Practice, 32*, 555–62.

Williams, K., & Johnson, V. W. (2002). Eliminating African-American health disparity via history-based policy. *Harvard Health Policy Review, 3*, 1–5. Retrieved January 30, 2009 from http://www.hcs.harvard.edu/~epihc/currentissues/fall2002.

Zhang, N., & Burkard, A. W. (2008). Client and counselor discussion of racial and ethnic differences in counseling: An exploratory investigation. *Journal of Multicultural Counseling and Development, 36*, 77–87.

SELF-CHECK EXERCISES

1. What are the arguments for and against expanding the definition of diversity beyond the category of race?

2. What is involved in practicing multicultural counseling?
3. What role does the Black church play in the lives of people of African descent?
4. How does diversity counseling differ from other types of counseling?

FIELD-BASED EXPERIENTIAL EXERCISES

1. Interview an older African American or person of African descent and discuss his or her role and position in the family with regard to advising and guidance.
2. Interview an African American counselor and a White counselor about the approaches he or she uses when working with clients of African descent.
3. Review counseling psychology, social work, or rehabilitation counseling curricula for inclusion of multicultural counseling instruction.

MULTIPLE-CHOICE QUESTIONS

1. To work effectively with clients counselors should have which specific multicultural competencies?
   a. Honesty, trust, and skills
   b. Awareness, knowledge, and skills
   c. Empathy, trust, and knowledge
   d. Research skills, empathy, and good eye contact
2. People of African descent are neglected by which type of research?
   a. Internal validity
   b. Site-based
   c. Evidence-based practice
   d. Structure analysis
3. The Black church is used to describe which type of faith?
   a. Strength-based
   b. Converted practice
   c. Many denominations
   d. Integrated
4. African Americans tend to have which type of locus of control?
   a. External
   b. Internal
   c. Singular
   d. Plural
5. African tradition has heavy emphasis on:
   a. The individual
   b. Western philosophic system
   c. Interdisciplinary system
   d. Collective destiny

Answers to the multiple-choice questions are provided at the back of the book

14 Resolving Conflict in Africa: In Search of Sustainable Peace

Joleen Steyn-Kotze and Gerrie Swart

OVERVIEW. Conflict is a normal part of human life. A person may argue with his or her life partner, parents, or friends. It is inevitable that at some point in time one will be in a conflicting situation with someone. Individuals have different ideas about how to do things and how to access and compete for scarce resources. In Africa social conflict and its resolution is the primary concern of this chapter. The chapter defines social conflict and discusses its associated theoretical paradigms and processes. It provides an assessment of conflict and explores holistic approaches to conflict resolution that go beyond negotiation and mediation. Lastly, the chapter highlights the role of counselors in constructing sustainable peace in Africa.

LEARNING OBJECTIVES

By the end of the chapter, the reader should be able to:

1. Define social conflict.
2. Analyze the phenomenon of social conflict according to its various theoretical paradigms.
3. Provide an assessment of social conflict in Africa (including traditional conflict management processes).
4. Highlight the role of social psychology in conflict resolution in Africa.

INTRODUCTION

Between 1946 and 2011 there were at least 276 armed conflicts worldwide. Nearly half of them occurred after 1989. No fewer than 116 of those – or just over half – occurred between 1989 and 2002 in seventy-nine different locations around the world. In 2002 alone, there were thirty-one active conflicts in twenty-four locations. Of the thirty-one active conflicts, thirteen took place in Africa. By the mid-1990s, the African continent appeared to be a chief beneficiary of the end of the Cold War. Wars that had been sustained by the Cold War, as well as by South African destabilization, were on the verge of ending (Wallensteen, 2007). The African continent experienced the greatest fluctuation in terms of the number of conflicts that have been experienced – from fourteen wars in 1989 and seventeen in 1990 and 1991 to nine in 1995, only to increase to fourteen in 1998. While the number of conflicts revealed an exponential decrease, the severity of these conflicts showed a rapid increase. From a lack of respect for the rule of law by some of the national governments, Africa's precarious security situation has provided an enabling environment for the continuation and exacerbation of conflict.

In Africa, the end of the Cold War led many of its proxy wars to come to an end. However, in its wake there was a new phenomenon of small-scale civil wars that have caused more casualties on the African continent over the last two decades than anywhere else on Earth. The intensity and severe costs attached to violence in Africa have reached alarming proportions. Conflicts in Africa cost the continent a staggering US$300 billion between 1990 and 2005 – an amount equivalent to all the international aid received by sub-Saharan Africa in the same period (Oxfam International, The International Action Network on Small Arms [IANSA] and Saferworld, 2007). Quite clearly, Africa's gross domestic product was impacted by these conflicts. The results of the study were released in October 2007 in a report by Oxfam International, IANSA, and Saferworld, which showed on a large scale, the effect of conflict on Africa's gross domestic product (GDP). The report, entitled "Africa's Missing Billions: International Arms Flows and the Cost of Conflict," compares the economies of countries at war with those of countries experiencing peace. According to the report on average the African economy shrinks by 15% and the continent loses about US$18 billion a year due to conflict. Nearly 38 percent of the world's armed conflicts continue to be fought on the African continent; and in 2006, almost half of all high-intensity conflicts were in Africa.

Conflict is a normal part of our daily engagement with other people and groups, and is not necessarily negative. Managed through discussion and negotiation, conflict facilitates social change and ensures that societies evolve to meet their needs. Through constructive interaction between different societal groups, problems are identified and the journey toward a sustainable solution becomes a reality. Each conflict is unique and is driven by its own characteristics, dynamics, and issues. No two conflicts will be exactly the same. There is no a *one-size-fits-all* solution to conflict resolution.

Perceptions are central to conflict. Bloomfield and Reilly (1998a) highlighted that two elements often combine in conflict: identity and distribution or the sharing of economic, social, and political resources within a society, which is central to understanding conflict in Africa. Most conflicts on the African continent are termed *intrastate conflict* in that these conflicts are in the form of civil wars or armed struggles within the boundaries of the state. Central to these conflicts are the identity perceptions of nation and nationalism rooted in a competition for resources, recognition, and power (Save-Soderbergh, 1998). Azar (1990) referred to these so-called *ethnic conflicts* as "protracted social conflict" in that these types of conflicts have several unique characteristics focusing on religious, cultural, or ethnic communal identities coupled with a dependence on the satisfaction of needs such as security, communal recognition, and distributive justice. Therefore, so-called *ethnic conflict* does not occur just because of diversity within society, but relates to institutions, recognition, and security needs of diverse groups within society. Azar (1990) asserts that "most contemporary conflicts are about developmental needs expressed in terms of cultural values, human rights and security" (p. 2). Therefore, conflict resolution is not impossible, but requires an active analysis to determine the factors involved in the conflict.

IMPORTANCE, DEFINITION, AND SCOPE OF KEY TERMS AND CONCEPTS

A conflict has its own life cycle. It appears, reaches an emotional, even (and often) violent climax, then tapers off, disappears – and more often than not reappears. The spiral of hatred and violence becomes a meta-conflict. Participants appear to be preoccupied with the goals of preserving and destroying themselves and each other. Meta-conflicts intensify, overshadowing the root conflict via incompatibility and contradiction. Galtung (2000) contended that a conflict develops an external character, vexing and waning, disappearing and reappearing. The original root of the conflict recedes into the background. Conflicts may combine, in series or parallel, into complex formations with many parties and many goals.

Typologies of Conflict

Coser (1956) cited in Anstey (2007) sees conflict as "a struggle over values and claims to scarce status, power and resources in which the aims of the opponents are to neutralise, injure or eliminate their rivals" (p. 5). A conflict involves two or more parties that perceive their goals and aims to be incompatible or perceive themselves as too different to coexist peacefully in meeting their unique needs through the redistribution of societal resources.

A distinction can be made between manifest and latent conflicts. Anstey (2007) argued that a latent conflict entails "conflict exists in a relationship when parties believe that their aspirations cannot be achieved simultaneously, or perceive a divergence in their values, needs or interests" (p. 6) whereas manifest conflict views that parties "purposefully employ their power in an effort to eliminate, defeat, neutralise, or change each other to protect or further their interests." A manifest conflict manifests itself in the use of force or violence leading to human casualties. Latent conflicts hide in societal cleavages, but have not broken into open confrontation. Analysts interested in conflict prevention tend to be especially concerned with these latent conflicts. Another distinction is between social cleavages involved in a conflict that are either vertical or horizontal. The former are based on ethnicity, race, or religion, whereas the latter are based on control of or access to economic resources (Hyden, 2006). Domestic political conflicts include a diverse amalgam of civil strife, ranging from protests, strikes, riots, plots, assassinations, coups d'état, to civil wars.

Social recognition needs are central to a peaceful society. By these needs, we mean a recognition of the needs of all groups residing within the society. In conceptualizing belonging needs, both Clark (1990) and Fisher (1990) highlight that central to a sustained peace is the right and need of recognition for different cultural–linguistic communities. He further argues that "individuals and social groups have undeniable needs and rights for dignity, respect, security and a 'place in the sun' in both physical and psychological terms – that is, identity, participation and adequate control over their own destiny" (pp. 93–4). Therefore, by placing identity needs central to conflict resolution, the politics of belonging and recognition come into play. This idea involves a delicate balancing act in an increasingly multicultural and diverse context, both globally and internally within states. In using this theory as central to conflict resolution, Clark (1990) outlines the following (see Table 14.1).

Approaches and Theories of Conflict

There are various theories and approaches to understanding conflict: micro and marco. Micro-theories consider conflict to arise from human aggression – whether learned or innate. Macro theories relate the causes of conflict to factors within society such as structures, institutions, and other relationships that constitute interaction and engagement in human society. These translate into two approaches to conflict: the psychological approach and the sociological approach.

Psychological Approach

The psychological approach to conflict is rooted in the assumption that conflict and aggression are innate to human behavior (Bradshaw, 2007). Table 14.2 shows the epistemology of conflict.

In the different psychological traditions, these theories are useful in understanding where aggression originates and how it can impact behavior in different scenarios. It fails, however, to provide an adequate explanation for protracted social conflict in Africa.

Table 14.1. Considerations and predictions in conflict resolution

Key considerations	Conflict resolution	Key questions	Predictions
Components of sacred meaning in various cultures and the manner in which they satisfy needs for people in a cultural–linguistic group. This will facilitate cross-cultural comparisons (including a variety of beliefs, rituals, and social institutions that provide sacred meaning and how to satisfy those needs.	Seek the means for evaluating sources of internal conflict	Which are due to social injustice? Which are due to a failure of compelling social norms? Which are due to ethnic divergence within a pluralistic society? Which have a long history of external interference?	Contrast the degree of social bondedness and sacred meaning that exist in Western societies with that of non-Western societies. Can assess the likely impact of, for example, economic failure, in order to assess the preserve of social bondedness to avert violent conflict and anarchy.
Need to determine the correlation between the apparent sufficiency of sacred meaning within various societies and their cultural homogeneity or disruption thereof.	Identify the potential for compromise; in other words, which issues will parties be willing to compromise on and which ones not?	What are the sacred remnants of social identity that will be clung to and will not be open to compromise? How are they perceived to be threatened?	We can assess the history of the conflict and how the historical context has shaped the current societal structure that may be conducive to the conflict.
Examine the artificial surrogates for social bondedness in different societies and determine how recognition and meaning needs are being "satisfied."	Determine what maintains or disrupts social cohesion and social bonding.	What processes of change will help most maintain social cohesion through the preservation of social bonding and sacred social meaning? When these were destroyed, what was the success in creating new social meanings?	Can determine the process of facilitating the creation of a new society based on common values and meanings in order to generate a sustainable peace where all groups are included and afforded some degree of recognition and belonging.

Sociological Approaches

Baaz (2005, pp. 1) states that

> there exists no society without conflicts; in each society there exists differences in circumstances, interests, and beliefs that can create friction between its members. Hence what differs [sic] a society from another is not the existence of conflicts but type of conflict, and how conflicts are dealt with.

Generally, sociological approaches to conflict concur that conflict is a natural phenomenon in any given society. Conflict drives processes of social change, but becomes negative when it becomes violent. The sociological approach views society from two main perspectives. The functionalist school argues that society must be understood in terms of its parts that constitute the whole, whereas conflict theorists argue that to understand society, one must conceptualize society as a struggle between groups (Anon, 2009; McMorrow-Hernandez, 2009; Vadelay, 2009). Functionalism looks at how social institutions facilitate change in society and how harmonious those institutions are, whereas conflict sociological approaches regard social change as a competition among different groups, classes, and cultural–linguistic communities. Group approaches regard social change as a result of different collectives, classes, and cultural-linguistic communities.

The primary differences between the psychological and sociological approaches to conflict are found in their unit of analysis. The psychological approaches focus on the person and seek the answer within the individual, whereas the sociological approach focuses on society and its makeup and seeks the answer from the manner in which society and its associated institutions are constructed. These theories are summarized in Table 14.3.

Most African conflicts cannot be reduced to a choice between psychological or sociological approaches, primarily because most contemporary conflicts are related to identity and distributive issues.

Burton's Human Needs Theory

All human beings and social groups seek recognition, and have the desire and need, to belong. Often, this desire and need to belong lead to social conformity of individuals and groups to prevalent social norms. If denied the need for recognition of culture, language, or existence, individuals and groups will *fight* to protect their identity and protect culture.

Ethnic conflict must be conceived as a process in which collective human needs and fears are acted out in powerful ways. Such conflict is typically driven by nonfulfillment or threats to the fulfillment of basic needs.

Table 14.2. Epistemological aspects in theories of conflict

Conflict theory	Theorist	Root of conflict	Reason for conflict
Biological/genetic explanations			
Ethology – We are born violent and aggressive	K. Lorenz	Aggression which is part of our genetic makeup	The aim of aggression is to win or control territory, increase solidarity between males and females, generate or preserve dominance, and natural selection through survival of the fittest
Psychotherapy approach to conflict	S. Freud and W. James	We are taught through biological, psychological, and social elements – aggression is part of our characters.	A destructive urge that when we redirect outward and not inward will lead to aggression and conflict
Sociobiology thesis	Fromm	The instinct to protect ourselves in dangerous circumstances and the will to survive through a process of natural selection	There is conflict because of the presence or collaboration of both aggression as instinct and aggression as learned.
Psychological/genetic explanations			
Frustration–aggression theory	Dollard	Frustration is the key to conflict – blocking the achievement of a goal	When a desired behavior is blocked, we will respond aggressively to remove the obstacle to what it is we want to do or achieve.
Alienation	Reich and Fromm	Social institutions tarnish human character in that we learn our characteristics from society	Societies are not static and change over time. This leads to unresolved conflicts within society and individuals. Exploitation of the individual and other outside factors triggers a conflict-filled personality with a predisposal to competition and violence. Society thus creates the consciousness.
Relative deprivation	Gurr	There are variances between expectations and the capacity to deliver on those expectations.	We experience the system as unfair, especially when we perceive to be disadvantaged. We have a sense of injustice when we compare ourselves to others. This frustration leads to conflict.

Constructed from Baaz (2005), Bradshaw (2007), Pruit (2006), and Rummel (1979).

Central needs include identity, security, recognition, autonomy, self-esteem, and a sense of justice (Kelman 2004, p. 60). Closely related to these central needs in intergroup conflict situations are fears about the denial of needs – focusing on perceived threats to security or identity. Needs for collective identity and security and the fears and concerns about survival associated with them, often are important causal factors in intergroup and intercommunal conflict (Kelman, 2004).

Needs theory and social institutions are linked on the basis of two primary themes: the need to belong or identity needs, and the need to maintain an acceptable standard of life necessary for survival or distributive needs. Indeed, if these two needs are not met, the potential for conflict increases, especially when needs deprivation is geared toward one community or cultural–linguistic group. In these cases, the opportunity for exploitation and manipulation by political leaders creates ethnic mobilization (Bloomfield & Reilly, 1998b, p. 9). In these scenarios, there is an extremely high potential for conflict because needs deprivation is linked to the group identity; and the cause of needs deprivation is linked to social institutions that discriminate against the group because of their cultural–linguistic origin. These areas of conflict are linked to economic factors such as financial hardships, unemployment, low wages, questions of culture (minority language-rights and religious freedoms), and territorial disputes (quests for self-determination, especially if there is a concentration of a cultural–linguistic community in a specific area) (Bloomfield, Ghai, & Reilly, 1998).

Cultural and ethnic claims to identity are not always negative; it is how identity needs and claims are channeled that will determine whether it is a destructive or constructive force. Fisher (1990) argues that assurances to group identity can lead to a sense of security necessary for sustainable peace. Indeed, diversity of culture, the right to different ways of life, and the right to tolerate

Table 14.3. Summary of theoretical issues in the genesis of conflict

Conflict theory	Theorist	Root of conflict	Reason for conflict
Economic/Structural theories			
Marxism	Karl Marx	The prevailing economic order and class system that determines access to scarce resources	Unequal and exploitative relationship between different classes in society causes conflict that will culminate with the replacement of the economic order with a more "suitable" one.
Resource competition theory	Coughlan and Samarasinghe Sumner	Group competition due to the distributive character of society	Increase in rivalry for scarce resources between different groups, whether gender groups, classes, or cultural–linguistic communities
Conflict sociology's primary assumptions			
Competition		Competition is the root of all conflict.	Conflict occurs because of a competition for scarce resources, without which survival will be minimal or quality of life will be negatively influenced.
Structural inequality		Domination	Power relationships are central to society. It is in the interest of those in power to maintain the current system and structure to ensure that they are able to enjoy the prestige, wealth, and power that they have.

Constructed from Anon. (n.d.), and Bradshaw (2007).

a different way of life informs many debates internally to a state. Knight (1982) notes that "ours is a cultural world ... But ours is also a political world..." (p. 514). Intrinsically the union between culture and politics is linked in that culture informs political life and vice versa. Morality and its associated analysis of right and wrong, good and evil, acceptable and unacceptable political and social behavior, equality, freedom, and sources of authority are influenced to a large extent by the cultural dimension. Therefore, societies must engage in behavior that can encompass a variety of claims to recognition and identity needs. It does not mean that all groups will necessarily agree with the perceived morality that other groups attach to various social and sacred rituals and meanings, but an acknowledgment that the right to culture and identity is necessary for sustainable peace.

THE PSYCHOLOGY OF CONFLICT

Conflicts do not start out violently; they gradually evolve to reach a violent climax. According to Draman (2003), typically a conflict evolves through five stages: pre-violence, escalation, endurance, de-escalation, and post-conflict.

Mitchell (1981) identified three factors that must be present for social conflict to exist: conflict situation, conflict attitudes, and conflict behavior. The conflict situation arises when parties perceive themselves to have incompatible goals (Tessendorf, 1991). Parties perceive certain resources as essential for survival or a sustainable future. They become frustrated at perceived actions that impede their efforts to gain access to those resources. Therefore, an element of frustration–aggression theory and human needs theory emerges. As the conflict continues to develop, a conflict attitude emerges as well.

Conflict attitudes are perceptions that each group holds of parties involved in the conflict. These include stereotypes, negative perceptions, and are characterized by mistrust and disdain. In addition, in-groups perceive themselves to be *better* than the other groups, who are increasingly painted in a negative light. Therefore, as the conflict escalates, "the opponents are classified according to intruder self-image which endorse the parties' right to act against those whom they perceive as 'aliens', or by purging dissendents from within their own group in terms of the 'traitor-in-our-midst' image" (Mitchell 1981, p. 101–2, cited in Tessendorf, 1991, p. 37). Indeed, as the conflict progresses, conflict attitudes will fuel perceptions of injustices (Tessendorf, 1991). The conflict attitude will determine how parties involved interpret and perceive each other's behavior and actions. As mistrust and contempt increase, they will interpret actions and behaviors of the out-group in an increasingly negative manner. Hence, one finds stronger in-group solidarity and cohesion geared toward unity and justice in achieving their goals and aims regardless of the cost. The conflict attitude provides the justification for actions taken in achieving the goals and aims of the different parties in the conflict. It is this *psychology of conflict* that is regarded as an exacerbating factor, arising through the stresses of being in a conflict, rather than being a prime cause of international disputes.

Conflict behaviors are actions taken by parties involved in the conflict geared toward realizing their goals. Tactics and strategies aim to obtain a more advantageous state of affairs for the parties (Mitchell, 1981, cited in Tessendorf, 1991). The use of tactics and strategies increases the

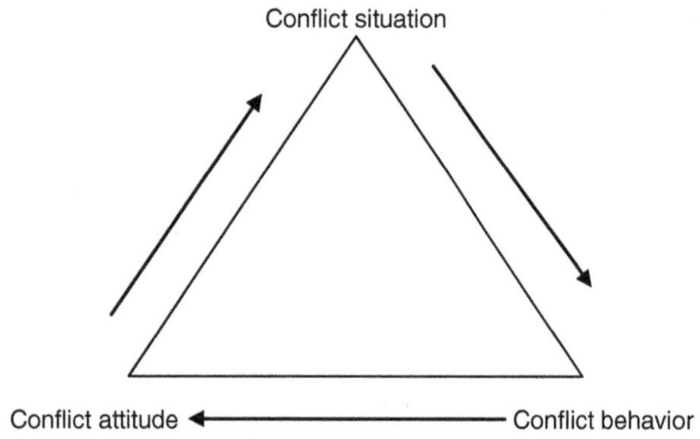

Figure 14.1. The cognitive elements of social conflict.

intensity of the conflict, and as the conflict progresses, parties lose sight of the original issue and the issues increase in number, further fueling the conflict.

Bloomfield and colleagues (1998) see social conflict as a triangle in that the conflict situation sets the stage, conflict behavior imprisons parties in cycle of action and reaction, and the conflict attitudes provide the psychological justifications for the conflict in that

> a belief that another group is less valuable than our own group, or that they are plotting our destruction, or that their own beliefs offend our moral code, or that they generally are a danger to us, will generate conflict between us and them. (Bloomfield, Ghai, & Reilly, 1998, p. 45)

The cognitive elements of social conflict are shown in Figure 14.1.

This process is reinforcing in that the actions taken by parties will reinforce the attitudes, perceptions, and stereotypes of other parties. Conflict behavior leads to the "injured" party feeling obliged to retaliate. This obligation, in turn, worsens the conflict situation in that, there is a massive increase in the issues that originally characterized the conflict. The consequences of a long-term violent conflict can be very devastating. Societies become militarized, violence becomes institutionalized and accepted, civilian casualties increase, rape and starvation become organized weapons of war, and noncombatants such as women and children bear the brunt of this dehumanizing process (Bloomfield & Reilly, 1998b). Consequently, "such communal trauma breeds deep and festering wounds and establishes heroes and martyrs on all sides whose memories and sacrifices serve to deepen the real and perceived divide between the conflicting identities" (Bloomfield & Reilly, 1998b, p. 11).

PEACE INTERRUPTED: AFRICA'S STRUGGLE TO END WAR

History of Research and Practice in Conflict Resolution

Successful conflict prevention has proven elusive. Research undertaken over 1945 to 1993 suggests that about half of all peace agreements fail in the first five years after they have been signed (Licklider, 1995). While the end of war can inaugurate a durable peace, the termination of one conflict often introduces a short interregnum until the outbreak of the next violent encounter. This reality has characterized many, if not all, of Africa's most brutal, violent, and protracted conflicts.

Often, conflict in Africa is embedded in highly complex *war networks* (or what can be described as a regional conflict complex), that straddle territorial boundaries, identity, and ethnic groups. The notion of purely civil or internal wars is no longer sustainable; most African wars are actually regional conflict formations, with added global connections and influences. Mary Kaldor (2006) refers to the emergence of "new wars," that is, a new type of organized violence that has developed, particularly on the African continent. Kaldor stresses that in most of the literature, these "new wars" are described as internal or civil wars or else as "low-intensity conflicts" (p. 2). Yet, although most of these wars are localized, they involve a myriad of transnational connections so that the distinction between internal and external, between aggression (attacks from abroad) and repression (attacks from inside the country), or even between local and global, are difficult to sustain (Kaldor, 2006, p. 3).

The purported aims of the protagonists in Africa's wars defy simple categorization. The multiplicity of participants translates into a multiplicity of objectives. While some groups may articulate genuine political grievances, or seek state power or self-determination, others pursue ethnonationalist or religious goals, such as ethnically or religiously pure political communities or the maintenance of elite power (Jackson, 2006). Simultaneously local actors may be engaged in struggles to gain access to critical resources, such as water, land, grazing rights, or security. In some instances, violence is transformed from instrument to objective, that is, from a means to an end, *to an end in itself*.

Another important characteristic of the so-called new wars as espoused by Kaldor (2006) is the changed mode of warfare – the means through which these new wars are fought. The strategies of the new warfare draw on the experience of both guerrilla warfare and counterinsurgency, yet they are quite distinctive. The new warfare borrows from counterinsurgency techniques of destabilization aimed at sowing "fear and hatred." This often involves population expulsion through various means such as mass killing and forcible resettlement, as well as a range of political, psychological, and economic techniques of intimidation (Kaldor, 2006).

The role of identity politics in Africa's wars form an important part of developing a greater understanding of the root causes of conflict and the driving factors that precipitate and exacerbate conflict (Jackson, 2006). There are a range of crucial variables in the construction of political conflict, such as the pervasive role played by elites as well as ethnic-local, national, political, military, and religious actors; the historical construction and maintenance

Discussion Box 14.1: War-child

The conflict in the Democratic Republic of the Congo (DRC) had resulted in what many analysts considered to be "Africa's First World War," embroiling the entire Great Lakes region in chaos, causing widespread instability, insurrection, violence, brutal conflict, the internal displacement of millions of innocent civilians and a staggering refugee crisis. The conflict has claimed nearly three million lives, and counting. It has been described as one of the most complex conflicts since the end of the Cold War.

As the conflict continues, the people most severely affected in the Democratic Republic of the Congo (DRC) are women and children. Children, especially, will lead their lives running from the conflict because of the possibility of kidnapping to serve as child-soldiers. Recruitment of children as soldiers into various armed groups is rampant in Masise in the Kivu region (Allen, 2006). Indeed, Allen conveys the story of Ndungutsa, recruited at age thirteen by militia. Ndungutsa witnessed the death of his brother who, refusing to join the militia, was shot. Ndungutsa was left with little choice as he did not want to die. This tragedy is not merely limited to boy-children, but girl-children are often abducted to become sex slaves and produce children. Some of the girls and boys are as young as ten years old. The DRC has one of the world's largest numbers of child soldiers. Allen notes that a third of the DR Congo's child soldiers will never be reintegrated back into their communities. In some cases because of the shame, in others, simply because their families can't afford to take them on. Also, there are the ever-present threats and intimidation. The ruthless exploitation of children by the leaders of armed forces to further their own material and political ends stands out as one of the most grotesque human rights abuses of this entire conflict (Amnesty International, 2003).

For further reading on child soldiers, please visit http://news.bbc.co.uk/2/hi/africa/5213996.stm.

For an eye-opening documentary visit YouTube and watch Children of Conflict – Congo Parts 1 and 2 at http://www.youtube.com/watch?v=kpd3ykS4QOQ.

Questions

1. Given the brutal history of the DRC, what are the likely impacts on society?
2. In your view, if this situation is not dealt with, what will be the most devastating impacts of the conflict on future generations?
3. What role do you think counselors can play in the healing process of the DRC?

of exclusive (and often antagonistic) identities by colonial and postcolonial ruling elites for the purposes of political and social control; the perceptions of insecurity between ethnic groups in situations of emergent anarchy or state failure; and the role of language, history, symbols and culture in fomenting interethnic rivalry (Jackson, 2006). In essence, it is argued that inflamed ethnic passions are the consequence of political conflict, not the cause. Dictators on the African continent fuel self-serving civil wars by arming ethnically based militias, propagating hate, fear, suspicion and damaging myths or stereotypes about political opponents.

The question is what makes ordinary people acquiesce to or participate in political violence directed against those with whom they once peacefully coexisted? The causes of war lie in the deliberate creation of a society-wide "conflict discourse" by political, military, and ethnic cultures (Jackson, 2006, p. 24). These self-interest groups monopolize politics, media, academia, religion, and popular culture, using them to reconstruct political and social discourses toward hatred, intergroup conflict, and ultimately war. The main features of these discourses include identity construction and the creation of an "other"; creating or drawing upon a discourse of victimhood and grievance; creating a discourse of imminent threat and danger to the political community; and overcoming social and cultural inhibitions and norms that prohibit interpersonal violence.

Influence of Culture

The Burundi conflict is an interesting case study on the role of culture in a conflict. Burundi can be classified as a real nation-state where social groups such as the Banganwa, Bahutu, Batutsi, and Bastwa occupy the same territory, speak Kirundi, share the same culture and the same socio-political organisation of the kind, the *Mwami* (Ntahombaye & Nduwayo, 2007).

This shared sense of identity rooted a shared identity for Burundians under the royal authority of the Mwami, thus creating a monarchical state. The traditional structure was regarded as an administrative structure represented as in Figure 14.2.

The traditional structure facilitated social cohesion and a collective identity and allowed each group to play a role. Much research conducted around the causes of the Burundian conflict highlight a multidimensional nature in that "... ideological, socio-cultural (degradation of

Discussion Box 14.2: The Rwandan Conflict

In the early 1990s, when the ruling Hutu clique faced growing political opposition, they sought to maintain their hold on power by rousing Hutu against an imminent Tutsi threat, fomenting a climate of fear and hatred. Ethnic antagonism had become a lethal weapon to inflict mass slaughter on a scale that had not been witnessed since the holocaust. Of grave concern was that ample evidence of the imminent disaster had presented itself. In a joint report released in December 1990, European ambassadors warned that "the rapid deterioration of the relations between the two ethnic groups, the Hutu and the Tutsi, runs the imminent risk of terrible consequences for Rwanda and the entire region" (Meredith, 2005, p. 495). Great effort had been expended to identify "the enemy." An army memorandum released in 1992 divided the enemy into two categories: the principal enemy – the Tutsi, extremist and nostalgic for power who have never recognized and will never recognize the realities of the 1959 social revolution, seeking to retain power by all means necessary, and the accomplices of the enemy – anyone who supported the principal enemy, namely the groups within which the enemy were said to recruit, including Tutsi refugees, Tutsis inside the country, and Hutu malcontents (Meredith, 2005). The central purpose of the propaganda had been to stir up fears that the Tutsi, to regain power, were prepared to slaughter Hutu en masse.

In April 1994, the downing of the aeroplane carrying Rwandan President Habyarimana (a Hutu) by unknown insurgents triggered a destructive and brutal genocide on a scale unseen since the Second World War. In a few short months, the Rwandan Army and Interahamwe militiamen had massacred more than 800,000 Tutsis and moderate Hutus. In response, Tutsi rebels, who had formed the Rwandan Patriotic Front (RPF), succeeded in overthrowing the (majority) Hutu regime in Kigali. More than 2 million Hutus, all of them fearing revenge killings and some of them participants in the genocide, fled to eastern Zaire, where many joined forces with the Interehamwe who had based themselves there (Swart & Solomon, 2004). The genocidaires were intent not only on retaking Rwanda. They set out to exterminate Tutsi groups living in Zaire.

Questions

1. Identify the conflict situation, attitude, and behavior that fueled the Rwandan conflict.
2. The Rwandan conflict escalated to a point of genocide. Track the escalation of the conflict by focusing on the issues that fueled the conflict.

As a counselor, what are your suggestions on the issues that need to be addressed to build a sustainable peace in Rwanda?

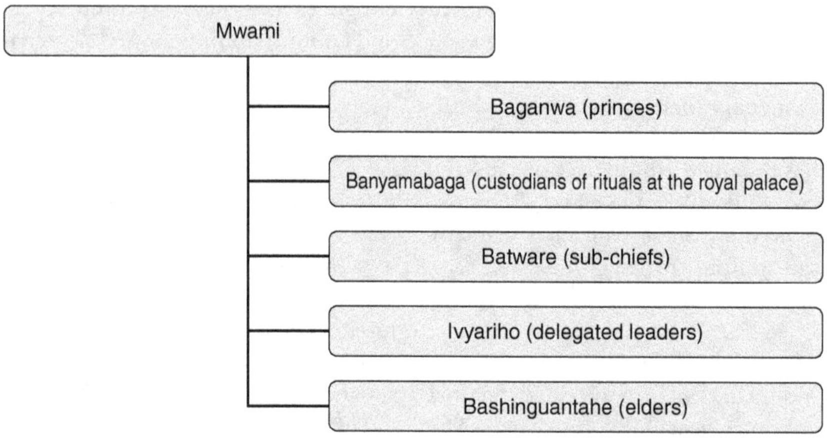

Figure 14.2. Burundi cultural–structural authority complex.

values), psychological (suspicion, fear), political (fight for power), and economic (unequal access to economic and social opportunities with regard to education, employment and health)" (Ntahombaye & Nduwayo, 2007). In Burundi, group identity essentially translates into one cultural–linguistic group, and the ethnic dimension to the Burundian conflict is difficult to understand. Colonial powers effectively divided a united territory by manipulating and creating ethnic groups on the basis of the racist ideologies that informed the divide and rule strategies of the colonial powers. Therefore, ethnicity was created in the minds of the people (Ntahombaye

& Nduwayo, 2007). At independence, many of these structures, perceptions, and attitudes remained. The colonial master–servant relationships remained and fueled conflict. Linked to these perceived divisions were access to scarce resources and benefits, which was not rooted in individual behavior, but linked to group identity. For that reason the Burundian conflict and the identities that fueled it is locked in "...economic interests and political strategies..." (Ntahombaye & Nduwayo, 2007, p. 249). Fear and reciprocal hatred were manifested through the perceived competition for power, and accordingly, then resources.

Political Leadership and the Predatory State

The African continent has given birth to the *Presidents-for-life* phenomenon. Amendments to the constitutions of states such as Nigeria, Namibia, and Zimbabwe allow presidents to leave office only once they have died. In many of the conflicts that plague the African continent, the state and its leadership has often become what is known as a predatory state: a state that exploits its people for the enrichment and benefits of political leaders and their allies.

Many African presidents, upon taking power, come from the liberation movement that had brought independence and freedom to the people and foster a perception that they are consequently entitled to power. Often corrupt and predatory regimes characterize these presidencies and conflict becomes rooted in ethnic mobilization and a glorification of the role they had played in bringing liberation to the people. At independence, a culture of political authoritarianism, coupled with a weak foundation of democracy and economic development, facilitated the entrenchment of political power into the presidency, fueling a political space of contestation, with more often than not violent interaction and oppression (Southall, Simutanyi, & Daniel, 2006). Indeed, Murithi (2006, p. 9) notes that

> if we are looking for reasons why these conflicts have plagued the African continent, we do not need to look further than the leadership of these countries. Competing self-interested political and military elites have made use of the divisions and legacies of colonialism and the illegitimate nature of the post-colonial African state to exacerbate tension and fuel conflict.

The most contemporary example is Mugabe's regime in Zimbabwe. A conflict in making since the early 2000s, it is only when Mugabe staged his one-man election in 2008 that the rest of the African continent finally condemned his behavior. With an economy that has virtually collapsed, and increased Western condemnation for his regime, Mugabe still manages to garner sufficient support for his regime among some of his African allies and economic and political elites within Zimbabwe. Capitalizing on liberation rhetoric and the brutal colonial history of the Smith regime, Mugabe played on the emotions of the people with specific reference to access to land. The sunset clauses of the Lancaster Agreement had effectively centralized commercial farming land in the hands of White farmers for approximately ten years. Sensing discontent among the people that could have threatened his position, Mugabe embarked on a radical policy of land grab that saw the eviction of farmers for redistribution of their land to the indigenous people of Zimbabwe. This radical move, condemned by the Western world, but silently supported by Mugabe's African contemporaries, saw the start of economic and political turmoil in Zimbabwe.

As the conflict progressed from forced land evictions to increased brutality against any form of opposition to the Mugabe regime, the African political leaders remained hauntingly silent. Partly, this silence is because of a bond rooted in a *brotherhood of arms* wherein African leaders assisted one another during their liberation struggles, the most notable ally being Thabo Mbeki. Nkrumah had poetically stated: *Own first the political kingdom and all other benefits will come unto you*. Public coffers had become a means for political elites and their allies to enrich themselves at the cost of human and economic development, effectively facilitating further violent competition for access to state power and its associated benefits. Many presidents had died in office, and it will not be surprising that Mugabe may very well join the ranks of the former presidents-for-life.

Current Practices in Conflict Resolution Counseling

Orthodox analyses of Africa's wars have been capable of providing only limited understandings of their causes and characteristics. Moreover as Jackson (2006) stresses that the failure of effective conflict analysis has too often resulted in remedial bankruptcy: misconceiving the deeper causes of Africa's wars. Practitioners have repeatedly applied unsuitable or ultimately damaging solutions to conflict settlements. The conceptual failure of conflict analysis has presaged the normative failure of conflict resolution. The true nature of Africa's wars suggests that conflict management has become wholly insufficient as a durable solution to endemic violence. What is required is the prioritization of preventive and transformative approaches to conflict resolution. The analysis of and resolution of conflict is impossible without a wide-ranging, or interdisciplinary, framework, making use of the insights provided by other social sciences.

Creating an African Peace

A fundamental problem, however, for parties employing coercive or persuasive strategies in a conflict is when to "make peace." While most studies on peaceful settlement of disputes see the substance of the proposals for a solution as the key to a successful resolution of conflict, a growing focus of attention, according to Zartman (2000), shows that a second and equally necessary key lies in the timing of efforts for resolution. Parties resolve their conflicts only when they are ready to do so – when alternative, usually unilateral means of achieving a satisfactory result are blocked and the parties feel that they are in an uncomfortable and costly stalemate (Zartman, 2000). The Constitution of UNESCO (1946) states in part that

> since wars begin in the minds of men, it is in the minds of men that the defences of peace must be constructed;.... And that a peace based exclusively upon the political and economic arrangements of governments would not be a peace which could secure the unanimous, lasting and sincere support of the peoples of the world...

The document further suggests that ignorance, misunderstanding, misperception, and mistrust lie at the roots of problems that arise among nations and through which their differences have all too often broken into war. The need to assess how conflict attitudes fuel and affect conflicts in the African context is crucial, as this appears to be an often overlooked dynamic in conflict resolution theory when addressing conflict situations on the continent, with frequent regression into all-out war.

Negative peace – absence of war – is invariably unsustainable and underpins the baleful statistic that half of Africa's wars have reignited within a decade of ending. Yet the construction of a positive peace that addresses the multifarious motivations of the combatants and addresses their residual mutual suspicion is a challenge that lies beyond existing economic and political capacity (Furley & May, 2006). The "psychology of conflict" is regarded as an exacerbating factor, arising through the stresses of being in a conflict, rather than being a prime cause of international disputes.

Restorative Justice and Traditional Approaches to Peace-making

Any form of sustainable peace in Africa is dependent upon Africans owning the peace-making process. These can range from traditional mechanisms of conflict resolution to institutions and processes of restorative justice. Indeed,

> traditional conflict resolution structures are closely bound with socio-political and economic realities of the lifestyles of African communities. These conflict resolution structures are rooted in the culture and history of African people, and are in one way or another unique to each community (Phalya, Adan, & Masinde, 2004, p. v).

For that reason Hagg and Kagwanja (2007) argue that intrastate conflicts based on identity politics requires a reconfiguration of existing conflict resolution mechanism and techniques where we need to reconceptualize identities as the building blocks for sustainable peace while incorporating traditional conflict resolution mechanisms. What is striking about incorporating traditional structures to conflict resolution is the increased legitimacy indigenous conflict resolution structures enjoy among these communities (Phalya, Adan, & Masinde, 2004).

Indigenous Approaches

An indigenous conflict resolution mechanism is one system that can aid in achieving sustainable peace in Africa. Hagman (2007) states that "in many African societies, elders play a crucial role in managing public affairs in their community, both with and in the absence of formal state recognition" (p. 31). In this sense, the elders are charged with the overall well-being of communities, including the social, political, economic, cultural, and spiritual welfare of the people (Hagman, 2007). Many conflict societies in Africa are characterized by the state institutions effectively losing control of a given part of their territory. In these instances, traditional authorities, customs, and practices fill the void of managing conflict instead of the state. This is contradictory to Western practices, which regard traditional authority as undemocratic owing to the hereditary nature of the institution. In addition, traditional Western mechanisms of conflict resolution may be completely inappropriate for conflict resolution in an African context in that the focus is on a reconciliatory environment as opposed to the Western models that tend to alienate and confuse (Choudree, 1999).

The context of Africa and its political life is very different from the Western experience. Choudree (1999) highlights Western and African approaches to conflict resolution (Table 14.4).

Although traditional authority structures were manipulated by the colonial powers, it is often the only *more* legitimate institution able to generate authority within a given community. However, Murithi (2006) warns that we need to guard against glorifying indigenous approaches as these approaches are generally exclusive, effectively excluding people based on gender. Given that women and children are the worst affected by conflict and at most times are central in community initiatives, the challenge is to find a balance between traditional conflict resolution strategies that incorporate all parties involved in the conflict.

In constructing peace, Murithi (2006) highlights the centrality of social solidarity as "... peace is not just the absence of violence, but the presence of social solidarity" (p. 13). Constructing social solidarity entails restoring the "humanness" of groups involved in the conflict so that parties in the conflict must start to focus on the common welfare of each other (Murithi, 2006). In this sense, *Ubuntu* plays a central role in constructing peace and social solidarity in that *Ubuntu* is considered as the essence of humanity. *Ubuntu* entails a world view that *I am because you are* or a person is a person through other people (Murithi, 2006). The concept of *Ubuntu* becomes central in constructing a sustainable peace in that "...the lessons for peace building ... is that by adopting and internalizing the principles of *ubuntu*, we can contribute toward creating healthy relationships based on recognition that within the web of humanity everyone is linked to everyone else" (Murithi, 2006, p. 17).

Table 14.4. Approaches to conflict resolution

	African approach to conflict resolution	Western approach to conflict resolution
Type of interaction	Face-to-face and community approach	Individual approach with third party involvement
Type of justice that underpins approach to conflict resolution	Coexistential justice	Contentious justice
Approach to the nature of the post-conflict relationship	Mending the relationship	Terminating the relationship
Dispute settlement by courts	Tendency to mediate and arbitrate	Tendency to adjudicate
Preference	Reconciliation	Impartial application of the rules
Type of environment	Informal and less intimidating	Foreboding and formal
Judge	Chief who is generally charismatic and familiar with the populace	Impartial and generally unknown to the parties involved
Role played by "judge"	Active and suggests mediation at almost any point	Inactive and does not become involved in the proceedings through making suggestions and mirrored in procedures and processes
Emphasis	Group relationships and rights	Individuals and individual rights

This is relevant when dealing with issues around transitional or restorative justice. By adopting and internalizing *Ubuntu*, principles of forgiveness and reconciliation create positive strategies for peace-building (Murithi, 2006). Any state emerging from a conflict will require a process of healing where victims are able to claim some form of justice. There are various institutions and processes that states may wish to follow. South Africa embarked on a process of healing through storytelling by adopting the Truth and Reconciliation Commission wherein public discourse was characterized by admitting to the crimes of Apartheid and seeking forgiveness. The Rwandan experience preferred traditional courts known as the Gacaca Tribunals. Osman (2006) highlights that

> The Rwandan genocide of 1994 heightened the need for justice for its victims. It signified the depth that human cruelty can descend towards the destruction of fellow humans. The act of genocide usually results from coordinated efforts perpetrated by its executors. These perpetrators were under the leadership of individuals from political, economic, and religious arena who used their power to persuade and mobilize the general public. The perishing of a million people in 100 days signifies the existence of well organized and meticulous planning and execution. With the end of the genocide came the need for justice for its victims of these atrocities (p. 1).

Any conflict society has demands for justice that must be dealt with. In executing their process of healing and restorative justice, the Rwandan case followed two approaches: the first approach, the United Nations tribunals in Arusha, saw the persecution of leaders who instigated the genocide, and the second approach, the GACACA, incorporated elements of the local traditional justice system (Osman, 2006). In this sense, the Rwandan experience married Western and traditional approaches in search of a sustainable peace through healing and restorative justice.

Any negotiated settlement that seeks to end violent and protracted conflict will need to incorporate elements of restorative justice to secure validity among the people and the elites. The process of restorative justice, however, must remain the decision of the communities and states involved. No outside, Western influence can dictate which approaches to healing and justice conflict states must undertake; Africa needs its own peace-making and healing processes in resolving its conflict. Reconstructing a nation and society, after a violent conflict, is a long process, and it is the responsibility of all stakeholders to be involved in that process. Restorative justice is merely one element of reconstructing the state, society, and the nation. An element of learning to live, work, and play together becomes central to a sustainable peace in that the stereotypes that fueled the conflict needs to be broken down. Ntahombaye and Nduwayo (2007) identify political and sociocultural initiatives that must be undertaken in searching for a sustainable peace as follows: these are "... advocacy on citizenry, participation in the culture of democracy, memory restitution through history, and depolitisation and demystification of ethnicity" (p. 240). Initiatives that these include are

> deepening dialogue and negotiation at all levels, rehabilitating the social and cultural values and customs likely to enhance social cohesion and peace ... incorporating peaceful conflict resolution mechanisms and human rights into the education system, designing an integrated national reconciliation programmes, providing support to the cultural organisations which promote peace and human rights, and advocating for media involvement in the above initiatives.

Social–Psychological Approaches

The social–psychological study of conflict is characterized not so much by the nature of the conflicting units it

Research Box 14.1: Religion and Conflict

Svensson, I. (2007). Fighting with Faith: Religion and conflict resolution in civil wars. *Journal of Conflict Resolution*, *51*, 930–49.

Objective: Svensson attempted to prove that the intrastate religious conflicts are more intractable and consequently difficult to settle than other forms of conflict. His objective was to explain why religious intrastate religious conflicts are perceived as more protracted than other forms of conflict and demonstrate the indivisible nature of religious armed conflict. The premise of the study was the state is the primary resource in civil conflicts, and when conflicting religious positions regarding the state emerge, the subjective value of the conflict increases. Once religion and subjective values increase, a perception that there is no alternative to the state emerges.

Method: The study was conducted on a dyadic level in which two measures of religious dimensions of armed conflicts were used. The researchers first measured whether religious identities are present in the combatants, and second, collected data on explicit demands that include religious dimensions in the conflict. The study included all armed conflicts from 1989 to 2003 using a probe analysis, an assessment of the likelihood that parties will sign a peace agreement, and manage incompatibility for a minimum of one year. The study examined religious incompatibility, religious dissimilarity, and civil war termination factors (which include territory, ethnicity, duration, and mediation).

Results: The study found that negotiated settlements are less likely if conflicts are fought with parties where at least one side has made explicit religious demands. Also, the study found that third-party involvement through mediation and guarantees is an important explanatory factor for negotiated settlements in armed conflicts. Conflicts with religious rather than territorial dimensions are least likely to result in agreed settlements.

Conclusions: The research produced four implications:

1. Religious aspects of armed conflicts are pivotal when negotiators need to gauge for peace.
2. Multifaith dialogue may not be the most important priority when seeking ways to reduce armed conflict. The assumption that religious dissimilarity further protracts a conflict is not necessarily correct.
3. Measures aiming to prevent conflict actors from expanding their demands into religious realms should be emphasized and developed.

Questions

1. Given the results of the research, what should future research priorities be?
2. Why may multifaith dialogue not be necessarily the most appropriate form of conflict resolution in religious conflicts? What should the focus be on?
3. Relate the research findings to the conflict in Darfur. Does the Darfur conflict support Svensson's findings?

studies as by its approach to conflict. This approach is distinguished by its focus on the interplay between psychological and social processes. It is concerned with the perceptions, beliefs, and values of the conflicting units as well as their actualities; these may or may not correspond. It is concerned with how the social realities of the parties in conflict affect their perceived and experienced realities and how the psychological realities of the conflicting parties affect the development of their social realities (Deutsch & Shichman, 1986).

The social–psychological perspective on conflict highlights the possibility of discrepancy between the objective and the perceived state of affairs. Recognition of this possibility suggests a typology of conflicts that emphasizes the relationship between the two. Such an emphasis leads to specification of the types of distortion that can occur, including the non-recognition of real conflicts of interest as well as their displacement and misattribution (Deutsch & Shichman, 1986). Under certain conditions a large conflict may seem so potentially dangerous that it exerts a strong pressure to reach agreement. To reduce the size and intensity of conflict, one may diminish the perceived opposition between the parties in values and interests through emphasizing common superordinate goals and through the techniques of controlled communication (Deutsch & Shichman, 1986). These techniques essentially assume that perceived opposition can be reduced if the conflicting parties can be led to see how much they have in common, if their differences can be seen in the context of their similarities and agreements. Commonly, they assume that perceived differences will decrease if misunderstandings are eliminated through improved, open, full, and direct communication between the parties. Sometimes, however, the removal of misunderstanding sharpens the awareness of conflicting interests or beliefs, an awareness that had been beclouded by benevolent misunderstandings (Deutsch & Shichman, 1986).

Understanding the Psychology of Conflict

Psychology plays two related but different roles in conflict resolution. Psychological factors influence what states or their leaders believe is important. In other words, during substantive negotiations psychology plays a decisive role in determining the objectives of the sides. An understanding of the other parties' perceptions and outlook can provide valuable insight into how to approach negotiations. Furthermore, nations, like individuals, possess their own characteristics, patterns of behavior, and historical context that in essence shapes the psyche of a nation. Therefore, states are inclined to react based on these inherent beliefs and perceptions that may or may not have been shaped by past experiences that were traumatic, caused trauma, fear, or considerable suspicion and enmity. Thus, what might seem to an outsider as a rational compromise that protects both sides' vital interests may well be perceived differently by the parties themselves (Seldowitz, 2004).

Psychologists and diplomats adopt a vastly different approach to abnormal behavior. The primary task of the diplomat in this respect is to ascertain whether the abnormal behavior is the product of a particular leader or reflects ideas shared by a large segment of the population (Seldowitz, 2004). When discussing the concept of conflict, perception should be included as a central concept because the conflicts and the opponent's intentions often are defined according to subjective perceptions. There could be an abundance of space for agreement in a conflict, but if the parties perceive the conflict as impossible to resolve or the opponent to be untrustworthy this might not help in resolving the conflict (Swanström & Weissman, 2005).

High-intensity social conflicts are of particular importance, wherein disputes have a tendency to expand and escalate so that they become independent of their initiating causes. A number of key elements include an anarchic social situation; a competitive orientation; internal conflicts that express themselves through external conflicts; and cognitive rigidity, misjudgments, and misperceptions that lead to distorted views that may perpetuate conflict (Crocker, Hampson, & Aall, 1999). Additionally, there may be unwitting commitments, whereby parties become overcommitted to rigid positions and committed unwittingly to the beliefs, defenses, and investments involved in carrying out their conflictual activities; self-fulfilling prophecies; vicious escalating spirals; and gamesmanship orientation, which turns the conflict away from issues of what in real life is being won or lost to an abstract conflict over images of power (Crocker, Hampson, & Aall, 1999).

The social–psychological approach to mediation centers on providing a forum in which parties can explore options and develop solutions, often outside the highly charged arena of a formal negotiating structure. The approach involves appeals to superordinate goals and values. It plays on the parties' aspirations for legitimacy and their desire to be part of the broader political community. In this approach, the use of moral suasion and symbolic rewards or gestures is important. To this school, the establishment of a dialogue, of a pattern of exchanges and contacts between and among official parties or other influential representatives, helps set the stage for a lasting peace built on an agreement developed by the parties in a collaborative process.

One of the driving assumptions behind the social–psychological approach is that although parties identify specific issues as the causes of conflict, conflict reflects subjective, phenomenological, and social fractures, and, consequently, analyzing "interests" can be less important than identifying the underlying needs that govern each party's perception of the conflict (Crocker et al., 1999). Because much of human conflict is anchored in conflicting perceptions and in misperception, the contribution of third parties lies in changing the perceptions, attitudes, values, and behaviors of the parties to a conflict.

Social–psychological approaches stress the importance of changing attitudes and the creation of new norms in moving parties toward reconciliation. Early intervention, according to this formulation, is preferable because once relations have deteriorated because of violence, and attitudes are embedded in "we–they" images of the enemy, it becomes much more difficult for mediators to move the parties toward sober reflection about their real-world choices and to change perceptions (Crocker et al., 1999).

It is clear that as the level of violence rises, the number of potential entry points in a conflict situation declines as perceptions and attitudes are hardening. The barriers to entry are increasing as parties perceive increasing risks of negotiation, coupled with status and legitimacy concerns. As a situation of high levels of violence transpires, the number of potential entry points into a conflict situation is even less, as "we–they" images of the enemy have hardened. Furthermore, the barriers to entry are high as parties are locked into a continuing struggle. Therefore, although a peace agreement has been formally signed, the underlying issues that led to conflict in the first place, as well as the accompanying tensions and suspicions and deeply entrenched hatreds and enmity amongst parties, may continue to persist.

There are few traditionally Western approaches that address the issue of dealing with the psychological origins of conflict and the "embedded enemy images" that are a serious obstacle to managing conflict and reducing tensions. Practitioners arguing for a greater consideration of psychological aspects argue that peace-building is about changing attitudes and that attitudinal change requires a change in the procedures, roles, and structures of the disputing parties, including the development of institutional capacity at the local or communal level for dealing with conflict (Hampson, 2001). Attitudinal change can be fostered through special problem-solving workshops and third-party assistance in developing and designing other kinds of dispute resolution systems that are compatible with local culture and norms and are directed at elites at different levels (top, middle range, and grassroots) in society.

The problem-solving workshop pioneered by John Burton and Herbert Kelman is based on the assumption that conflict is a subjective, phenomenological, and social process. It takes issue with the ripeness thesis about hurting stalemates on the grounds that, because conflict is essentially a matter of perceptions, third parties have to work on changing the perceptions, attitudes, values, and behaviors of the parties to a conflict. Ripeness, in other words, does not emerge automatically. It has to be cultivated with the assistance of third parties who help the parties involved to reach a better understanding of the conflict's dimensions and the joint strategies required for a mutually acceptable solution (Hampson, 2001, p. 396). The problem-solving workshop attempts to change the process of interaction among conflicting parties. Problem-solving seeks to open channels of communication between the parties, allowing both sides to see their respective intensions more clearly and to be more aware of their own reactions to the conflict.

LEGAL AND PROFESSIONAL ISSUES

The search for a sustainable peace is still an ongoing endeavor in Africa. Central to the African Union is the generation of sustainable and lasting peace. There have been various conventions and resolutions such as the United Nations Peace Building Commission and the African Union Post-Conflict Reconstruction and Development Policy Framework. These conventions seek to facilitate the creation of a sustainable peace through donor and foreign aid, stand-by forces, and the establishment of headquarters to observe peace-building efforts.

The Darfur conflict has demonstrated the limited scope of the sustainability of attempts to generate lasting peace of the African Union and the United Nations. There is a lack of buy-in from the role players in the conflict, as evident in the ceasefire violations that have occurred. Also, in attempting to settle the conflict, the International Criminal Court (ICC) warrant for arrest further increased the stakes of the conflict as the perception of persecution dictates. Issues surrounding state sovereignty emerge. The challenge for sustainable peace remains rooted on three pillars: inclusivity of all role players in generating an acceptable, and not perfect, peace-building solution, stronger action against violations of ceasefire and other agreements, and clarity on the role of international peacekeeping forces, and the ICC. Therefore, the challenge remains a fine balance among punitive measures, humanitarian interests, and not alienating the role players in the conflict.

Other obstacles to sustainable peace-building relate to financial and human resources. Many African economies are weak and unable to bear the cost of peace-building missions and initiative. The result is that some richer states like South Africa carry most of the cost associated with peace-building efforts. Increased international aid and assistance for peace-building becomes essential as a lack of resources will invariable lead to a lack of sustainable peace.

Conflict resolution and mediation is a sensitive process that must be done, at least in some part, in secret. This secrecy is essential so that perceptions of failing constituents do not obstruct peace-building efforts through negotiation. Many former African leaders such as Nelson Mandela and Thabo Mbeki have consolidated their roles as mediators of conflicts on the African continent, to some extent as the result of the successful negotiations ending the South African conflict. However, no negotiation can take place without the assistance of a team able to identify the root causes of the conflict, as well as the dynamics of the state. Therefore, sustainable peace-building requires an interdisciplinary approach to conflict resolution wherein a team and not an individual is able to drive the search for a sustainable peace.

ISSUES FOR RESEARCH AND OTHER FORMS OF SCHOLARSHIP

Peace-building, in an African context, requires a multi- and interdisciplinary approach. Scholarship must attempt to generate sufficient academic collaboration among, for example, political scientists, sociologists, anthropologists, and psychologists in generating knowledge for sustainable peace. No peace agreement can attempt to claim sustainability if a holistic approach is not undertaken. Similarly, no post-conflict society can be rebuilt without an interdisciplinary approach to a sustainable peace.

This approach must focus on the generation of social cohesion sufficient to generate some sense of national solidarity that can facilitate the generation of a national identity. South Africa, for example, has embraced a diversity of unity identity, and the United States an approach of solidarity as *a big melting pot*. Whichever approach a post-conflict society decides upon, central to it is the generation of national solidarity. If divisions and exclusion persist in a post-conflict society, the search for a sustainable peace will remain elusive.

SUMMARY AND CONCLUSION

Very little research has been conducted on how psychological variables, particularly conflict attitudes such as negative images, attitudes, perceptions, and conflict behavior, can fuel and exacerbate a conflict situation, especially conflicts in Africa, and how this may derail the success of preventive diplomacy in resolving such severe conflicts. Tetlock and Goldgeier (2000) argue that any approach that fails to consider psychological factors is incomprehensive. Psychological research focuses on the role of cognitive factors, individual and cultural characteristics, and motivational factors affecting judgments, actual negotiation behaviors, and outcomes of negotiations. The need to incorporate psychological negotiation research as a salient tool to provide for a more coherent understanding of diplomatic negotiations aimed at ending conflict is crucial to design peace agreements that are durable.

In creating a sustainable peace in Africa, it becomes essential to take into consideration the pscychology of conflict and the incorporation of an understanding of identity and recognition rights. In addition to the pscychological aspects, there is a need to incorporate traditional conflict resolution mechanisms and approaches to conflict resolution strategies and engagements. As war starts in the *minds of men*, constructing peace must commence with a process that is known and respected by the people. Owning the peace process will generate commitment to its implementation and it is this sense of ownership that will facilitate a positive, cooperative, and sustainable peace.

REFERENCES

Allen, K. (2006). Bleak future for Congo's children. Retrieved May 16, 2009 from online at http://news.bbc.co.uk/2/hi/africa/5213996.stm.

Amnesty International. (2003). Democratic Republic of the Congo: Children at war. Retrieved May 16, 2009 from http://www.amnesty.org/en/library/info/AFR62/034/2003.

Anon. (n.d.). Sociological perspective. Retrieved May 14, 2009 from http://www.public.asu.edu/~zeyno217/301/socprspctvs.htm

Anon. (2009). The conflict perspective. Retrieved May 14, 2009 from http://socialsciences.cypresscollege.edu/~rrhymes/pdf/socialtheories.pdf

Anstey, M. (2007). *Managing change: Negotiating conflict*. Cape Town: Juta & Co.

Azar, E. (1990). *The management of protracted social conflict*. Hanover, NH: Darmouth.

Baaz, M. (2005). Conflict theory. Retrieved May 15, 2009 from http://www.mah.se/upload/IMER/kurser/Peace%20and%20Conflict%20Studies/conflict%theory/202.ppt.

Bloomfield, D., & G. Reilly. (1998a). Overview. In G. Reilly & P. Harris (Eds.), *Democracy and deep rooted conflict: Options for negotiators* (pp. 2–6). Stockholm: IDEA.

Bloomfield, D., & Reilly, G. (1998b). The changing nature of conflict and conflict management. In G. Reilly & P. Harris (Eds.), Reilly, *Democracy and deep rooted conflict: Options for negotiators* (pp. 7–28). Stockholm: IDEA.

Bloomfield, D., Ghai, Y., & Reilly, G. (1998). Analysing deep-rooted conflict. In G. Reilly & P. Harris (eds)., *Democracy and deep rooted conflict: Options for negotiators* (pp. 29–36). Stockholm: IDEA.

Bradshaw, G. (2007). *Conflict management for South African students: Theory and application*. Port Elizabeth: Peacemakers Conflict Management Services.

Choudree, R. (1999). Traditions of conflict resolution in South Africa. *Journal of Conflict Resolution*, *1*(11), 9–27.

Clark, M. (1990). Meaningful social bonding as a human need. In J. Burton (Ed.), *Conflict: Human needs theory* (pp. 34–59). London: Macmillan.

Coser, L. (1956). *The functions of social conflict*. London: Routledge and Kegan Paul.

Crocker, C., Hampson, F., & Aall, P. (1999). *Herding cats: Multiparty mediation in a complex world*. Washington, DC: United States Institute of Peace Press.

Deutch, M., & Shichman, S. (1986). Conflict: A social psychological perspective. In G. Hermann (Ed.), *Political psychology: Contemporary problems and issues*. London: Jossey-Bass.

Draman, R. (2003). Conflict prevention in Africa: Establishing conditions and institutions conducive to durable peace. In D. Carment & A. Schnable (Eds.), *Conflict prevention: Path to peace or grand illusion?* (p. 234). Toyko and New York: United Nations University Press.

Fisher, R. (1990). Needs theory, social identity and conflict. In J. Burton (Ed.), *Conflict: Human needs theory* (pp. 89–111). London: Macmillan.

Furley, O., & R. May (2006). Introduction. In O. Furley &. R. May (Eds.), *Ending Africa's wars: Peace and conflict, development and civilisation*. London: SAGE Publications.

Galtung, F. (2000). *Conflict transformation by peaceful means: The Transcend method*. New York: Transcend (A peace and development network and United Nations Disaster Management Training Programme).

Hagg, G., & Kagwanja, P. (2007). Identity and peace: Reconfiguring conflict resolution in Africa. *African Journal of Conflict Resolution*, *7*(2), 9–35.

Haggman, T. (2007). Bringing the Sultan back in: Elders as peacemakers in Ethopia's Somali region. In L. Buur & M. Kyed (Eds.), *State recognition and democratization in sub-Saharan Africa: A new dawn for traditional authorities?* London: Palgrave: Macmillan.

Hampson, F. (2001). Parent, midwife, or accidental executor? The role of third parties in ending violent conflict. In C. Crocker, F. Hampson, & P. Aall (Eds.), *Turbulent peace: The challenges of managing international conflict*. Washington, DC: United States Institute of Peace Press.

Hyden, F. (2006). *African politics in comparative perspective*. New York: Cambridge University Press.

Jackson, R. (2006). Africa's wars: Overview, causes and the challenges of conflict transformation. In O. Furley & R. May (Eds.), *Ending Africa's wars – Progression to peace*. Surrey, England: Ashgate Publishing.

Kaldor, M. (2006). *New and old wars: Organized violence in a global era*. Cambridge: Polity Press.

Kelman, H. (2004). The nature of international conflict: A social-psychological perspective. In H. J. Langholtz & C. E. Stout (Eds.), *The psychology of diplomacy*. Westport, CT: Praeger Publishers.

Knight, D. (1982). Identity and territory: Geographical perspectives on nationalism and regionalism. *Annals of the Association of American Geographers*, *72*(4), 514–31.

Licklider, R. (1995). The consequences of negotiated settlements in civil wars 1945–1993. *American Political Science Review*, *89*(3), 681–90.

McMorrow-Hernandez, J. (2009). Functionalist and conflict theorist views of social change: Two prominent perspectives on the issue of social change. Retrieved May 15, 2009 from Associated Content: http://www.associatedcontent.com/pop_print.shtml?content_type=article&content

Meredith, M. (2005). *The state of Africa: A history of fifty years of independence*. Cape Town & Johannesburg: Jonathan Ball Publishers.

Mitchell, C. (1981). *The structure of international conflict*. London: Macmillan.

Murithi, T. (2006). African approaches to building peace and solidarity. *African Journal of Conflict Resolution*, *6*(2), 9–34.

Ntahombaye, P., & Nduwayo, F. (2007). Identity and cultural diversity in conflict resolution and democratisation for the African Renaissance. *African Journal of Conflict Resolution*, *7*(2), 239–73.

Osman, A. (2006). Post genocide justice in Rwanda UN Tribunal and Gacaca. *International Studies Association*. Retrieved 15 May, 2009 from All Academic: http://www.allacademic.com/meta/p_mla_apa_research_citation/0/9/9/6/8/p99688_index.html

Phalya, R., Adan, M., & Masinde, I. (2004). Indiginous democracy: Traditional conflict resolution mechanisms – Pokot, Turkana, Samburu and Marakwet. Eastern Africa: Intermediate Technology Development Group.

Pruit, D. (2006). Some research frontiers in the study of conflict resolution. In M. P. Deutsch (Ed.), *The handbook of conflict resolution: Theory and practise* (2nd ed.). London: Jossey-Bass.

Rummel, R. J. (1979). Understanding conflict and war, Vol. 3. Retrieved May 15, 2009 from http://www.hawaii.edu/powerkills/NOTE12.htm

Save-Soderbergh, D. (1998). Preface. In Reilly, G. & P. Harris (Eds.), *Democracy and deep rooted conflict: Options for negotiators* (pp. v – vi). Stockholm: IDEA.

Seldowitz, S. (2004). The psychology of diplomatic conflict resolution. In H. Langholtz & C. Stout (Eds.), *The psychology of diplomacy*. Westport, CT: Praeger.

Southall, R., N. Simutanyi, & J.Daniel. (2006) Former African Presidents. In R. Southall & H. Melber (Eds.), *Legacies of power: Leadership change and former African presidents in African politics*. Cape Town: Human Science Research Council.

Svensson, I. (2007). Fighting with faith: Religion and conflict resolution in civil wars. *Journal of Conflict Resolution*, *51*, 930–49.

Swanström, N., & Weissman, M. (2005). *Conflict, conflict prevention and conflict management and beyond: A conceptual exploration*. Washington & Upsala: Central-Asia Caucasus Institute and Silk Road Studies Programme.

Swart, G., & Solomon, H. (2004). *Conflict in the DRC: A critical assessment of the Lusaka Ceasefire Agreement*. Johannesburg: South African Institute of International Affairs.

Tessendorf, H. (1991). *A theoretical overview of the causes of the Natal conflict*. Unpublished honours treatise, University of Port Elizabeth.

Tetlock, P. E., & Goldgeier, J. (2000). Human nature and world politics: Cognition, influence, and identity. *International Journal of Psychology*, *35*, 87–96.

UNESCO. (1945, November 16). Constitution. Adopted in London.

Vadelay, R. (2009). Sociological pespective: Functionalism. Retrieved May 14, 2009 from Associated Content: http://www.asssociatedcontent.com/pop_print.shtml?content_type=article&content

Wallensteen, P. (2007). *Understanding conflict resolution*. London: SAGE Publications.

Zartman, I. (2000). Ripeness: The hurting stalemate and beyond. In P. Stern & D. Druckman (Eds.), *International conflict resolution after the Cold War*. Washington, DC: National Academies Press.

SELF-CHECK EXERCISES

1. Characterize the nature and causes of conflict in Africa.
2. Discuss a theory of conflict you perceive to be relevant to the African context. Cite an example of a conflict you are familiar with to illustrate your point.
3. Choose any conflict on the African conflict and determine the conflict situation, conflict attitudes, and conflict behavior.
4. What role could indigenous African conflict resolution strategies play in building sustainable peace on the continent? What are the opportunities and threats to using such approaches? Discuss with reference to a particular conflict.
5. What role can counselors play in constructing a sustainable peace in Africa?
6. Describe Western approaches to conflict resolution and evaluate how these may apply to African settings.

FIELD-BASED EXPERIENTIAL EXERCISES

1. Interview two or three people from a conflict territory in Africa. Discuss the issues and the factors that they think fuels their conflict. Compare and contrast their responses.
2. Interview a negotiator and determine which approach to conflict resolution is used.

MULTIPLE-CHOICE QUESTIONS

1 Conflict is defined as:
   a. Violence
   b. Arguing
   c. Competition over scarce resources and the politics of belonging
   d. Domination and culture

2 Conflict is:
   a. Positive in that it facilitates social change
   b. Always negative
   c. Always present where one finds diversity
   d. Found only in societies that are diverse

3. Human needs theory stresses that institutions are:
   a. Quick to adapt to the changing nature of human needs
   b. Fair and reasonable in the distribution of scarce resources
   c. Slow to adapt to the changing nature of human needs
   d. Can effectively manage conflict

4. Traditional African approaches to conflict resolution focuses on:
   a. The individual and third-party involvement in a formal environment that seeks retribution and termination of the relationship
   b. A community-based approach that seeks to adjudicate and terminate the relationship
   c. A community-based approach focusing on face-to-face interaction in an informal environment that seeks to mend the relationship

   d. The individual and his/her rights in getting justice

5. Ubuntu means
   a. I am the most important
   b. Greetings in the name of peace
   c. We owe society nothing
   d. I am because you are

6. An important new characteristic of the so-called new wars as espoused by Kaldor (2006) are:
   a. The accelerating costs of warfare
   b. The changed mode of warfare
   c. The new stages of warfare
   d. The outcomes of warfare

7. Mitchell (1981) identified three key factors that must be present in order for social conflict to exist: They are:
   a. Conflict parties, conflict causes, and conflict manifestations
   b. Conflict situation, conflict attitudes, and conflict behavior
   c. Conflict triggers, conflict motivations, and conflict behavior
   d. Conflict factors, conflict perceptions, and conflict issues

Answers to the multiple-choice questions are provided at the back of the book

PART 3
COUNSELING APPLICATIONS

Section Editor
Elias Mpofu

15 Counseling for Trauma

David J. A. Edwards and Linda Eskell Blokland

OVERVIEW. Very intense emotions can be evoked in individuals who experience traumatic events such as being assaulted or raped, seeing a murder, being involved in a motor vehicle accident, or having one's home washed away in a flood. In this chapter, we focus on how counselors can recognize when clients have been exposed to trauma and the common symptoms they may display. We also look at how the kind of help counselors can give depends on the circumstances and the context in which the client is seen for counseling. We review a range of interventions from immediate help in stabilizing individuals in the immediate aftermath to the treatment of posttraumatic stress disorder (PTSD) that persists months or even years after the traumatic event took place, and how these interventions have been used in African contexts.

LEARNING OBJECTIVES

By the end of the chapter, the reader should be able to:

1. Identify and describe the kinds of traumatizing events that give rise to stress reactions such as PTSD.
2. Explain the range of typical psychological effects of being exposed to such traumatizing events.
3. Discuss individual differences among people in the way they are affected by traumatic events.
4. Critically discuss different ways that counselors can help people experiencing the immediate or long-term effects of exposure to traumatizing events.
5. Critically discuss the role of trauma interventions in communities exposed to man-made or natural disasters.

INTRODUCTION

Although difficult and upsetting situations are a normal part of everyday life, some events are so extreme that they trigger overwhelmingly intense emotions that push people beyond the limits of what they can deal with. These *traumatizing* events include motor vehicle accidents, industrial accidents (such as mine disasters), domestic accidents (such as fires), exposure to criminal violence, sexual molestation or rape, and other tragedies such as drownings or attacks by animals. Witnessing or even hearing about these kinds of events is also traumatic. Thus, those who know someone affected by such events or who see someone being assaulted, murdered, injured in a motor vehicle or industrial accident, or drowned may often be deeply affected as well (Edwards, 2005b).

People vary a great deal in their reactions to trauma, with many factors impacting on individual responses, including cultural influences. However, affected individuals often respond with "intense fear, helplessness or horror" (American Psychiatric Association, 2000, p. 467). This was the case with Amos (described later in Case Study 15.1), who felt paralyzing fear when he witnessed the shootings in the street. This prevented him from acting rationally in the moment, and he was unable to focus on what was happening around him. In the immediate aftermath of a traumatic event, individuals can experience intense anxiety responses such as muscle tension, shallow breathing, hyperventilation, and palpitations, but other emotions may also be experienced (Caffo, Forresi, & Lievers, 2005). These symptoms are what the ICD-10 (World Health Organization [WHO], 1992) terms an *acute stress reaction* (ASR). Typically, people in trauma first feel dazed and disoriented, and may have difficulty focusing on what is happening around them. They may experience a variety of intense emotions that may shift unpredictably and in ways that vary from person to person: "... depression, anxiety, anger, despair, overactivity and withdrawal may all be seen but no one type of symptom pre-dominates for long" (WHO, 1992, p. 147). For most people, these reactions settle down quite quickly, within a few hours or days. Others do not experience such intense reactions at all and carry on as if nothing extreme had happened. Some, who show no marked signs of psychological distress at the time, may develop symptoms months or years later. This kind of *delayed onset PTSD* is common after disasters such as floods or earthquakes (Njenga, Nguithi, & Kang'ethe, 2006).

We illustrate this chapter with several case examples from our own files. Except where specifically noted, all clients are Black Africans living in South Africa. Case Study 15.1 gives four examples of the kinds of crisis a counselor might encounter in individuals exposed to various traumatizing events.

Case Study 15.1: The Many Faces of Post-Traumatic Stress Disorder

1. Amos (age twenty-five), who had witnessed a shooting on the side of the road, turned and began to run, apparently aimlessly, into oncoming traffic. He needed to be guided to a room where he was offered a chair, and someone stayed with him, repeatedly asking him simple questions about himself until he calmed down and regained orientation to his situation.
2. Nomsefo (age ten) kept herself isolated from other children at school and was frequently irritable or tearful. Sometimes, she was disruptive in class. At home, she could not sleep alone. She was clinically depressed and had posttraumatic stress disorder (PTSD). She had been five years old when her fifteen-year-old half-brother began to sexually molest her. In due course, he started to rape her. Although she told her mother, no action was taken and it was only when she was seven years old that friends who had noticed blood on her underwear urged her to tell her mother. Eventually, she was sent to a foster home in another town while her half-brother was prosecuted, and after about three years, jailed. Her mother sometimes visited her; but Nomsefo remained with the foster family even after the end of the trial. She was so traumatized that she could hardly speak to the psychologist who was helping her; and this silence continued for many sessions (Edwards, Sakasa, & van Wyk, 2005).
3. Grace (age twenty-two), a Zimbabwean, went to see a student counselor at her university after she became so depressed she could not concentrate on her academic work. It was only in the third session that the counselor identified what had precipitated her problems. A few months earlier, she had become pregnant when her fiancé had visited from Zimbabwe. She told him about it over the phone, but could not easily discuss it. She had had an abortion a few weeks later (Boulind & Edwards, 2008). Once the counselor realized this, she carefully questioned her further and found that Grace was also suffering from PTSD.
4. Karabo (age twelve) was referred for counseling for behavioral problems. According to his teachers, his mood fluctuated. At times, he was lively and engaging, but at others, he was withdrawn and morose. He was uncooperative in the classroom, acted aggressively, and bullied other children. However, psychological assessment identified a significant contribution of trauma in causing and maintaining these problems. He told of how, when he was eight, he had witnessed the slow and painful death of his mother from AIDS. He still often experienced disturbing dreams about this. His family had few resources and almost no money, so after his mother's death, he was left largely in the company of his older cousins. They were members of a gang involved in criminal activities and became role models for antisocial behavior.

Questions

1. Identify symptoms from each case.
2. Return to these cases once you have covered the section on Importance and Definition of Key Terms. Identify the symptoms that indicate traumatic effects in the individuals and fit them into one of the three classes discussed. Can you explain how these symptoms fit into known conditions?

IMPORTANCE, DEFINITION, AND SCOPE OF KEY TERMS AND CONCEPTS

A number of conditions and formal diagnoses are associated with trauma experiences and symptoms. This section examines major conditions while drawing from examples of cases to illustrate these.

A diagnosis of PTSD is given to individuals who still display symptoms of trauma a few weeks after the precipitating event. Although affected individuals may show a range of symptoms, counselors should be particularly watchful for the three classes of symptoms that are normally used to define PTSD, which are explained using cases described in various sections of this chapter.

Symptoms of Traumatic Experience

Reexperiencing symptoms are caused by the activation of the trauma memory and include intrusive images of the traumatic event, nightmares, and the feeling of being back in the traumatic situation, as if it is happening all over again. Langu (see Case Study 15.3) had frequent images of his brother's burned body. Zanele (see Case Study 15. 2) would see the rapist's face when she looked at a Black man, which resulted in her running out of the classroom when the teacher was a man. She also reexperienced being hit on the head with a screwdriver. Langu, Zanele, and Grace (see Case Study 15.1) all experienced disturbing dreams related to their traumas. These phenomena are sometimes referred to as *flashbacks*.

Avoidance symptoms include being cut off from feelings, actively avoiding thinking about the trauma, or avoiding that which reminds them of the trauma, such as newspaper stories or news broadcasts about similar traumatic events. Langu, Zanele, Grace, and Nomsefo (see Case Study 15.1) felt unable to speak with their families about what had happened to them. Grace and Langu deliberately avoided thinking about their traumas and focused on their work. Nomsefo isolated herself from other children. To control her *nightmares*, Zanele

Case Study 15.2: Depression, PTSD, and Traumatic Grief

Langu (age twenty-one) had been affected by a series of motor vehicle accidents involving him and his family (Karpelowsky & Edwards, 2005). The first had left his father unconscious for several hours. He and his father were in the second accident, although neither was injured. In the third accident, Langu was badly shaken when his car rolled several times. The fourth accident involved his brother and uncle, who died and were burned after their car caught fire. Langu had to identify his brother's body, which was badly burned and hardly recognizable. He was a student and returned to university after the funeral. However, he could not focus on his academic work. The counselor he consulted made a diagnosis of severe depression and ASD (it was still less than four weeks since his brother died). During the next fifteen months, she assessed and treated him over twenty-two sessions. Two aspects that the therapy focused on were the horror of seeing his brother's badly burned body in the mortuary and the traumatic grief resulting from his death.

Question

1. Engage in a discussion with peers around the complexity of the diagnosis made above and discuss the possible implications for treatment and recovery.

would try to keep awake at night, resulting in severe loss of sleep.

Hyperarousal symptoms result from overactivation of the sympathetic nervous system. This overactivation results in anxiety symptoms such as elevated heart rate, sweating, or feeling hot, and/or easily startled. Individuals may be *hypervigilant*, as if expecting something bad to happen at any moment. They may also be *irritable* and prone to sudden outbursts of anger. Langu experienced regular episodes of intense anxiety. Zanele was easily startled even in situations where she knew she was safe, and she lived in constant fear. Grace experienced an intense and unexpected *panic attack* several months after the abortion.

Formal Diagnostic Classifications

The *DSM-IV* (American Psychiatric Association, 2000) specifies that there must be at least one reexperiencing symptom, three avoidance symptoms, and two arousal symptoms for the diagnosis of PTSD to be made, but the ICD-10, which is used by medical schemes in South Africa, does not specify the numbers of symptoms. In many cases, the symptoms subside within a few weeks. For example, in a study of rape survivors in the United States, the DSM criteria for PTSD were met by 94 percent after two weeks, but by only 65 percent at one month, 53 percent at two months, and 47 percent at three months (Foa & Rothbaum, 1998). For this reason, a diagnosis of PTSD is not given in the first month after the trauma.

A very severe response in the immediate aftermath of a trauma is described by the diagnosis of acute stress disorder (ASD) in the DSM-IV. This diagnosis is quite different from the ICD-10's ASR, as it includes all the symptoms of PTSD as well as at least three symptoms of *dissociation*: emotional numbing, reduced awareness of surroundings, derealization (experiencing the world as if it is not real), depersonalization (feeling as if one is no longer a person), and amnesia (inability to remember a significant part of the trauma, not caused by concussion). There are two reasons for the addition of the dissociative symptoms. First, it was believed that people who experienced them at the time of the trauma were more likely to develop chronic PTSD. However, subsequent research has challenged this belief (Edwards et al., 2005). Second, individuals who did not experience such a severe immediate reaction to trauma would not receive a diagnosis at all, and this has the advantage of recognizing that some form of distress in response to trauma is quite normal.

LASTING EFFECTS OF TRAUMA

It is perhaps not surprising that the more severe the trauma, the more likely are individuals to develop PTSD. The most traumatizing events are genocide and warfare, followed, in order, by sexual assault, physical assault, terror directed at an individual or a small group of people, accidents, technological disasters, and natural disasters. There is a greater likelihood of PTSD symptoms in individuals who suffer serious injury or financial loss. Among victims of assault, those threatened with deadly weapons or with death are more likely to exhibit PTSD symptoms than those not so threatened (Staab, Fullerton, & Ursano, 1999).

Unfortunately, even when the trauma is over, people may continue to experience negative after-effects, sometimes for the rest of their lives. For this reason, counselors are concerned not only with recent events. Traumatic situations that happened years or even decades ago can lie at the root of a person's current psychological difficulties. Many individuals with PTSD related to sexual abuse during childhood receive therapeutic help only as adults.

The effects of trauma go beyond the main symptoms of PTSD, and it is important for counselors to be aware of a range of possible emotional responses (Edwards, 2005c). Some of these are illustrated in the text that follows using the cases referred to in this chapter.

1. *Guilt*: Langu felt guilty that he had survived, but his brother died. Grace felt guilty that she had taken the life of her unborn child.

Discussion Box 15.1: Cultural Bias in Psychiatric Diagnosis

Critics have questioned whether the use of diagnostic categories, such as PTSD, is appropriate at all. They argue that because PTSD is a normal response to trauma, it should not be thought of as a disease or disorder. For example, Hirschowitz and Orkin (1997) found that between 78 percent and 85 percent, of persons who had been exposed to violence, had at least one symptom of PTSD. Other critics argue that PTSD is a Eurocentric diagnosis that may not be appropriate for persons of African descent (Edwards, 2005a). Summerfield (2001) argues that PTSD is an invention of Western psychiatry that places too much focus on individuals and their symptoms and not enough on the broader context that is creating the distress. When a large number of people are in distress, as result of war or disaster, it is not appropriate to respond by offering everyone treatment for PTSD. However, despite these objections, PTSD is regularly seen in Africa and is clearly recognizable to clinicians there (Eagle, 1998, 2000; Edwards, 2005b; Ensink, Robertson, Zissis, & Leger, 1997; Leibowitz-Levy, 2005). Furthermore, there are effective ways of helping people who have PTSD symptoms. So there is real practical value in being able to recognize it. At the same time, as we discuss in this chapter, it is important to recognize that (1) not all those exposed to trauma develop PTSD, (2) treating PTSD symptoms is not the only focus of intervention after a traumatic event, and (3) repeated exposure to trauma can result in many other psychological problems. Thus, counselors may have a range of roles to play in helping in the aftermath of a traumatic event and should not dismiss the concerns of people exposed to trauma whose symptoms do not fit a typical PTSD profile.

Question

1. With reference to the community in which you live, how useful do you think the concept of PTSD would be in helping to identify people who need help and in channeling appropriate support to them?

2. *Shame*: Langu felt ashamed that he was no longer coping with his work. Nomsefo and Zanele felt ashamed about being sexually assaulted. Zanele felt embarrassed because the rapist had taken her panties and she felt ashamed that others might see them (see Lee, Scragg, & Turner, 2001 for the significance of guilt and shame in PTSD).
3. *Helplessness and defeat*: Zanele felt helpless and completely overpowered by the rapist.
4. *Disgust*: Zanele felt disgust at the experience of feeling dirty and smelling unpleasant after the rape. Langu felt disgust at the sight of his brother's burned body.
5. *Anger*: Nomsefo felt angry not only with her half-brother for raping her, but also with her mother for protecting him, and so neglecting and betraying her. Langu felt angry that his brother had died and that he had had to be the one to identify the body. Grace felt angry that her fiancé had not understood what she was going through or participated more in the decision to have the abortion.
6. *Sadness*: Langu, Zanele, Grace, and Nomsefo felt sad because they felt socially isolated and it seemed that no one understood what they were going through. Nomsefo had lost her family, as her mother seldom visited her and her half-brother was in jail.
7. *Grief*: Langu felt grief for his dead brother. Grace felt grief for the child she never gave birth to.

Several of these experiences (especially sadness, grief, shame, and helplessness) also make individuals vulnerable to *depression*. Furthermore, PTSD is itself so distressing that it can disrupt people's lives. Sufferers may become irritable with their families and friends or withdraw from them completely. The reexperiencing of symptoms and hypervigilance may interfere with their ability to work. As a result, like Zanele, Langu, and Nomsefo, they may become depressed because they become pessimistic about ever being able to function again at the level they did before the trauma.

Resilience in the Face of Trauma

Critics have warned that counselors may focus too much on the distressing symptoms that result from exposure to trauma and easily forget that many individuals are *resilient* and cope remarkably well in response to extreme events (see Case Study 15.4). Gist and Woodall (1999) remind us that "adversity can, and in fact most commonly will, provide challenges from which character and resilience are built." Resilient individuals have stability and the capacity to adapt well in the face of adversity or trauma (Yehuda, Flory, Southwick, & Charney, 2006). Individual differences in resilience can be seen from research on soldiers and emergency workers showing that those who coped well with stressful situations at first were likely to continue to cope well in the future, while those who coped poorly in their first encounter with a traumatic event were likely to continue to cope poorly (Staab et al., 1999).

Factors Associated with Resilience

Social Support

Having supportive friends or family helps individuals cope with traumatizing events (Yehuda et al., 2006). Institutions such as clubs or churches may also be an important

Case Study 15.3: Individual Differences in Response to Trauma

Those involved in a traumatic event may react in quite different ways, as is shown by three cases from the files of the second author. The home of a South African Indian family was burglarized twice while the whole family was at home; and the members were seen for counseling. On both occasions, the parents displayed clear PTSD symptoms at first consultation and also at follow-up, while neither of the two young adult children (ages seventeen and twenty-three) showed any marked symptoms at all. In the second case, a father and daughter from a South African Colored family were at home when their home was robbed. The intruders shot and injured both of them. The father continued to show marked symptoms of PTSD up to eighteen months later, while his daughter (eighteen years) experienced symptoms initially, but these abated after about three months. In a third case, there had been several armed robberies in the home of a Black South African family from a middle-class suburban area. A number of family members spoke with strong feelings of anger and shock about what had happened, but one member, a middle-aged woman, displayed no obvious emotional distress and chose not to come for follow-up counseling. Each time, she saw the absurdity in what had happened and how it had happened. She seemed to have a high estimation of her own efficacy in such situations and laughingly described her own efforts to outwit the attackers.

Question

1. Discuss what factors you might expect could have played a role in both the resilience and vulnerabilities demonstrated in the cases above. You are not given background details, but consider the possibilities.

source of support. However, just having other people around may not be enough by itself. If friends or family are to be helpful, they need to be sensitive to the needs of the traumatized person. After a trauma, some people want to be left alone, while others want company. Some people want to talk, and others want to reflect quietly. At the same time, if traumatized individuals withdraw and become depressed, they may need caring people to encourage them to become more active and engage socially. They may also need guidance and mentorship about the best ways to cope and solve problems in the aftermath of the trauma. Traumatized individuals also need empathy and understanding, and friends or family who cannot offer this may make matters worse. Usually the process of recovery from a traumatic event involves talking to others about what happened and one's experience. This communication helps the affected individual to engage with the memory of what happened and put it in perspective. Therefore, having friends one can talk to about what happened can make a great difference (Litz, Gray, Bryant, & Adler 2002; Masten & Coatsworth, 1998).

Emotional Stability, Well-being, and Optimism

A resilient person is more sociable and extroverted, with a good level of self-confidence and self-esteem, and is more flexible, easygoing, optimistic, with a positive outlook on life (Masten & Coatsworth 1998; Strümpfer, 2003; Yehuda et al., 2006). People with these characteristics are less vulnerable to developing PTSD (Staab et al., 1999).

Engagement and Meaningfulness

The meaning individuals give to what has happened to them is also a large factor in determining how they will cope. Contrast the attitude of a person who believes "I am a helpless victim and can do nothing about what happens to me" with that of another person who thinks, "this is a big challenge and I must find a way through it." It is not difficult to see that the second person will likely be more resilient. Finding constructive meaning in what happened is a large factor in enabling individuals to cope well without showing evidence of long-term negative effects (Herbert & Sageman, 2004). Spiritual beliefs or religious affiliation can contribute here, as they can be an important source of meaning in the face of suffering (Masten & Coatsworth, 1998; Peterson & Roy, 1985). Those who can give meaning to their lives are more able to engage with facing and dealing with their problems and to tackle them in a sustained and committed manner (Strümpfer, 2003).

Composite Resilience Concepts

Two terms that have been used to conceptualize resilience are *sense of coherence* (SOC) (Eriksson & Lindström, 2005) and *hardiness* (Kobasa, Maddi, & Kahn, 1982). Each of these combines several of the factors examined in the preceding text. SOC includes three factors: experiencing change as a meaningful challenge, comprehensibility (events are experienced as structured, predictable, and explicable), and manageability (believing one has the resources to cope). In a study of Swiss victims of serious accidents, Schnyder and Moergeli (2003) found that the higher SOC scores were, the lower were PTSD symptoms. In a study of South African journalists, the SOC dimensions of manageability and comprehensibility were associated with lower PTSD symptoms (Marais & Stuart, 2005). Hardiness also has three components: a sense of control over one's fate (also called internal locus of control), a sense of commitment, and seeing change as a challenge. King, King, Fairbank, Keane, and Adams (1998) studied male and female U.S. soldiers who had served in Vietnam, of whom 18 percent had PTSD. The lower the hardiness, the greater was the likelihood of experiencing PTSD symptoms. The authors found that hardiness and social support worked together, since hardy individuals seemed to be good at building networks of social support.

Differences in Response to Trauma

Resilience and Vulnerability

As discussed previously, many people seem to cope well despite high levels of exposure to traumatizing events. After a traumatic event such as an assault or a rape, some people may show little or no psychological disruption, or if they do, it lasts a few days at most. About half of those who have PTSD symptoms soon after a trauma no longer have significant symptoms a few months later (Harvey & Bryant, 2002). Many people believe that the best way to cope with a traumatic event is to "put it behind you and move on." Indeed, some people seem to be able to do this. Otherwise, they would not be able to cope with occupations, for example, in the police or military, where trauma exposure is routine. Nevertheless, following any kind of trauma, there is at least a minority who show the full symptom profile of ASD and who continue to experience PTSD for several months or even years. In seeking to understand individual differences in response to trauma, psychologists continue to investigate *protective factors, like those summarized above*, that make people resilient in the face of trauma, as well as *vulnerability factors* that make individuals more likely to develop psychological problems, as well.

Prolonged or repeated exposures to traumatizing events are important vulnerability factors. Some exposure to adversity can foster resilience, but the more prolonged the exposure to trauma, the more likely it is that there will be negative psychological effects (Seery, Holman, & Silver, 2010). A study of military veterans showed that the more combat exposure they had had the more likely they were to have PTSD (Boscarino, 1995). This effect is illustrated by a case involving a Black South African police officer who experienced PTSD symptoms after he was called to a motor vehicle accident in which two people were killed. He had more than twelve years' experience as a police officer and had been present at fatal accidents on many previous occasions, as well as at scenes of shootings, murders, knife violence, bloody motor vehicle accidents, and aggressive assaults. He had never before experienced disturbing flashbacks of any of these memories before; but now, he told the counselor, since this latest accident, he was troubled by intrusive images of many of these earlier traumatic events.

Evidence for the traumatizing effects of repeated exposure comes from the Adverse Childhood Experiences study (the ACE study) conducted in the United States over an extended period (Chapman, Dube, & Anda, 2007). The researchers concluded that repeated trauma in childhood is "vastly more common than recognized or acknowledged" (van der Kolk, 2005, p. 402) and is associated with increased vulnerability to mental health problems in adulthood including depression, suicide attempts, alcoholism, drug abuse, sexual promiscuity (and sexually transmitted diseases), domestic violence, obesity, and physical inactivity. Trauma has a damaging effect on normal child development as it leads to "a breakdown in [the] capacity to process, integrate, and categorize what is happening… [which results in] a breakdown in the capacity to regulate internal states" (van der Kolk, 2005, p. 403). This breakdown means that children fail to learn how to manage their emotions and behavior and become vulnerable to extreme and intense emotional states. Ongoing exposure to trauma and adversity has not only psychological effects. The ACE study has shown that it also increases vulnerability to physical health problems such as heart disease, cancer, stroke, diabetes, skeletal fractures, and liver disease (van der Kolk, 2005).

Gender

Gender is also a vulnerability factor. Being able to cope with trauma is often seen as a masculine trait. Mamphela Ramphele (1995, p. 33), a former vice chancellor of the University of Cape Town, recollects hearing her father say, "*moshimane ke draad, ga a lle ge a e kwa bohloko*" ("a boy is like a piece of wire and should not cry"). By contrast, there is an expectation that women are more vulnerable to trauma and more likely to break down emotionally. Evidence that PTSD is more common in females than in males is presented below. However, this finding should not be interpreted as an all or none effect of gender. There is evidence that the majority of men have a breaking point if exposed to multiple traumas, for example, in military combat, and many men develop PTSD after exposure to a single traumatic event. While women do show more symptoms of psychological distress following trauma, many women cope with persistent adverse life circumstances as well as or better than the men around them. Indeed, in many communities characterized by poverty and lawlessness, there are women who hold families together and support children while many men abandon their families and cope by abusing alcohol.

There is also some association between *vulnerability and age*. Old people become more vulnerable because they are physically less able to protect themselves in an emergency than younger adults. Aging also increases the risk of neurological problems such as strokes or dementia, and these can precipitate delayed PTSD in survivors of severe trauma who were not previously troubled by PTSD symptoms (Grossman, Levin, Katzen, & Lechner, 2004). Very young children may not fully understand the significance of traumatic events unless they are personally injured or their caretakers injured or killed. Their reaction is often determined by that of the adults around them. In South Africa, under apartheid, the negative impact of state repression in the townships was more severe in children whose mothers coped poorly with trauma (Dawes, Tredoux, & Feinstein, 1989; Swartz & Levett, 1989).

Case Study 15.4: A Raped Teenager Receives Counseling

Zanele (age fifteen) experienced states of intense panic at school and on several occasions ran from the classroom. She was having flashbacks of the face of a man who had twice raped her. These flashbacks were triggered by looking at the teacher (Payne & Edwards, 2009). Her mother had divorced her father because he was physically abusive and wasted money on alcohol. She lived with her father and other relatives and on two occasions she was waylaid not far from their home by a man who assaulted and raped her. When a relative realized something was wrong, the rapes were reported to the police and a social worker referred her to a psychologist. She was assessed and treated over twenty-three sessions. Zanele was suffering from depression and PTSD, but her depression remitted very quickly once she realized the therapist could help her. After a few weeks, the rapist was released by the police and no charge was brought against him. A few weeks later, a medical check revealed that Zanele had been infected with several sexually transmitted diseases, including HIV. Despite these complications, Zanele's PTSD largely remitted after about fifteen sessions. The therapist provided a great deal of psychoeducation about PTSD symptoms associated trauma and about living with HIV infection. Treatment was largely based on cognitive therapy and also included building social support within Zanele's family.

Questions

1. In this case, the therapist did not have to address Zanele's depression directly and was able to concentrate on treating the PTSD. What do you think was the reason?
2. Why is it likely to be important for a woman who has been raped to know that the rapist is in custody or serving a jail term?

A more recent study in Soweto also found that the better mothers coped with difficult life circumstances, the less vulnerable were their children to psychological problems (Barbarin, Richter, & de Wet, 2001).

HISTORY OF RESEARCH AND PRACTICE IN TRAUMA COUNSELING IN AFRICAN SETTINGS

The Impact of Trauma: Universal or Culturally Shaped?

Researchers have often asked whether working with trauma in Africa or with Black Africans is likely to be different from working with trauma in other cultures and contexts. It is widely acknowledged that ASD and PTSD as defined in the ICD-10 (WHO, 1992) and *DSM-IV* (American Psychiatric Association, 2000) are quite recognizable in African communities (Musisi, 2004; Njenga et al., 2006; Onyut et al., 2005; Seedat, 2004). Clinical experience in South Africa also provides evidence that the kinds of approaches to treatment developed internationally are appropriate and effective with Black African clients (Eagle, 2004; Edwards, 2009, 2010; Leibowitz-Levy, 2005). Several researchers note that PTSD is not the only kind of diagnosis seen in Africa as a consequence of trauma. Depression, other anxiety disorders, and dissociative and somatoform disorders are also seen. However, this is true of most parts of the world and, as we saw earlier, prolonged exposure to trauma can give rise to a wide range of psychological problems. There is some evidence that dissociative and somatoform disorders are more common in Africa than in Western societies (Hirschowitz & Orkin, 1997), and Musisi (2004) discusses the possibility of a distinct culture-bound trauma syndrome characterized by somatization symptoms. Nevertheless, other studies suggest that cultural factors play little detectable role in determining the nature of trauma symptoms (Monnier, Elhai, Frueh, Sauvageot, & Magruder, 2002; Njenga et al., 2006). For example, Nagel, Matsuo, McIntyre, and Morrison (2005) found that socioeconomic variables tended to override racial and cultural factors in determining responses to sexual victimization.

In many cases, the effects of culture are likely to be more subtle (see Research Box 15.1). Some African clients may attribute their symptoms to being bewitched (Eagle, 2004), but this specific belief can usually be addressed through psychoeducation. In any counseling situation, counselors need to be aware of local contextual factors to understand the world and experience of the client. This understanding enables them to be responsive to the specific needs and situations each client brings (Stiles, Honos-Webb, & Surko, 1998). The research we review in this chapter is consistent with the view that there are universal, psychological (and physiological) processes underlying psychological problems associated with exposure to trauma, as well as general principles that counselors can draw on in whatever cultural context they work. At the same time, traumatized individuals do not live in a vacuum, and counselors need to be able to apply these general principles in a way that is informed by and sensitive to a variety of contextual factors. Without local knowledge, counselors will not understand the significance of specific beliefs, attitudes, or social practices or the nature of the kinds of obstacles to recovery that individuals face, and this may well prevent them from effectively putting the more general principles into practice.

With regard to the effects of *prolonged exposure to trauma*, especially in childhood, there is no reason to think that the situation is any different, in Africa, where adversity in childhood is commonplace (e.g., Dawes & Donald, 1994; Seedat et al., 2004). In a study of sixty children in Khayelitsha in South Africa, many had been the targets of assault themselves, more than half had seen someone stabbed, and 45 percent had seen someone killed. One witnessed a fight between gang members in which the heads of two men were hacked off. Another saw community members beat to death a man who had previously killed a woman by slitting her throat (Ensink et al., 1997). Children born into such troubled communities are likely to have ongoing exposure to trauma over months and years, and counselors in Africa can expect that the psychological problems and troubled behavior they see in some clients have their origin in such prolonged exposure.

Several studies comparing the effects of trauma on women and men have shown that, after exposure to a traumatic event, females are more likely to have posttraumatic symptoms than males (Stein, Walker, & Forde, 2000; Caffo et al., 2005; Edwards et al., 2005). Innate psychological factors may play a role as, throughout the evolution of our species, women have needed to specialize in giving birth and nurturing and rearing children, while men have often engaged in dangerous activities such as hunting and defense of the community. However, social attitudes also play a role. In many societies, men have been more powerful than women, and widespread victimization of women and girls has been routine. In many African communities, women and children, especially girls, are among the most vulnerable to violence-induced trauma (Hamber, 2004). During peace time, women and girl children are most likely to be traumatized from violence in the home at the hands of family members or close family associates (Rasool, Vermaak, Pharoah, Louw, & Stavrou, 2002). As a result, women are still widely stereotyped as "more helpless" than men. Females are therefore more likely to have internalized an identity of being less able to cope with extreme events. In addition, as a result of victimization, they may have experienced feelings of powerlessness, which increases their vulnerability to distress following trauma.

Effects of Trauma Experienced in Childhood

Persons exposed to trauma and abuse as children are likely to be more vulnerable to developing PTSD if exposed to trauma later in life. In a study of women who were seeking treatment for PTSD and who had been sexually abused in childhood, a very high degree of vulnerability was found. In some cases, events that were not life-threatening like losing a job, or relatively minor events like conflict with a partner or criticism from a family member were enough to precipitate PTSD symptoms (Koopman, Gore-Felton, Classen, Kim, & Spiegel, 2001). Those who have experienced at least one traumatic event before the age of thirteen years are also more vulnerable to major depression in later years (Caffo et al., 2005).

Exposure to prolonged or repeated trauma can have pervasive effects on psychological functioning that are different from PTSD. Children brought up in unsafe communities or abusive homes or exposed to sexual abuse in the family, or living in a war zone may experience one trauma after another over months or years. They may develop personality characteristics that are a result of this prolonged exposure. For example, they may be suspicious and mistrusting, or overly inhibited and socially withdrawn. They may also be very volatile, exhibiting sudden shifts in emotional state. Sometimes these shifts are the result of reexperiencing symptoms caused by the triggering of traumas they were exposed to in the past. This has been called "complex PTSD" (Herman, 1995, 2001; Williams & Sommer, 2002) or "developmental trauma disorder" (van der Kolk, 2005).

The Impact of Trauma on Individuals, Families, and Communities

Traumatizing events are common in all societies. They are particularly frequent where there is social breakdown and poverty. Africa has been rocked by warfare for decades while famine, disease, flooding, and drought are frequent sources of mass disaster on the continent, which has few resources to deal with the dire aftermath (Edwards, 2005b; Njenga et al., 2006). During destabilizing events such as these, civilians are exposed to threats, assaults, rapes, murders of loved ones, imprisonment, torture, and loss of their homes. Some occupations expose their members to traumatic situations as a matter of course. For example, those who work in the military may witness the deaths of enemies and friends and, after injuring or killing others, often feel deeply shocked by their own violent behavior (Edwards, 2005b). Emergency services workers (Ward, Lombard, & Gwebushe, 2008), police (Jones & Kagee, 2005; Kopel & Freidman, 1997, 1999), and even journalists (Marais & Stuart, 2005) also have a very high level of exposure to trauma.

Violent crime is another source of trauma prevalent in many urbanizing African communities. For example, from April, 2007 to March, 2008, 18,487 murders were reported to the South African Police Services. The number of attempted murders was similar, and in addition 36,190 rapes, 14,481 residential robberies, 198,049 incidents of common assault (which includes domestic violence), and 237,853 burglaries at residences were reported (South African Police Service, 2006). These figures do not include crimes not reported to the police at all. Estimates of just how many people have been exposed to traumatic violent events vary. Data from one survey (South African Advertising Research Foundation, 2006) suggested that 11.6 percent of adults were victims of violent crime in South Africa in a one-year period. In another South African study, Hirschowitz and Orkin (1997, p. 169) estimated that "approximately five million adults (23 % of the

Discussion Box 15.2: Practitioners at the Front Line

The sweeping statistics that summarize just how many children and adolescents experience trauma fail to convey the painful realities of the lives of those exposed. But counselors, psychologists, and other practitioners come face to face with these realities on a daily basis. Smith and Holford (1993) examined some of the experiences of thirty-five children and adolescents seen at the Child and Adolescent Family Unit at the University of the Witwatersrand in South Africa. A brother (age fifteen) and sister (age fourteen) watched as their father shot their mother, who slowly bled to death. A six-year-old girl was raped by her father and later found his dead body; he had also raped a fourteen-year-old boy and then shot himself. In other cases, six children had been raped and another three had witnessed someone close to them being raped. A four-year-old girl had watched as intruders beat her mother to death and beat her father unconscious; they then locked her, her father, and sister in a cupboard for four hours. Practitioners are faced with the challenge of responding sensitively and meaningfully to children and adolescents with experiences like these.

Questions

1. What are the risks that counselors face when dealing with cases such as these?
2. How do you think counselors may need to address these risks?

population aged 16 to 64 years) had been exposed to one or more violent events" and that "78% of those who had experienced at least one traumatic event had one or more symptoms of PTSD."

The families of members of the police, military, primary response health care workers, and emergency service personnel have been found to have particularly high levels of domestic violence. Particularly, in African countries, these groups of workers are often badly affected. As a result of the impact of their experiences at work, frequently on a daily basis, they may be found to be prone to road rage, common assault, aggravated violent crime, and alcohol- or substance-induced violence. These high levels of violence have been attributed to frequent and often untreated exposure to trauma in the line of duty (Hamber, 2000, 2004). Media use of phrases such as "the war against crime" or criminals "waging a war against society" point to the similarity between low-intensity warfare and ongoing criminal activity and remind us of the endemic traumatizing environments in which many people in Africa live. The exposure to trauma, when untreated, often begets more trauma. Low tolerance of frustration and high irritability, which are common effects of exposure to trauma, contribute to the high levels of domestic violence that is common within many communities. Furthermore, some of those distressed in the aftermath of trauma may seek relief from tension, anxiety, and irritability through the use of illegal drugs or alcohol. Such self-medication may only lead to further problems in the future because abuse of illegal drugs and alcohol can in turn promote aggression and violence as well as crime, contributing to an ongoing cycle in which violence and trauma are perpetuated.

Other African countries may be just as violent or even more so. In a study of adolescents at schools in Nairobi and Cape Town, 80 percent had experienced at least one traumatic event, and the average number of traumas experienced was 2.5. More than half had witnessed street violence, a third had been robbed or mugged, and about 25 percent in South Africa and 15 percent in Kenya had been in serious accidents. Although South Africa has a reputation for its culture of violence, witnessing violence, being physically beaten by a family member, or being sexually assaulted were actually more frequent in Kenya than in South Africa (Seedat, Nyamai, Njenga, Vythilingum, & Stein, 2004). Other research in Kenya found that 38 percent of children are sexually abused by an adult before the age of eighteen and that among girl victims of violence (sampled from a children's home and the police), 70 percent had been sexually abused, mostly by family members and caretakers (Amunga, Maiyoa, Achokaa, & Ashioya, 2009).

Such ongoing community violence may be an aftermath of war or political conflict (Edwards, 2005b). Frequently political groups in Africa try to achieve political objectives by means of what has been termed "low-intensity" warfare using youth militia or even soldiers. This aims at destabilizing populations by targeting civilians rather than soldiers. Typically, once war has finished, those involved in it direct violence toward members of their own society, especially those most vulnerable such as women and children. There is a shift from military violence to criminal violence (Turshen, Meintjies, & Pillay, 2001). In addition, conflicts between rival political groups can lead to violent acts against political rivals, which in turn invite retaliation from those affected. Social or commercial conflicts can also lead to violence. For example, passengers may demonstrate about poor train services or taxi operators fight over the control of lucrative routes or gangs fight over the control of the trade in illegal drugs. Even organized demonstrations and marches can go out of control and result in demonstrators damaging cars and property and attacking police or other demonstrators. These factors can lead to an ongoing cycle of violent acts that can include "murder, bomb blasts, 'necklacing', burning of property [and] police brutality" (Hirschowitz & Orkin, 1997, p. 169).

During war itself, thousands of people are exposed to extreme and often repeated traumas. Accounts of the civil war in Nigeria between 1966 and 1970 (Odejide,

Discussion Box 15.3: Severe and Prolonged Trauma: The Challenge for Counselors

A counselor in a refugee camp worked with a shy fifteen-year-old boy from Somalia (Onyut et al., 2005). At the age of nine, he had witnessed the shooting and death of both his parents during the civil war. He became separated from his younger brother and sister and lost all contact with them. He fled and survived for several years, until, at the age of fourteen, he found his way to the refugee camp. King (2002) describes how, during the genocide in Rwanda in 1994, she fled into the bush and on several occasions just avoided being seen by Hutu militia who might well have raped and killed her. In the end, she and fourteen others were captured and marched away. Only half of the group survived. By the time the war was over, many of her relatives had died, including two brothers; and she had watched numerous people being killed, many of whom she knew.

Questions

1. Consider the challenges that would be faced by the counselor in wanting to reintegrate the boy back into his community. Discuss what some of these might be.
2. Suggest some long-term planning to assist this community.

Research Box 15.1: Individualism versus Collectivism: Does It Make a Difference in Response to Trauma?

Jobson, L., & O ' Kearney, R. T. (2009). Impact of cultural differences in self on cognitive appraisals in post-traumatic stress disorder. *Behavioural and Cognitive Psychotherapy*, *37*, 249–66.

It has often been argued that African culture fosters collectivism and interdependence, while Western cultures foster individualism and independence. It has also been suggested that these different cultural values could affect ways in which people experience personal distress. Some evidence for this was found by Jobson and O'Kearney (2009) in Australia. They conducted their study in a community with many immigrants, including those who had fled from political repression. Individuals who had experienced a trauma were classified as being from an independent (Australia, United States, Western Europe) or an interdependent culture (Asia, Africa, Middle East). About half of the participants, in each group, had marked PTSD symptoms. Furthermore, the independent group did not differ from the interdependent group in the number of PTSD symptoms. However, the researchers did find a difference with respect to "self-defining memories." These are "...memories that you feel convey powerfully how you have come to be the person you currently are" (p. 99). Participants were asked to write down five of these memories. In the interdependent group, the memory content did not differ between those with PTSD and those without. However, in the independent group, those with PTSD recorded more trauma-related memories than those without PTSD. One possible explanation for this difference is that it is more difficult for people from interdependent cultures to define themselves as people who had been traumatized because it does not accord with the communal identity.

Question

1. Consider the implication of the results of this research for counseling. How might a counselor adjust his or her approach to accommodate for these findings?

Sanda, & Odejide, 1998) and the civil war in Mozambique that ended in 1992 (Peltzer & Chongo, 2000), document exposure to violence on a massive scale. In these kinds of conflicts, millions of people lose their homes, often in violent circumstances. There is killing, rape, assault, torture, and brutality on a massive scale.

The negative effects of trauma from war or civil conflicts can persist for generations and manifest in the form of psychological and behavioral disturbances as well as undermining the general health of those affected. A "culture of violence" (Hamber, 2004) emerges, in which individuals automatically seek to resolve conflicts or solve problems by violent means. In such circumstances, there is an increase in substance abuse as a means of coping, and increased vulnerability to the spread of disease. In many parts of Africa, researchers have shown that areas affected by war are particularly vulnerable to the spread of epidemics such as HIV/AIDS and the Ebola virus. This in turn has a negative influence on socioeconomic development (Musisi, 2004).

COUNSELING PROCEDURES AND INTERVENTIONS

Models for trauma intervention generally include providing opportunities for those affected to talk about what happened to them and to feel the intense emotions often associated with trauma. Sometimes the discussion is with an individual counselor, especially for individuals who feel embarrassed about sharing their experiences with others. Sometimes this is done in groups, which can have the advantage that hearing others describing their experiences can help other group members and result in the members offering each other support afterwards as well. However, some people do not feel safe in groups because they mistrust others, while some vulnerable individuals risk becoming so emotionally overwhelmed that group members or group leaders are unable to reach out to them. Therefore, individuals should never be compelled to participate in a group against their will. Also, different kinds of intervention may be necessary at different stages of the process, which also differs from individual to individual. The section that follows examines various interventions and influencing factors which may be preferable in particular circumstances.

Help in the Immediate Aftermath of Traumatic Events: Trauma Support

Helpers on the scene of a traumatic event or counselors called to assist shortly afterwards need to assess the situation before making active interventions. The kind of emotional support that counselors are trained to give may not be the first priority. For example, it is particularly important to identify individuals who require medical attention. Many of those affected need practical support, for example, the provision of warmth, liquids, or sustenance, or assistance in contacting friends and relatives or getting home or to a hospital. When people are in a state of acute and extreme shock, they can become disorientated. Individuals may need to be assisted with some very basic tasks and helped to stay focused when in this state. Sometimes simple activities such as showing them where to sit, giving them something to hold onto, and asking basic questions, such as their names and addresses, can help them to stay focused until further help is available.

For example, a Black African woman involved in a road accident while traveling in a taxi was herself physically unharmed; but she frantically wanted to find her young child who had been thrown from the vehicle. This was her first priority. Until she knew where the child was, she could not focus on what anyone was saying to her. Another example illustrates the large individual differences in response to a traumatic event. A young man caught and injured in an armed robbery at his workplace became hysterical when the attackers tried to force him into a back room. His head was streaming with blood after he was struck with the butt of gun; and he began to scream loudly. An older woman colleague, recognizing his complete loss of control and inability to hear what anyone was saying to him, wrapped her arms around him and held him until he quieted down. Then, he was able to focus on regaining his composure. In providing this kind of practical support, those on the scene will function best if, like the woman we have just described, they are warm and friendly, clear headed, and, where individuals are confused or very distressed, firm and authoritative.

Two skills in which counselors are trained may be of particular help to people in the aftermath of trauma. The first is *psychoeducation*, which involves providing information about the psychological effects of trauma and ways of coping. This information helps affected individuals understand that their reactions are normal and guides them with respect to how best to cope in practical ways. Most people can benefit from this kind of intervention. The second counseling skill involves *encouraging people to tell the story* of the traumatic event and to express and understand their emotional responses. However, not all those exposed to trauma need this kind of intervention and resilient individuals often recover on their own. Trying to impose this kind of counseling can therefore be unwelcome and even harmful (Bonanno, 2004). However, it does not mean that this kind of counseling has no place in the aftermath of a trauma and it is important to identify individuals who may need further psychological help as early as possible (van Wyk & Edwards, 2005).

Counseling interventions in the early stages have often been termed *debriefing*, a word that originates in the military context where individuals may not want to be thought of as needing counseling. Debriefing refers to a range of interventions designed to help individuals come to terms with traumatic events because there is the risk that those exposed to repeated traumas and who do cope by avoiding thinking about them may eventually crack, as in the case of the policeman described earlier in this chapter. A particularly comprehensive program was developed for emergency services personnel by Mitchell and Everly (1995) and more recently a similar approach called "post-traumatic stress management" (PTSM) was developed by Macy, Behar, Paulson, Delman, Schmid, and Smith (2004) for intervention on a community-wide basis in Boston in the United States of America.

Assessment and Treatment of Persons Negatively Affected by a Traumatizing Event

As we have seen, the majority of those affected by trauma may not need specialized treatment but those who have severe symptoms can benefit from systematic psychological intervention. Edwards (2009) observes that counselors, who look at the literature, may be confused by what appears to be a bewildering array of treatment approaches. They may read about "psychodynamic therapy," "narrative therapy," "eye-movement desensitization and reprocessing," "exposure therapy," "cognitive therapy," and "cognitive–behavior therapy." However, Edwards argues that over the past twenty years, there has been considerable integration of different treatment techniques in most of the main approaches, so that what is more striking is the commonalities between the different approaches rather than the differences between them. On

Case Study 15.5: Trauma Support after an Industrial Accident

Workers at a factory in South Africa were thrown into shock when a fellow worker's head was blown off in an accidental explosion. The counselor called to assist started by carefully assessing the needs of staff at different levels of the organization. As an initial response to the trauma, psychological interventions were planned to take place over five sessions. Most members were given psychoeducation about the effects of such a trauma in the form of a group presentation. However, senior management not only had to deal with their own trauma; but they also had to handle official legal processes and facilitate a supportive process for their employees. Therefore, they received separate psychoeducation, some of which was given individually, on how to respond to the needs of their staff and workers. There were marked differences in how individuals were affected. Not surprisingly, those who had witnessed the accident or knew the victim well were more vulnerable; several individuals were very strongly affected emotionally and some were given sick leave. By contrast, many employees adopted a supportive and caring role toward those who were showing distress. An important aspect, of response to the event, was a memorial service held in the factory and the presence of senior management at the funeral of the dead man held in his rural home district. As a result of these absences, the factory was partially closed down for several days and production gradually resumed as staff returned. Counseling was offered both in groups and individually. It was voluntary, and those who attended expressed appreciation and found it helpful. One of the senior managers felt particularly responsible for what had happened, although there was no evidence that he had been negligent, or that his feelings of guilt were reality based. He continued in counseling for several months after the accident.

Question

1. Consider how each of the following might make a different kind of contribution to helping people cope with a situation like this: (a) individual counseling, (b) holding a memorial service, and (c) a psychoeducational presentation on the normal typical ways in which people respond to a trauma.

this basis, he proposed an integrative model that we present at the end of this chapter.

Appraising the Situation: Psychological Assessment

Before proceeding with treatment, it is useful to do a thorough psychological assessment to gain a full understanding of the difficulties the client is facing and his or her links to past traumatic events. This can take several hours, as will the treatment, so it is important to establish that the client understands this and is motivated to come for several visits. A diagnostic assessment is needed to determine whether clients have PTSD and what symptoms they have. This calls for direct and careful questioning, as they will not normally list their symptoms in the way they appear in the *DSM-IV* or ICD-10. It is also important to check whether clients are also depressed. A large proportion of clients with PTSD also suffer from depression and the hopelessness, helplessness, and inactivity associated with this will need to be addressed in treatment planning. It is also important to check whether the client is suicidal and to do crisis intervention if he or she is. Additionally, it is important to investigate whether there were psychological problems before the trauma, as this will mean that treatment will probably be longer and more complex. In particular, clients should be questioned about previous abuse and trauma, previous episodes of depression, and alcohol or drug dependence or abuse.

Furthermore, it is important to establish the personal meanings associated with the traumatic event, as these vary from person to person. *Peritraumatic appraisals* are those experienced while the trauma is taking place. For a woman who has been raped, for example, these might include, "I am completely helpless," "I am dirty and contaminated," "It's my own fault, I asked for it." During a hijacking, a man might think, "I am going to die," "I am not safe anywhere," "I am not the man I thought I was," "It's my fault that I did not look out more carefully." "I want to kill him (the hijacker)." *Posttraumatic appraisals* are thoughts and attitudes that clients have about themselves now, in the aftermath of the trauma. Some of these appraisals are in response to the symptoms of PTSD and depression they are dealing with. These might include thoughts like, "There's something wrong with me," "I'm not normal," "I should be over this by now," "I am going mad," "My life is over," or "I'll never be the same again." These appraisals underlie the range of different emotions associated with PTSD that we reviewed earlier. Knowing the link between an emotion and the associated appraisal makes it easier to target it in planning the treatment.

Posttraumatic appraisals may be easier to access than peritraumatic appraisals because the peritraumatic appraisals are embedded in the memory of the trauma that clients may be suppressing. These appraisals can be accessed in two ways: first, when the memory is involuntarily triggered and gives rise to reexperiencing, and second by having the client relive the traumatic event in the session. This means asking them to tell the story, with eyes closed, visualizing events and feeling the associated emotions. Some clients are able to do this quite early in the assessment. However, some may not be ready until the treatment is well underway. Many clients experience great relief after doing the reliving, as it shows them that they can tolerate the memory and survive it. However, it can be emotionally overwhelming and if not carefully managed, could result in a client leaving treatment altogether. Clients who are not ready for reliving can first be asked to tell the story in an emotionally detached manner. However, for some people, telling the story itself triggers reexperiencing.

Reliving allows the counselor to identify the most emotionally charged aspects of the memory. These "hotspots" are the key to treatment because the appraisals associated with them contribute to maintaining the PTSD. The reliving also provides an opportunity to assess whether there are any gaps in the trauma memory. Often clients will skip past the most intense moments and need to be brought back and asked to go over that section slowly. Sometimes, an intense part is dissociated and the client will appear not to remember it all. As these are the most intense hotspots, it is essential to recover them if treatment is to be successful (Grey, Holmes, & Brewin, 2001; Grey, Young, & Holmes, 2002).

Support and Trust in Treatment

Assessment and treatment are demanding for clients and it is important to assess how much social support they have. Ask whether they have friends or family members who are supportive, caring, and capable of empathy for what they are going through. If they have, you know that when they leave the session, they are going to a supportive setting. Those with little or no support may find it harder to cope between sessions. Find out, too, the extent to which they feel supported by you, the counselor. Usually it takes time for clients to learn they can trust the counselor to understand their experience without being judgmental or overwhelmed by the intensity of the trauma. The assessment process is not only about obtaining information, but also about building a working relationship with the client. Clients can only develop trust in counselors who are genuinely trustworthy. When working with trauma, counselors need to have real commitment to the client and be prepared to manage crisis situations if they arise. To work effectively with trauma, counselors need their own support systems, which need to include regular supervision and even their own personal therapy (Eagle, 2005).

Treatment Basics: The Role of Memory and Reintegration

Treatment usually involves reengaging with the emotionally distressing memory of the trauma. Unless this is done, the individual will continue to be vulnerable to PTSD symptoms in the future because of the nature of an important aspect of memory, called autobiographical memory. This complex cognitive structure encodes our life experience as an ongoing story. It includes some specific episodes that are important for our understanding of who we are, but much of it is abstracted and simplified and organized as a set of generalizations about how the world works and our place within it. Autobiographical memory gives us an ongoing sense of who we are, where we have come from, and where we are going. Most everyday events are automatically incorporated into autobiographical memory because they fit in with our ongoing story, or, if they don't fit in easily, we discuss them with friends and family until we can make some sense of them. But extreme events are not easily incorporated. They violate our assumptions about how the world works, and the associated emotions are so intense that we try to avoid thinking about them. They get dissociated, which means they are left out of autobiographical memory. But, they are not erased. Instead, the split-off memory is easily triggered by reminders of all sorts and it is this that gives rise to reexperiencing symptoms and the sense that the event is still alive in the present. Unless they can be integrated into autobiographical memory, individuals remain vulnerable to developing PTSD, and avoidance has the effect of maintaining the problem indefinitely (Ehlers & Clark, 2000).

The goal of treatment is to facilitate the integration of the trauma memory into autobiographical memory so it can take its place there as another event that happened in the past. Clients must give up all avoidances (thought suppression, avoiding triggers, etc.). They are therefore asked to tell the therapist the whole story of what happened. They may also write it down as a narrative between sessions. They are encouraged to do a reliving of the trauma to ensure that all hotspots are identified and understood. Where appropriate, the therapist may go with them to where the trauma occurred so they can reconstruct it in detail (Ehlers, Clark, Hackmann, McManus, & Fennell, 2005). Specific exercises can be given to reduce the power of triggers. Zanele's (see Case Study 15.2) therapist brought a man into the session so that his presence would trigger her images of her rapist. Zanele was then encouraged to look carefully and see that it was not the rapist but a completely different person. This helped to eliminate intrusions at school.

Individualizing the Treatment

In addition, the meaning behind each of the intense emotions (fear, anger, guilt, shame, etc.) must be identified and altered in a more realistic and positive direction. In the process of reliving, some disturbing emotions may resolve themselves automatically. For example, a client who had a motor vehicle accident will recognize that much of the time it is safe to travel in a car. A man who was hijacked will recognize that if he takes care, most of the time he will be safe. However, some meanings need active work if they are to shift. If a rape survivor feels guilty that maybe she invited the rape by the way she dressed, the counselor

Case Study 15.6: Children's Accelerated Trauma Treatment (CATT) for PTSD in Rwanda

As an eighteen-year-old, Jean-Claude, a Rwandan teacher, witnessed a horrifying atrocity in which four close relatives were killed. Several years later, he attended a Luna Children's Charity training week on addressing PTSD, which is still widespread there, following the 1990 genocide. Although wanting to help others, he still suffered PTSD himself. After receiving psychoeducation on the effects of trauma on children, he was invited to experience the CATT technique, which involves playing out the whole episode very rapidly using toys and figures that participants make themselves. Using a truck, a boy figurine from the toy box, and four characters made of craft materials, leaves, and dried grass, Jean-Claude played out the events. Hutu militia had hoisted him onto a truck, tied up his relatives with rope, and transported them all to a trench. Jean-Claude was thrown off the truck and watched as his relatives were chopped in half with machetes and hurled into the trench. He ran until he realized he was safe. In playing out his story, his heart rate increased at the point where they were killed, but his intense focus on playing out what happened protected him from being overwhelmed; and he continued to a point where he realized that he had survived. Next, he played the episode backwards from the point he had survived to a point where he was with his family and nothing terrible had yet happened. This process involved sticking the broken figures back together and transporting them back to how they were at the beginning! Rewinding his story at speed inhibited his emotions so he did not become overwhelmed. Asked to repeat the process again, once forwards and again backwards, Jean-Claude now told the story in quite a philosophical way, with little emotion. The intervention had enabled him to incorporate what had happened into autobiographical memory, so that he now experienced it as in the past, and knew that he was alive and able to carry on with his life.

Later, workshop participants spoke together about their stories. For some, it was the first time they had described the traumatizing events they had been through without experiencing flashbacks and being overwhelmed. Afterwards, they were able to use CATT with children and adolescents in their local areas and reported extremely successful results.

Contributed by Carly Raby, Founder of Luna Children's Charity www.lunachildren.org.uk

Questions

1. How much training do people need to offer counseling to those with PTSD; and what factors would be important in training?
2. Why might using play materials be of value in working with PTSD?

needs to challenge this perception actively and remind her that men have no right to force themselves on women and when they do it is a criminal offense. If she feels shame, it will be important to affirm that she has nothing to be ashamed of; it is the rapist who committed the shameful act. If she feels a helpless victim, it will be important to help her to look after herself in the future by becoming more assertive or even taking self-defence classes. Langu felt angry about his brother's death and the therapist actively worked to help him to accept that there are some things over which he had no control and to start to mourn for his dead brother. In such cases, psychological interventions for working with bereavement (Boelen, van den Hout, & van den Bout, 2006; Shear, Frank, Houck, & Reynolds, 2005) can be incorporated into treatment.

Because these interventions can evoke intense distress, it is important that the counselor attends to three factors to manage it. First, a great deal of psychoeducation must be given about PTSD and the healing process so clients can understand how this painful process will help them recover. Second, clients need to have control over the pace of exposure to the traumatic material. They can be told what options there are and be invited to choose one they feel they can handle. For example, some willingly do a reliving early in the process. Others need to tell the story in a more detached manner before being ready to evoke all the intense emotions. Third, clients need to learn that they can trust the counselor to remain empathic, to care for them, and to guide them from one step to another (Ehlers et al., 2005).

Finally, the goal of therapy is for clients to rebuild their lives and see a meaningful future. Those who have withdrawn from friends or hobbies should be encouraged to reengage. Where the trauma has left individuals disabled, they may need to be guided to adjust to their disability. Where a loved one has died, as in the case of Langu, they may need help to mourn them. At the end of therapy, the counselor can feel pleased if, instead of saying, "I'll never be the same again," the client can say, as Grace did to her therapist, something like: "I've grown from this. Because of what happened I am a more mature and stronger person." This is called posttraumatic growth (Calhoun & Tedeschi, 2006).

An Integrative Model for Guiding Intervention

Trauma counseling is a complex field because of the wide range of traumatizing events, the large individual differences in how individuals respond to them, and the fact that sometimes counselors deal with individuals in the immediate aftermath of a trauma while at others they may help those suffering the effects of trauma experienced months or years before. This means that there is no fixed way for counselors to respond when helping a traumatized person. What will be appropriate and helpful depends on the circumstances and context.

However, the literature contains many useful guiding principles that Edwards (2009, 2010) has synthesized into the model in Figure 15.1, based on work in South Africa with Black Africans. It is drawn from experience with treating and supervising cases like that of Langu, Grace, and Zanele referred to earlier. It is also compatible with the experiences reflected in the international literature on trauma. It is based on two central ideas. First, there are stages in addressing trauma. This insight goes back as far as the French psychologist Janet a century ago, who identified three stages: (1) stabilization and symptom-oriented treatment, (2) exploration of traumatic events, and (3) personality reintegration and rehabilitation (Herman, 2001). Modern trauma experts describe very similar stages (Ford, Courtois, Steele, van der Hart, & Nijenhuis, 2005; Herman, 2001; Phillips & Frederick, 1995). In the model, the three levels represent stages: (1) crisis intervention and stabilization; (2) promoting engagement with treatment; and (3) selection, sequencing, and timing of active treatment interventions. The second idea is that there are different areas of clinical focus (CF) that may be appropriate when working with trauma survivors. In the model, there are seven CFs in the numbered boxes.

Depending on circumstances, counselors need to move responsively between these CFs, and although the model does not tell counselors exactly when to move from one to another, it can guide them in two important ways. First, it reminds them that the kind of intervention they should be focusing on depends on the level or stage. Second, it reminds them that resolving problems at the lower levels provides a foundation for work at the higher levels. For example, the difficult work of retelling or reliving a trauma (CF6) and reevaluating problematic appraisals requires a foundation of stability (Level 1), an understanding on the part of the client of the reason that this is likely to be helpful, and trust in the counselor (Level 2). Where these foundations are established, traumatized individuals can sometimes move to Level 3 quite quickly. Where there is an inadequate foundation at Levels 1 and 2, it is difficult to be effective in the healing and rebuilding work of Level 3, and embarking on it may even be counterproductive.

The model incorporates elements emphasized by differing approaches to trauma counseling. Thus, Level 1 incorporates what we have learned about crisis intervention and trauma support (van Wyk & Edwards, 2005). At Level 2, CF5, with its focus on the relationship, is an area that psychodynamic therapists have focused on a great deal (Schottenbauer, Glass, Arnkoff, & Gray, 2008). At Level 3, CF6, which involves using interventions designed to promote the integration of the trauma memory into autobiographical memory, allows for a wide range of methods for achieving this, including not only telling the trauma narrative and reliving the trauma, but also drawing, painting, and other expressive methods.

ISSUES FOR RESEARCH AND OTHER FORMS OF SCHOLARSHIP

A growing awareness of and interest in trauma and its psychological impact has led to a number of institutes and organizations dedicated to research and practice in the field, many of them in Africa. The classification of PTSD and similar conditions within medical diagnostic systems such as the DSM and ICD has led to an intensification of research into its effects on health and well-being. Research in Africa could best focus on how local contextual social and cultural factors affect behavior and experience after exposure to single or repeated traumatizing events.

An important research area is how people are affected by trauma and how they cope. Qualitative studies that investigate individuals' experiences in depth are more likely to yield information useful to counselors than quantitative multivariate studies that often yield results that are too generalized to be applied directly. Of particular importance is the study of the impact of trauma on vulnerable groups such as children and women. Gender-based violence is a widespread problem, and groups like Black lesbian women are often brutally victimized (Arndt & Hewat, 2009). Many groups of children in Africa and the African Diaspora are vulnerable. Thus, a study in the Western Cape of South Africa of the relative impact on children of witnessing a crime, being victim of crime, and perpetrating a crime found that the majority of children had experiences in more than one category (Nadasen & Pierce, 2009). There is considerable scope for documenting children's responses to domestic abuse, to continuing violence in schools from peers and from teachers, and more extreme situations such as military involvement. The negative psychological impact of cultural practices such as female genital mutilation, circumcision (which can be botched), and child marriage also deserves more research attention (Rembe & Odeku, 2009).

There is a need for local studies on the effectiveness of different kinds of intervention ranging from public and social interventions and brief counseling, to more structured psychotherapy. Internationally, there is no shortage of authoritative guidelines for treatment. Extensive guidelines published in 1999 stimulated further research that led to publication of further treatment guidelines by the International Society for Traumatic Stress Studies, most of which are based on professional practice and research in Western contexts between 2000 and 2007 (Courtois & Ford, 2009). Particularly challenging is research on assessment and intervention for complex traumatic stress disorders where the effects of prolonged trauma are very pervasive and management and treatment very resource

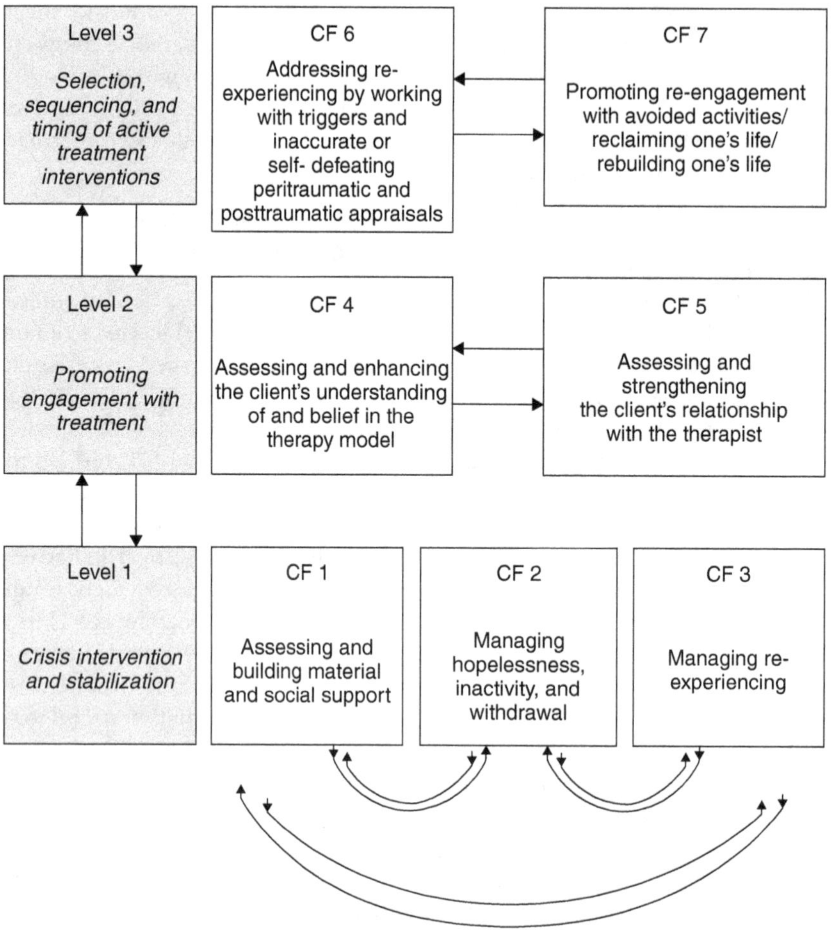

Figure 15.1. A model for evidence-based responsive treatment planning for PTSD. (First published in the *Journal of Psychology in Africa* [Edwards, 2009] and reproduced with permission.)

intensive (Courtois & Ford, 2009). Research on developing and evaluating training programs for counselors in different local contexts would also be of value.

SUMMARY AND CONCLUSION

People vary considerably in their responses in the immediate aftermath of traumatic events, as well as in the ensuing months and years. However, there are broad patterns of response that provide the basis for such diagnostic categories as ASR or PTSD, although comorbid disorders, especially depression, are common. Some people show remarkable resilience in the face of traumatic events and may even grow stronger and more mature as a result of extreme experiences (posttraumatic growth). It is important for counselors to be aware of the different kinds of intervention that might be appropriate in different contexts, ranging form crisis intervention and trauma support in the immediate aftermath of a trauma to long-term psychotherapy for individuals who have longstanding problems related to exposure to multiple traumatic events. Where large numbers are affected as a result of such events as natural disasters, large-scale accidents that affect whole communities, or civil war or civil disturbance, helping responses need to be planned on a community-wide basis, not just directed at individuals.

When working with individuals, there is a great deal of information in the literature to guide assessment and the planning of interventions, some of which is summarized in the present chapter. There is considerable evidence for the successful application of these approaches in Africa. Where individuals show the classic signs of PTSD with reexperiencing, avoidance, and hypervigilance, this indicates that the trauma memory has not been integrated into autobiographical memory and interventions are designed to correct this. However, other factors also need to be addressed such as inactivity, avoidance, social isolation, and mistrust. In particular, if individuals are to come to terms with the suffering caused by trauma, they often need to form a trusting relationship with a counselor who can guide them through what is often a painful and challenging process.

REFERENCES

American Psychiatric Association (2000). *DSM-IV-TR: Diagnostic and statistical manual of mental disorders (4th ed.): Text revision*. Washington, DC: Author.

Amunga, J., Maiyoa, J., Achokaa, J., & Ashioya, I. (2009). Violence against children and the effect on education. *Journal of Psychology in Africa, 19*, 119–22.

Arndt, M., & Hewat, H. (2009). The experience of stress and trauma: Black lesbians in South Africa. *Journal of Psychology in Africa, 19*, 207–12.

Barbarin, O. A., Richter, L., & de Wet, T. (2001). Exposure to violence, coping resources, and psychological adjustment of South African Children. *American Journal of Orthopsychiatry, 71*, 16–25.

Boelen, P. A., van den Hout, M. A., & van den Bout, J. (2006). A cognitive-behavioural conceptualization of complicated grief. *Clinical Psychology: Science and Practice, 13*, 109–28.

Bonanno, G. (2004). Loss, trauma and human resilience: Have we underestimated the human capacity to thrive after extremely aversive events? *American Psychologist, 59*(1), 20–8.

Boscarino, J. A. (1995). Post-traumatic stress and associated disorders among Vietnam veterans: The significance of combat exposure and social support. *Journal of Traumatic Stress, 8*, 317–66.

Boulind, M., & Edwards, D. J. A. (2008). The assessment and treatment of post-abortion syndrome: A clinical case study from Southern Africa. *Journal of Psychology in Africa, 18*, 539–48.

Caffo, E., Forresi, B., & Lievers, L. S. (2005). Impact, psychological sequelae and management of trauma: Impact and psychological sequelae. *Current Opinion in Psychiatry, 18*(4), 422–8.

Calhoun, L. G., & Tedeschi, R. G. (2006). *Handbook of posttraumatic growth: Research and practice*. Mahwah, NJ: Lawrence Erlbaum.

Chapman, D. P., Dube, S. R., & Anda, R. F. (2007). Adverse childhood events as risk factors for negative mental health outcomes. *Psychiatric Annals, 37*(5), 359–64.

Courtois, C. A., & Ford, J. D. (Eds.). (2009). *Treating complex traumatic stress disorders: An evidence-based guide*. New York: Guilford Press.

Dawes, A., & Donald, D. (Eds). (1994). *Childhood and adversity: Psychological perspectives from South African research*. Cape Town: David Philip.

Dawes, A., Tredoux, C., & Feinstein, A. (1989). Political violence in South Africa: Some effects on children of the violent destruction of their community. *International Journal of Mental Health, 18*, 16–43.

Eagle, G. T. (1998). An integrative model for brief term intervention in the treatment of psychological trauma. *International Journal of Psychotherapy, 3*, 1–11.

Eagle, G. T. (2000). The shattering of the stimulus barrier: The case for an integrative approach for short-term treatment for psychological trauma. *Journal of Psychotherapy Integration, 10*, 301–24.

Eagle, G. T. (2004). Therapy at the cultural interface: Implications of African cosmology for traumatic stress intervention. *Psychology in Society, 30*, 1–22.

Eagle, G. T. (2005). Grasping the thorn: The impact and supervision of post-traumatic stress therapy in the South African context. *Journal of Psychology in Africa, 15*(2), 197–207.

Edwards, D. J. A. (2005a). Critical perspectives on research on post-traumatic stress disorder and implications for the South African context. *Journal of Psychology in Africa, 15*(2), 117–24.

Edwards, D. J. A. (2005b). Post-traumatic stress disorder as a public health concern in South Africa. *Journal of Psychology in Africa, 15*(2), 125–34.

Edwards, D. J. A. (2005c). Treating PTSD in South African contexts: A theoretical framework and a model for developing evidence-based practice. *Journal of Psychology in Africa, 15*(2), 209–20.

Edwards, D. J. A. (2009). Treating posttraumatic stress disorder in South Africa: An integrative model grounded in case-based research. *Journal of Psychology in Africa, 19*(2), 189–98.

Edwards, D. J. A. (2010). Using systematic case studies to investigate therapist responsiveness: Examples from a case series of PTSD treatments. *Pragmatic Case Studies in Psychotherapy, 6*, Module 4, Article 3, 255–75. Retrieved from http://pcsp.libraries.rutgers.edu/index.php/pcsp/article/view/1047/2459

Edwards, D. J. A., Sakasa, P., & van Wyk, G. (2005). Trauma, resilience and vulnerability to PTSD: A review and clinical case analysis. *Journal of Psychology in Africa, 15*(2), 143–53.

Ehlers, A., & Clark, D. M. (2000). A cognitive model of posttraumatic stress disorder. *Behaviour Research and Therapy, 38*, 319–45.

Ehlers, A., Clark, D. M., Hackmann, A., McManus, F., & Fennell, M. (2005). Cognitive therapy for post-traumatic stress disorder: Development and evaluation. *Behaviour Research and Therapy, 43*, 413–31.

Ensink, K., Robertson, B. A., Zissis, C., & Leger, P. (1997). Posttraumatic stress disorder in children exposed to violence. *South African Medical Journal, 87*, 1526–30.

Eriksson, M., & Lindström, B. (2005). Validity of Antonovsky's Sense of Coherence scale: A systematic review. *Journal of Epidemiology and Community Health, 59*, 460–6.

Foa, E. B., & Rothbaum, B. O. (1998). *Treating the trauma of rape: Cognitive-behavioral therapy for PTSD*. New York: Guilford Press.

Ford, J. D., Courtois, C. A., Steele, K., van der Hart, O., & Nijenhuis, E. (2005). Treatment of complex traumatic self-dysregulation. *Journal of Traumatic Stress, 18*, 437–47.

Gist, R., & Woodall, S. J. (1999). There are no simple solutions to complex problems: The rise and fall of critical incident stress debriefing as a response to occupational stress in the fire service. In R. Gist & B. Lubin (Eds.), *Response to disaster: Psychosocial, community, and ecological approaches* (pp. 211–35). New York: Brunner Mazel.

Grey, N., Holmes, E., & Brewin, C. R. (2001). Peritraumatic emotional 'hotspots' in memory. *Behavioural and Cognitive Psychotherapy, 29*, 357–62.

Grey, N., Young, K., & Holmes, E. (2002). Cognitive restructuring within reliving a treatment for peritraumatic emotional "hotspots" in posttraumatic stress disorder. *Behavioural and Cognitive Psychotherapy, 30*, 37–56.

Grossman, A. B., Levin, B. E., Katzen, H. L., & Lechner, S. (2004). PTSD symptoms and onset of neurologic disease in elderly trauma survivors. *Journal of Clinical and Experimental Neuropsychology, 26*, 698–705.

Hamber, B. (2000). Have no doubt it is fear in the land: An exploration of the continuing cycles of violence in South Africa. *South African Journal of Child and Adolescent Mental Health, 12*(1), 5–18.

Hamber, B. (2004). The impact of trauma: A psychosocial approach. Keynote address to conference, *A shared practice – victims work in action*, April 7–8, 2004, Radisson Roe Park Hotel, Limavady, Northern Ireland.

Harvey, A. G., & Bryant, R. A. (2002). Acute stress disorder: A synthesis and critique. *Psychological Bulletin, 128*, 886–902.

Herbert, J. D., & Sageman, M. (2004). "First do no harm": Emerging guidelines for the treatment of posttraumatic reactions. In G. M. Rosen (Ed.), *Posttraumatic stress disorder: Issues and controversies* (pp. 213–32). New York: John Wiley & Sons.

Herman, J. L. (1995). Complex PTSD: A syndrome in survivors of prolonged and repeated trauma. In G. S. Everly & J. M. Lating (Eds.), *Psychotraumatology: Key papers and core concepts in post-traumatic stress* (pp. 87–100). New York: Plenum Press.

Herman, J. L. (2001). *Trauma and recovery: From domestic abuse to political terror*. London: Pandora.

Hirschowitz, R., & Orkin, M. (1997). Trauma and mental health in South Africa. *Social Indicators Research, 4,1* 169–82.

Jobson, L. & O' Kearney, R. T. (2009). Impact of cultural differences in self on cognitive appraisals in post-traumatic stress disorder. *Behavioural and Cognitive Psychotherapy, 37*, 249–66.

Jones, R., & Kagee, A. (2005). Predictors of post-traumatic stress symptoms among South African police personnel. *South African Journal of Psychology, 35*, 209–24.

Karpelowsky, B. J., & Edwards, D. J. A. (2005). Trauma, imagery and the therapeutic relationship: Langu's story. *Journal of Psychology in Africa, 15*(2), 185–95.

King, L. A., King, D. W., Fairbank, J. A., Keane, T. M., & Adams, G. A. (1998). Resilience/recovery factors in posttraumatic stress disorder among female and male Vietnam veterans: Hardiness, postwar social support and additional stressful life events. *Journal of Personality and Social Psychology, 74*, 420–34.

King, R. U. (2002). Trauma, healing and reconciliation in Rwanda. *International Journal of Disability, Community and Rehabilitation, 1*(3). Retrieved August 10, 2009 from http://www.ijdcr.ca/VOL01_03_CAN/articles/king.shtml

Kobasa, S. C., Maddi, S. R., & Kahn, S. (1982). Hardiness and health: A prospective study. *Journal of Personality and Social Psychology, 42*, 168–77.

Koopman, C., Gore-Felton, C., Classen, C., Kim, P., & Spiegel, D. (2001). Acute stress reactions to everyday stressful life events among sexual abuse survivors with PTSD. *Journal of Child Sexual Abuse, 10*, 83–99.

Kopel, H., & Friedman, M. (1997). Posttraumatic stress symptoms in South African police exposed to violence. *Journal of Traumatic Stress, 41*, 307–17.

Kopel, H., & Friedman, M. (1999). Effects of exposure to violence in South African police. In J. M. Violanti & D. Paton (Eds.), *Police trauma: Psychological aftermath of civilian combat* (pp. 99–112). Springfield, IL: Charles C Thomas.

Lee, D. A., Scragg, P., & Turner, S. (2001). The role of shame and guilt in traumatic events: A clinical model of shame-based and guilt-based PTSD. *British Journal of Medical Psychology, 74*, 451–66.

Leibowitz-Levy, S. (2005). The role of brief term interventions with South African child trauma survivors. *Journal of Psychology in Africa, 15*(2), 155–63.

Litz, B. T., Gray, M. J., Bryant, R. A., & Adler, A. B. (2002). Early intervention for trauma: Current status and future directions. *Clinical Psychology: Science and Practice, 9*, 112–34.

Macy, R. D., Behar, L., Paulson, R., Delman, J., Schmid, L., & Smith, S. F. (2004). Community-based acute posttraumatic stress management: A description and evaluation of a psychosocial-intervention continuum. *Harvard Review of Psychiatry, 12*, 217–28.

Marais, A., & Stuart, A. D. (2005). The role of temperament in the development of post-traumatic stress disorder amongst journalists. *South African Journal of Psychology, 35*, 89–105.

Masten, A. S., & Coatsworth, J. D. (1998). The development of competence in favorable and unfavorable environments: Lessons from research on successful children. *American Psychologist, 53*, 205–20.

Mitchell, J. T., & Everly, G. S. (1995). Critical incident stress debriefing [CISD] and prevention of work related traumatic stress among high-risk occupational groups. In G. S. Everly & J. Lating (Eds.), *Psychotraumatology: Key papers and core concepts* (pp. 159–69). New York: Plenum Press.

Monnier, J., Elhai, J. D., Frueh, B. C., Sauvageot, J. A., & Magruder, K. M. (2002). Replication and expansion of findings related to racial differences in veterans with combat-related PTSD. *Depression and Anxiety Journal, 16*(2), 64–70.

Musisi, S. (2004). Mass trauma and mental health in Africa. *African Health Sciences, 4*(2), 80–2.

Nadasen, K., & Pierce, L. (2009). Relative impact of victimization and witnessing violence. A comparison of the effects of witnessing community violence and direct victimization among children in Cape Town, South Africa. *Journal of Interpersonal Violence, 24*(7), 1192–1208.

Nagel, B., Matsuo, H., McIntyre, K. P., & Morrison, N. (2005). Attitudes towards victims of rape. *Journal of Interpersonal Violence, 20*(6), 725–37.

Njenga, F. G., Nguithi, A. N., & Kang'ethe, R. N. (2006). Mental health consequences of war: A brief review of research findings. *World Psychiatry, 5*(1), 38–9.

Odejide, O. A., Sanda, O. A., & Odejide, I. O. (1998). Intergenerational aspects of ethnic conflict in Africa. In Y. Danieli (Ed.), *International handbook of multigenerational legacies of trauma* (pp. 373–85). New York: Plenum Press.

Onyut, L. P., Neuner, F., Schauer, E., Ertl, V., Odenwald, M., Schauer M., & Elbert, T. (2005). Narrative exposure therapy as a treatment for child war survivors with posttraumatic stress disorder: Two case reports and a pilot study in an African refugee settlement. *BMC Psychiatry, 5*(7). Retrieved August 5, 2009 from http://www.biomedcentral.com/1471-244X/5/7/

Payne, C. & Edwards, D. J. A. (2009). What services and supports are needed to enable trauma survivors to rebuild their lives? Implications of a systematic case study of cognitive therapy with a township adolescent girl with PTSD following rape. *Child Abuse Research in South Africa, 10*, 27–40.

Peltzer, K., & Chongo, A. (2000). Trauma and the rehabilitation of torture and violence victims in Mozambique. In S. N. Madu, P. K. Baguma, & A. Pritz (Eds.), *Psychotherapy and African reality* (pp. 74–94). Pietersburg: UNIN Press.

Peterson, L. R., & Roy, A. (1985). Religiosity, anxiety, and meaning and purpose: Religion's consequences for psychological well-being. *Review of Religious Research, 27*, 49–62.

Phillips, M., & Frederick, C. (1995). *Healing the divided self: Clinical and Ericksonian hypnotherapy for posttraumatic and dissociative conditions*. New York: W. W. Norton.

Ramphele, M. (1995). *Mamphela Ramphele: A life*. Cape Town: David Philip.

Rasool, S., Vermaak, K., Pharoah, R., Louw, A., & Stavrou, A. (2002). *Violence against women: A national survey*. Pretoria: Institute for Security Studies.

Rembe, S., & Odeku, K. (2009). Violation of children's rights by traditional cultural practices and the responses by states in Eastern and Southern Africa. *Journal of Psychology in Africa, 19*, 63–70.

Schnyder, U., & Moergeli, H. (2003). The course and development of early reactions to traumatic events: Baseline evidence from a non-intervention follow-up study. In R. Orner & U. Schnyder (Eds.), *Reconstructing early intervention after trauma* (pp. 106–17). Oxford: Oxford University Press.

Schottenbauer, M. A., Glass, C. R., & Arnkoff, D. B. (2008). Contributions of psychodynamic approaches to treatment of PTSD and trauma: A review of the empirical treatment and psychopathology literature. *Psychiatry: Interpersonal and Biological Processes, 71*, 13–34.

Seedat, S. (2004). Trauma exposure and post-traumatic stress symptoms in urban African schools: Survey in Cape Town and Nairobi. *The British Journal of Psychiatry*, *184*, 169–75.

Seedat, S., Nyamai, C., Njenga, F., Vythilingum, B., & Stein, D. J. (2004). Trauma exposure and post-traumatic stress symptoms in urban African schools: Survey in Cape Town and Nairobi. *British Journal of Psychiatry*, *184*, 169–75.

Seery, M. D., Holman, E. A., & Silver, R. C. (2010). Whatever does not kill us: Cumulative lifetime adversity, vulnerability, and resilience. *Journal of Personality and Social Psychology*, *99*(6), 1025–41.

Shear, M. K., Frank, E., Houck, P. R., & Reynolds, C. F. III. (2005). Treatment of complicated grief: A randomized controlled trial. *JAMA*, *293*, 2601–8.

Smith, C., & Holford, L. (1993). Posttraumatic stress disorder in South Africa's children and adolescents. *Southern African Journal of Child and Adolescent Psychiatry*, *5*, 57–69.

South African Advertising Research Foundation. (2006). All Media and Product Study Survey. Retrieved June 3, 2009 from http://www.saarf.co.za

South African Police Service Statistics. (2006). Retrieved April 23, 2009 from http://www.saps.gov.za/dynamicModules/internetsite/wphome.asp

Staab, J. P., Fullerton, C. S., & Ursano, R. (1999). A critical look at PTSD: Constructs, concepts, epidemiology, and implications. In R. Gist & B. Lubin (Eds.), *Response to disaster: Psychosocial, community, and ecological approaches* (pp. 101–27). New York: Brunner Mazel.

Stein, M. B., Walker, J. R., & Forde, D. R. (2000). Gender differences in susceptibility to posttraumatic stress disorder. *Behaviour Research and Therapy*, *38*, 619–28.

Stiles, W. B., Honos-Webb, L., & Surko, M. (1998). Responsiveness in psychotherapy. *Clinical Psychology: Science and Practice*, *5*, 439–58.

Strümpfer, D. J. W. (2003). Resilience and burnout: A stitch that could save nine. *South African Journal of Psychology*, *33*, 69–79.

Summerfield, D. (2001). The invention of post-traumatic stress disorder and the social usefulness of a psychiatric category. *British Medical Journal*, *322*, 95–8.

Swartz, L., & Levett, A. (1989). Political repression and children in South Africa: The social construction of damaging effects. *Social Science and Medicine*, *28*, 741–50.

Turshen, M., Meintjies, S., & Pillay, A. (Eds.). (2001). *Aftermath: Women in post-conflict transformation*. London: Zed.

van der Kolk, B. (2005). Developmental trauma disorder: Towards a rational diagnosis for children with complex trauma histories. *Psychiatric Annals*, *35*(5), 401–8.

van Wyk, G., & Edwards, D. J. A. (2005). From trauma debriefing to trauma support: A South African experience of responding to individuals and communities in the aftermath of traumatizing events. *Journal of Psychology in Africa*, *15*, 135–42.

Ward, C. L., Lombard, C., & Gwebushe, N. (2008). Critical incident exposure in South African emergency services personnel: Prevalence and associated mental health issues. *British Medical Journal*, *23*, 226–31.

Williams, M. B., & Sommer, J. J. (2002). *Simple and complex post-traumatic stress disorder: Strategies for comprehensive treatment in clinical practice*. New York: Guilford Press.

World Health Organization (WHO). (1992). *The ICD-10 classification of mental and behavioural disorders: clinical descriptions and diagnostic guidelines*. Geneva: Author.

Yehuda, R., Flory, J. D., Southwick, S., & Charney, D. S. (2006). Developing an agenda for translational studies of resilience and vulnerability following trauma exposure. *Annals of the New York Academy of Sciences*, *1071*, 379–96.

SELF-CHECK EXERCISES

1. Distinguish between acute stress disorder (ASD) and posttraumatic stress disorder (PTSD).
2. Give four examples of intense anxiety responses.
3. Distinguish between the criteria used by the ICD-10 and the DSM in their classification of psychological responses to a traumatizing event.
4. Mention three types of symptoms that may persist beyond the initial intense stress response.
5. Give three reasons to explain why civil unrest may increase trauma incidences.
6. Mention five possible emotional responses to trauma.
7. Mention at least three factors that make a person vulnerable to developing PTSD.
8. What is delayed onset PTSD and when is it likely to appear?
9. Briefly describe the symptoms of dissociation and mention five examples.
10. What are some of the possible results of prolonged exposure to trauma for adults and for children?
11. Mention at least three factors that promote resilience in people exposed to trauma.
12. What is the difference between peritraumatic and posttraumatic appraisals?
13. Mention two differences that could be seen in persons of non-Western culture experiencing PTSD.
14. Mention two skills that can be used in the immediate aftermath of a traumatic incident when treating persons affected.
15. Mention two ways in which peritraumatic appraisals may be accessed if they become suppressed.
16. What are the two central ideas upon which Edwards based his model for PTSD treatment?
17. List the stages of trauma treatment of Edwards' model.
18. Without looking at your textbook, draw a diagram illustrating Edwards' evidence-based responsive treatment planning for PTSD.

FIELD-BASED EXPERIENTIAL EXERCISES

1. Volunteer at a local organization caring for children or young people in need such as street children and HIV/AIDS orphans or place of safety. You will need to work within the limitations of the regulations of the law and of the organization. Keep a journal of your experiences and reflections on your interactions and observations.
2. Take out and watch one or more of the following movies portraying PTSD or psychological effects of traumatic events:
   Hotel Rwanda
   Birdy

Fearless
The Fisher King
Once Were Warriors
Blue
Empire of the Sun
Sophie's Choice
In the Valley of Elah
The Deer Hunter
Thin Red Line

Identify traumatizing events for the character(s). Identify stress reactions within the affected character(s) in the film. Relate these to the symptoms and diagnoses discussed in the chapter.

3. Search the same three local or national daily newspapers for a week. Note any reports about events that you believe could have produced posttraumatic stress symptoms for the persons involved. Keep a record of how many incidents are reported. Note the language used by the reports describing the events. Draw up a table of statistics of your own showing the frequency of different types of incidents.
4. Contact a local branch of a crisis center and ask permission to interview the manager or one of the counselors. Find out about the types of crises that present at the center. Ask about debriefing and follow-up procedures for both the clients and also for any counselors who feel burnt out or affected by the work they do.
5. Some police stations and also some emergency service providers allow persons to spend a day with them "on duty" to observe the work they do. Contact your local service points of your choice and find out if this is possible. If you do this task, reflect on your experiences in a journal.

MULTIPLE-CHOICE QUESTIONS

1. The major difference between ASD and PTSD is:
   a. ASD is part of the ICD-10 classification system whereas PTSD is part of the DSM.
   b. ASD is a severe response in the immediate aftermath of a trauma.
   c. ASD does not include dissociative symptoms.
   d. PTSD includes reexperiencing, withdrawal, and somatoform disorders.
2. Civil unrest may increase trauma incidences because:
   a. Warfare is always traumatic.
   b. Civil unrest, by nature, is accompanied by violence.
   c. Social structures are interrupted.
   d. People become more vulnerable to trauma during civil unrest.
3. Some of the emotional responses to trauma can leave a victim of trauma:
   a. Vulnerable to depression
   b. With long-term memory loss
   c. Vulnerable to psychosis
   d. Physically ill
4. Studies in *resilience* show that those who coped well with stressful situations at first, were *likely* to:
   a. Continue to cope poorly
   b. Continue to cope well in the future
   c. Develop delayed onset PTSD
   d. Have recovered well from PTSD in the past
5. Delayed onset PTSD occurs more *typically*:
   a. After natural disasters
   b. As a result of childhood trauma
   c. In people with a history of resilience
   d. In cases of sexual assault
6. During the treatment process of reliving the traumatic event, a "hotspot" refers to:
   a. The client's exhaustion point in therapy
   b. An emotionally charged theme in the memory
   c. Sign that a memory is being suppressed
   d. The point in the trauma story at which the client should begin
7. Sometimes peritraumatic appraisals are difficult to access because:
   a. Clients confuse them with posttraumatic appraisals.
   b. The treatment is focused on the here and now.
   c. They are embedded in the memory of the trauma that clients may be suppressing.
   d. They can emerge only in dreams.
8. One of the major goals of PTSD treatment is to:
   a. Integrate distressing memories into autobiographical memory
   b. Relive the event before it is integrated into autobiographical memory
   c. Effectively dissociate distressing memories
   d. Recover all dissociated memories
9. *Posttraumatic growth* refers to:
   a. An increased intensity in trauma symptoms
   b. The noted increase in traumatic incidences in the world
   c. A statistical change in traumatic events reported
   d. A sense of having become stronger from the experience of trauma
10. Edwards' model of treatment for PTSD is based on two central ideas which are that:
    a. There are different stages in addressing trauma; there are several different areas of potential clinical focus
    b. Posttraumatic memories need to be uncovered; peritraumatic memories are embedded in autobiographical memory
    c. Dissociated memories need to be triggered; peritraumatic memories need to be integrated into autobiographical memory
    d. The therapist proceeds sequentially through areas of clinical focus; triggers for reexperiencing need to be extinguished

Answers to the multiple-choice questions are provided at the back of the book

16 HIV and AIDS Counseling

Lisa Lopez Levers, Elias Mpofu, Ronél Ferreira, and Joseph M. Kasayira

OVERVIEW. All African countries and communities currently face the challenge of dealing effectively with the HIV and AIDS pandemic. Despite countless efforts and initiatives to support communities in dealing with this challenge, African communities often are characterized by a lack of sufficient services and outside support. This chapter provides an overview of typical ways of counseling people infected with and affected by HIV and AIDS in the African context. The role of community-based resources, including governmental and nongovernmental organizations (NGOs), is surveyed. HIV and AIDS counseling roles that go beyond voluntary testing and counseling (VTC) are explained, such as the provision of support to vulnerable individuals, families, and communities. The chapter also highlights a variety of formal and informal actors who potentially may fulfill a counseling role; these include teachers, nurses, family members, spiritual leaders, village chiefs, and people in other helping professions. An overview of leading themes in HIV and AIDS research is presented, including typical practices in HIV and AIDS counseling in the African context.

LEARNING OBJECTIVES

By the end of the chapter, the reader should be able to:

1. Outline the counseling needs of those infected with and affected by HIV and AIDS in the sub-Saharan African context.
2. Compare and contrast traditional and contemporary responses to the HIV and AIDS pandemic, with specific reference to African communities.
3. Explain the extent and nature of support required by people living with HIV and AIDS.
4. Describe the various roles that professional counselors might fulfill in providing care and support to people living with HIV and AIDS.
5. Discuss the major behavioral and social science trends in research concerning HIV and AIDS.
6. Identify other professionals or paraprofessionals who readily might be positioned to assume some counseling-related duties as "lay counselors."

INTRODUCTION

The ripples of HIV and AIDS have reached nations across the globe. Sayson and Meya (2001, p. 542) summarized the global impact of the pandemic in the following way: "As when a stone is dropped into a pool, ripples from AIDS move to the very edge of society, affecting first just one person in a family, then the entire family, then the community, and finally the nation." Sub-Saharan Africa has been hardest hit by the multiple ripples of the pandemic.

According to the UNAIDS' (2008) report, by the end of 2007, approximately 22 million people were living with HIV in the sub-Saharan region of Africa. This number accounts for two-thirds (67 percent) of the global total (32.9 million) of people living with HIV in the year 2007. During that same year (UNAIDS), an estimated 1.9 million people, in the region, were infected with HIV. Sub-Saharan Africa has the highest number of children living with HIV; 2 million of the world's 2.1 million children living with HIV at the end of 2007 lived in the region (World Health Organization [WHO], 2009). Also, sub-Saharan Africa has the highest number of children orphaned by AIDS, approximately 11.6 million children younger than the age of eighteen, who have lost one or both parents to AIDS (UNAIDS).

There were 1.5 million deaths in sub-Saharan Africa, during 2007, and that could be ascribed to AIDS-related illnesses; this accounts for 75 percent of the AIDS-related deaths, worldwide, in 2007 (UNAIDS, 2008). In 2003, more than 400,000 children younger than the age of fifteen died of AIDS in sub-Saharan Africa (Cabassi, 2004; Tindyebwa et al., 2004; UNAIDS/UNICEF/USAID, 2002; UNAIDS/WHO, 2005). Thus, the HIV and AIDS pandemic can be regarded as a cross-sectoral issue, having an impact on and posing challenges at numerous social service levels: health, economics, education, and agriculture, as well as in the private and public sectors (Brookes, Shisana, & Richter, 2004; Smart, 2003b).

Significant socioeconomic vulnerability has resulted from HIV and AIDS for many Africans (Lwanda, 2005; Republic of Malawi, 2004; University of Zimbabwe, 2003). The University of Zimbabwe publication (2003, p. 1) defined socioeconomic vulnerability "as a process in which people are subjected to economic and social re-engineering in such a manner that they are left with little or no options of pursuing sustainable socio-economic survival strategies."

Facing the challenges associated with HIV and AIDS necessitates responses on various levels and calls for the availability of support and counseling for individuals, within families, and within communities. The challenges posed by HIV and AIDS require a multisectoral, integrated response involving international, national, and regional actors from as many sectors of society as possible, including local communities.

National governments, NGOs, public sector, private sector, and people living with HIV and AIDS can complement their mutual initiatives and operate in a consolidated way, while protecting the human rights and dignity of the people involved (Brouard, Maritz, Pieterse, van Wyk, & Zuberi, 2005; Cabassi, 2004; Department of Economic and Social Affairs of the United Nations, 2005). However, despite the need for counseling, many people living with HIV and AIDS in sub-Saharan Africa experience difficulty in accessing support services in the form of professional counseling. As a result, family members and friends often need to respond immediately to the distress of significant others by providing first-level paraprofessional or informal counseling. In addition to family members, professionals such as teachers, community health workers, pastors, and other health-related personnel might take on the role of counseling, acting as lay counselors. This role is especially true in countries and communities with limited resources and external support, such as rural and informal settlement communities. Although well intended, such first-level responders often lack the adequate skills, knowledge bases, and technologies necessary to address the psychosocial needs of people living with HIV and AIDS. In counseling interventions to treat HIV and AIDS in African settings, both technical knowledge and cultural sensitivity are of paramount importance.

IMPORTANCE, DEFINITION, AND SCOPE OF KEY TERMS AND CONCEPTS

The ability to cope with and manage the various aspects of HIV and AIDS is essential to an effective community response to the pandemic. In this section, we briefly explain key concepts in understanding the psychosocial aspects of HIV and AIDS counseling. We consider, among other terms, concepts such as people infected with and affected by HIV and AIDS, vulnerability in the context of HIV and AIDS, psychosocial interventions to treat HIV and AIDS, and counseling that enhances strategies for coping.

People Infected with HIV and AIDS

The term "people infected with HIV" refers to people who are living with the human immunodeficiency virus. This virus actively infects certain protective cells (CD4-receptor cells, also called T-helper cells or CD4+ lymphocytes) that are a part of the body's immune system, by attaching to the cell, replicating, and going on to infect other cells. As the body's defense against infectious diseases becomes compromised, the immune system is rendered increasingly more "deficient." Generally, this process takes at least several years to progress. HIV is the retrovirus that causes AIDS; it is called a retrovirus because it replicates itself as part of the host cell's DNA.

Although early symptoms of HIV infection can mimic flulike symptoms, for most people, HIV infection is not apparent. In addition, a person can be HIV positive long before developing the symptoms associated with AIDS. As the virus progresses, the immune system is weakened and becomes vulnerable to opportunistic infections. To be diagnosed with AIDS, a person typically must have a T4 cell (CD4 cell) count of less than 200 per cubic millimeter of blood. A number of AIDS-associated diseases may affect the respiratory system, the gastrointestinal system, the central/peripheral nervous system, and the skin. A person can become infected through unsafe sex practices or as a result of unsafe health practices; these typically involve coming into direct contact (unprotected by a prophylactic, such as a condom during sex or gloves when caring for an infected person) with bodily fluids (blood or sexual fluids).

The biophysiological aspects of living with HIV and AIDS are numerous and well documented. From a behavioral or social science perspective, the psychosocial effects of living with HIV and AIDS are numerous, but have not been as definitively delineated, especially in relationship to African settings. One problem is that many (if not most) interventions have been based on Western biomedical paradigms, without giving sufficient consideration to the importance of local cultures.

People Affected by HIV and AIDS

The term "people affected by HIV and AIDS" refers to people whose lives have been touched, influenced, or changed in some way by another who is HIV-positive or who has AIDS. Often the consequences of HIV and AIDS are negative or harmful to another. For example, when an HIV-positive parent becomes ill, young children or other family members may need to take on additional responsibilities. Individuals, families, and communities may be affected by HIV and AIDS on a direct level by means of daily contact with HIV-infected people, by sharing their homes with orphaned children, or by way of participation in community programs addressing the needs of those infected with and affected by HIV and AIDS. On an indirect level, people are affected by the socioeconomic factors of the pandemic, such as weakening levels of education, health care, and social services. As a result, people from uninfected households in affected communities are inevitably affected by the HIV and AIDS pandemic, whether directly or indirectly.

Vulnerability

People who are living with or are affected by HIV and AIDS may experience vulnerability on multiple levels.

Information Box 16.1: Transmission of HIV

Please read the following two excerpts, and then address the questions and activities at the end of the information box.

Source A: Centers for Disease Control and Prevention (CDC). (2007). *HIV and its transmission*. Retrieved from http://www.cdc.gov/hiv/resources/factsheets/transmission.htm

The CDC states the following in its discussion, located on the CDC website, regarding the transmission of HIV:

HIV is spread by sexual contact with an infected person, by sharing needles and/or syringes (primarily for drug injection) with someone who is infected, or, less commonly (and now very rarely in countries where blood is screened for HIV antibodies), through transfusions of infected blood or blood clotting factors. Babies born to HIV-infected women may become infected before or during birth or through breastfeeding after birth.

Source B: Bernard, E. J. (2008, 16 May). *Texas jury concludes saliva of HIV-positive man a 'deadly weapon,' sentenced to 35 yrs jail*. Reported at aidsmap News. Retrieved September 7, 2009, from http://www.aidsmap.com/en/news/57E118E4-CC57-4C0E-A200-E7709A67AF1F.asp

The following excerpt is taken from a news report at aidsmap:

A forty-two-year-old HIV-positive man from Texas who spat at a police officer, during his 2006 arrest for being drunk and disorderly, has been sentenced to thirty-five years in prison by a Dallas court and must serve at least half of his sentence before being eligible for parole because the jury found that his saliva was a deadly weapon.

The case, which was reported by more than 175 news outlets yesterday, has outraged UK HIV organizations, particularly since only three reports – from *The New York Times*, *USA Today*, and the Mississippi *Clarion-Ledger* – actually mention that HIV cannot be transmitted via spitting.

"It is shocking that in the same country which has some of the most advanced research into HIV and its treatments, there can be such ignorance within the legal system as to how HIV is transmitted," said Deborah Jack, Executive Director of the National AIDS Trust. "This is not justice but a victory for fear, myth and prejudice. Such a verdict – contradicted by all the science – must constitute a breach of Mr Campbell's right to a fair trial."

Lisa Power, Head of Policy at Terrence Higgins Trust, added: "The saliva of someone with HIV is not a deadly weapon. Putting someone with HIV in a situation where they cannot access condoms, treatment is poor and they may have little choice about sexual activity is a far more dangerous thing to do, and US clinicians need to tell the Texas legal system so."

Questions

1. Discuss the ways identified by the CDC for transmission of HIV. How do these compare with the misunderstandings in the legal case?
2. How does such stigma and misinformation relate to counseling issues?
3. Identify and discuss some of the ways that professionally trained counselors can advocate for the rights of people living with HIV, especially in terms of accurate information.

Physical vulnerability is associated with painful symptoms and feelings of discomfort due to the disease. *Personal vulnerability* relates to an individual's experiences and emotional pain based on feelings such as anger, fear, loss, grief, denial, mood swings, low self-worth, powerlessness, and even depression. Finally, the fear of disclosing an HIV status, due to stigmatization and potential discrimination and isolation, often results in *social vulnerability*. The vulnerability experienced personally or socially can be as overwhelming as the physical vulnerability of the disease process, and in some instances, more so.

Children Affected by HIV and AIDS

As noted previously, the countries in sub-Saharan Africa, particularly in the southern region, have some of the highest prevalence rates of HIV and AIDS in the world. The HIV/AIDS pandemic has affected Africa's economic and social structures in multifaceted ways. One significant outcome of a pandemic, in which so many adults of child-bearing age have become ill or have died, is the number of children affected. Many children have been orphaned and left behind in varying degrees of vulnerability. Some have been left to live in poverty, some have become street children, and many are forced to live in deleterious circumstances where they are maltreated or otherwise exploited; these are highly vulnerable children who are also at risk of contracting HIV, and thus perpetuating the pandemic. An argument can be made that all children in African settings have been left vulnerable, as a consequence of the pandemic, and that they are all at high risk. This risk is compounded by certain cultural factors within various African societies, such as the proclivity for parents not to speak to children about matters regarding illness, death, and sexuality, as well as the proclivity for children not to speak to adults about any type of abuse.

Interventions

Community-focused interventions seem to be more robust in their effects than single-problem-focused interventions; yet, little research has been toward developing and applying such models (see Catalano, Berglund, Ryan, Lonczak, & Hawkins, 2004; National Research Council and Institute of Medicine, 2002). In this regard, interventions that focus on both reducing risks and enhancing protective factors appear to hold great promise. HIV and AIDS counseling interventions with people in sub-Saharan Africa must be designed to be socioculturally sensitive to be credible (Lynch & Levers, 2007).

Counseling people living with HIV and AIDS implies guidance and support on various levels. Professional counselors are expected to assist clients in dealing with their vulnerabilities and in coping with psychosocial challenges such as feeling incompetent to perform on expected levels, overcoming feelings of inadequacy, frustration and insecurity, fear, facing the possibility of death, and financial strain, to mention but a few. Based on the level of emotional and psychological stress people living with HIV and AIDS experience, they require care and support in the form of professional counseling; however, they may need continued support, additionally, which may take the form of lay or paraprofessional counseling.

Lay counselors

Lay counselors are people other than those primarily trained to provide such a service. Within the context of an indigenous community, any community member can fulfill a supportive role and provide assistance to others in need. Any activity that supports a person living with HIV and AIDS, in whichever manner is useful to the person, can be regarded as lay counseling. This lay counseling can include support in the form of merely listening and displaying empathy toward those in need. Also, it can include directed support initiatives such as organizing and facilitating a community support group for people facing challenges like HIV and AIDS. For many Africans, local traditional healers serve as de facto lay counselors (Levers, 2006; Levers & Maki, 1995; see also Chapter 1, this volume).

Anyone working as a lay counselor needs to possess accurate information about HIV and AIDS, which must be viewed as a prerequisite for taking up the role of a lay counselor. Fundamental information includes (1) both humane and hygienic ways of dealing with AIDS-related conditions, (2) facts regarding HIV transmission, (3) disease-specific nutritional concerns, (4) basic listening and communication skills, (5) emotional support, and (6) an understanding of available community resources.

Coping

Coping with HIV and AIDS implies an ability to deal with the various challenges related to the pandemic, such as grieving the loss of loved ones, as well as the physical and psychosocial symptoms associated with the condition. Furthermore, families living with HIV and AIDS need to cope with additional financial burdens placed upon them when individuals can no longer earn an income and have higher expenses due to treatment and basic health care (Nnko, Chiduo, Wilson, Msuya, & Mwaluko, 2000; Swanepoel, 2005).

Within the context of HIV and AIDS, coping implies a process whereby people are continually required to manage the challenges related to the pandemic – both the challenges experienced internally (such as feelings and perceptions) and those on an external level (like stigmatization and discrimination by other community members). Social support is a key concept in coping, as people facing challenging situations often rely on the support of others to cope. The construct of social support is thought to comprise three main areas: (1) concrete, tangible, and practical forms of support; (2) instrumental or informational support, in the form of advice; and (3) emotional support (Dillon & Brassard, 1999; Dirkzwager, Bramsen, & Van der Ploeg, 2003; Greenglas, 2002). The latter two facets of support in turn relate to counseling, which in many instances takes on the form of lay counseling by family members and friends, who are interdependent with others.

According to the interdependent-self approach to coping (Johnson & Johnson, 2002), individuals are involved in networks of reciprocal relationships with family members, friends, other community members (e.g., people at church and people in other walks of life such as teachers and other service personnel). When faced with stress, people rely on these social networks for support and the provision of resources. In this manner, coping is regarded as a joint process of problem solving with social support from networks of other people.

HISTORY OF RESEARCH AND PRACTICE IN HIV AND AIDS COUNSELING

When HIV and AIDS first emerged, African governments were slow to acknowledge the problem and take appropriate action, a clear indication that at least several African countries were unaware of the danger the disease caused to public health (AVERT, 2009; Lwanda, 2005; University of Zimbabwe, 2003). Discussion of HIV and AIDS was minimal, and government officials rarely addressed the subject in speeches. The traditions of silence and taboos surrounding issues related to HIV and AIDS, and the fact that the governments initially viewed the pandemic as a wholly medical problem, delayed early preventive education. For instance, Malawi's first short-term plan to combat HIV was designed mainly to ensure the screening of blood before transfusion. The country's first ten-year plan-of-action for medical research included sexually transmitted diseases (STDs) in priority areas, but did not mention HIV and AIDS at all (Lwanda, 2005).

The history of counseling research and practice associated with HIV and AIDS counseling is a brief one. As noted previously, in the past three decades, much of the HIV and AIDS research focused on etiology and aspects of medical treatment and care. Relatively little research addressed counseling issues, especially regarding the efficacy of modern counseling practices. However, in the past decade, there has been an impressive range of studies on the particular psychosocial constructs in prevention and care (e.g., Parker, Easton, & Klein, 2002; Quinn & Overbaugh, 2005; Uwimana & Struthers, 2007).

A full review of the entire spectrum of associated research is beyond the scope of this chapter; however, a perusal of the most frequently cited research literature in the behavioral and social sciences, related to HIV and AIDS in African settings, revealed the following themes: (1) Risk Behaviors and Contextual Factors; (2) Gender, Sexuality, and Sexual Violence; (3) Impact on the Family and Lifespan Issues; (4) Health Communication; (5) Prevention Programming; (6) Voluntary Counseling and Testing; (7) Stigma and HIV and AIDS; and, (8) Policy, Development, and Politics. The focus in this section is on providing an overview of these current research trends.

Risk Behaviors and Contextual Factors

The advent of HIV has caused decreasing life expectancy in countries throughout sub-Saharan Africa, with the high mortality burden expected to continue until a vaccine becomes available or changes occur in sexual habits (Walker, Walker, & Wadee, 2005). As early as 1990, researchers began to identify existing gaps in knowledge regarding the sociocultural concerns related to HIV and AIDS. According to Akeroyd (1997), many of the research priorities for behavioral and social aspects of HIV and AIDS in Africa were determined by the Global Program on AIDS, largely reflecting the interests of biomedical researchers, and thus limiting the range of areas explored. A major critique was that social and behavioral scientists often were relegated to data production rather than assisting with establishing important research agendas. Akeroyd called for a broader array of research methods capable of framing personal and social risk factors and other vulnerabilities that might be associated with the transmission of HIV.

Aggleton, O'Reilly, Slutkin, and Davies (1994) and Simbayi et al. (2007) reviewed research that examined the determinants of risk-related sexual behavior as these relate to the incidence of new cases of HIV. The studies revealed individual and social factors that influence risk taking. For instance, Aggleton et al. observed that educational and community-based interventions appeared to reduce the risk for HIV. Simbayi et al. noted that a high percentage of HIV-positive persons in South Africa did not disclose their status to their sexual partners, which increased risk to partners.

Although interventions that address risk behaviors are important, Cunha (2007) contended that the context in which such behaviors occur is vitally important. She examined literature reviews and identified three major determinants that have shaped the AIDS pandemic in developing country contexts: poverty, mobility, and gender inequity. Sociocultural biases toward females place them at risk for HIV from being coerced into unsafe sexual practices by male partners. Also, casual sex is a major risk for contracting HIV (Bunnell et al., 2006; Stoneburner & Low-Beer, 2004).

Influence of migration and interregional trade

According to AVERT (2009), the world's first known heterosexually spread instance in the HIV epidemic occurred in Kinshasa, the capital city of the Republic of the Congo, in the early 1980s. However, HIV and AIDS first reached epidemic level in east Africa, especially areas bordering Lake Victoria. By the end of the decade, HIV infection had been identified in all of the Central to East African states. Groups of people identified to have facilitated the initial rapid spread of HIV-1 included truck drivers and migrants such as soldiers, traders, and miners. In 1988, the second highest prevalence rate of HIV in all of Africa was found on the road linking Tanzania and Zambia. The Tanzania–Zambia road and other internal trade routes from Congo and Kenya were considered to be possible avenues through which HIV entered into some southern African countries such as Malawi and Zimbabwe (AVERT, 2009; Lwanda, 2005). The first HIV case in Zambia was reported in 1984, while the first HIV cases in Botswana, Malawi, and Zimbabwe were reported in 1985. By the end of the decade, the southern African countries of Malawi, Zambia, Zimbabwe, and Botswana joined East Africa in being the focus of the global HIV pandemic.

The association between migration and HIV and AIDS was a well documented phenomenon long before the underlying behavioral and social mechanisms were understood. In an examination of migration patterns in Kenya, Brockerhoff and Biddlecom (1999) found migration to be a critical factor in high-risk sexual behavior, in that migrants were more likely to engage in casual sex with multiple partners. Campbell (1997) investigated migrant workers in South African gold mines and reported findings similar to those for studies on migrant workers in Kenya.

Influence of transactional sex

Transactional sex has placed women at increased risk for HIV and has been associated with gender-based violence, substance use/abuse, and socioeconomic disadvantage (Dunkle et al., 2004). Nearly thirty different studies, in the United States and sub-Saharan Africa, provided evidence for several different links between the epidemics of HIV and violence (Maman, Campbell, Sweat, & Gielen, 2000). A number of risk factors have been viewed as relative

Case Study 16.1: Sex Work

Source: UNAIDS. (n.d.). *Sub-Saharan Africa*. Retrieved from http://www.unaids.org/en/countryresponses/regions/subsaharanafrica.asp

Sex work is an important factor in many of West Africa's HIV epidemics. More than one-third (35 percent) of female sex workers, surveyed in 2006 in Mali, were living with HIV, and infection levels exceeding 20 percent have been documented among sex workers in Senegal and Burkina Faso. Sex work plays an important, but less central, role in HIV transmission in southern Africa, where an exceptionally high background prevalence results in substantial HIV transmission during sexual intercourse unrelated to sex work.

Questions

1. Discuss the possible drivers of the high rate of HIV infection among female sex workers reported above.
2. What types of psychoeducational programming could help in decreasing the rate of HIV infection among female sex workers in sub-Saharan Africa?

Case Study 16.2: Heterosexual Intercourse Related to Serodiscordant Couples

Source: UNAIDS. (2008). *Report on the Global AIDS Epidemic (Sub-Saharan Africa)*. Retrieved May 17, 2010 from http://www.unaids.org/en/countryresponses/regions/subsaharanafrica.asp

According to Demographic and Health Surveys in five African countries (Burkina Faso, Cameroon, Ghana, Kenya, and the United Republic of Tanzania), two-thirds of HIV-infected couples were serodiscordant, that is, only one partner was infected. Condom use was found to be rare; in Burkina Faso, for example, almost 90 percent of the surveyed cohabiting couples said they did not use a condom the last time they had sex.

A separate, community-based study in Uganda has shown that, among serodiscordant heterosexual couples, the uninfected partner has an estimated 8 percent annual chance of contracting HIV. Strikingly, in about 30 to 40 percent of the serodiscordant couples surveyed, the infected partner was female. Indeed, it appears that more than half of the surveyed HIV-infected women, who were married or cohabiting, had been infected by someone other than their current partner.

Questions

1. Discuss the high rate of couples not using condoms.
2. What factors explain the high rate of HIV-infected women in the Ugandan study?

to gender and sexuality, and these are considered in the next section.

Gender, Sexuality, and Sexual Violence

A number of studies and theoretical papers have pointed to the special vulnerabilities of women relating to HIV and AIDS (e.g., Gilbert & Walker, 2002; Maman et al., 2000; Quinn & Overbaugh, 2005). Jewkes, Levin, and Penn-Kekana (2003) conducted an epidemiological study of gender-based violence, by investigating the associations among a range of markers of gender inequity. The study's findings suggest that women experienced difficulties discussing HIV prevention with partners, including suggesting the use of condoms.

As complex as gender issues have been for adults, sexual decision-making, exploration, and negotiation in the midst of HIV and AIDS among youth is fraught even more with conflict, uncertainty, misperception, and manipulation by power or control (Aarø et al., 2006; Eaton, Flisher, & Aarø, 2003; Klepp, Flisher, & Kaaya, 2007; Varga, 1997). MacPhail and Campbell (2001) found that South African youth were less likely to use condoms. However, young men and women belonging to sports clubs were less likely to be HIV-positive and more likely to use condoms than nonmembers (Campbell, Williams, & Gilgen, 2002). Peltzer, Pengpid, and Mashego (2006) have emphasized that the sexual behaviors of youth are socially influenced by peer networks and perceived permissive community attitudes toward casual sex. Several other studies (e.g., Ahmed, Flisher, Mathews, Mukoma, & Jansen, 2009; Helleve et al., 2009; Mukoma, et al., 2009; Peltzer, 2001) have investigated HIV and AIDS prevention interventions in African schools and reported modest positive effects of risk reduction.

Early clinical studies indicated a lower risk of HIV infection among circumcised males in Africa. One investigation found that male circumcision reduced HIV seroprevalence

Discussion Box 16.1: Norms for Condom Use

Heterosexually transmitted HIV infection is high among youth in South Africa. The literature tells us that knowledge levels about HIV is high in this group, but that perceived vulnerability and reported use of condoms are low. MacPhail and Campbell (2001) conducted a focus group study with South African youth, both male and female, in an age range of thirteen to twenty-five years. They concluded that condom use among the youth was influenced by their:

- Lack of perceived risk
- Peer norms
- Condom availability

Question

1. Explain the paradox between high knowledge of HIV and high-risk behavior among the youths.

rates by almost 60 percent (Auvert et al., 2005; Bongaarts, Reining, Way, & Conant, 1989; Weiss, Quigley, & Hayes, 2000). However, there was increased risk in women whose circumcised partners resumed sexual activity before healing occurred. Baeten, Celum, and Coates (2009, p. 183) pointed out that while the risk of HIV infection is not reduced for females whose circumcised partners are HIV-positive, "...women will benefit from male circumcision programmes. Wide-scale roll-out of male circumcision is expected to lead to decreasing HIV prevalence in communities over 10–20 years, in both men and women, by averting new infections in men and onward transmission to their partners."

Impact on the Family and Life Span Issues

Much of the published research regarding the psychosocial implications of HIV and AIDS has focused on the individual; yet the most proximal system in which most individuals participate on a daily basis is the family (Letamo, 2008). Bor, Miller, and Goldman (1993) examined the impact of HIV and AIDS on the family system. They identified the following initial areas of concern: social stigma, isolation and secrecy, stress and coping, social support, communication and disclosure, and responses to illness. Ankrah (1993) observed that the AIDS epidemic had negatively affected the ability of the African family to respond to members afflicted with HIV and AIDS.

Orphaned children

Researchers have begun to detail the phenomenon of the many child-headed households, due to the AIDS pandemic, in sub-Saharan Africa (e.g., Mutepfa et al., 2008; Ushamba & Mupedziswa 2008). With the high prevalence of orphanhood in sub-Saharan Africa from the HIV pandemic, children have been forced by circumstances to take on adult responsibilities. Strengthening the social and civil institutions charged with caring for and protecting vulnerable children is a priority for national and regional bodies in sub-Saharan Africa. The interruption of typical childhood and adolescent trajectories of development, as well as the potential for exploitation and abuse, have placed these children at high risk (Li et al., 2008).

Health Communication

The manner in which health- and mental health-related information is conveyed has been shown to have an impact on the efficacy of the intervention. For example, successful mitigation of HIV and AIDS in Uganda is explained in part by the fact that information about HIV was communicated via social networks perceived to be credible by the audience participants (Stoneburner & Low-Beer, 2004). Entertainment-education was used to increase audience members' knowledge, attitudes, and behavior adoption concerning HIV prevention activity (Vaughan, Rogers, Singhal, & Swalehe, 2000). However, competing governmental bureaucracies in some African countries have not effectively harmonized their HIV and AIDS control programs, thus obscuring communication that is necessary to stakeholders (Richey, 2003).

Prevention Programming

Social science research in the first decade of the epidemic focused on behavioral determinants of HIV infection and failed to investigate broader contextual factors (Parker, 2001). The scope of prevention efforts has since moved beyond individuals and families to the community (van Wyk, Strebel, Peltzer, & Skinner, 2006). The major approaches to developing HIV prevention programs within communities are (1) participatory approaches that develop a program from the bottom up and begin with the community as the starting point; and (2) theoretical approaches that follow a predetermined course of action or way of interpreting community behavior.

Voluntary Counseling and Testing

Voluntary counseling and testing (VCT) combines HIV testing with counseling, information, and support. Nearly all countries in sub-Saharan African have VCT services,

Research Box 16.1: Sexual Risk with Antiretroviral Therapy

Bunnell, R., et al. (2006). Changes in sexual behavior and risk of HIV transmission after antiretroviral therapy and prevention interventions in rural Uganda. *AIDS*, *20*(1), 85–92.

Objective: The impact of antiretroviral therapy (ART) on sexual risk behavior and HIV transmission among HIV-infected persons in Africa was unknown. The study assessed changes in risky sexual behavior and estimated HIV transmission from HIV-infected adults after six months of ART.

Method: A prospective cohort study was performed in rural Uganda, involving 926 HIV-infected adults. A home-based ART protocol included prevention counseling, voluntary counseling and testing (VCT) for cohabitating partners, and the provision of condoms. Baseline and follow-up data included participants' HIV plasma viral load and assessment of partner-specific sexual behaviors (e.g., risk behaviors).

Results: Six months after initiation of ART, risky sexual behavior was reduced by 70 percent. More than 85 percent of the risky sexual acts occurred within married couples. The estimated risk of HIV transmission from cohort members declined by 98 percent, from 45.7 to 0.9, per 1,000 person-years.

Conclusions: The provision of ART, prevention counseling, and partner VCT was associated with reduced sexual risk behavior and estimated risk of HIV transmission among HIV-infected Ugandan adults, during the first six months of therapy. The researchers suggested that integrated ART and prevention programs may reduce HIV transmission in Africa.

Questions

1. Explain the apparent success of the ART in reducing risky sexual behavior.
2. What is your opinion about the finding that more than 85 percent of the risky sexual acts occur within marriage?

and a majority of these are funded by the U.S. government and the European Union. For example, VCT was introduced to Malawi at two sites in 1992 and became more widespread in 1995, when the Malawi AIDS Counseling Resource Organization (MACRO) was founded. More VCT centers have been established since, and antiretroviral drugs (ARVs) have been made available to many people infected with HIV. In 2004, as the result of a grant from the Global Fund to fight AIDS and TB, 13,000 Malawians infected with HIV were receiving ARVs. The number rose dramatically to 29,000 at the end of 2005, and to 101,000 by the end of 2007.

Painter (2001) examined the literature regarding relationships between the members of couples who tested for HIV and recommended that increased attention to couples-focused VCT may provide a higher leveraged HIV prevention intervention for African couples. MacPhail, Pettifor, Coates, and Rees (2008) examined the attitudes of parents and youth regarding the use of VCT. The youth reported experiencing stigma and discrimination in association with the use of VCT. They rarely referred to the community (or, by extension, community-based services) as a source of support. The researchers concluded that there is a pressing need for youth-friendly VCT services. Stigma influenced people not to engage in VCT because they feared that the cost of a positive result would be social rejection (Parker & Aggleton, 2003; Kalichman & Simbayi, 2003). Nyblade, Pande, Mathur, MacQuarrie, and Kidd (2003, p. 44) defined stigma as "a complex phenomenon that is deeply intertwined with social values, fears around sex and death, and gender and social inequity." Clacherty and Associates (2002) reported that stigma and discrimination extended to children and youth infected with and affected by HIV and AIDS.

Policy, Development, and Politics

A number of authors have highlighted the political dimensions of the AIDS pandemic (e.g., Boone & Batsell, 2001; Butler, 2005; Fassin & Schneider, 2003; Johnson, 2004). For example, Boone and Batsell (2001) suggested the following five policy focus areas for Africa: (1) variations in state response to the pandemic, (2) relationships between governments and NGOs, (3) the AIDS challenge to neo-liberalism, (4) North–South collaboration regarding AIDS, and (5) connections between AIDS and international security issues. For instance, Gauri and Lieberman (2006) examined the question of why some national governments have acted more aggressively than others in addressing the HIV and AIDS pandemic. They argued that lack of synergy between government departments in their HIV and AIDS counseling interventions reduced overall impact. When results have been less than optimal, there is be a tendency to blame other government departments rather than providing effective policies and practices. Hyder et al. (2007) explored the interface between research and policymaking in low-income countries, emphasizing the importance of engaging key stakeholders and creating a system that enhances accountability.

Research Box 16.2: Effects of Voluntary Testing and Counseling on Sexual Risk Behavior

Kalichman, S. C., & Simbayi L. C. (2003). HIV testing attitudes, AIDS stigma, and voluntary HIV counseling and testing in a black township in Cape Town, South Africa. *Sexually Transmitted Infections*, *79*, 442–7.

Objective: In the face of a lack of awareness of voluntary counseling and testing (VCT) opportunities among South Africans, this study sought to examine relationships among HIV testing history, attitudes toward testing, and AIDS stigma.

Method: The researchers surveyed 224 men and 276 women living in a Black township in Cape Town. Of the respondents, 98 percent were Black, and 74 percent were thirty-five years of age or younger.

Results: Those who had been tested for HIV comprised 47 percent of the respondents. The researchers found that risks of exposure to HIV were comparably high among those who tested and those who did not. The researchers reported that attitudes toward VCT showed (1) that individuals who had not tested, as well as those who had tested and did not know their results, held significantly more negative testing attitudes than those who had tested and knew their results; and (2) that compared to those who had tested, those who did not test demonstrated significantly greater AIDS-related stigma – they attributed more shame, guilt, and social disapproval to people living with HIV than did the study respondents who had tested.

Conclusions: Given the suggested connection between negative testing attitudes and stigma, the researchers supported public education about the benefits of VCT that includes stigma reduction. They recommended structural and social marketing strategies targeting AIDS stigma reduction as a way to decrease resistance to VCT.

Questions

1. Explain the contradictory evidence that people who tested for HIV carried the same risk profile as those who did not seek testing.
2. How may not having been tested for HIV influence stigma toward those diagnosed and people living with HIV?

CURRENT PRACTICES IN HIV AND AIDS COUNSELING

Efforts to prevent the spread of HIV in sub-Saharan Africa have been spearheaded by the civil societies (such as National AIDS Council, National AIDS Commission, NGOs, and religious and academic organizations) that are involved with HIV and AIDS counseling in their various capacities (O'Manique, 2004). Thus, current HIV and AIDS counseling has focused on individual and community-based educational interventions, voluntary counseling and testing (VCT), prevention of mother-to-child transmission (PMTCT), encouragement for condom use, provision of psychosocial support, and availability of antiretroviral drugs (ARVs) (as previously discussed). In the following subsections, these issues are discussed in terms of the following topical areas: (1) global and regional responses, (2) community-based interventions, (3) counseling OVC, (4) counseling children and adolescents within the school context, (5) supporting people living with HIV and AIDS, (6) lay counseling for family members, and (7) counseling for vulnerability due to HIV and AIDS.

Global and Regional Responses

A number of global responses to the AIDS pandemic have been successful in drawing attention to important issues; these, in turn, have influenced productive regional programming in areas where need is great. An example of a global response is the *Framework for the protection, care, and support of orphans and vulnerable children living in a world with HIV and AIDS* that was endorsed by USAID, UNICEF, and UNAIDS in 2003, as part of the *Children on the Brink* series (UNAIDS/UNICEF/USAID, 2002). The framework identified five strategies in support of children infected with and affected by HIV and AIDS, which have been adopted internationally, nationally, and locally (Richter, Manegold, & Pather, 2004; Tindyebwa et al., 2004; USAID, 2005). The first strategy involves strengthening and supporting the capacity of families to protect and care for orphaned and vulnerable children in the form of, for example, economic and psychosocial support, improving access to basic services and education, increasing agricultural productivity, improving access to employment and markets, and providing additional ways of generating income. In addition, support can take the form of basic care for those with AIDS, or assistance to parents in drawing up wills, planning for the future of their children, and discussing it with them.

Second, community-based responses were targeted to be mobilized and supported. Communities are regarded as the second safety net for orphaned and vulnerable children and for vulnerable households, as community members might identify vulnerable children and families, assist them first-hand, or direct them to local or outside resources. Strengthening community-based responses has taken the form of developing community gardens, organizing youth groups and recreational activities, and encouraging schools to exempt children from school fees.

The third identified strategy centers on strengthening of the capacity of children and young people to address their own needs worldwide, by ensuring access to essential services. Support initiatives aim at keeping vulnerable children in school, preparing them for the future, and enabling them to provide for their own needs. Interventions focus on school attendance, access to basic health and nutrition services, safe water and sanitation, protection of vulnerable children, and placement where needed.

Some regional responses have been based on the *Framework for the protection, care, and support of orphans and vulnerable children living in a world with HIV and AIDS* (UNAIDS/UNICEF/USAID, 2004) and aimed at ensuring that governments develop policies and essential services to protect vulnerable children. As a fourth strategy, governments are required to take action and ensure that children, families, and communities are able to cope, for example, by further developing, implementing, and enforcing laws to protect vulnerable children, and by making sure that those who do not have the support of family or community members are provided with essential social services. Strategies include the development of national action plans to guide programming; the development of Children's Acts and protection services; as well as the delivery of education, health, and other essential services, by collaborating with international organizations, NGOs, religious groups, donors, and the private sector.

Finally, regional initiatives complement national and community counseling to raise HIV and AIDS awareness at the various levels of society. An awareness of the impact of the pandemic was identified as something that continually needs to be encouraged among community leaders, policy makers, organizations, and the general public, in order to establish a shared sense of responsibility. Initiatives focus on aspects such as stigma, discrimination, and social mobilization, as well as involving the media, faith-based groups, and other stakeholders (Richter et al., 2004; Tindyebwa et al., 2004; UNAIDS et al., 2002).

Community-based Interventions

According to Geballe, Gruendel, and Andiman (1995), Lucas (2004), Mallmann (2002), and Van Dyk (2001), communities should take control over their own well-being. Any response to HIV and AIDS should be guided by the experiences of community members on ground level, as they are the people who feel the impact of the pandemic and who need to find ways of facing the challenge. Community-based coping supports the *Ubuntu* principle – a philosophy characteristic of African indigenous communities that emphasizes the importance of community and collectivism. Thus, in African communities, broad community involvements and support to one another in the micro- and meso-systems (including churches, local organizations, schools, and teachers, for example) can be regarded as a culturally embedded strength (Snow, 2001). As such, the possibility of actors like nurses, volunteer workers, teachers, NGO officials, church ministers, and others fulfilling the role of lay counselors lies at the core of African people facing challenging times.

Community-based responses to HIV and AIDS, within African indigenous communities, often are mediated by so-called social capital. This response entails establishing networks that community members might rely on in order to work together to address challenges, thereby strengthening the community and enhancing a sense of belonging. In this manner, social capital facilitates people to support one another and provide lay counseling to each other in difficult times. Subsequently, communities with a high level of social capital, including lay counseling by community members – often those in helping professions such as social workers, nurses, and teachers – may be able to cope more easily with social challenges (Lucas, 2004; Ngcobo, 2001). As a result, the responsibility of these actors generally goes beyond their initial calling. For example, within the context of care and support, the task of a teacher may go beyond the children in the classroom; the task may extend to the families of the children in the classroom and if needed, their neighbors or other community members.

Some community members might be hesitant to become involved in caring for and supporting people living with HIV and AIDS, based on myths and misconceptions, especially relating to the transmission of the virus (Clacherty & Associates, 2002; Ferreira, 2008). People who are willing to act as lay counselors often perceive it as being their responsibility to correct myths and misconceptions, as these can be regarded as preventative factors for community members providing efficient support to others. In addition, a correction of misconceptions implies the potential of reducing stigmatization, thereby encouraging other community members to support those living with HIV and AIDS.

Counseling Orphaned and Vulnerable Children

Although caregivers of orphaned and vulnerable children differ across regions, the surviving parent or extended family still seems to form the primary basis of care to these children in African cultures (Amoateng, Richter, Makiwane, & Rama, 2004; Gilborn, Nyonyintono, & Jagwe-Wadda, 2001; Miamidian, Sykes, & Bery, 2004; Monasch & Boerma, 2004; Winkler, Modise, & Dawber, 2004). Grandparents and relatives caring for orphaned and vulnerable children are, however, often old or impoverished. As a result, they typically turn to other community members for support. In the case of relatives or community members not being available or able to take orphaned children into their care, children might end up in child-headed households, placed in institutions (the last resort), or living homeless on the street (International Social Service & UNICEF, 2004; Linsk & Mason, 2004; Nyambedha, Wandibba, & Aagaard-Hansen, 2003; Ratsaka-Mothokoa, 2001; Richter et al., 2004).

In addition to relatives and other community members, governments often fulfill a role with regard to orphaned children and families taking care of them. For example, national governments may offer financial assistance in the form of grants, food support for impoverished families, free health care for children, exemption from school fees, and free vocational training for young people (Meintjes, Budlender, Giese & Johnson, 2003; Ngcobo, 2001; Richter et al., 2004). Furthermore, schools typically seem to play a role in supporting communities coping with children infected with and affected by HIV and AIDS, specifically in communities characterized by limited resources. School-based support includes identifying children infected with and affected by HIV and AIDS early, addressing their special educational needs, referring and monitoring of vulnerable children, teaching learners life skills, providing school-based nutrition programs, offering pastoral care and counseling, financially assisting children who need it, involving caregivers and guardians, and supporting children living with HIV and AIDS.

Supporting People Living with HIV and AIDS

Within African indigenous communities and against the background of the *Ubuntu* principle, support to people living with HIV and AIDS implies a variety of acts. First, the acceptance of people who are infected is regarded as important, thereby not rejecting or isolating them. Second, African communities typically provide material support to others in need, in the form of financial support, food parcels, and supplements. In addition, advice is given and recommendations made with regard to influencing people to have healthier lifestyles. Finally, community members demonstrate care by, among other things, regularly visiting individuals infected with HIV and counseling them when needed (Ferreira, 2006). Religion and prayer generally informs part of any support and counseling act. In addition, hope is typically emphasized when informally counseling people living with HIV and AIDS, thereby providing emotional and spiritual support. Due to the stigma often attached to psychological services in some African cultures, formal counseling services might at times not be accessed, despite the availability thereof (Ferreira, 2006; Loots, 2005; Kelly, 2001).

INFLUENCE OF CULTURE

Current practices in HIV and AIDS counseling in sub-Saharan Africa can be understood better when reviewed in the context of traditional African views of disease and medicine. One common belief is that some outbreaks of disease are caused by other people or witchcraft, while other outbreaks are caused by ancestral spirits or God (Lyons, 1992). When witchcraft is adopted as explanatory, it absolves the family and the patient of responsibility for acquiring HIV. Therefore, when the Western concept of AIDS causation is adopted, the patient becomes stigmatized as someone who sought the disease (Lwanda, 2005). However, even with clear instances of mortality from AIDS, patients are presumed to have died from works of witchcraft or angered ancestral spirits (see also Chapter 1, this volume). Illness and mortality from HIV and AIDS is less likely to be publicly acknowledged by family, although admitted in private among the members.

ISSUES FOR RESEARCH AND OTHER FORMS OF SCHOLARSHIP

Despite legal and policy frameworks having been put into place over the past couple of decades to support HIV and AIDS counseling (Birdsall & Kelly, 2005; Giese, Meintjes, Croke, & Chamberlain, 2003; Smart, 2003a), it seems clear that the intended intervention initiatives are not reaching all communities. Examples of communities that frequently do not benefit from programs put into place include poor, rural, and informal settlement communities. It also seems clear that well-intended intervention initiatives sometimes lack sufficient cultural sensitivity, and this may compromise their effectiveness. Several of the most relevant research issues are identified and briefly discussed in the following subsections.

Psychosocial and Cultural Aspects of HIV and AIDS

Much of the research that has examined the myriad of issues concerning the effects of HIV and AIDS has been biomedical in nature and conducted primarily from a positivist orientation. The psychosocial effects of living with HIV and AIDS are equally important, and in need of in-depth investigation. For instance, research on the role of African traditional healers in treating HIV promises to yield important insights into beliefs that influence response to HIV and AIDS as a public health issue (Levers, 2006; Levers & Maki, 1995; see also Chapter 1, this volume). The constructs such as vulnerability, coping, and psychosocial support important to HIV and AIDS counseling need to be investigated in African cultural settings. For example, research should examine the mechanisms for coping with and managing the various aspects of HIV and AIDS so counselors are better equipped in building such constructs into culturally sensitive interventions. Also, the impact of HIV and AIDS on families needs to be addressed in a more systematic manner. Letamo (2008, p. 362) has identified specific research areas ripe for investigation concerning the "links between reproductive health, sexuality, HIV and AIDS, and the family," as well as for the development of intervention strategies, public policies, and therapeutic programs that address family issues.

Therapeutic and Training Aspects of HIV and AIDS

More research needs to be conducted that is specific to the professional counseling interventions that are appropriate to working with persons living with HIV and AIDS.

As best practices continue to be identified, the efficacy of these counseling interventions needs to be robustly investigated. For example, a better understanding of the role of personal decision making relating to VCT, disclosure of seropositive status, and uptake of circumcision or other risk reduction issues is needed for the design of more efficacious interventions. Motivation may be a construct worthy of in-depth investigation as it pertains to making healthy and productive personal decisions when living with HIV and AIDS. Such research could inform counselors' interventions in profound ways. Counselors need codified practice, which are grounded both in research and in an ethics of care, to help clients.

More pedagogy-based research is needed to develop critical AIDS-related aspects of the pre-service education of professional counselors, as well as the training of paraprofessional counselors. Ways of integrating useful knowledge into a variety of curriculum levels need to be tested and refined. Creative ways of sensitizing and conscientizing human service workers, quickly and effectively, need to be investigated so that capacity can be built for much-needed counseling services for people affected by HIV and AIDS throughout Africa and the Diaspora.

Being Informed as Prerequisite to Being a Lay Counselor

Paraprofessionals often display a lack of self-confidence and thus need to be informed on HIV- and AIDS-related issues, before becoming involved in supporting others living with HIV and AIDS. Their aspiration to be knowledgeable is generally based in their desire to be able to answer the questions of colleagues and other community members. Basic required information includes that on nutrition and treating AIDS-related conditions and individuals infected with HIV. Other important aspects include providing emotional support for a person living with HIV and AIDS, including addressing the challenge of stigmatization (Clacherty & Associates, 2002; Ferreira, 2006; Odendaal, 2006). Lay counseling needs to be backed by more scholarship.

Some community members might be hesitant to become involved in caring for and supporting people living with HIV and AIDS, based on myths and misconceptions, especially relating to the transmission of the virus (Clacherty & Associates, 2002; Ferreira, 2008). As such, people who are willing to act as lay counselors often perceive it as their responsibility to correct myths and misconceptions, as these can be regarded as preventative factors for community members providing efficient support to others. Correction of misconceptions regarding HIV and AIDS has the potential of reducing stigmatization, thereby encouraging other community members to support those living with HIV and AIDS, but more research is needed.

Generally, African communities cope with the challenges associated with HIV and AIDS by relying on themselves, their own abilities, and the resources available in the immediate local community, of which schools, churches, and other support services typically fulfill a primary role. Yet, these same natural resources also offer opportunities for learning more about the context. Generally, teachers and nurses, for example, are in an optimal position to provide care and support to other community members, but they often know which households are severely affected by poverty and the pandemic, what kind of help is needed, who might be dying of AIDS, who is taken care of by relatives or other community members, and who is living on his or her own.

SUMMARY AND CONCLUSION

The purpose of this chapter was to examine the psychosocial impacts of HIV and AIDS on people in African settings, as well as to explore the types of interventions used by counselors with their clients in African settings. The pandemic has affected people at individual, couple, family, community, and national levels; many challenges have emerged that have altered people's lives.

The history of research and practice in HIV and AIDS counseling revealed trends in the following focus areas: risk behaviors and contextual factors; gender, sexuality, and sexual violence; impact on the family and life span issues; health communication; prevention programming; voluntary counseling and testing; stigma and HIV and AIDS; and, policy, development, and politics. Current practices have included global and regional responses, community-based interventions, counseling OVC, counseling children and adolescents in schools, support counseling for people living with HIV and AIDS, lay counseling for family members, and counseling for vulnerability due to HIV and AIDS.

Counselors possess the capacity to assist people living with HIV and AIDS to cope better with stressors and to better manage their responses to a variety of aspects of the situation. Counselors have the potential to mitigate the effects of cultural and environmental factors in ways that allow people to empower themselves in taking the best actions to enhance their own lives.

REFERENCES

Aarø, L. E., Flisher, A. J., Kaaya, S., Onya, H., Fuglesang, M., Klepp, K-I., & Schaalma, H. (2006). Promoting sexual and reproductive health in early adolescence in South Africa and Tanzania: Development of a theory- and evidence-based intervention programme. *Scandinavian. Journal of Public Health, 34*(2), 150–8.

Aggleton, P., O' Reilly, K., Slutkin, G., & Davies, P. (1994). Risking everything? Risk behavior, behavior change, and AIDS. *Science, 265*, 341–5.

Ahmed, N., Flisher, A. J., Mathews, C., Mukoma, W., & Jansen, S. (2009). HIV education in South African schools: The dilemma and conflicts of educators. *Scandinavian. Journal of Public Health, 37*, 48–54.

Akeroyd, A. V. (1997). Sociocultural aspects of AIDS in Africa: Occupational and gender issues. In G. C. Bond, J. Kreniske,

I. Susser & J. Vincent (Eds.), *AIDS in Africa and the Caribbean* (pp. 11–30). Boulder, CO: Westview Press.

Amoateng, A. Y., Richter, L. M., Makiwane, M., & Rama, S. (2004). Describing the structure and needs of families in South Africa: Towards the development of a national policy framework for families. A report commissioned by the Department of Social Development. Pretoria: Child, Youth and Family Development, Human Sciences Research Council.

Ankrah, E. M. (1993). The impact of HIV/AIDS on the family and other significant relationships: The African clan revisited. *AIDS Care*, *5*(1), 5–22.

Auvert, B., Talijaard, D., Lagarde, E., Sobngwi, J., Sitta, M., & Puren, A. (2005). Randomized, controlled intervention trial of male circumcision for reduction of HIV-infection risk: The ANRS 1265 trial. *PLoS Med*, *2*, 1112–2.

AVERT. (2009). *The history of AIDS in Africa*. Retrieved August 29, 2009 from http://www.avert.org/history-aids-africa.htm

Baeten, J. M., Celum, C., & Coates, T. J. (2009). Male circumcision and HIV risks and benefits for women. *The Lancet*, *374*, 182–4.

Birdsall, K., & Kelly, K. (2005). *Community responses to HIV/AIDS in South Africa: Findings from a multi-community survey*. Johannesburg: Centre for AIDS Development, Research and Evaluation (CADRE).

Bongaarts, J., Reining, P., Way, P., & Conant, F. (1989). The relationship between male circumcision and HIV infection in African populations. *AIDS*, *3*, 373–7.

Boone, C., & Batsell, J. (2001). Politics and AIDS in Africa: Research agendas in political science and international relations. *Africa Today*, *48*(2), 3–33.

Bor, R., Miller, R., & Goldman, E. (1993). HIV/AIDS and the family: A review of research in the first decade. *Journal of Family Therapy*, *15*(2), 187–204.

Brockerhoff, M., & Biddlecom, A. E. (1999). Migration, sexual behavior and the risk of HIV in Kenya. *International Migration Review*, *33*, 833–56.

Brookes, H., Shisana, O., & Richter, L. (2004). *The national household HIV prevalence and risk survey of South African children*. Cape Town: HSRC Press.

Brouard, P., Maritz, J., Pieterse, J., van Wyk, B., & Zuberi, F. (2005). *HIV/AIDS in South Africa 2005: Course companion to the CSA entry level course and general information source*. Pretoria: Centre for the Study of AIDS.

Bunnell, R. Ekwaru, J. P., Solberg, P., Wamai, N., Bikaako-Kajura, W., Were, W., ... Mermin, J. (2006). Changes in sexual behavior and risk of HIV transmission after antiretroviral therapy and prevention interventions in rural Uganda. *AIDS*, *20*(1), 85–92.

Butler, A. (2005). South Africa's HIV/AIDS policy, 1994–2004: How can it be explained? *African Affairs (London)*, *104*, 591–614.

Cabassi, J. (2004). Renewing our voice: Code of good practice for NGOs responding to HIV/AIDS. Geneva: The NGO HIV/AIDS Code of Practice Project.

Campbell, C. (1997). Migrancy, masculine identities and AIDS: The psychosocial context of HIV transmission on the South African gold mines. *Social Science & Medicine*, *45*, 273–81.

Campbell, C., Williams, B., & Gilgen, D. (2002). Is social capital a useful conceptual tool for exploring community level influences on HIV infection? An exploratory case study from South Africa. *AIDS Care*, *14*(1), 41–54.

Catalano, R. F., Berglund, M. L., Ryan, J. A., Lonczak, H. S., & Hawkins, J. D. (2004). Positive youth development in the United States: Research findings on evaluations of positive youth development programmes. *The Annals of the American Academy of Political and Social Science*, *591*, 98–124.

Clacherty & Associates. (2002). The role of stigma and discrimination in increasing the vulnerability of children and youth infected and affected by HIV/AIDS – Report on participatory workshops. Report for Save the Children (UK), South Africa Programme. Arcadia, South Africa: Save the Children.

Cunha, M. (2007). South African politics, inequalities, and HIV/AIDS: Applications for public health education. *Journal of Developing Societies*, *23*, 207–19.

Department of Economic and Social Affairs of the United Nations. (2005). *Population, development and HIV/AIDS with particular emphasis on poverty: The concise report*. New York: United Nations Publication.

Dillon, D. H., & Brassard, M. R. (1999). Adolescents and parental AIDS death: The role of social support. *OMEGA*, *39*(3), 179–95.

Dirkzwager, A. J. E., Bramsen, I., & Van der Ploeg, H. M. (2003). Social support, coping, life events, and posttraumatic stress symptoms among former peacekeepers: A prospective study. *Personality and Individual Differences*, *34*(8), 1545–59.

Dunkle, K. L., Jewkes, R. K., Brown, H. C., Gray, G. E., McIntryre, J. A., & Harlow, S. D. (2004). Transactional sex among women in Soweto, South Africa: Prevalence, risk factors and association with HIV infection. *Social Science & Medicine*, *59*, 1581–92.

Eaton, L., Flisher, A. J., & Aaro, L. E. (2003). Unsafe sexual behaviour in South African youth. *Social Science & Medicine*, *56*, 149–65.

Fassin, D., & Schneider, H. (2003). The politics of AIDS in South Africa: beyond the controversies. *British Medical Journal*, *326*, 495–7.

Ferreira, R. (2006). *The relationship between coping with HIV&AIDS and the asset-based approach*. Unpublished doctoral thesis, University of Pretoria.

Ferreira, R. (2008). Culture at the heart of coping with HIV&AIDS. *Journal of Psychology in Africa*, *18*(1), 97–104.

Geballe, S., Gruendel, J., & Andiman, W. (Eds.) (1995). *Forgotten children of the AIDS epidemic*. New Haven: Yale University Press.

Giese, S., Meintjes, H., Croke, R., & Chamberlain, R. (2003). The role of schools in addressing the needs of children made vulnerable in the context of HIV/AIDS. Paper in preparation for the Education Policy Round Table (July 28–29, 2003), Children's Institute, University of Cape Town.

Gilborn, L. Z., Nyonyintono, R. K., & Jagwe-Wadda, G. (2001). *Making a difference for children affected by AIDS: Baseline findings from operations research in Uganda*. New York: The Population Council Inc.

Greenglas, E. R. (2002). Proactive coping and quality of life management. In E. Frydenberg (Ed.), *Beyond coping: Meeting goals, visions, and challenges* (pp. 37–62). Oxford: Oxford University Press.

Helleve, A., Flisher, A. J., Onya, H., Kaaya, S., Mukoma, W., Swai, C., & Klepp, K-I. (2009). Teachers' confidence in teaching HIV/AIDS and sexuality in South African and Tanzanian schools. *Scandinavian. Journal of Public Health*, *37*, 55–64.

International Social Service & UNICEF. (2004). Improving protection for children without parental care – Care for children affected by HIV/AIDS: The urgent need for international standards. New York: UNICEF.

Jewkes, R. K., Levin, J. B., & Penn-Kekana, L. A. (2003). Gender inequalities, intimate partner violence and HIV preventive practices: Findings of a South African cross-sectional study. *Social Science & Medicine*, *56*, 125–34.

Johnson, D. W., & Johnson, R. T. (2002). Teaching students how to cope with adversity: The three Cs. In E. Frydenberg (Ed.), *Beyond coping: Meeting goals, visions, and challenges* (pp. 195–217). Oxford: Oxford University Press.

Johnson, K. (2004). The politics of AIDS policy development and implementation in postapartheid South Africa. *Africa Today*, *51*(2), 107–28.

Kalichman, S. C., & Simbayi, L. C. (2003). HIV testing attitudes, AIDS stigma, and voluntary HIV counselling and testing in a black township in Cape Town, South Africa. *Sexually Transmitted Infections*, *79*, 442–7.

Kelly, M. J. (2001). *The great challenge: HIV/AIDS and development in Africa*. Paper presented at the Education for Development and Democracy Initiative (EDDI) International Conference (May 28–June 1, 2001), Benin.

Klepp, K-I., Flisher, A. J., & Kaaya, S. F. (Eds). (2007). *Promoting adolescent sexual and reproductive health in east and southern Africa*. Uppsala, Sweden: Nordic Africa Institute.

Letamo, G. (2008). Reproductive health, sexuality, and HIV and AIDS in Botswana: The family connection? In T. Maundeni, L. L. Levers & G. Jacques (Eds.), *Changing family systems: A global perspective*. Gaborone, Botswana: Bay Publishers.

Levers, L. L. (2006). Traditional healing as indigenous knowledge: Its relevance to HIV/AIDS in southern Africa and the implications for counselors. *Journal of Psychology in Africa*, *16*, 87–100.

Levers, L. L., & Maki, D. R. (1995). African indigenous healing, cosmology, and existential implications: Toward a philosophy of ethnorehabilitation. *Rehabilitation Education*, *9*, 127–45.

Li,X.,Naar-King,S.,Barnett,D.,Stanton,B.,Fang,X.,&Thurston,C. (2008). A developmental psychopathology framework of the psychosocial needs of children orphaned by HIV. *Journal of the Association of Nurses in AIDS Care*, *19*(2), 147–57.

Linsk, N. L., & Mason, S. (2004). Stresses on grandparents and other relatives caring for children affected by HIV/AIDS. *Health & Social Work*, *29*(2), 127–36.

Loots, M. C. (2005). *Exploring teachers' mobilisation of assets in support of community-based coping with HIV & AIDS*. Unpublished master's dissertation, University of Pretoria.

Lwanda, J. (2005). *Politics, culture and medicine in Malawi: Historical continuities and ruptures with special reference to HIV/AIDS*. Zomba: Kachere.

Lucas, S. (2004). *Community, care, change, and hope: Local responses to HIV in Zambia*. Washington, DC: Social & Scientific Systems, Inc./The Synergy Project.

Lynch, M. F., & Levers, L. L. (2007). Ecological-transactional and motivational perspectives in counseling. In J. Gregoire & C. Jungers (Eds.), *Counselor's companion: Handbook for professional helpers* (pp. 586–605). Mahwah, NJ: Lawrence Earlbaum.

MacPhail, C., & Campbell, C. (2001), 'I think condoms are good but, aai, I hate those things': Condom use among adolescents and young people in a southern African township", *Social Science and Medicine*, *52*, 1613–27.

MacPhail, C. L., Pettifor, A., Coates, T., & Rees, H. (2008). "You must do the test to know your status": Attitudes to HIV voluntary counseling and testing for adolescents among South African youth and parents. *Health Education & Behavior*, *35*(1), 87–104.

Mallmann, S. (2002). *Building resiliency among children affected by HIV/AIDS*. Windhoek: Catholic AIDS Action.

Maman, S., Campbell, J., Sweat, M. D., & Gielen, A. C. (2000). The intersections of HIV and violence: Directions for future research and interventions. *Social Science & Medicine*, *50*, 459–78.

Meintjes, H., Budlender, D., Giese, S., & Johnson, L. (2003). Children 'in need of care' or in need of cash: Questioning social security provisions for orphans in the context of the South African AIDS pandemic. Working paper by the Children's Institute, and the Centre for Actuarial Research, University of Cape Town.

Miamidian, E., Sykes, A., & Bery, R. (2004). *Economic strengthening to improve the well-being of orphans and vulnerable children*. Workshop report (working draft) (June 14–16, 2004), Dar es Salaam, Tanzania. Washington, DC: Bureau for Africa, USAID.

Monasch, R., & Boerma, J. T. (2004). Orphanhood and childcare patterns in sub-Saharan Africa: An analysis of national surveys from 40 countries. *AIDS*, *18*(2), S55–S65.

Mukoma, W., Flisher, A. J., Ahmed, N., Jansen, S., Mathews, C., Klepp, K-I., & Schaalma, H. (2009). Process evaluation of a school-based HIV/AIDS intervention in South Africa. *Scandinavian. Journal of Public Health*, *37*, 37–47.

Mutepfa, M. M., Phasha, N., Mpofu, E., Tschombe, T., Mamwenda, T., Kizito, S., et al. (2008). Child-headed households in sub-Saharan Africa. In T. Maundeni, L. L. Levers & G. Jacques (Eds.), *Changing family systems: A global perspective*. Gaborone, Botswana: Bay Publishers.

National Research Council and Institute of Medicine. (2002). *Community programs to promote youth development*. Division of Behavioral and Social Sciences and Education. Washington, DC: National Academies Press.

Ngcobo, M. P. J. (2001). *Explaining positive responses to AIDS: A study of the Mophela community and their responses to the care of orphans*. Unpublished master's dissertation, University of Natal, Durban.

Nnko, S., Chiduo, B., Wilson, F., Msuya, W., & Mwaluko, G. (2000). Tanzania: AIDS care – Learning from experience. *Review of African Political Economy*, *27*(86), 547–57.

Nyambedha, E. O., Wandibba, S., & Aagaard-Hansen, J. (2003). Changing patterns of orphan care due to the HIV epidemic in western Kenya. *Social Science & Medicine*, *57*, 301–11.

Nyblade, L., Pande, R., Mathur, S., MacQuarrie, K., & Kidd, R. (2003). *Disentangling HIV and AIDS stigma in Ethiopia, Tanzania and Zambia*. Washington, DC: International Center for Research on Women [ICRW] (USAID Cooperative Agreement No. HRN-A-00–98–00044–00).

Odendaal, V. (2006). *Describing an asset-based intervention to equip educators with HIV and AIDS coping and support competencies*. Unpublished master's thesis. Pretoria: University of Pretoria.

O'Manique, C. (2004). *Neoliberalism and AIDS crisis in sub-Saharan Africa*. Hampshire, UK: Palgrave Macmillan.

Painter, T. M. (2001).Voluntary counseling and testing for couples: A high-leverage intervention for HIV/AIDS prevention in sub-Saharan Africa. *Social Science & Medicine*, *53*, 1397–1411.

Parker, R. (2001). Sexuality, culture, and power in HIV/AIDS research. *Annual Review of Anthropology*, *30*, 163–79.

Parker, R., & Aggleton, P. (2003). HIV and AIDS-related stigma and discrimination: A conceptual framework and implications for action. *Social Science & Medicine*, *57*, 13–24.

Parker, R. G., Easton, D., & Klein, C. H. (2002). Structural barriers and facilitators in HIV prevention: A review of international research. *AIDS*, *14*, S22–S32.

Peltzer, K. (2001). Factors affecting behaviors that address HIV risk among senior secondary school pupils in South Africa. *Psychological Reports*, *89*, 51–56.

Peltzer, K., Pengpid, S., & Mashego, T-A. B. (2006). *Youth sexuality in the context of HIV/AIDS in South Africa*. New York: Nova Science.

Quinn, T. C., & Overbaugh, J. (2005). HIV/AIDS in women: An expanding epidemic. *Science*, *308*, 1582–3.

Ratsaka-Mothokoa, M. H. (2001). *The impact of HIV/AIDS on children and their families*. Unpublished master's dissertation, University of the Witwatersrand.

Republic of Malawi Government. (2004). *Behavioral surveillance survey report: Malawi 2004*. Lilongwe: Author.

Richey, L. A. (2003). HIV/AIDS in the shadows of reproductive health interventions. *Reproductive Health Matters*, *11*(22), 30–5.

Richter, L., Manegold, J., & Pather, R. (2004). *Family and community interventions for children affected by AIDS*. Cape Town: HSRC Press.

Sayson, R., & Meya, A. F. (2001). Strengthening the roles of existing structures by breaking down barriers and building up bridges: Intensifying HIV/AIDS awareness, outreach, and intervention in Uganda. *Child Welfare League of America*, *80*(5), 541–50.

Simbayi, L. C., Kalichman, S. C., Strebel, A., Cloete, A., Henda, N., & Mqeketo, A. (2007). Disclosure of HIV status to sex partners and sexual risk behaviours among HIV-positive men and women, Cape Town, South Africa. *HIV/AIDS*, *83*, 29–34.

Smart, R. (2003a). Children affected by HIV/AIDS in South Africa: A rapid appraisal of priorities, policies and practices. Pretoria, South Africa: Save the Children (UK).

Smart, R. (2003b). *Policies for orphans and vulnerable children: A framework for moving ahead*. South Africa: Futures Group International and the Centre for Development and Population Activities.

Snow, L. K. (2001). *Community transformation: Turning threats into opportunities*. A community building workbook from the Asset-Based Community Development Institute. Chicago: ACTA Publications.

Stoneburner, R., & Low-Beer, D. (2004). Population-level HIV declines and behavioral risk avoidance in Uganda. *Science*, *304*, 714–18.

Strand, K., Marullo, S., Cutforth, N., Stoecker, R., & Donohue, P. (2003). Principles of best practice for community-based research. *Michigan Journal of Community Service Learning*, *9*(3), 5–15.

Swanepoel, A. (2005). *Exploring community volunteers' use of the memory box making technique to support coping with HIV and AIDS*. Unpublished master's dissertation. University of Pretoria.

Tindyebwa, D., Kayita, J., Musoke, P., Eley, B., Nduati, R., Coovadia, H., et al. (2004). *Handbook on paediatric AIDS in Africa*. Kampala, Uganda: African Network for the Care of Children Affected by AIDS (ANECCA).

UNAIDS (Joint United Nations Programme on HIV/AIDS). (2008). *2008 Report on the global AIDS epidemic*. Geveva: World Health Organization.

UNAID/UNICEF/USAID. (2004, July). *Framework for the protection, care, and support of orphans and vulnerable children living in a world with HIV and AIDS*. Retrieved September 7, 2009 from http://www.unicef.org/aids/files/Framework_English.pdf.

UNAIDS/UNICEF/USAID. (2002). *Children on the brink 2002: A joint report on orphan estimates and program strategies*. Washington, DC: TvT Associates.

UNAIDS/WHO. (2005). *AIDS epidemic update December 2005: Special report on HIV prevention*. Geneva: UNAIDS.

USAID. (2005). *USAID Project profiles: Children affected by HIV/AIDS*. Washington, DC: USAID.

University of Zimbabwe. (2003). *Zimbabwe Human Development Report 2003, redirecting our responses to HIV and AIDS: Towards reducing vulnerability – the ultimate war for survival*. Harare: Poverty Reduction Forum, Institute of Development Studies, University of Zimbabwe.

Ushamba, A., & Mupedziswa, R. (2008). A generation on the edge of a precipice?: HIV/AIDS and child-headed households in Zimbabwe. In T. Maundeni, L. L. Levers & G. Jacques (Eds.), *Changing family systems: A global perspective*. Gaborone, Botswana: Bay Publishers.

Uwimana, J., & Struthers, P. (2007). Met and unmet palliative care needs of people living with HIV/AIDS in Rwanda. *Journal of Social Aspects of HIV/AIDS Research Alliance*, *4*, 575–85.

Van Dyk, A. C. (2001). *HIV/AIDS care and counselling: A multidisciplinary approach*. Kaapstad: Pearson Education South Africa.

van Wyk, B., Strebel, A., Peltzer, K., & Skinner, D. (2006). *Community level behavioural interventions for HIV prevention in sub-Saharan Africa*. Cape Town, RSA: HRSC Press.

Varga, C. A. (1997). Sexual decision-making and negotiation in the midst of AIDS: Youth in KwaZulu-Natal, South Africa. *Health Transition Review*, 7(Supplement 3), 45–67.

Vaughan, P. W., Rogers, E. M., Singhal, A., & Swalehe, R. M. (2000). Entertainment- education and HIV/AIDS prevention: A field experiment in Tanzania. *Journal of Health Communication*, *5*, 81–100.

Walker, A. R. P., Walker, B. F., & Wadee, A. A. (2005). A catastrophe in the 21st century: The public health situation in South Africa following HIV/AIDS. *The Journal of the Royal Society for the Promotion of Health*, *125*, 168–71.

Weiss, H. A., Quigley, M. A., & Hayes, R. J. (2000). Male circumcision and risk of HIV infection in sub-Saharan Africa: A systematic review and meta-analysis. *AIDS*, *14*, 2361–70.

Winkler, G., Modise, M., & Dawber, A. (2004). All children can learn: A handbook on teaching children with learning difficulties. Cape Town: Francolin Publishers.

World Health Organization (WHO). (2009). Paediatric HIV and treatment of children living with HIV. Retrieved September 7, 2009 from http://www.who.int/hiv/topics/paediatric/en/

SELF-CHECK EXERCISES

1. What are some of the contextual factors that have been associated with the spread of HIV and AIDS in sub-Saharan Africa?
2. How has the AIDS pandemic affected the family system in sub-Saharan Africa? How does such knowledge inform the work of a professional counselor?
3. Discuss the impact of HIV and AIDS on African children, especially those who have lost one or both parents. What kinds of services are needed to assist orphans and other vulnerable children?
4. How are cultural influences relevant to HIV and AIDS counseling in sub-Saharan Africa?
5. Identify the major research trends concerning HIV and AIDS for the practice of counseling in sub-Saharan Africa.

FIELD-BASED EXPERIENTIAL EXERCISES

1. Interview two or three community members on their knowledge of counseling services available to people infected with and affected by HIV and AIDS.
2. Interview a lay counselor focusing on the support he or she provides to people living with HIV and AIDS in the community. Discuss the experiences of the person you interview in terms of personal challenges and potential value of becoming involved in other contexts.
3. Find at least three articles in the newspaper that reflect stigmatizing or discriminating attitudes concerning HIV and AIDS. With a student peer, identify the attitudes, and discuss strategies that a community-based counseling organization might use to address such discrimination.
4. Identify one or two popular songs with lyrics that touch on HIV and AIDS in a nonstereotypical way. Write down the lyrics and examine them for the positive message that is conveyed. Identify ways in which the use of positive messages can assist a professional counselor in working with HIV-positive clients.
5. Visit a community-based organization that provides HIV and AIDS services. Ask to interview someone about counseling services, and take notes. After you leave the site, write a summary page about the activities there.

MULTIPLE-CHOICE QUESTIONS

1. Responding to and dealing with the HIV and AIDS pandemic on ground level should be driven by:
   a. The World Health Organization and UNAIDS
   b. Local governments
   c. Nongovernmental organizations
   d. Communities themselves
   e. Individuals who volunteer to take the lead
2. People living with HIV and AIDS are often socially vulnerable because of:
   a. Unhealthy eating habits and a lack of medical care
   b. A lack of support within the immediate family
   c. Discrimination and stigmatization associated with the pandemic
   d. Inability to earn an income
   e. Uncertainty in terms of spiritual fulfilment
3. In dealing with children orphaned by HIV and AIDS, the following people/institutions usually fulfill the most central role:
   a. Family members
   b. Friends and neighbors
   c. Schools and teachers
   d. Churches and ministers
   e. Government institutions and children's homes
4. Which one of the following is *not* provided by teachers, nurses, social workers, and other people in helping professions when fulfilling the role of lay counseling?
   a. Spiritual support in terms of prayer and home visits
   b. Material support in terms of food parcels and supplements
   c. Social support by means of home visits and support group meetings
   d. Medical support in the form of antiretroviral treatment
   e. Emotional support in terms of acceptance, basic care, and support
5. Which one of the following descriptions best describes community-based coping with HIV and AIDS?
   a. Spontaneously dealing with challenges by relying on available support and existing resources within the community
   b. Relying on other communities and examples of best practice to cope with challenges in the community
   c. Identifying and actively pursuing external agencies that could provide support and financial assistance to cope with challenges faced by the community
   d. Passively awaiting external assistance while coping with challenges on an individual basis
   e. Nominating a few competent individuals in the community to initiate projects that could assist other community members to cope with the challenges they face

Answers to the multiple-choice questions are provided at the back of the book

17 Substance Use Disorder Counseling

Monika M. L. dos Santos, Solomon T. Rataemane, Elias Mpofu, and Andreas Plüddemann

OVERVIEW. Substance use disorders cover a range of problems associated with using and abusing psychoactive substances such as alcohol, cannabis, cocaine, heroin, benzodiazepines, as well as a variety of other substances taken to affect thoughts, feelings, and behavior. Interventions may include a "mix" of approaches, both modern and indigenous, including assessment and diagnosis, self-help intervention, outpatient, diversion and restorative justice approaches, residential care, and harm-reduction tactics. In this chapter, various substance use disorder concepts, the history of substance use disorder practice and research, substance use disorder recovery theories, legal and professional issues related to substance use disorders, as well as issues for further research and scholarship in Africa are examined. Cultural issues that affect and influence the use and treatment of substances use disorders within the African context are also explored.

LEARNING OBJECTIVES

By the end of the chapter, the reader should be able to:

1. Define key concepts relevant to substance use disorders.
2. Outline core African indigenous and modern practices used to treat or counsel clients with substance use disorders.
3. Discuss the rationale of major recovery theories and psychosocial theories relating to substance use disorder counseling.
4. Discuss legal and professional issues related to substance use disorders within the African context.
5. Identify prospective areas of research that would advance the knowledge of substance use disorder intervention and scholarship within the African context.

INTRODUCTION

Substance use is perhaps as old as the history of mankind; for example, ancient societies used mind-altering substances for a variety of purposes, including trade and war, love and religion (Rudgley, 1998). Most indigenous African communities continue to believe in and use certain substances, including alcohol and tobacco, for ritualistic purposes. The extent to which the use of mind-altering drugs by indigenous African communities results in dependence is unknown. It is possible that social sanction in these communities restrict the use of psychoactive or mind-altering substances to "privileged" others believed to be leaders in spiritual health or mediation (Sobiecki, 2008). A psychoactive substance is defined as a drug that alters the state of consciousness of the user (Rudgley, 1998). Reber (1985) characterizes psychoactive substances as a generic term for any drug that affects the consciousness, mood, and awareness.

In contemporary Africa, use of psychoactive substances is increasingly prevalent in the younger generations, mostly for recreational purposes. Recreational substance use refers to the use of psychoactive drugs for recreational purposes rather than for work or approved medical or spiritual purposes, although the distinction is not always clear (often spiritual use is considered recreational use) (Rudgley, 1998). Sociocultural pressures associated with transition to modernization in predominantly tradition-led African communities, may encourage the recreational use of substances, where traditional use of substances for therapeutic, ritual, or religious reasons has been replaced by socially detrimental substance abuse and dependence (Boone, 2001). The modern-day African suburbs are likely to be emotionally alienated jungles, just as any squatter camp, township, or slum in which the individual must fight to survive. It has been suggested that, among other things, low self-esteem and poor ego development frequently underlie the need to seek a pseudo-identity in alcohol, prescription/over-the-counter medication, or within the illicit drug subculture. Alcohol or a drug use can reduce psychological or physical pain, fill a spiritual void, confer an identity, or kill time, but only up to a point and at a price. In most cases, the substance user perceives the substance as providing the most convenient and effective means of filling a dominant need and providing immediate gratification, and has no initial strong disincentives against filling it in this way. Some may be unable for one reason or another to find a meaningful and supportive relationship within their family networks or in orthodox society. An illicit psychoactive substance, for example, may be sought because it represents something recognizable and carries with it a sense of importance. This is reinforced by all the introverted ritual, sexual symbolism, jargon, and paraphernalia of the "scene" (Dos Santos & Van Staden, 2008; McIntosh & McKeganey, 2002).

Table 17.1. Summary of studies of injection drug use in Africa

Country	Area	Population	Sample size	IDUs (%)	IDUs sharing needles (%)
Egypt	Country	Drug users	636	16.40	30.8 (ever)
	Cairo	Drug users	431	92.8	59.1 (ever)
Kenya	Country	General	1420	23	26.7–81.0 (ever)
	Nairobi	Heroin users	348	44.8	27.5–43.1 (past 6 months)
Mauritius	Country	School students	380	1.2	–
	Country	Tertiary students	100	4.3	–
	Country	Drug users	100	91.0	80.0 (past 3 months)
	Country	Juvenile offenders	50	17.4	–
	Country	Adult offenders	150	49.7	30.5 (ever)
	Country	Sex workers	100	74.5	76.7 (ever)
Nigeria	Lagos	Heroin users	398	20.6	11.0–15.0 (past 6 months)
South Africa	Cape Town	Heroin users	250	23.0	86.0 (past 30 days)
Tanzania	Dar es Salaam	IDUs	51	100.0	31.1 (ever)

Dewing, S., Plüddemann, A., Myers, B. J. & Parry, C. D. H. (2006).

IMPORTANCE, DEFINITION, AND SCOPE OF KEY TERMS AND CONCEPTS

In this section, substance use, as an important social concern, and the definition of some commonly used terms for substance use disorders are addressed, followed by the social importance of substance use and definition of key terms and concepts.

Importance

Substance use disorders are unique among contemporary problems in the breadth of their social impact. No other condition has mobilized such a range of institutional responses, nor involved so many professions and disciplines, for example, medicine, mental health, public health, education, legislature, the judiciary, law enforcement, and foreign affairs. These disorders have also, unfortunately, inspired irrational fear in the general public. Substance use disorders have become a symbol of the social disorder of the times, associated with materialism, poverty, crime, the problems of societies in transition, the disadvantaged, the affluent, the inner cities, and the rural communities.

Sociocultural Influences

In the African context, the problems of illiteracy, high unemployment rates, AIDS, poverty, and crime exacerbate the problem (United Nations Office on Drugs and Crime, 2007). Furthermore, some treatment procedures, such as detoxification and rehabilitation, can be especially expensive, and there is a large disparity between the services of the private and public health and welfare sector. There are warning signs that Africa is under attack, targeted by cocaine traffickers from the West (Colombia) and heroin smugglers in the East (Afghanistan). This threat needs to be addressed rapidly to eradicate drug-related crime, money laundering, and corruption, and to prevent the spread of drug use that could cause havoc across a continent already plagued by other tragedies (United Nations Office on Drugs and Crime, 2007).

Intravenous Drug Use

The growing number of intravenous drug users (IDUs) in Africa also has the potential to provide a significant contribution to the spread of HIV/AIDS on this continent, arising within a context of an established and growing HIV epidemic. IDU has become the primary mode of HIV transmission in certain regions of North Africa, Asia, the Middle East, and South America (Ball, 1999). This mode of HIV transmission is a concern given that the efficiency per injection is six-times higher than for heterosexual acts. IDU-driven epidemics tend to spread much more rapidly than those driven by sexual transmission (United Nations Office on Drugs and Crime, 2005); the prevalence of HIV/AIDS among IDUs can reach more than 50 percent of a given population, sometimes up to 90 percent within very short periods of time. Such rapid transmission has been observed in both industrialized and developing countries (Des Jarlais, McKnight, & Milliken, 2004). Sub-Saharan Africa contains only 10 percent of the world's inhabitants, yet is home to more than 60 percent of the global HIV-infected population (UNAIDS, 2005).

Although the AIDS epidemic in sub-Saharan Africa is currently driven by heterosexual transmission, there are indications that both IDU and non-IDU are becoming increasingly important modes of transmission in certain sub-Saharan African countries as the problem continues to grow (Adelekan & Stimson, 1997; Needle, Ball, Des Jarlais, Whitmore, & Lambert; 2000). However, there is little information on IDU in Africa not only because it is a relatively new phenomenon in this region, but also because many African countries simply lack the funds required to monitor drug use trends in a systematic way (Affinnih, 2002). Of particular relevance is the increasing use of heroin throughout Africa (Adelekan & Stimson, 1997; International Narcotics Control Board, 2004; United

Discussion Box 17.1: Are Substance Use Disorders Diseases?

If substance dependence is indeed a "disease," it is not a typical one. A disease seems, at base, to have three characteristics. First, it is something that is bad to have and would be good to have go way or be cured. Second, it must be a condition over which the sufferer has no control of at the time – even though some diseases, such as gonorrhea or syphilis, may have been originally brought on by the sufferer's own "misbehavior." Finally, a disease is a condition that is regarded primarily within the domain of the medical profession to try to cure or alleviate (Kaplan, 1983). It remains unclear as to whether or not substance use disorders meet the first criterion of a disease. Although it is often taken for granted that sufferers wish to be cured, this is not always the case; however, many want to have the circumstances surrounding their lives – such as police harassment, changed. The second criterion for a disease is that the condition, regardless of what brought it on, once established, is beyond the control of the sufferer. With respect to substance dependence, this also raises problems. Certainly some sufferers act as if they cannot control themselves, yet others manage quite well, once they decide they want to. Nor does the third criterion for a disease seem to be any more applicable to substance use disorders.

Questions

1. Explain the disease concept of substance use disorders.
2. Identify alternative concepts that may substantiate or discount the disease hypothesis of substance use disorders.

Nations Office on Drugs and Crime, 2007). While other drugs are commonly injected among some populations; heroin is the drug that is perhaps most widely injected around the world (McCurdy, Williams, Ross, Kilonzo, & Leshabari, 2005). Because the use of opiates is not indigenous to Africa, the diffusion of heroin use across the continent is a direct consequence of drug trafficking. Weak detection controls and porous borders along the eastern, western, and northern coasts of Africa have facilitated the safe transport of heroin originating in Afghanistan, Pakistan, and Southeast Asia en route to Europe and the United States. The transhipment of heroin through Africa has increased dramatically since 1990 and this has been accompanied by the development of a local market for heroin in many African countries where it did not exist before. In general, the literature review indicates the common occurrence of high-risk behavior such as needle sharing and unsafe sex within the IDU populations surveyed in Africa, necessitating the consideration of employing harm-reduction strategies such as needle-exchange programs, as well as diversion/restorative justice programs of heroin-dependent criminal offenders (Dewing, Plüddemann, Myers, & Parry, 2006).

Substance Use Disorder Concepts

The *DSM-IV-TR* (American Psychiatric Association, 2000) is widely held to be authoritative in defining key terms in substance use disorder and other mental health conditions. However, mental health concepts and healing practices in African cultures and their clinical implications are an evolving project (Haque, 2008). The extent to which *DSM-IV-TR* criteria for mental health conditions apply to African settings is unknown. Nonetheless, we briefly define terms associated with psychoactive substance use referencing the *DSM-IV-TR*, while also mindful of the potential limitations of that document in non-Western settings.

Substance Dependence, Abuse, Intoxication, and Withdrawal

Individuals who develop a substance use disorder often go through unpleasant and potentially terrifying experiences or consequences, which can be extremely difficult to escape from.

According to the American Psychiatric Association (2000), the essential feature of *substance dependence* is a cluster of cognitive, behavioral, and physiological symptoms indicating that the individual continues use of the substance despite significant substance-related problems. There is a pattern of repeated self-administration that can result in tolerance, withdrawal, and compulsive substance use behavior. An individual is said to have developed substance dependence when there is a strong, compelling desire to continue taking it. This desire may derive from a wish either to experience its effects or to avoid or escape the aversive experiences produced by its absence. Dependence on a substance may be largely psychological or physiological in origin.

DSM-IV-TR addresses the concept of *substance abuse* by defining it by how significantly the use of the substance interferes with a person's life (American Psychiatric Association, 2000). Substance abuse is used only for cases in which there has been relatively long-term abuse (i.e., longer than a month), leading to impaired social or occupational functioning (Reber, 1985).

Substance intoxication is often associated with substance abuse or dependence. Evidence of recent intake of the substance can be obtained from the history, physical examination (e.g., smell of alcohol on the breath), or toxicological analysis of body fluids (e.g., urine or blood). Any possible maladaptive behavior change induced by a substance depends on the social and behavioral context, and may place the individual at significant risk for adverse effects, for example, legal problems, disruption in social and family relationships, and financial difficulties (American Psychiatric Association, 2000).

Most individuals with *substance withdrawal* have a craving to readminister the substance in order to reduce the adverse symptoms. The dose and duration of use and other factors such as the presence or absence of additional illnesses also affect withdrawal symptoms. Withdrawal develops when doses are reduced or stopped, whereas signs and symptoms of intoxication decrease, in some cases gradually, after dosing stops (American Psychiatric Association, 2000).

Essentially, substance dependence is strongly associated with *psychological dependence*. Psychological dependence refers to a phenomenon that can vary in intensity from mild involvement with a behavior to a dependence that seriously restricts the individual's other behavioral options. The term is thus used to describe a rather pervasive drive to obtain and take a substance (Krivanek, 1988). The term is usually defined by exclusion; in other words, it is used for dependencies on substances whose action does not produce fundamental biochemical changes such that continued doses of the substance are required for normal functioning. Substances such as cannabis are commonly cited as ones likely to produce psychological dependence with habitual use (Reber, 1985).

The idea of *relapse*, or the return to substance use after a period of abstinence, is the breaking of a commitment to abstinence, by even a single use of the substance of choice, or the use of any psychoactive substance whatsoever, including alcohol, after a period of abstinence. Relapse can also be understood as a breakdown in abstinent thinking and lifestyle, long before the actual breaking of the commitment to abstinence. Determinants of relapse are identified as psychological (emotional) or physical (urges and cravings) events, interpersonal factors such as social pressure or interpersonal conflict, and nonpersonal environmental events such as financial loss, accidents, and unemployment (Marlatt & Gordon, 1985).

Correlates of Substance Use Disorders

Epidemiological studies have shown that between 30 and 60 percent of all substance dependents have comorbid mental health diagnoses, including major depression, schizophrenia, bipolar disorder, anxiety disorders, post-traumatic stress disorder (PTSD), and personality disorders (Karam, Yabroudi, & Melham, 2002; Rodrigues-Llera et al., 2006; Vasile, Gheorghe, Civrea, & Paraschiv, 2002). Epidemiological studies are those that attempt to link human health effects, by means of statistical studies on human populations, to a specified cause. A concurrent mental disorder can complicate substance use disorder treatment in a multitude of ways; for example, clinically depressed individuals have an exceptionally hard time resisting environmental cues to relapse. People with heroin dependence and mental illness comorbidity, for example, are more likely to engage in behaviors that increase the risk of HIV/AIDS, and injecting heroin dependents with antisocial personality disorder more frequently share needles (Leshner, 1999). Heroin is a highly addictive substance derived from morphine. It produces an immediate rush if injected and a sense of calm in the user. Users can become preoccupied with the feelings the drug produces and getting their next dose. Opiates, such as codeine and morphine, are natural or synthetic derivatives of opium that have similar analgesic and sedative effects. Misuse of opiates alone has been associated with a fourteen-fold increase in risk of suicide, the same order of increase that is found in severe mental illness (Leshner, 1999).

HISTORY OF SUBSTANCE USE: COUNSELING, PRACTICE, AND RESEARCH IN INDIGENOUS AND MODERN AFRICA

The history of substance use disorder intervention has repeatedly been characterized by fads and fashions. Some of the treatments that have been used have been at best ineffective, and at worst harmful and occasionally even dangerous. It is a distressing reflection upon the field that practices and procedures for the treatment of substance use disorders can so easily be introduced and applied without (or even contrary to) evidence. This is illustrated by the extraordinary range of interventions that have been used to detoxify heroin dependents. Several of these treatments have been more dangerous than the untreated withdrawal syndrome (Kleber, 1981). We briefly consider the history of research and practice in substance abuse in the African context.

Precolonial Period

In addition to alcoholic drinks (especially beer which has a very long history in Africa), cannabis, tobacco, and other substances of intercontinental importance, Africa has numerous psychoactive plants, many of which have been used by indigenous cultures. Unlike in other areas of the world, such as Amazonia and Mexico, the use of hallucinogenic and narcotic plants in sub-Saharan Africa has received very little attention from researchers. According to a 1658 entry in the diary of Jan van Riebeeck (who was the first governor of a Dutch settlement at the Cape of Good Hope), the Hottentots of southern Africa make use of "a dry powder which... (they) eat and which makes them drunk." This powder was probably derived from Leonotis leonorus, the leaves of which were also smoked alone or in conjunction with tobacco. The Basarwe of Botswana use a local plant they call kwashi (a bulbous perennial,

Case Study 17.1: Adam and Eve

They appeared to be young naive teenagers in love, but the murder they committed was one of the most gruesome South Africa has seen. Why did they do it? What turned them into killers? On a Tuesday night in July 2001, a good Samaritan picked up two young hitchhikers in Pretoria West. Little did he know whom he was inviting into his car. In fact, the story started five days earlier in a block of flats where the two youngsters – she was fifteen at the time, he was seventeen – ended an afternoon of sex and drugs with a bloody, gruesome murder. Captain Bernice Cronje stated "The whole flat was full of blood." They stabbed her thirty-seven times in the back and the chest. The whole house was in a mess, because the people who did it stayed there for three days. Dr. Irma Labuscagne, a forensic criminologist, was intimately involved with the case. Irma believes that things went completely haywire for the two as they grew into adolescence. They were both latchkey kids who found solace among peers with destructive habits. The boy and girl found an anchor in one another. They dubbed themselves "Adam and Eve." Diaries and love letters paint a picture of obsessive infatuation between them. Irma says the girl toyed with the idea of murder long before it happened. She says they tried out sizes of knives a month before they did it. The frenzied violence of the two shocked officials on the case, but more scandalous were letters left at the scene, detailing the gory aftermath of the crime. For three days, they stayed cooped up with the bloody body, eating and having sex, until the botched hijack led to their arrest. The young couple cooperated fully with police; ten months later the case came to court in Pretoria and they pleaded guilty to all charges. They were sentenced to twenty years' imprisonment, with no possibility of parole before fifteen years.

Source: (De Chaud, 2002).

Questions

1. Discuss any possible psychiatric comorbidity that the drug-dependent perpetrators may have presented with.
2. Examine the potential life-history/life-world circumstances that may have contributed toward the crime taking place.
3. Identify and discuss all prospective interventions that may be undertaken in an attempt to rehabilitate the perpetrators.

Pancratium trianthum) as a hallucinogen. By rubbing the bulb into cuts in the head, visions are reportedly seen. The hallucinogenic bulb of the *Boophane disticha* has been used traditionally by the Basuto people of South Africa in male initiation rites, as it is believed to aid communication with the ancestors. The Basuto also use its bulb in their medicine, as an arrow poison and even as a way of committing suicide. Its use as a hallucinogen for contacting the spirits or ancestors is reported from Zimbabwe. The consumption of cannabis in the Binga District, an area of land bounded by a line drawn from a point on the Zimbabwe–Zambia international boundary, has been described as traditional in precolonial times, and is considered to be an integral part of the Tonga culture (Arnett, 2007; Zeleza & Dickson 2003). In Zaire a plant named *niando* (*Alchornea floribunda*) is used for its aphrodisiac, stimulant, and narcotic properties. It is also used as a hallucinogen by the members of the Gabonese Byeri cult (Rudgley, 1998).

Modern Period

Reports on the use of traditional substances such as alcohol, cannabis, and khat remain prevalent in contemporary Africa. The introduction of prescription drugs to Africa drastically increased the availability and use of psychoactive substances. This notwithstanding, alcohol, cannabis, and khat still remain the most common substances of abuse in Africa. Khat is an evergreen shrub (*Catha edulis*) native to tropical East Africa, having dark green opposite leaves that are chewed fresh for their stimulating effects. More recently, trafficking in heroin and cocaine has made narcotic drugs easily available across Africa, despite the existing legal control measures. Complications arising from the use/abuse of psychoactive substances often draw public attention to their deleterious effects, which culminate in drug control policy formulation. The contribution of poverty, political instability, social unrest, and refugee problems to the rapid spread of psychoactive substance use/abuse in Africa, particularly among the youth, remains a concern. The possible linkage between psychoactive drug use and HIV infection has already been discussed (Odejide, 2006).

Using data from the World Health Organization Global Alcohol Database (GAD), Roerecke, Obot, Patra, and Rehm (2008) found considerable variation in levels of overall per capita alcohol consumption among sub-Saharan countries, ranging from an overall adult per capita recorded and alcohol consumption for the year 2002 estimated in Uganda (18.6 L), Nigeria (14.1 L), Burundi (14.0 L), Zimbabwe (13.5 L) to Mauritania (0.01 L), Niger (0.1 L), and Guinea (0.2 L). The population-weighted average adult per capita alcohol consumption in sub-Saharan Africa was 7.4 L, slightly above the global level of 6.2 L, and in terms of average consumption per drinker, sub-Saharan Africa was with 19.5 L, far above the worldwide estimate

Discussion Box 17.2: Impact on South Africa: Society and Community

South Africa's unique history and distinctive cultures have resulted in a local drug scene unlike any other in the world. Apartheid ensured that patterns of drug consumption and distribution remained highly segmented along ethnic and regional lines. While many of these apartheid-era divisions persist, the drug scene in South Africa is becoming increasingly difficult to compartmentalize. Social fragmentation, poverty, and a youthful population are three factors that contribute to South Africa's crime problem in general and to its drug problem in particular. The mass relocations during apartheid shredded the delicate social fabric for many people and destroyed the greatest crime prevention tool of all – familial and community accountability. South Africa experiences one of the highest levels of income inequality in the world. In the past, poverty actually militated against the consumption of drugs within the black majority population. White South Africans, by contrast, have always consumed the widest variety of drugs and seem to be the first to experiment with any new substance entering the country, largely because of their economic advantage, international exposure, and youth identification with European and American cultural trends. Curiously, colored gangs closely parallel those found in the United States, with all the turf wars, hand signs, tattoos, initiation rites, and drug dealing that are part of the "thug" life. Apartheid did produce some unintended positive results. Cocaine and heroin, although present in small amounts before the 1994 elections, took off only once South Africa was allowed to emerge fully in international commerce and travel once again. In their place, however, certain substances enjoyed a popularity seen nowhere else in the world – Mandrax and Wellconol. There is also evidence that the apartheid state promoted the drug use as a form of chemical warfare against the democratic resistance (Leggett, 2001). With the coming of democracy in South Africa, the borders were opened to immigrants from the rest of the continent, especially countries that assisted in the struggle against apartheid. Nigeria, in particular, played an important part in assisting with the birth of democracy in South Africa. It is generally agreed that the present wave of Nigerian immigrants first made their appearance in Johannesburg since the early 1990s, peaking in the inner-city residential hotels of Hillbrow, Yeoville, and Berea. Hillbrow's sleazy hotels are notorious crime hotspots. Unfortunately, Nigerian syndicates are known internationally for their involvement in heroin and cocaine trafficking (Baynham, 1998; Leggett, 2001).

Questions

1. Explore and discuss the factors that may influence substance misuse in countries that experience rapid political and social transformation.

of 13.9 L (Roerecke et al., 2008). According to WHO (2000) estimates, the eastern and southern African regions have the highest consumption of alcohol per drinker in the world (World Health Organization [WHO], 2004). In addition, the prevalence of hazardous drinking patterns in the region, such as drinking a high quantity of alcohol per session, or being frequently intoxicated, is second only to that in Eastern Europe. Consumption of commercial beverages is expected to rise in the coming years as economic conditions continue to improve in some countries and as a result of increasing marketing and promotion activities by the industry (WHO, 2004).

Significant ethnic differences in illicit drug use is evident in the United Kingdom. Compared with white British adolescents, cannabis use is significantly higher among black Caribbean adolescents and young people of mixed ethnicity, but is lower among Bangladeshi, Indian, and Pakistani adolescents. Lifetime cannabis use is also significantly higher among Black Caribbeans and young people of mixed ethnicity, but lower among Bangladeshi, Indian and Pakistani adolescents. Living in the United Kingdom for five years or less markedly reduces the risk of lifetime and recent cannabis use when controlled for ethnicity and social class. Glue or solvent use was reported in 3.2 percent of adolescents, with use significantly higher among Bangladeshi young people. Further research is needed in understanding culture-specific risk and protective factors in different ethnic groups, and the importance of cultural identity in mediating health risk behaviors. The high use of solvents by Bangladeshi young people poses a public health problem that may require targeted interventions (Jayakody et al., 2005).

During 2004, there was extensive community concern around the use of methamphetamine (known locally as "tik") in certain suburbs of Cape Town, South Africa, particularly due to the rapid escalation in the use of the substance by adolescents and young adults (Plüddemann et al., 2007). Methamphetamine is an amphetamine derivative used in the form of a crystalline hydrochloride; it is used as a stimulant to the nervous system and as an appetite suppressant. The issue received considerable media attention. In response, the provincial government appointed a task team in one of the most affected areas to deal with the problem. A special session was also called in the provincial legislature and experts and community representatives were invited to give their input on the problem. Data collected by the South African Medical Research Council from specialist substance abuse treatment centers

Discussion Box 17.3: Treatment Demand Trends (selected sites in South Africa): Methamphetamine (%) as the Primary Drug and Secondary Substance of Abuse

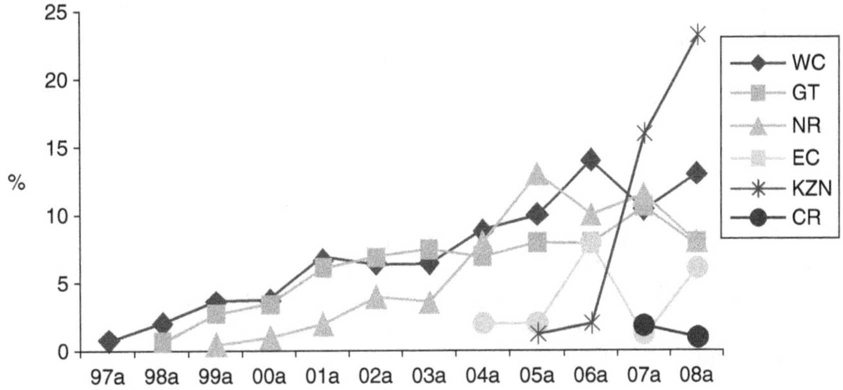

Source: Plüddemann, Parry, Cerff, Bhana, Potgieter, Gerber, Mohamed, Petersen & Carney, 2007.

Questions

1. Discuss how the escalation of the use of a new drug in a community might impact on those providing counseling, treatment, and rehabilitation services.
2. If you were the provincial director for Mental Health & Substance Abuse services in your province, what measures would you have taken, given the above situation, to assist staff in substance use disorder counseling and rehabilitation facilities?

in Cape Town (as part of the South African Community Epidemiology Network on Drug Use (SACENDU) project) also indicated a sharp increase in the proportion of patients reporting methamphetamine as a primary substance of abuse and an increase in the overall proportion of patients who report methamphetamine as a primary or secondary substance of abuse. In the first half of 2002, only 4 of 1,608 patients (0.2 percent) reported methamphetamine as a primary substance of abuse, compared to 1,166 of 2,862 (41 percent) in the first half of 2007.

Because of the many negative side effects of methamphetamine, treatment services have been particularly challenged in Cape Town, as a high proportion of methamphetamine users experience a methamphetamine-induced psychosis, requiring psychiatric intervention (often not readily available at outpatient services). Thus, methamphetamine poses new challenges to the substance use disorder counseling and rehabilitation centers and their staff in Cape Town, requiring additional training and strategic planning (Plüddemann et al., 2007).

CURRENT INTERVENTIONS IN AFRICAN SETTINGS

Current interventions for substance use disorders in African settings cover collaborative efforts between modern mental health/health professionals and indigenous healers, as well as the full range of modern psychotherapies within the context of African indigenous healing practices. The section concludes by considering various theories of substance use disorder recovery.

Collaborative Efforts

Typically, people with substance use disorders in Africa seek help from mental health/health practitioners and indigenous healers (Robertson, 2006). Generally, there is no formal referral system for patients from experts in the formal health sector (e.g., psychiatrists, psychologists) to those in the nonformal health sector (i.e., indigenous healers) or vice versa (Mpofu, 2003). It is, however, estimated that 70 percent of South Africans consult indigenous healers, who include diviners, herbalists, faith healers, and traditional birth attendants, and 61 percent of psychiatric patients had consulted indigenous healers during the past twelve months in a study by Robertson (2006). Indigenous healers' interpretations appear to be intuitive, rather than based on phenomenological or physiological evidence of dysfunction (Kruger, 1981). In the study by Robertson (2006), a client consulting an indigenous healer for alcohol dependence was diagnosed as having *amafufunyane* (possession by evil spirits), while another was told that his beer had been poisoned, making him lose control over his drinking (*idliso*). Some of the treatment measures prescribed by indigenous healers make "medical sense," whereas others appear to work on suggestion.

The motivation for corroboration is put forward, as indigenous healers have been serving African communities since time immemorial, because these healers understand the belief system of their people, and enjoy a respected place in their society. By understanding and entering African religious and therapeutic expressions through its own language, important underlying, and possibly historic, commonalities and connections can be identified. The basis for variants and transformations can also be established more intelligibly (Janzen, 1992).

It also appears that in indigenous healing the locus of control is often externalized and intervention can only be through medication offered by the *amagqira*, which seems to be in contradiction with some of the Western approaches to the treatment of substance use disorders, for example, by mental health practitioners. Some traditional healers consider substance dependence as a spiritual house arrest that restricts creativity and enforces the substance dependent to ignorantly misuse the gift of creativity. Anyone, regardless of race, creed, color, social, ethnic, or cultural background, who has reached the stage where he or she sincerely desires to be free from substance dependence can find an answer in the power of the heart. The key solution to healing lies in the understanding that every problem humans experience is in fact a spiritual "fire alarm" warning one to change one's ways and to vacate all forms of destructive behavior. The way to heal is through the heart, not through the head. Modern medicine insists on trying to treat disease without understanding the spiritual cause. It is argued that the allopathic approach merely diverted each disease and caused it to morph and reappear in a slightly different guise (Serva-Dei, 2000).

Unfortunately, Western medicine often ridicules this simple knowledge, and many people suffer and die each year just to sustain an allopathic industry that is specifically designed to sustain the illusion of healing (Serva Dei, 2000). Notwithstanding, more knowledge needs to be gained, widely shared, and debated, specifically about how indigenous healers practice, and what form of collaboration would be most appropriate. To proceed in any other way would be a disservice to clients and to the health profession in general (Robertson, 2006).

Psychotherapy and Recovery Theories

Key psychotherapies in counseling substance use disorders, such as psychodynamic psychotherapy, transpersonal psychology and family therapy, are considered in this subsection, as well as theories of recovery from substance use disorders such as the maturing out hypothesis, contextual factors, and stages of recovery models.

Psychodynamic psychotherapy is a form of depth psychology, the primary focus of which is to reveal the unconscious content of a substance dependent's psyche in an effort to alleviate psychic tension (Aziz, 1990). Most psychodynamic approaches are centerd on the idea that some maladaptive functioning is in play, and that this maladaption is, at least in part, unconscious. The presumed maladaption develops early in life, and it is posited that in later years, the client will begin to feel some dissonance in his or her day-to-day lives as a function of this paradigm. It is accepted that what modern man thinks and talks about, preliterate man acts out in his dancing, singing, rituals, and ceremonies, and much can be learned about the African society and ourselves by an understanding of the deeper meaning of these rituals and ceremonies. To counteract the tendency of Western man to rely too much on his thinking and intellectual functions, most schools of depth psychology encourage their clients to paint, model with clay, sculpture, or dance their dreams and fantasies where it seems appropriate. Such methods can make material that often seems chaotic available, and thus more concrete and easier to relate to. This may assist the client to accept and integrate what often seems foreign into the conscious mind, where it can be subjected to scrutiny and assessment. By giving external and concrete form to fantasy and dream images they become meaningful and in most instances less threatening. The cosmology of the *amagqira* relates to Jung's phenomenological attitude to unknown psychic material, that is, allowing material from the unconscious depth of the psyche to manifest itself without control or interference from the ego (Bührmann, 1984). The psychodynamic therapist first intervenes to treat the discomfort associated with the poorly formed function, and then helps the substance-dependent individual acknowledge the existence of the maladaption, while working to develop strategies for change (Aziz, 1990, 2007). Psychodynamic psychotherapy demands considerable introspection and reflection on the part of the client. It also relies on the substance dependent's desire to be helped to support its effectiveness, as well as the client's willingness to reveal him- or herself, and his or her level of insight. Consequently, the individual must possess enough resilience and ego strength to manage the strong emotions this form of therapy may provoke (Bernard, 2004).

The emergence of *transpersonal psychology*, however, seems to offer more synergy with the central tenets of African cosmology and healing (Tart, 1975). Transpersonal psychology is a school of psychology that studies the transpersonal, self-transcendent, or spiritual aspects of the human experience. Issues considered in transpersonal psychology include spiritual self-development, peak experiences, mystical experiences, systemic trance, and other metaphysical experiences of living. Transpersonal psychology attempts to unify modern psychology theory with frameworks from different forms of mysticism. These vary greatly depending on the origin but include religious conversion, altered states of consciousness, trance, and other spiritual practices.

Transpersonal psychology is at the forefront of a shift in psychology away from reductionistic methods based on positivism toward a human science based on holism in understanding the full range of human experiences. Despite the advances in mental health care, there is a relationship between transpersonal psychology and African traditional healing. The solution associated with these differences emerges from encouraging African health care systems and conventional psychological healing systems to function in a complementary fashion.

Case Study 17.2: Kagiso Maifadi

At the age of nineteen, Kagiso Maifadi presented for his second residential psychiatric drug treatment program. Kagiso's story illustrates a history of substance dependence starting with cannabis at the age of thirteen. Kagiso grew up in a township in South Africa. He was well liked at school, and started experimenting with illicit substances while mixing with "the wrong crowd." Five years after he began abusing cannabis, Kagiso also started to smoke heroin or what the South African township youth call *nyaope*, and ultimately developed a dependence on heroin. As typical of many youth misusing heroin, Kagiso failed a grade at school and started to get involved in petty crime because of his heroin dependence, culminating in his arrest. Luckily, he was only fined for his misdemeanors. Like many modern-day heroin users, Kagiso came from an intact family, being the eldest of two children, with both parents married; he described stable family relationships. Kagiso booked himself voluntarily into a psychiatric drug rehabilitation program and verbalized his "rock bottom" as occurring when he heard that he had failed his final grade at school. Kagiso also presented with depression comorbidity. He responded positively toward therapeutic directives during the course of his residential treatment.

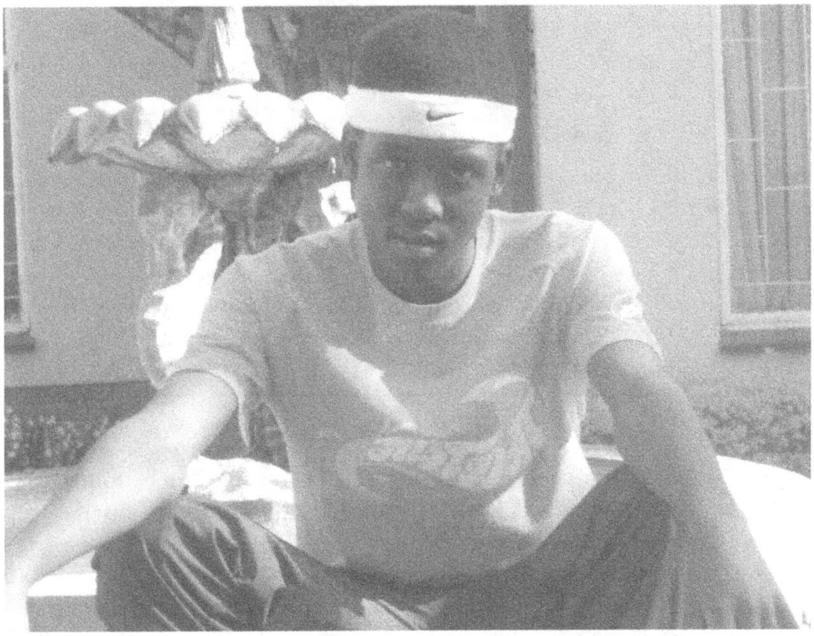

(Photo) Kagiso Maifadi pictured at Vista Clinic (South Africa) where he underwent residential psychiatric care due to his heroin dependence.

Questions

1. Describe the full constellation of circumstances presumed to be involved in the client's problems.
2. Explain all mental health concepts related to the client's presenting problem.
3. How would symptom relief and intervention be explained from a secular Western perspective?

Family therapy offers a way to view clinical problems within the context of a family's transactional patterns. Family therapy also represents a form of intervention in which members of a family are assisted to identify and change problematic, maladaptive, self-defeating, enabling, and repetitive relationship patterns. Unlike individual focused therapies, in family therapy, the identified patient (the family member considered to be the problem in the family) is viewed as a symptom bearer, expressing the family's disequilibrium or current dysfunction. The family system itself is the primary unit of treatment and not the identified patient. Helping families change leads to improved functioning of individuals as well as families (Corsini & Wedding, 1995). Some form of family intervention is now standard for both residential and outpatient treatment of substance use disorders. Successful outcome to intervention is related to family stability and support (Donoghoe et al., 1987; Gleeson, 1991; Sandoz, 1991; Sheridan, 1994).

In traditional African belief systems, illness is thought to be caused by disturbed social relationships that create imbalances in the form of mental and physical problems. Mental illnesses, such as substance use disorders, are regarded as a sign of a lack of harmony between the person and the environment (Cassell, 1994; Karim, Ziqubu-Page & Arendse, 1994). This harmony, in most

Research Box 17.1: Heroin Dependence Recovery

Dos Santos, M., & Van Staden, F. (2008). Heroin dependence recovery. *Journal of Psychology in Africa*, *18*(2), 327–38.

Objective: This descriptive study explored the factors that are important in achieving abstinence, in allowing recovery to be maintained in the long term, and in potentially allowing an eventual exit from heroin dependence, from the experiences and suggestions of forty long-term voluntarily abstinent heroin dependents.

Method: A mixed design, making use of qualitative analyses of in-depth case-study interviews, as well as quantitative analyses of data from the cross-sectional survey regarding the sample profiles, was adopted for the study. Information was collected from forty participants, thirty-one of whom remained voluntarily abstinent from heroin for over a year, meeting the *DSM-IV-TR* criteria for Opioid Dependence Sustained Full Remission (American Psychiatric Association, 2000). The remaining nine participants fulfilled the *DSM-IV-TR* criteria for Opioid Dependence Early Partial Remission (American Psychiatric Association, 2000).

Results: Findings revealed that behavior modification and the promotion of recovery occurred mostly through interventions, producing a range of positive effects that facilitated natural recovery processes.

Conclusion: Clear support was obtained for the "maturing out" hypothesis of heroin dependence.

Questions

1. What were the reflections of long-term voluntarily abstinent heroin dependent participants concerning the recovery process they underwent?
2. In what respect may the biographic and sociodemographic backgrounds of the long-term voluntarily abstinent heroin dependent participants have contributed toward or influenced their recovery?
3. What are the long-term voluntarily abstinent heroin dependent participant perspectives' regarding intervention within their recovery process? How does this enhance your understanding of indigenous and modern substance use disorder intervention modalities?

African communities, is controlled by the ancestors and thus affects traditional African belief systems; for example, the majority of Shona people in Zimbabwe believe that illnesses, such as substance dependence, may come from the ancestor spirits, angry spirits, or even alien spirits (Pelzer & Ebigbo, 1989). Indigenous healers usually work successfully with illness that has high emotional content, which is known as psychosomatic illness in allopathic medicine, and psychological illness. They believe they receive healing powers from the ancestors (Hewson, 1998). To this end, family therapy can be used, in a complementary manner within the African indigenous context, to address ancestral, family and social dynamics.

Maturing Out Approaches

One of the earliest and most widely quoted accounts of giving up opiates is the *"maturing out" hypothesis* of Winick (1962). Winick advanced the theory that opioid dependence is a self-limiting process and that most opiate dependents mature out of their use naturally. Based on a study of 7,234 arrestee records of opiate dependents in the United States, which showed that as age increased, the number of people being arrested for drug-related offences decreased, he concluded that two-thirds of opiate dependents "mature out" of their syndrome in their mid-thirties.

The maturing out hypothesis consisted of more than a trend to cessation of opiate use within a specified age group. Winick (1962) proposed a psychodynamic explanation. He speculated that substance abusers begin taking opiates as a method of coping with the challenges and problems of early adulthood. Years later, as a result of some process of emotional homeostasis, the stresses and strains of life become sufficiently stabilized so that the individual can face them without the support provided by opiates. Waldorf (1983) argued that, besides the "maturing out" of opioid dependence and death, individuals can also "drift" out of use, become alcoholic or mentally ill, give up because of religious/political conversion, "retire" by giving up the substance while retaining certain aspects of the lifestyle, or change because their situation or environment has changed.

Young African males are turning to substances such as heroin at an alarming rate. In a sense, substances such as heroin, are replacing the traditional "manhood" rituals and initiation rites of the indigenous African culture. Traditional initiation schools, for example, may also be unfamiliar with the heroin/drug dependence and withdrawal syndromes, and the specialized care that such syndromes necessitate. This phenomenon may highlight the significant role that the reinstilling of traditional rites may have in averting such dependencies, and in helping African substance dependents "mature-out" of their syndromes (Dos Santos, 2009).

Contextual Factors

Changes in the socioemotional context of a substance abuser can also lead to complete remission. For instance, Robins (1993) proposed that a change in environment for many servicemen returning from the Vietnam War resulted in remission, indicating the important role that social context may play in dependence and recovery. The second factor is very severe dependence, which seems paradoxical, but evidence suggests that severity – getting tired/hitting rock bottom – may be favorable for recovery. The third factor is the fortuitous occurrence of life experiences, which disrupt entrenched habits and minimize relapse. These experiences include acquiring a substitute behavior that competes with the dependence, encountering compulsory supervision, discovering new sources of hope and an improved self-esteem, and finding new people to love to whom the dependent is not "in debt." Several studies have also shown that the influence of significant others, such as partners or children, can be important in the decision to quit (Frykholm, 1985; Simpson, Joe, Lehman, & Sells, 1986; Smart, 1994; Waldorf, 1983). Another important factor reported to be influential in the decision to stop is deteriorating health or the fear of health problems (Simpson et al., 1986; Valliant, 1983; Waldorf, 1983), as well as the occurrence of more general negative events such as a period in prison or the overdose or death of drug-using friends/associates (Edwards, Oppenheimer, & Taylor 1992; Shaffer, 1992; Shaffer & Jones, 1989).

Phases of Recovery

Frykholm (1985) proposed three phases of addiction recovery, referred to as experimental, adaptation, and compulsive, and three phases of deaddiction, wherein the process of becoming addicted is reversed. According to Frykholm, the first phase of deaddiction involves a period of ambivalence, during which the negative effects of substance use are increasingly felt, resulting in a gradual desire to stop using substances. This is generally offset by a continuation of pleasurable effects of substances and a physical dependence on substances. In contrast, in the treatment phase, attempts at detoxification become more sustained and substance-free periods grow longer. In this phase, the substance dependent perceives a need for external control and support and so seeks help, and may also undergo a radical reorientation in which he or she suddenly experiences a desire to fulfill the role of ex-addict. The final stage is referred to as emancipatory, and involves the period following detoxification when the substance dependent effectively becomes an ex-addict and can remain "clean" without external assistance (Frykholm, 1985). Although Frykholm (1985) provided a useful model of substance dependence, his work has been criticized for not allowing for spontaneous recovery from dependence. As previously noted, spontaneous recovery from substance use is possible from personal and contextual influences.

LEGAL AND PROFESSIONAL ISSUES

Key legal and professional considerations, in understanding substance use counseling in African settings, are regulation criteria, access to treatment, and professional skill development. Each one of these aspects is discussed in turn.

Regulation

In the not so distant past, almost anyone in South Africa, for example, could open a drug rehabilitation center, offer rehabilitation services, and ask a fee for these services – regardless of his or her professional training or background. These facilities are able to fall outside the ambit of the *Mental Health Act* (Act 17 of 2002) and the *Prevention and Treatment of Drug Dependency Act* (Act 20 of 1992) by calling themselves "care centers." Such facilities are thus not regulated by the National Departments of Health or Social Development. Numerous unregistered examples of such centers still prevail in South Africa, and various human rights violations have been reported (Bateman, 2006). This situation has also arisen due to the state's closure of several long-established centers and a reduction in subsidies for organizations such as the South African National Council on Alcoholism and Drug Dependence (SANCA).

Psychiatric facilities, registered by the National Department of Health, most often treat substance use disorders as secondary symptoms. However, there has been a recent inclination in psychiatric facilities to open specialized substance use disorder units. Only recently the *Minimum Norms and Standards for Substance Dependence Inpatient Centres* has been issued by the National Department of Social Development (2005). These norms and standards outline the criteria for the registration of residential rehabilitation facilities in South Africa. However, the manpower to monitor the standards set is likely to be deficient (Bateman, 2006; Leggett, 2001). The Minimum Norms and Standards for Outpatient Treatment are currently under review by the National Department of Social Development.

Access to Treatment

Research indicates that patients who receive residential care are more likely to succeed than those who do not, and the probability of success rises with the length of stay in residential treatment (Gossop, 2003). Substance dependents do not have equal access to residential care; probably the single most compelling reason for redundancy of adequate substance use disorder interventions in Africa is the lack of affordable treatment centers to which clients may actually be directed, though there is a trend to open up state-subsidized beds in some African countries (Bateman, 2006). It is also clear that there is an important interaction between the characteristics of the client and the type of intervention. Therapeutic success depends on matching client and therapy (Krivanek, 1988; National Drug Master Plan: Republic of South Africa, 1999). Regrettably, the period between a young substance user's first experience with the substance and first treatment consultation is often several years, by which time successful treatment is likely to be more complicated.

Professional Skills Development

A lack of general training on the part of program personnel makes assessment and intervention redundant (Bateman, 2006, Gossop, 2003; Krivanek, 1998). Counseling interventions are also now provided by a wide range of personnel with differing training backgrounds, and in a wider range of settings. The processes of recovery from a substance use disorder are not always gradual and incremental, but they often reflect sudden changes in beliefs and behaviors. Recovery may also be highly idiosyncratic. Counseling is not an impersonal process offered by neutral agents. For the client it can be an important life event, and the relationship between patient and therapist can have great emotional and psychological significance. It is surprising that substance use disorder research has paid very little attention to the role of therapist characteristics and skills and their influence on treatment outcome (Dos Santos & Van Staden, 2008; Gossop, 2003).

At present, there are techniques and tools that provide individuals with useful assistance and knowledge on how to stop using and refrain from returning to substance use. It is no longer acceptable to simply do what feels right. Organizations and professionals who specialize in treating substance use disorders are an accepted part of the health care delivery system. As in all other areas of health care, there is a rapidly increasing dependence on the use of scientific information to shape and improve the future of the field. Within the past decade, psychiatrists, medical doctors, psychologists, social workers, family therapists, nurses, and other allied health professionals have all incorporated knowledge about the identification and treatment of substance use disorders into categories of licensure and certification requirements. It is the ethical responsibility of the clinical practitioner in the substance use disorder intervention field, as in other fields (i.e., cancer and heart disease), to stay informed about new and more effective clinical procedures. The field of substance use disorder treatment is becoming increasingly professional, and those who are part of the system need to continue to stay abreast of new developments. New techniques and tools can be used to make a difference in promoting successful recovery for individuals currently unsuccessful with existing treatments (Coombs, 2004). As new approaches with sound scientific support emerge, methods may be revised and new treatment options added. Although some of the elements of effective treatment intervention have been defined in this chapter, there is much to learn and much room for improvement.

ISSUES FOR RESEARCH AND SCHOLARSHIP

In this subsection, various issues for substance use disorder counseling and research are explored. These concerns address the limited evidence base for substance use disorder interventions, the poor regulations of substance use disorder interventions, and the lack of infrastructure and resources of substance use disorder interventions. Interdisciplinary collaboration between professionals and indigenous healers is also discussed.

Limited Evidence Base

Most research indicates a need for some level of social support or therapeutic intervention for substance dependents, and a number of models and programs have been developed to help them. Unfortunately, most interventions remain input orientated and little is done to measure their impact and effectiveness. However, just because a program has not been subjected to the scrutiny of research does not mean it does not work, but the sheer number of people receiving services of unknown value for substance use disorders is cause for concern (Barlow & Durand, 1995). Collaboration with indigenous healers is important and more knowledge needs to be gained about how indigenous healers and mental health services in the formal health sector can work together. Criteria of efficacy in substance use disorder counseling need to be formulated, both in terms of specific therapies and interventions found in indigenous and in modern practice, in terms of the more general question of whether, and how, they may contribute to substance use disorder recovery. Both individual (psychological, symbolic, pharmacological) as well as social mechanisms (entering and extending a network, creating support groups and redistributive chains, social competence) need to be studied as therapeutic mechanisms that may have generalizable qualities.

Regulation Criteria

Different parties are involved or have a strong interest in substance abuse intervention services. These include the *individual patients* entering treatment; the *clinical programs* that offer different types of services; *family members* or others who are personally involved with those receiving treatment; third-party *treatment purchasers and funders* (national, regional, and local); and various types of *regulatory agencies* who oversee, evaluate, or enforce legal or clinical standards. There are also other concerned individuals and agencies that have personal or professional relationships with substance dependents in treatment. All of these groups tend to have different expectations about intervention and about what should count as a successful intervention outcome. An effective response to substance misuse and dependence cannot be regarded as the sole responsibility of treatment services. Other services will necessarily come into contact with people with substance dependence problems, and the responsibility for engaging with these problems should be spread more widely. Although collaboration between mental health practitioners and traditional healers may also appear to be warranted, evidence is currently lacking to support collaboration between the two groups as full-fledged medical partners (Robertson, 2006).

Lack of Infrastructure and Resources

Rocha-Silva (1998) notes that matters are further complicated by the lack of integrated information needed for the effective intervention for substance dependents in Africa. She cites the lack of "infrastructure," in developing countries, that generally facilitates long-term comprehensive and integrated information gathering. Unlike other sub-Saharan countries, however, South Africa is unique in that it now has a well-developed capacity for surveillance and research on drug-related problems. The primary resource of this information is the South African Community Epidemiology Network on Drug Use (SACENDU) project, which currently monitors alcohol and other drug use trends in South Africa (Parry & Pithey, 2006).

Despite growing evidence of and association between African substance abusers' use of indigenous and supplementary modern treatment services (such as psychosocial and pharmacological/medical care) and treatment outcomes, substance dependence treatment programs in Africa generally fail to meet international research-based treatment standards; for example, detoxification services are provided for by fewer than half of all facilities in Cape Town (Myers & Parry, 2002). Emerging standards for substance use disorder treatment have called upon treatment providers to enhance traditional addiction services with services that address clients' psychosocial needs.

Interdisciplinary Collaboration

Since the problem of substance use disorder intervention and recovery is everyone's concern, substance use disorder research reflects the preconceptions of the variety of researchers who have studied it. The clinical psychologist may view substance dependence as a character disorder that may be addressed by the facilitation of the identity restructuring of the personality. The economist may see substances as commodities and study their marketing systems in terms of supply and demand measured by cost and purity of the substance. In a similar way, pharmacologists, anthropologists, and other specialists bring their own skills and special points of view to substance dependence and recovery. Interdisciplinary collaboration would contribute to more effective interventions for substance use treatment in African settings.

SUMMARY AND CONCLUSION

With the increase in our knowledge of human chemistry and psychodynamics, specialization has tended to dismember human beings. Observation and treatment in bits and pieces can mean that the total person is lost sight of and becomes no more than the sum of his or her symptoms. Substance use disorder recovery is more likely to be successful if it is multisystemic and multidisciplinary in approach, and when it addresses clients' functioning in a number of contexts and from the viewpoint of people familiar with those contexts. An intervention team should comprise members with unique expertise and insight into the contexts in which the recovering substance dependent will ultimately function. Although professionals are encouraged to work with people with experiences and expertise outside their customary comfort zones (e.g., indigenous healers) who may be significant to the client's world view, integrating such systems will not be easy (Mpofu, 2003). It is not just the beliefs of the patient that are important in a doctor–patient relationship but those of the doctor or therapist as well.

The field of substance use disorder intervention worldwide has been "in transition" for some time; in terms of theory and practice, the field is less in transition now than it was a few years ago. Many interventions and procedures have begun to be integrated routinely into clinical practice. In particular, motivational and cognitive–behavioral approaches, following the surge of interest in these approaches in research studies, have made great inroads into practice at the grassroots level. Pharmacological approaches have been updated to include the latest advances in the pharmacological treatment of substance use disorders. The use of medications specific to the treatment of substance use disorders, despite reasonably strong research evidence for their efficacy, has not become widespread in practice in Africa. Pharmacological interventions remain one of the most fervently researched and heavily funded of all approaches to substance dependence intervention (Rotgers, Morgenstern, & Walters, 2003).

Assessing, diagnosing, and counseling a substance abuser can be quite complicated. Substance use disorders involve biological, psychological (including behavioral, cognitions, spirituality, and emotions), and environmental factors that influence its onset, course, maintenance, and treatment. Because of the interactions of biological, psychological, and environmental factors there can be great differences between presentations of substance dependence in different users. There is a great variation between individuals and no single pathway into dependence or to recovery. Conversely, research has made many advances in the past few years and there have been some promising interventions developed for people who are substance dependent.

REFERENCES

Adelekan, M. L., & Stimson, G. V. (1997). Problems and prospects of implementing harm reduction for HIV and injecting drug use in high-risk sub-Saharan African countries. *Journal of Drug Issues*, *27*, 315–23.

Affinnih, Y. H. (2002). Revisiting sub-Saharan African countries' drug problems: Health, social, economic costs, and drug control policy. *Substance Use and Misuse*, *37*, 265–90.

American Psychiatric Association. (2000). *Diagnostic and statistical manual of mental disorders – text revision* (4th ed.). Washington, DC: Author.

Arnett, J. J. (2007). *International encyclopedia of adolescence: A historical and cultural survey of young people around the world*. New York: Routledge.

Aziz, R. (1990). *C.J. Jung's psychology of religion and synchronicity*. Albany, NY: The State University of New York Press.

Aziz, R. (2007). *The syndetic paradigm: The untrodden path beyond Freud and Jung*. Albany, NY: The State University of New York Press.

Barlow, D. H., & Durand, V. M. (1995). *Abnormal psychology: An integrated approach*. Pacific Grove, CA: Brooks/Cole.

Bateman, C. (2006). Illegal addiction treatment centres 'mushrooming.' *South African Medical Journal*, *96*(5), 379–81.

Baynham, S. (1998). The Nigerian nexus. In The South African Institute of International Affairs. *The illegal drug trade in Southern Africa: International dimensions to a local crisis*. Johannesburg: Jan Smuts House.

Bernard, B. (2004). *Resiliency: What we have learned*. San Francisco: West Ed.

Boone, R. (2001). Update from UNODCCP. In A. Plüddemann, S. Hon, C. Parry, A. Bhana, S. Matthysen, & W. Gerber (Eds.). *South African Community Epidemiology on Drug Use (SACENDU): Monitoring alcohol and drug abuse trends (phase 9)* (pp. 3–7). Cape Town, South Africa: Medical Research Council.

Bührmann, M. V. (1984). *Living in two worlds: Communication between a white healer and her black counterparts*. Cape Town, South Africa: Human & Rousseau.

Cassell, E. J. (1994). *The nature of suffering and the goals of medicine*. New York: Oxford University Press.

Coombs, R. E. (2004). *Handbook of addictive disorders: A practical guide to diagnosis and treatment*. Hoboken, NJ: John Wiley & Sons.

Corsini, R. J., & Wedding, D. (1995). *Current psychotherapies* (5th ed.). Itasca, IL: F. E. Peacock.

De Chaud, N. (2002). Adam & Eve. Carte Blanche. Retrieved August 18, 2002 from http://beta.mnet.co.za/carteblanche/Article.aspx?Id=2043&ShowId=1

Des Jarlais, D. C., McKnight, C., & Milliken, J. (2004). Public funding of US syringe exchange programs. *Journal of Urban Health: Bulletin of the New York Academy of Medicine*, *81*, 118–21.

Dewing, S., Plüddemann, A., Myers, B. J., & Parry, C. D. H. (2006). Review of injecting drug use in six African countries: Egypt, Kenya, Mauritius, Nigeria, South Africa and Tanzania. *Drugs: Education, Prevention & Policy*, *13*(2), 121–37.

Donoghoe, M., Dorn, N., James, C., Jones, S., Ribbens, J., & South, N. (1987). How families and communities respond to heroin. In N. Dorn & N. South (Eds.), *A land fit for heroin? Drug policies, prevention and practice*. Houndsmill Basingstoke, England: Macmillan.

Dos Santos, M. (2009). *Defeating the dragon: Heroin dependence recovery*. Saarbrücken, Germany: VDM Verlag Dr. Müller Aktiengesellschaft & Co. KG.

Dos Santos, M., & Van Staden, F. (2008). Heroin dependence recovery. *Journal of Psychology in Africa*, *18* (2), 327–38.

Edwards, G., Oppenheimer, E., & Taylor, C. (1992). Hearing the noise in the system: Exploration of textual analysis as a method for studying change in drinking behaviour. *British Journal of Addiction*, *87*, 73–81.

Frykholm, B. (1985). The drug career. *Journal of Drug Issues*, *15*, 333–46.

Gleeson, A. (1991). Family therapy and substance abuse. *Australian and New Zealand Journal of Family Therapy*, *12*(2), 91–8.

Gossop, M. (2003). *Drug addiction and its treatment*. Oxford: Oxford University Press.

Haque, A. (2008). Culture-bound syndromes and healing practices in Malaysia. *Mental Health, Religion & Culture*, *11*(7), 685–96.

Hewson, M. G. (1998). Traditional healers in Southern Africa. *Annals of Internal Medicine*, *128*(12), 1029–34.

International Narcotics Control Board. (2004). Report on the International Narcotics Control Board for 2004.

Janzen, J. M. (1992). *Ngoma: Discourses of healing in central and southern Africa*. Berkeley: University of California Press.

Jayakody, A. A., Viner, R. M., Haines, M. M., Bhui, K. S., Head, J. A., Taylor, S. J. C., et al. (2006). Illicit and traditional drug use among ethnic minority adolescents in East London. *Public Health*, *120*(4), 329–38.

Kaplan, J. (1983). *The hardest drug: Heroin and public policy*. Chicago: University of Chicago Press.

Karam, E. G., Yabroudi, P., & Melham, N. M. (2002). Comorbidity of substance abuse and other psychiatric disorders in acute general psychiatric admissions: A story from Lebanon. *Comprehensive Psychiatry*, *43*(6), 463–8.

Karim, S. S. A., Ziqubu-Page, T., & Arendse, R. (1994). The traditional healing process – bridging the gap. *South African Medical Journal*. *84*(3), 328–32.

Kleber, H. (1981). Detoxification from narcotics. In J. Lowinson & P. Ruiz (Eds.), *Substance abuse*. Baltimore: Williams & Wilkins.

Krivanek, J. (1988). *Heroin: Myths and reality*. Sydney, Australia: Allen & Unwin.

Kruger, D. (1981). *An introduction to phenomenological psychology*. Pittsburgh, PA: Duquesne University Press.

Leggett, T. (2001). Rainbow vice: The drugs and sex industries in the new South Africa. Claremont, South Africa: David Philip.

Leshner, A. I. (1999). Drug abuse and mental disorders: Comorbidity is reality. *NIDA Notes*, *14*(4), 3–4.

Marlatt, A., & Gordon, J. (1985). *Relapse prevention*. New York: Guilford Press.

McCurdy, S. A., Williams, M. L., Kilonzo, G. P., Ross, M. W., & Leshabari, M. T. (2005). Heroin and HIV risk in Dar es Salaam, Tanzania: Youth hangouts, *mageto* and injecting practices. *AIDS Care*, *17*, S65–76.

McIntosh, J., & McKeganey, N. (2002). *Beating the dragon: The recovery from dependent drug use*. Harow, UK: Prentice Hall.

Mental Health Act (Act 17 of 2002). *Government Gazette*. Cape Town: Republic of South Africa.

Mpofu, E. (2003). Conduct disorders: Presentation, treatment options and cultural efficacy in an African setting. *International Journal of Disability*, Community and Rehabilitation, 2(1). Retrieved August 19, 2009 from http://www.ijdcr.ca/VOL02_01_CAN/articles/mpofu.shtml.

Myers, B., & Parry, C. D. H. (2002). *Report on audit of substance abuse facilities in Cape Town*. Cape Town, South Africa: Medical Research Council.

National Department of Social Development. (2005). *Minimum Norms and Standards for Inpatient Treatment Centres*. Pretoria, South Africa: Author.

National Drug Master Plan: Republic of South Africa 2006–2011. Pretoria, South Africa: Drug Advisory Board.

Needle, R. H., Ball, A., Des Jarlais, D. C., Whitmore, C., & Lambert, E. (2000). The global research network on HIV prevention in drug-using populations (GRN) 1998–2000: Trends in the epidemiology, ethnography, and prevention of HIV/AIDS in injection drug users. Paper presented at the Third Annual Global Research Network Meeting on HIV Prevention in Drug Using Populations. Durban: South Africa.

Odejide, A. O. (2006). Status of drug use/abuse in Africa: A review. *International Journal of Mental Health and Addiction*, *4*(2), 87–102.

Parry, C. D. H., & Pithey, A. L. (2006). Risk behaviour and HIV among drug using populations in South Africa. *African Journal of Drug & Alcohol Studies*, *5*(2), 140–57.

Peltzer, K., & Ebigbo, P. O. (1989). *Clinical psychology in Africa: South of the Sahara, the Caribbean and Afro-Latin American*. Nigeria: Chuka Printing Company.

Plüddemann, A., Parry, C. D. H, Cerff, P., Bhana, A., Potgieter, H., Gerber, W., et al. (2007). Monitoring alcohol and drug abuse trends in South Africa (July 1996–June 2007). *SACENDU Research Brief*, *10*(2), 1–12. Medical Research Council of South Africa.

Prevention and Treatment of Drug Dependency Act (Act 20 of 1992). *Government Gazette*. Cape Town: Republic of South Africa.

Reber, A. S. (1985). *The penguin dictionary of psychology*. London: Penguin Books.

Robertson, B. A. (2006). Does the evidence support corroboration between psychiatry and traditional healers? Findings from three South African studies. *South African Psychiatry Review*, *9*, 87–90.

Robins, L. (1993). Vietnam veterans' rapid recovery from heroin addiction: A fluke or normal expectations? *Addiction*, *88*, 1041–54.

Rocha-Silva, L. (1998). The nature and extent of drug use and the prevalence of related problems in South Africa: A national surveillance. Pretoria, South Africa: HSRC Press.

Rodrigues-Llera, M. C., Domingo-Salvany, A., Brugal, M. T., Silva, T. C., Sanchez-Niubo, A., & Torrens, M. (2006). Psychiatric comorbidity in young heroin users. *Drug and Alcohol Dependence*, *84*(1), 48–55.

Roerecke, M., Obot, I., Patra, J., & Rehm, J. (2008). Volume of alcohol consumption, patterns of drinking and burden of disease in sub-Saharan Africa, 2002. *African Journal of Drug and Alcohol Studies*, *7*(1), 1–17.

Rotgers, F., Morgenstern, J., & Walters, S. T. (2003). *Treating substance abuse*. London: Guilford Press.

Rudgley, R. (1998). *The encyclopaedia of psychoactive substances*. New York: St Martin's Press.

Sandoz, C. J. (1991). Locus of control, emotional maturity and family dynamics as components of recovery in recovering alcoholics. *Alcoholism Treatment Quarterly*, *8*(4), 17–31.

Serva Dei, S. J. (2000). A pathway to freedom: Freedom from ad-dictions. God's instruction book for the mind opened and explained. Johannesburg, South Africa: SilverBird Electronic Publications.

Shaffer, H. (1992). The psychology of stage change: The transition from addiction to recovery. In J. Lowinson, P. Ruiz, R. Millman, & J. Langrod (Eds.), *Substance Abuse: A Comprehensive Textbook*. Baltimore, MD: Williams & Wilkins.

Shaffer, H., & Jones, S. (1989). *Quitting cocaine: The struggle against impulse*. Lanham, MD: Lexington Books.

Sheridan, M. J. (1994). A proposed intergenerational model of substance abuse, family functioning, and abuse/neglect. *Child Abuse & Neglect*, *19*(5), 519–30.

Simpson, D., Joe, G., Lehman, W., & Sells, S. (1986). Addiction careers: Etiology, treatment and 12 year follow up outcomes. *The Journal of Drug Issues*, *16*(1), 107–21.

Smart, R. (1994). Dependence and correlates of change: A review of the literature. In G. Edwards & M. Lader (Eds.). *Addiction: Processes of change*. Oxford: Oxford University Press.

Sobiecki, J. F. (2008). A review of plants used in divination in southern Africa and their psychoactive effects. *South African Humanities*, *20*, 333–51.

Tart, C. T. (1975). *Transpersonal psychologies*. London: Routledge/Kegan Paul.

UNAIDS. (2005). Fact sheet.

United Nations Office on Drugs and Crime. (2005). *World Drug Report 2005*. Vienna: Author.

United Nations Office on Drugs and Crime. (2007). *World Drug Report 2007*. Vienna: Author.

Vaillant, G. (1983). *The natural history of alcoholism*. Cambridge, England: Harvard University Press.

Vasile, D., Gheorghe, M. D., Civrea, R., & Paraschiv, S. (2002). Antisocial Personality Disorder – heroin dependence comorbidity. *European Neuropsychopharmacology*, *12* (Supplement 3), 392.

Waldorf, D. (1983). Natural recovery from opiate addiction: Some social-psychological processes of untreated recovery. *Journal of Drug Issues*, *13*(2), 237–80.

Winick, C. (1962). Maturing out of narcotics addiction. *UN Bulletin on Narcotics*, *14*, 1–7.

World Health Organization (WHO). 2004. *Global Status Report on Alcohol, 2004*. Geneva: Author.

Zeleza, T., & Dickson, E. (2003). *Encyclopedia of twentieth-century African history*. New York: Taylor & Francis.

SELF-CHECK EXERCISES

1. Define the various diagnostic categories of substance use disorders.
2. Outline the core theories regarding substance use disorder recovery that may influence African indigenous healing practices.
3. Describe any three major approaches to counseling intervention for substance use disorders with promise in African settings. What is the rationale of each of these methods? Speculate on how they are likely to achieve their therapeutic effects within the African context.
4. Discuss the extent to which individuals, groups (including families) and communities have access to interventions for substance use disorders.
5. Outline the extent and impact of information, education, and communication as a means of preventing substance use disorders.

FIELD-BASED EXPERIENTIAL EXERCISES

1. Interview a substance-dependent individual who is undergoing residential treatment. Determine his or her perceptions with regards to the effective treatments/interventions that are most conducive toward recovery for the syndrome that he/she presents with. How are his or her perceptions explained by indigenous and modern concepts of substance use disorder recovery?
2. Consult with three different substance dependents with similar profiles undergoing residential treatment and compare their responses.

3. Interview a mental health professional who specializes in the treatment of substance use disorders, with regard to (a) etiology of the condition, (b) view of effective counseling interventions, (c) role of pharmacotherapy, (d) views on indigenous healing practices, and (e) view with regard to harm-reduction intervention.
4. Observe a mental health substance use disorder specialist in practice to discover the process of assessing, diagnosing, and formulating an individual treatment care plan for an individual presenting with a substance use disorder.
5. Information on the prevalence of drug abuse and particularly IDU in Africa is limited due, in part, to poorly developed gathering systems. Discuss.
6. Discuss the piloting, evaluation, and development of harm-reduction polices and outreach programs (e.g., needle exchanges) within the African context.

Reproduced from Dewing, Plüddemann, Myers, & Parry, 2006.

MULTIPLE-CHOICE QUESTIONS

1. A phenomenon that can vary in intensity from a mild involvement with a behavior to an addiction that seriously restricts an individual's other behavioral options is referred to as:
   a. Physiological dependence
   b. Obsessive–compulsive disorder
   c. Substance dependence
   d. Psychological dependence
   e. Bipolar disorder
2. The "maturing out" hypothesis of substance dependence was first developed by:
   a. Ellis
   b. Biernacki
   c. Waldorf
   d. Jung
   e. Winick
3. A mode of HIV transmission that is six times higher than for heterosexual acts:
   a. Homosexual acts
   b. Blood transfusions
   c. Sex work
   d. Intravenous drug use
   e. Physical contact
4. The most compelling reason for redundancy of adequate substance use disorder interventions in Africa is due to:
   a. The lack of trained staff
   b. The lack of affordable treatment centers to which clients may be directed.
   c. The lack of education amongst substance dependents
   d. A high level of illiteracy
   e. A high level of HIV/AIDS among substance dependents
5. A mental illness that is concurrent to a substance use disorder is referred to as:
   a. Codependence
   b. Comorbidity
   c. Depression
   d. Personality disorder
   e. Bipolar disorder
6. A controversial social policy based on the philosophy of harm-reduction:
   a. Illicit drug contol
   b. Incarceration
   c. Needle exchange programs
   d. Diversion programs
   e. Rehabilitation
7. A behavioral procedure based on the principle of encouraging previously agreed behavior patterns by offering positive reinforcers when they occur, and by punishing the individual if they do not, or if other undesirable behavior patterns occur (such as substance use):
   a. Cognitive–behavioral therapy
   b. Operant conditioning
   c. Classical conditioning
   d. Relapse prevention
   e. Contingency management
8. The concept used for substance dependents facing criminal charges that are diverted from the criminal justice system to a means of making suitable restitution to specific victims and society in general, effectively given a choice between incarceration and rehabilitation:
   a. Dual diagnosis
   b. Restorative justice
   c. Comorbid
   d. Probation
   e. State patient
9. A form of depth psychology, the primary focus of which is to reveal the unconscious content of a substance dependent's psyche in an effort to alleviate psychic tension, relying heavily on the interpersonal relationship between the substance dependent and therapist:
   a. Psychoanalysis
   b. Rational–emotive therapy
   c. Psychodynamic psychotherapy
   d. Cognitive–behavioral therapy
   e. Multimodal therapy
10. The first line of intervention for an individual presenting with a substance use disorder should be:
    a. Pharmacological
    b. Indigenous healing
    c. Psychotherapeutic
    d. Assessment
    e. Psychiatric

Answers to the multiple-choice questions are provided at the back of the book

18 Career Counseling People of African Ancestry

Mark Watson, Mary McMahon, Nhlanhla Mkhize, Robert D. Schweitzer, and Elias Mpofu

OVERVIEW. One of the most important challenges facing the career counseling profession is developing effective strategies to counsel racially diverse individuals. Understanding the role of racial factors in career counseling requires an understanding of the impact of race on the development and identification of career concerns (Leong & Hartung, 1997). This chapter invites an understanding of career counseling with a focus on people of African ancestry. There is scant literature on the career development and career counseling of people of African ancestry including African Americans. This paucity of literature is explained, in part, by the fact that people of African ancestry have unique histories of being excluded from a broad range of human services, including career counseling.

This chapter considers career counseling with people of African ancestry. First, the chapter explores how the African cultural belief of *Ubuntu* may influence individuals and then considers its possible influence on career counseling. Second, the chapter considers how cultural contexts may impact the career counseling of individuals of African ancestry, specifically African Americans and African immigrants. Finally, social justice and narrative approaches to career counseling are examined as a means to address the needs of people of African ancestry in a range of cultural settings.

LEARNING OBJECTIVES

By the end of the chapter, the reader should be able to:

1. Demonstrate an understanding of the evolving nature of career counseling and of the culture of people of African ancestry.
2. Show how career counseling may be culturally influenced.
3. Critique the construct of *Ubuntu* as it applies to the career development of people of African ancestry.
4. Discuss career development from a group identity development perspective.
5. Discuss career counseling from a social justice perspective.
6. Evaluate narrative theory as an approach to the career counseling of people of African ancestry.

INTRODUCTION

In the context of a rapidly changing world, career counseling is unique in that it serves as an "interface between personal and societal needs, between individual and opportunity structures, between private and public identities" (Watts, 1996, p. 229). Thus, career counseling may be viewed as a process that is undergoing revision and redefinition to remain relevant and responsive to career development issues and concerns of the twenty-first century. For instance, there have been a number of calls in the literature to reinvent career counseling by incorporating indigenous psychologies, social constructionist, and hermeneutic and narrative approaches, among other possibilities (Collin & Young, 1992; Kuit & Watson, 2005; Mkhize, 2005; Mkhize & Frizelle, 2000).

Fundamental to the process of revising and redefining career counseling is a recognition of its historical roots in social justice (McMahon, Arthur, & Collins, 2008a). Over time, career counseling evolved away from these roots toward a more individualized, Westernized, middle-class perspective of career development. This evolved career theory and practice has been adopted and adapted in countries and cultures where its relevance is questionable (Stead & Watson, 2006). For example, career counseling theory and practice in South Africa and, one might add, Africa in general, has been critiqued for its over-reliance on imported theoretical and conceptual frameworks (Stead, 1996; Stead & Watson, 1998; Watson & Stead, 2002). Similarly, the scarcity and validity of frameworks for the career counseling of minority groups such as African Americans has been questioned (Brown & Pinterits, 2001; Leong & Hartung, 1997; Mpofu, 2005). However, people of African ancestry comprise a heterogeneous group, and attempts to present career counseling strategies for them run the risk of misrepresenting their experiences as individuals or stereotyping individuals from a particular population group.

Recently, there has been a greater emphasis in career counseling theory and practice that accommodates holistic, contextual perspectives that are reflected in Wolf and Kolb's (1980) longstanding definition of career development as involving

> one's whole life, not just occupation. As such, it concerns the whole person ... More than that, it concerns him or her in the ever-changing contexts of his or her life. The environmental pressures and constraints, the bonds

> that tie him or her to significant others, responsibilities to children and aging parents, the total structure of one's circumstances are also factors that must be understood and reckoned with. In these terms, career development and personal development converge. Self and circumstances – evolving, changing, unfolding in mutual interaction – constitute the focus and the drama of career development (pp. 1–2).

IMPORTANCE, DEFINITION, AND SCOPE OF KEY TERMS AND CONCEPTS

In essence, Wolf and Kolb's (1980) definition suggests the significant role of an individual's context in career development, one aspect of which could be an individual's cultural ancestry. Just as career counseling theory and practice may be regarded as an evolving process, so too may recent conceptualizations of culture be viewed as an evolving, contextualized process located within individuals (Stead, 2004). By way of example, people of African ancestry are now found in diverse cultural contexts ranging from traditional lifestyles and family structures, to African industrialized and Westernized cities, to those living as minority groups in majority societies of countries other than that of their African ancestry such as the United States.

THE TRADITIONAL CULTURAL VALUE OF *UBUNTU*

The African cultural concept of *Ubuntu* provides an example of how a cultural belief system can impact on our understanding of the career counseling process. The concept of *Ubuntu*, a Nguni term found in Southern Africa, is found in a number of African cultures and has salience across much of Africa. For instance, similar terms are used in Kenya, Tanzania, Uganda, Rwanda, Burundi, Mozambique, Egypt, and the Democratic Republic of the Congo (Karenga, 2004). The concept of *Ubuntu* is also evident in wisdoms and sayings found in African literature. Thus, Nelson Mandela refers to the proverb "*Umuntu ngumuntu ngabantu*," which may be translated as "A person is a person because of other people" or, as an alternative translation, "You can do nothing if you don't get the support of other people" (Sampson, 1999).

Despite the widespread usage of the concept, *Ubuntu* is a complex term that is difficult to limit to a single definition. Common features among definitions of *Ubuntu* are respecting the human dignity of others, treating and respecting others as human beings, group solidarity, human interdependence, and caring, and sensitivity to others' needs. In essence, *Ubuntu* refers to our common humanity, our interconnectedness, and our spiritual connectedness. Thus, the notion of *Ubuntu* provides a perspective on help seeking, caring, or counseling relationships involving people from diverse African ancestry.

This perspective suggests process implications illustrated by Dandala's (1996) definition of *Ubuntu* as the process of becoming a fully human, i.e., moral, person. Such a process leads to the attainment of ethical and moral sensibilities that define oneself as a truly human person (*Umuntu*). Thus, according to *Ubuntu*, individuals are defined by their practices within the context of their relationships (Karenga, 2004). These practices include the ethical obligation to respect the dignity of others and also to make a positive contribution toward the well-being of one's family and community (Mkhize, 2004). Several authors (e.g., Kamwangamalu, 1999; Mkhize, 2004; Ramose, 1999) point to the fact that an etymological analysis of the word *Ubuntu* would support this process view of becoming a person. In this regard, Ramose (1999) argues that "*Umuntu* ... is an activity rather than an act. It is an ongoing process impossible to stop unless motion itself is stopped" (p. 41). The process dimension of *Ubuntu* and *Umuntu* is reflected in the aBantu languages' root word "unu" meaning personhood and signifies the importance of becoming in all human activities (Mpofu, Gudyanga, & Ngara, 2007).

If *Umuntu* is not a static trait but a gradual process of becoming, how, then, is this to be achieved? To understand this process, it is important to turn to the role of the community as the context for the realization of both *Umuntu* and *Ubuntu* (Mnyaka & Motlhabi, 2005). The process of becoming a person does not occur in isolation from the community. Rather, the community plays a critical role in molding individuals into the best that they can be. This is premised on the idea of human interconnectedness: the view that humans do not exist alone, that their well-being is intimately interwoven with the well-being of others. *Ubuntu*, therefore, emphasizes the principle of human interdependence, and thus *Umuntu* views individuals as being in constant dialogue with other humans and the surrounding environment (Manganyi, 1973). This means that mature personhood is attained through participation in a community of other moral selves, that is, *Abantu* (Mkhize, 2004).

The concept of *Ubuntu* challenges Westernized conceptions of self-definition and identity. From the perspective of *Ubuntu*, individuals cannot be defined solely with reference to their internal psychological attributes such as thoughts and emotions. Rather, the community provides an important dimension of self-definition or identity. Mnyaka and Motlhabi (2005) argued that the growth of individuals takes place within the community; it is the community that opens up possibilities for individuals to realize their potential and, in turn, contribute to the good of others in the community. This stands in stark contrast to the autonomous view of self, wherein self is understood as being independent of others, trusting one's own judgment, and acting so as to maximize one's own interests (Mnyaka & Motlhabi, 2005).

From an *Ubuntu* perspective, career development includes all the activities a person engages with for the collective good or toward the betterment of the human condition. Edwards, Makunga, Ngcobo, and Dhlomo

(2004) provide a phenomenological explanation of five aspects of *Ubuntu*: (1) the meaning of life through human relations; (2) the meaning of life emerging from the quality of human relatedness; (3) communal spirituality and ceremony; (4) the humanity of caring, helping, and healing; and finally (5) the centrality of essentially human and humanly essential relationships. Each of these aspects is described below.

1. *The meaning of life through human relations*. Meaning in life as implied in the notion that *Ubuntu* is possible only through human relations. This position is consistent with that of modern interpersonal theorists who base their understanding of what it means to be human on the concept of interpersonal relatedness (Benjamin, 2003) and contemporary social identity theorists who argue that the self in the context of a group is more important than individual characteristics.

2. *The meaning of life emerging from the quality of human relatedness*. The meaning of life is dependent on the quality of human relationships and their authenticity. For instance, within traditional African communities, the everyday Zulu greeting of *sawubona*, the Ndebele greeting of *sabona*, and the Xhosa term *molo* can be translated to *we see you*. Similarly, a Zulu or Ndebele speaking person may ask "*Kunjani*" (i.e., how are you) in the sense of engaging in a genuine dialogue. A Zulu-speaking respondent may answer "*sihambanakho*," which implies we are going/living with it (e.g., as part of life's everyday survival struggle), "*sikhona*" (we are existing and present), "*siyaphila*" (we are alive, healthy, and well), "*siyaphila kakhulu*" (we are very well), or "*siphilile*" (we experience being sound, complete, and whole). Among the Ndebele speakers, the response would be "*sikona*," meaning "I am here" or "I am well." In common with many African language groups, the Ndebele response varies according to the relationship between the greeter and the respondent, that is, a younger person will always say *linjani* while an older person will say *kunjani*. Thus, there is a hierarchy in greetings based on age and the notion of respect for elder people.

3. *Communal spirituality and ceremony*. Communal spirituality, as reflected in *Ubuntu*, is most commonly expressed in traditional ceremonies and rituals (Edwards et al., 2004) that are based on the relationship between the individual, ancestors, self, and community. Rituals play a key role in maintaining health and well-being and take place within the public areas of the community, and they will always begin by acknowledging the ancestors in some form. Thus, the ancestors as well as members of the family or clan and the community are all involved in ritual. For instance, among the traditional Xhosa-speaking people, the first drop of home-brewed beer is "given" to the ancestors with the words "*Camagu*."

Notions of health and well-being are inextricably linked to the person's relations with the ancestors, with God (*Utixo*), and with members of the family or clan. Ill health within a traditional belief system may well result directly from the actions of a sorcerer but indirectly result from the individual being vulnerable and "open" to the influence of sorcery through the neglect of custom, which often refers to the neglect of family. Thus, issues of loyalty and obligation are paramount in human relationships.

4. *The humanity of caring, helping, and healing*. *Ubuntu* implies human involvement in caring, helping, and healing. In this sense, humanity is understood broadly and refers to the relationship between the community and the healer. In traditional and in contemporary communities, people are able to recognize and acknowledge "healers" as opposed to charlatans in the sense that genuine healing is characterized by the *Ubuntu* of committed, human care as opposed to the potentially corrupt influences of self-interested charlatans.

The "sacred" nature of healing, sometimes referred to as the "numinous" (Buhrmann, 1984) is revealed through the process whereby a person is "called" in traditional societies to become a healer. The traditional healer's special relationship with the ancestors is evident in the diagnostic process in which the healer "tells" clients the reason for their distress, thus encouraging clients to seek assistance. For instance, in a traditional community, distress may be related to the neglect of the ancestors, which may have left the individual vulnerable to negative influences. Again, this aspect of *Ubuntu* underpins the importance of loyalty and obligation in human affairs.

5. *The centrality of empathic human relationships*. *Ubuntu* implies essential ingredients of authentic human relationships that may be likened to Rogers' (1980) necessary conditions of empathy, warmth, respect, genuineness, immediacy, and concreteness. Within a traditional cosmology, these conditions are likened to the meaning-making aspects of relationships and particularly the notion of empathic understanding. This notion is well expressed by traditional healers who talk about their ability to "know" what is going on in the other person, through the sense of bodiliness, that is, the notion of *umbilini* (Xhosa term that refers to both intestines and also a feeling).

UBUNTU AND CAREER COUNSELING

Cultural issues can impact on the career counseling process in a number of ways. One such way is how the cultural beliefs of both the counselor and the client may influence the career counseling process. A related cultural influence on career counseling may be the definition and expectation of the roles within this process. We begin with an examination of the influence of cultural beliefs on the career counseling process.

Current approaches to career counseling have not fully exploited the emancipatory possibilities inherent in the idea of *Ubuntu*. In line with the process view of the self, career development becomes an ongoing process orientated toward maximizing the possibilities of the emerging self (*Umuntu*). This view of career development is mirrored in the African naming process, wherein great care is taken in the naming of the child, as it is believed that the child will take after his or her name. Likewise, in the event of death, funeral oration rituals take place to highlight the deceased's lived experience and the extent to which he or she fulfilled his or her social obligations to his or her family and the wider community. This ritual is referred to as the reciting of *inkambo ka mufi*, which literally can be translated as the deceased's journey, the sum total of the person's career.

The emergent view of the self makes it possible for the career counselor and the client to participate creatively in mapping out the possibilities inherent in *Umuntu* (developing as an individual who is always oriented toward other individuals). This mapping out involves the past, current, and future selves and is consistent with narrative approaches to career counseling that view counseling as a meaning-making process involving the rewriting of selves (Mkhize & Frizelle, 2000). Such meaning-making processes could involve eliciting stories from the client, along the following lines:

- How would you like to be remembered as a human being (e.g., by your family, community, religious congregants, and fellow workers)?
- Why is it important for you to be remembered like that?
- What do you need to do to be remembered that way?

Given that the community provides a context for the actualization of the individual, it is inconceivable within an African context that an individual's career can be realized independently of the community that "provides meaning and anchors in life for people" (Adonisi, 1994, p. 311). Thus, career counseling should aim at maximizing an individual's participation in social and communal life. It should enable the individual to strengthen community bonds in order to advance the community to a higher level of development than before. At the same time, the community should nourish the individual by opening up possibilities for the advancement of the self. This is consistent with understanding human existence as a dialogue between the individual and everything the individual stands in relation to (Manganyi, 1973; Mkhize, 2004).

While the process of becoming *Umuntu* suggests a balance between individuals and their social and environmental contexts, the reality is that social inequities impede opportunities to participate meaningfully in social and communal life and mitigate against *Umuntu* (the emergence of an ethical–moral self). Such societal inequities include violence, poverty, discrimination, oppression, lack of access to resources, and self-deprecating views about the self (Schiele, 1996; Speight & Vera, 2004). In addition, there are many issues in the work environment that people of African ancestry may face such as biased hiring and promotion practices, tokenism, isolation, or estrangement (Brown & Pinterits, 2001). Further, marked inequalities in learning and educational environments preclude full participation and progression for people of African ancestry (Akhurst & Mkhize, 2006; Nicholas, Naidoo, & Pretorius, 2006).

A view of counseling that is informed by the perspective of *Ubuntu*, therefore, means that a career counselor cannot view the client's situation from a detached, objective perspective informed by the theories of his or her discipline. Instead, recognizing that career counseling is not a value-free process, the counselor adopts a caring, relational, nondisciplinary stance toward the client. Thus, an *Ubuntu*-based approach to career counseling assumes a similar stance to the social justice perspective (Arthur, 2005; McMahon et al., 2008a; Nelson, Prilleltensky & MacGillivary, 2001; Speight & Vera, 2004) that calls for career counselors to also be agents of social change. An *Ubuntu*-based approach goes beyond the call for the adequate distribution of resources in society; it also calls on us to realize our moral and social responsibilities to others. This approach requires a move away from the tendency to conceptualize human problems in individualistic, intrapsychic terms and to take greater cognizance of the inescapably social and moral dimensions of career development.

We now turn our attention to an examination of the influence of culture on the definition and expectation of roles within the career counseling process. The influence of culture on the roles within the career counseling process raises awareness of interesting contradictory positions for those trained in Westernized approaches. For example, career counseling has been widely criticized for assuming an expert-driven process predicated on assessment. More recently, constructivist influences have seen less emphasis on the expert role and greater use of more collaborative approaches that value the knowledge of clients as experts in their own lives. However, many traditional communities in Africa are hierarchical and reinforce the notion of the expert being able to provide expert guidance and advice. He or she is also an expert in the culture and the views of the expert are respected. As an example, a healer asked of one of the authors, "what is so clever about the white doctors, they ask the patient what is wrong, then tell the patient what is wrong, that is, what they have been told. We look at the person and tell him/her what is wrong." This example suggests that there is still a place in career counseling to accommodate the more directive approaches that have been somewhat maligned in recent literature. Thus, career counselors need to be flexible enough in their practice to move between directive roles and facilitative, collaborative roles according to the needs of their clients.

Consideration of the expert role in career counseling draws our attention to the constructivist notion of agency, that is, clients' capacity to think and act for themselves. In a relationship where clients, given their cultural beliefs, seek an expert, fostering client agency may not be appropriate. The concept of agency is further compounded by the constructivist notion of context. Take, for instance, a career counseling client's traditional African family situation wherein loyalty and obligation may be both subtle and powerful. The family will go to great efforts to ensure that the oldest male or the oldest child receives a good education and every opportunity to achieve his or

Case Study 18.1: Chiluba

Chiluba, the eldest of four children, was born in a village in the Northern Province of Zambia, where her father worked for the local government. Her parents made every effort to send her to school and later to train as a teacher. She began working as a teacher, and after her father died, Chiluba took responsibility for educating her three siblings, who in turn achieved well. This involved purchasing uniforms, paying all school fees, and, as the siblings grew older and moved out of the family home; she also covered their living expenses. As her mother aged, Chiluba offered to bring her mother to the city in which she lived. However, her mother chose to remain in the village, where she had social support from the extended family. Nevertheless, Chiluba continued to provide her mother with financial support.

Questions

1. In what aspects does the case of Chiluba characterize career development from an *Ubuntu* perspective?
2. Consider the extent to which Chiluba's engagement with family in her career participation is typical of your culture of origin.

her career aspirations. Together with the efforts that the family makes, there is the expectation that the child will, in return, offer something back to his or her siblings and to the family in general. This becomes even more important as the parents age and the child then feels obliged to take care of the parents, even though the obligation is never spoken of.

The sense of obligation is a two-way process insofar as children of African descent describe a sense of responsibility to be academically successful as an expression of honor or gratitude to their parents for the sacrifices made by parents to offer them the opportunities that have often been at the expense of their own needs and means. Thus, the concept of agency may be redefined in the context of family and cultural belief systems. Let us illustrate this dynamic in Case Study 18.1.

Case Study 18.1 illustrated the interdependence that may be found in families of African ancestry. From a caring perspective, the notion of the family is broad, with parents, grandparents, aunts, and uncles all being involved in family relationships and feeling an obligation for each other. For instance, in Zimbabwe, the mother's younger sister is referred to as *umamo mutsane*, meaning small mother, while *umamo mukulu* means big mother and refers to the mother's older sister. Similar terminology applies to uncles, who are referred to as *ubaba mutsane* or *ubaba mukulu*. These close relationships extend to nephews, nieces, cousins, and in-laws.

Discussion of the cultural values of loyalty, obligation, and interdependence raises questions about the purpose of a fulfilling career self-actualization in the context of *Ubuntu*. These questions lie at the heart of what individuals do with their lives within the context of their extended communities and thus are central to career counseling. The notion of career self-actualization may well have different meanings across different cultural contexts. Within an African context, we would argue that critical aspects of career self-actualization cannot be separated from the *Ubuntu*-related experiences of obligation, loyalty, and interdependence. Thus, career counselors need to be aware of the possibility of tensions between individuals and their community (Mkhize & Frizelle, 2000) and assist individuals to navigate these tensions as well as other aspects of social life.

Extended family structure may even be evident in the context of international migration where groups of people from similar cultural backgrounds will take responsibility for new arrivals in order to assist each other. As a result, the extended family may play a key role in the education of all its children and may also influence the career choices of younger members of the extended family group. Indeed, the education of even one child is highly valued and is seen as contributing to the extended community. As a result, parents will make sacrifices to enable their children to benefit from educational opportunities in the hope that their children will "have a better life than we did." The previous discussion on *Ubuntu* strongly suggests the need for career counseling and career research that is contextualized in African settings and for African populations.

RESEARCH INTO CAREER COUNSELING OF PEOPLE OF AFRICAN ANCESTRY

In a seminal article on career research in South Africa, Stead and Watson (1998) examined the research literature over nearly two decades to establish what the career research challenges for the future should be. The authors concluded that most research conducted in South Africa has been largely guided by American theory and research trends. There has been little effort to research the appropriateness of such a career foundation in the African context and even less attempt to develop indigenous theories and instrumentation that are contextually sensitive to the African context.

Stead and Watson (2006) have more recently suggested that career research and practice needs to be "firmly rooted in Africa" (p. 181) and caution against the

Research Box 18.1: Holland's Hexagon Model and Black South African Adolescents

Watson, M. B., Stead, G. B., & Schonegevel, C. (1998). **Does Holland's hexagon travel well?** Australian *Journal of Career Development*, 7(2), 22–26.

Objective: John Holland's career theory and his interest typology were developed in America and have influenced the practice of career psychology for several decades. Holland believes that people can be classified as belonging predominantly to one of six personality types, each of which represents a preference for working in a matching environment. These six personality types are structured within a hexagonal model, with recent research questioning the cross-cultural and gender equivalence of this hexagonal model. The research compared the interest structure of Black South African disadvantaged adolescents with the hexagonal model proposed by Holland. In addition, the interest structure of males and females, as well as lower and middle socioeconomic status groups, was examined to determine the level of fit of their interest structures to Holland's theoretical model.

Method: A descriptive survey, correlational approach was used to compare the structure of interests of 529 Black South African disadvantaged adolescents with Holland's hexagonal interest structure to determine the extent to which they were the same.

Results: The results demonstrated that the Black South African adolescents' interest structure did not provide an acceptable level of fit to Holland's hexagonal structure. These results were consistent across gender and socioeconomic status groups.

Conclusion: The research suggests that career counselors should be cautious in the use of career theories and assessment tools that have been developed in specific cultural contexts.

Questions

1. How can career counselors accommodate contextual factors when using career assessment tools?
2. What are the implications of these research findings for the career counseling of minority and disadvantaged client groups?
3. What is the challenge to career counselors of the notion that "one size fits all"?

trend of career researchers and practitioners "embracing Euro-American perspectives as the touchstones for the advancement of a contextually appropriate career psychology" (p. 181). There has been some effort in recent times to address this concern. For instance, Maree and Molepo (2006) have proposed that career research on the refinement and development of postmodern narratives in diverse contexts would make a significant impact on the career counseling profession in South Africa. In this regard, Maree (2007a) has suggested steps for the development of an interest inventory that would facilitate narrative career counseling. Similarly, theoretically derived assessment processes that are applicable in the context and culture of people of African ancestry have been developed (e.g., McMahon, Patton, & Watson, 2005a, 2005b; McMahon, Watson, & Patton, 2010a, 2010b). This reflects the need for theoretical models that are more contextually sensitive as demonstrated by the research of Watson, Stead, and Schonegevel (1998) in Research Box 18.1.

African Refugees

Research with refugees of African ancestry living in Australia found that the respondents experienced hardships living in an adopted country but justified migrating in terms of the benefits for their children (Tlhabano & Schweitzer, 2007). This research on Somali and Sudanese refugees sensitizes career service providers to the specific needs of young African refugees in terms of their educational and career aspirations and is described in Research Box 18.2.

African Americans and Career Counseling

The issue of migration recognizes the relocation of people of African ancestry to settings other than the African continent. Indeed, even within the African continent, globalization is bringing about rapid change that sees culture and racial identity as evolving processes. While our discussion has been focused to this point on the traditional African cultural context and the value of *Ubuntu*, consideration needs to be given to people of African ancestry living in less traditional and more Westernized contexts. African Americans are a case in point. In this regard, there is literature descriptive of racial identity in terms of developmental statuses, specifically (1) pre-encounter, (2) encounter, (3) immersion–emersion, and (4) internalization (Cross, 1985; Helms, 1990). Progress through these statuses is hierarchical, with less healthy racial identity statuses (i.e., pre-encounter, encounter) preceding healthier racial statuses (i.e., immersion–emersion, internalization). Racial status development may be dependent on context and specific life events, with resultant minicycles in which individuals of higher racial identity status may

Research Box 18.2: Career Aspirations of Resettled Young Sudanese and Somali Refugees

Tlhabano, K. & Schweitzer, R. (2007). A qualitative study of the career aspirations of resettled young Sudanese and Somali refugees. *Journal of Psychology in Africa*, 17, (1–2), 13–22.

Objective: Australia is a major resettlement country for refugees from around the world. Since the mid-1980s, Australia has accepted a significant proportion of refugees from Africa, including people from Somali, Ethiopia, Eritrea, Sudan, Liberia, Sierra-Leone, the Congo, and more recently, Burundi. The largest group is from the Sudan, with approximately 25,000 people from the Sudan now resident in Australia. Resettlement is not without its problems, which include high unemployment, housing issues, language issues, the effects of trauma, and general health issues. The research cited aimed to document and explicate the experiences and aspirations of recently arrived young people from Africa.

Method: Semistructured interviews were conducted to examine the experiences of a sample of fourteen young resettled African refugees in Brisbane, Australia. Adopting a qualitative methodology, the interviews explored the participants' aspirations.

Results: The participants expressed high ambitions despite their experiences of pre-resettlement school disruption and post-resettlement language difficulties. The situation in their country of origin emerged as influential on their aspirations in both pre- and post-resettlement life. English language difficulties emerged as the most common consideration.

Pre-resettlement themes included school disruption and its influences on aspirations, particularly in terms of education. The experience of adverse events such as civil war had a significant impact on the participants' access to education. Post-resettlement themes comprised the expression of career aspirations, the experience of language difficulties, and influences on career aspirations. Participants experienced difficulties in adjusting to a new culture but nevertheless continued to have aspirations, some of which were different from their original aspirations. The use of English posed specific difficulties in terms of achieving their aspirations. A percentage of respondents were influenced by their experiences of hardship and became altruistic in their career choices.

Conclusion: The findings revealed that even in situations of chaos and potential trauma, young African people who have a history of valuing education will continue to desire to achieve academically and vocationally against all odds. Service providers need to recognize that young people from refugee backgrounds may benefit from educational services that address their expressed needs including language skills and community building.

Questions

1. What are the values of young people from Africa who have faced adverse circumstances that have forced them to seek refuge in a new country?
2. What are the challenges facing people entering a new country from a refugee background?
3. How might people who have been forced to migrate best achieve their aspirations in a new country?

function temporarily at a lower racial status level. Each of these statuses is now briefly described.

1. Pre-encounter

At the pre-encounter status level, African Americans may have a low racial identity salience or even subscribe to an "aracial" or color-blind world view. They may fail to perceive any obstacles or challenges to their career opportunities from belonging to a racial minority. For example, they are less likely to perceive discriminatory practices that impact on their career opportunities and may self-blame for others' racial actions that impede their career development (Sue & Sue, 2003).

2. Encounter

At the encounter status level there are two substages, those of racial identity crisis and racial identity search. A racial identity crisis occurs when an African American client experiences a profound crisis or event that challenges a previously held "aracial" world view. For example, an African American client may be denied a career opportunity and strongly suspect racial discrimination. This may make the individual ambivalent about career options or the individual could even disengage from job-seeking behavior (Mpofu, Crystal, & Feist-Price, 2000). A racial identity search is a consequence of the racial identity crisis. This search may be reflected in an interest in career services and career choices that would support an emerging sense of Black identity (Mpofu & Harley, 2006).

3. Immersion–Emersion

At the immersion–emersion status level, a high level of Black racial identity salience, centrality, and ideology emerges. While this may include the development of "Black pride" (Cosby, 1999), such positive feelings about racial identity are not internalized. For example, African

Discussion Box 18.1: The Use of Interest Inventories

Providing career counseling to people of African ancestry such as African Americans requires creativity with regard to matching one's personality characteristics, interests, skills, and abilities to the best occupational choices. Harrington (1991, p. 297) identified three logical questions that must be addressed when using interest inventories for cross-cultural counseling:

1. Do people (clients) have familiarity with the activities on the surveys?
2. Is the image of a job's functions the same from one culture to another?
3. Are the assumptions of the constructs on which an interest inventory is developed valid across cultures?

Several studies of the Strong Interest Inventory (SII) profiles suggest that African Americans have a higher preference for occupations in the Social, Enterprising, and Conventional typologies, while Asian Americans are higher in Investigative and Realistic typologies and Caucasians in Investigative, Realistic, and Artistic typologies. These different typological preferences have been explained in terms of differences in meanings of occupation with regard to racial groups and perceived opportunity structure. For example, occupational typologies in which minority groups have historically been involved may be better known to these minorities, have more minority role models, and thus be more meaningful to such minority groups. Consequently, while interest inventories can provide some insight, thorough interviews with African Americans would be the best indicators of future career success. Clearly, when working with African Americans, qualitative data may be more practical than quantitative data.

Questions

1. What does a career counselor need to consider when using interest inventories with clients of African ancestry?

Americans may grapple with understanding the ways in which similar others achieve meaningful participation despite the challenges of racial prejudice and discrimination, and they may seek employment that limits contact and interaction with a dominant White culture.

4. Internalization

At the internalization status level, African Americans have the healthiest level of racial identity development (Cross & Strauss, 1998; Pillay, 2005). This status level is characterized by a realistic positive regard of one's racial group as well as an acceptance of racially diverse others. African Americans at the internalization racial identity status level have feelings of inner security and satisfaction associated with being African American. Their racial ideology about how members of their own group should behave is less prescriptive than that of people at earlier racial identity status levels. As a result, African Americans at this status level may participate successfully in career environments that include racially different others, while at the same time maintaining their sense of identity as African Americans. For example, they may exhibit: the ability to contextualize experiences in relation to career goals; the ability to engage effective career-related problem-solving behaviors that counter programmatic, attitudinal, and environmental inequities; a developed racial identity that augments positive self-feelings in the face of perceived career barriers; and successful exploration of resources and social networks for career participation.

Clearly, such a range of social identity statuses suggests that a "one size fits all" Westernized approach to career counseling with African Americans may not be appropriate. Indeed, the need for career counselors to be sensitive to the relevance of the career models and measures available to them is evidenced in the example described in Discussion Box 18.1.

CURRENT ISSUES IN COUNSELING PEOPLE OF AFRICAN ANCESTRY

While Discussion Box 18.1 relates to African Americans, similar considerations may apply to career counseling with the broader population of individuals of African ancestry. Stead and Watson (2006) have questioned the appropriateness of using Westernized career approaches with Black South Africans and have called for the development and use of career theories, models, and techniques that originate in Africa. In this regard, Maree and Molepo (2006) discussed the use of narrative approaches to career counseling as being appropriate in a South African context.

In addition, career counselors may have to be sensitized to the needs and cultural context of their clients. For example, in job seeking and placement interventions for African Americans, clients may be assisted if career counselors inform them of the potential barriers in the labor market and assist them to develop strategies in overcoming such barriers. Thus, an advocacy role on the part of career counselors may involve educating employers about the benefits of employing their clients. Further, career development counseling with people of African ancestry can be significantly advanced by applying a social justice perspective and also by the use of narrative approaches.

Discussion Box 18.2: Social Justice Competencies of Career Development Practitioners

An Australian study (McMahon, Arthur, & Collins, 2008b) that investigated career development practitioners' perceptions and experiences of social justice found a micro-focus on intervention between practitioners and their individual clients, with few practitioners identifying a macro-focus on broader levels of intervention. This finding reflects the traditional focus of career development on individuals and may also indicate the limited focus in the professional training of practitioners on more macro-systemic interventions (Helms, 2003; Toporek & Williams, 2006).

The career development practitioners were able to describe several roles that they adopted in their social justice interventions. Again, these roles related predominantly to micro- rather than macro-systemic intervention levels. Such findings have implications for training career development practitioners in social justice intervention, particularly in terms of a more active role for intervention at macro-systemic levels, such as organizational, community, or political levels.

The importance of intervention at the macro-systemic level was illustrated by the fact that career development practitioners identified barriers to socially just career counseling as being predominantly at the macro-systemic level such as government and organizations. The findings suggest that, while career development practitioners can identify macro-systemic problems that individual clients face, they are less able to intervene at these levels. Thus, in some ways, the career development practitioners themselves face systemic barriers that restrict their effectiveness in dealing with the limitations that social injustices may impose on their clients' career development.

Questions

1. Why might career counselors find it difficult to intervene at macro-systemic levels such as organizations, communities, and government departments?
2. What are the macro-systemic barriers that clients may face in their career development?
3. How might training better prepare career counselors for macro-systemic socially just interventions and what could be the content of such training?

We now explain how these approaches could enhance career counseling for people of African ancestry.

Social Justice and Career Counseling

A social justice perspective invites career counselors to "work with broader systems and contexts to create more humane and equitable schools, universities, and work environments" (Hartung & Blustein, 2002, p. 45). This perspective suggests broader roles for career counselors and multiple levels of intervention (see Arthur & McMahon, 2005; McMahon et al., 2008a) if the needs of clients of African ancestry are to be adequately addressed. Among suggested roles for career counselors is that of advocacy, which leads us to a discussion of a social justice approach toward career counseling. The potential influence of *Ubuntu* on career counseling discussed earlier in this chapter suggests a number of similarities with the social justice perspective. Indeed, the International Competencies for Educational and Vocational Guidance Practitioners (Repetto, Malik, Ferrer-Sama, Manzano, & Hiebert, 2003) include social justice as a foundation competency.

Although the field of career counseling had its origins in the social justice movement (McMahon et al., 2008a), it has been suggested that social justice has been more implicit than explicit in the field, and that there is a lack of clarity about the nature of competence in social justice (Toporek & Chope, 2006; Toporek, Gerstein, Fouad, Roysicar, & Israel, 2006). In this regard, Arthur (2008) identifies five broad areas in which social justice competencies for career counselors could be developed. These include the career counselor: knowing the potential impact of systemic forces (e.g., oppression) on clients; consulting local community groups to plan career development services; including multiple roles and multiple levels in career development interventions; increasing access and availability of culturally appropriate career services and resources; and developing professional competencies related to social justice and career development. Reflecting these broad areas, Arthur (2005) lists seventeen social justice competencies that suggest multiple roles and levels of intervention for career counselors (Arthur & McMahon, 2005).

In essence, assuming a social justice perspective locates client issues in context, and to achieve socially just outcomes for clients, career counselors may need to assume roles such as advocate and intervene at levels such as communities and organizations. Such interventions represent a shift away from the traditional skill base of career counselors and the individual nature of career intervention. In advocating the development of social justice competencies, Arthur (2008) raises questions about whether career counselors have been adequately prepared to conduct social justice interventions as, to date, training has focused on intervention with individuals and not at systemic levels. Some insight into career counselors' views and experiences of social justice in their practice has been examined in Australia as described in Discussion Box 18.2.

A social justice position does not suggest the abandonment of current approaches to career counseling that have proven useful across a variety of settings. Rather, it challenges career counselors to reexamine and justify the approaches and frameworks within which they work in relation to the needs of individual clients located within their broader cultural context. One development that currently offers promise in addressing the shortcomings of traditional career counseling frameworks is the narrative approach.

Narrative Approaches

A more recent trend that has emerged in career counseling in general and career counseling in African settings specifically is the use of approaches informed by the principles of constructivism. For example, in South Africa, a number of authors (e.g., Eloff, 2002; Fritz & Beekman, 2007; Maree & Beck, 2004; Maree, Bester, Lubbe, & Beck, 2001; Maree & Molepo, 2006, 2007; Patton, McMahon, & Watson, 2006) have written on the application of narrative approaches to career counseling with people of African ancestry. A further example of the growing influence of narrative approaches in the South African context is evident in a Special Section of the journal *Perspectives in Education*, where Watson and McMahon (2005) suggested that narrative approaches may help address fundamental challenges facing career counselors in the construction of a new identity for career practice in the twenty-first century. In addition, drawing on the work of international and national specialists in the field of narrative counseling, the first South African text on narrative approaches to career counseling has been published (Maree, 2007b).

Narrative career counseling has the capacity to address some of the shortcomings of traditional approaches. For example, narrative approaches consider the contextual and cultural location of career issues and encourage clients to actively engage in an interactive and dynamic process in which they construct their own reality within the environments in which they live (Watson, 2006). However, a criticism of constructivist and narrative approaches is that they have not necessarily provided practical guidelines for career counselors (Patton & McMahon, 2006; Reid, 2006). In the South African context, there have been recent attempts to address this criticism. For example, a qualitative career assessment process has been developed and trialed with a diverse range of client groups in settings including South Africa (McMahon et al., 2005a, 2005b; McMahon, Watson, & Patton, 2010a, 2010b). Patton and colleagues (2006) have described the use of this qualitative career assessment process in a storied or narrative approach to career counseling with a client of African ancestry. This nascent movement toward more narrative approaches to career counseling may help to provide a tentative answer to the question posed by Watson and McMahon (2005) about what constitutes a good narrative for career counseling in the twenty-first century and a culturally sensitive approach for dealing with people of African ancestry.

SUMMARY AND CONCLUSION

This chapter has considered career counseling with people of African ancestry. In particular, career counseling has been considered both from the perspective of the traditional African cultural value of *Ubuntu* and in relation to African Americans. A social justice approach to career counseling offers a way forward that may accommodate both traditional and cultural beliefs as well as the needs of people of African ancestry in transitional and diverse cultural contexts. In this regard, career counselors need to be sensitive to the cultural contexts of their clients and how such contexts may be experienced and interpreted by the client. Further, career counselors are urged to reflect on their own personal and professional cultural values and how these may impact on effective career counseling with people of African ancestry.

REFERENCES

Adonisi, M. (1994). The career in community. In P. Christie, R. Lessem, & L. Mbigi (Eds.), *African management: Philosophies, concepts and applications* (pp. 309–14). Randburg, South Africa: Knowledge Resources.

Akhurst, J., & Mkhize, N. J. (2006). Career education in South Africa. In G. B. Stead & M. B. Watson (Eds.), *Career psychology in the South African context* (2nd ed., pp. 139–53). Pretoria, South Africa: Van Schaik.

Arthur, N. (2005). Building from diversity to social justice competencies in international standards for career development practitioners. *International Journal for Educational and Vocational Guidance*, *5*, 137–48.

Arthur, N. (2008). Qualification standards for career practitioners. In J. Athanasou & R. Van Esbroeck (Eds.). *International handbook of career guidance* (pp. 303–23). Dordrecht, The Netherlands: Springer.

Arthur, N., & McMahon, M. (2005). Multicultural career counseling: Theoretical applications of the Systems Theory Framework. *The Career Development Quarterly*, *53*, 208–22.

Benjamin, L. S. (2003). *Interpersonal diagnosis and treatment of personality disorders* (2nd ed.). New York: Guilford Press.

Brown, M. T., & Pinterits, E. J. (2001). Basic issues in the career counselling of African Americans. In W. B. Walsh, R. P. Bingham, M. T. Brown, & C. M. Ward (Eds.), *Career counselling for African Americans* (pp. 10–25). Mahwah, NJ: Lawrence Erlbaum.

Buhrmann, V. (1984). *Living in two worlds: Communication between a white healer and her black counterparts*. Cape Town: Human and Rousseau.

Collin, A., & Young, R. A. (1992). Constructing career through narrative and context: An interpretive perspective. In R. A. Young & A. Collin (Eds.), *Interpreting career: Hermeneutical study of lives in context* (pp. 1–12). London: Praeger.

Cosby, M. C. (1999). The influence of racial identity development and locus of control on career self-efficacy of African American adolescents. *Dissertation Abstracts International*, *60*, 6-B.

Cross, W., Jr. (1985). Black identity: Rediscovering the link between personal identity and reference group orientation. In

M. B. Spencer, G. K. Bookins, & W. R. Allen (Eds.), *Beginnings: The social and affective development of Black children* (pp. 93–122). Hillsdale, NJ: Lawrence Erlbaum.

Cross, W. Jr., & Strauss, L. (1998). The everyday functions of African American identity. In J. K. Swim & C. Stangor (Eds.), *Prejudice: The target's perspective* (pp. 268–79). New York: Academic Press.

Dandala, H. M. (1996). Cows never die: Embracing African cosmology in the process of economic growth. In R. Lessem & B. Nussbaum (Eds.), *Sawubona Africa: Embracing four worlds in South African management* (pp. 69–85). Sandton, South Africa: Zebra Press.

Edwards, S. D., Makunga, N. V., Ngcobo, H. S. B., & Dhlomo, R. M. (2004). Ubuntu: A fundamental method of mental health promotion. *International Journal of Mental Health Promotion, 6*(4), 16–21.

Eloff, I. (2002). Narrative therapy as career counselling. In J. G. Maree & L. Ebersöhn (Eds.), *Lifeskills and career counselling* (pp. 129–38). Sandown, South Africa: Heinemann.

Fritz, E., & Beekman, L. (2007). Engaging clients actively in telling stories and actualising dreams. In K. Maree (Ed.), *Shaping the story: A guide to facilitating narrative counselling* (pp. 163–75). Pretoria, South Africa: Van Schaik.

Harrington, T. F. (1991). The cross-cultural applicability of the Career Decision-Making System. *The Career Development Quarterly, 39*, 295–301.

Hartung, P. J., & Blustein, D. L. (2002). Reason, intuition and social justice: Elaborating on Parson's career decision-making model. *Journal of Counseling and Development, 80*, 41–7.

Helms, J. E. (1990). *Black and white racial identity: Theory, research and practice*. Westport, CT: Greenwood.

Helms, J. E. (2003). A pragmatic view of social justice. *The Counseling Psychologist, 31*, 305–13.

Kamwangamalu, N. M. (1999). Ubuntu in South Africa: A sociological perspective to a pan-African concept. *Critical Arts: A South-North Journal of Cultural & Media Studies, 13*(2), 24–41.

Karenga, M. (2004). *Maat: The moral ideal in Ancient Egypt: A study in classical African ethics*. New York: Routledge.

Kuit, W., & Watson, M. (2005). Postmodern career counselling, theory and training: Ethical considerations. *Perspectives in Education, 23*(2), 29–37.

Leong, F. T. T., & Hartung, P. (1997). Career assessment with culturally different clients: Proposing an integrative-sequential conceptual framework for cross-cultural career counseling research and practice. *Journal of Career Assessment, 5*, 183–202.

Manganyi, N. C. (1973). *Being-black-in-the-world*. Johannesburg: Spro-Cas/Ravan.

Maree, K. (2007a). First steps in developing an interest inventory to facilitate narrative counselling. In K. Maree (Ed.), *Shaping the story: A guide to facilitating narrative counselling* (pp. 176–205). Pretoria, South Africa; Van Schaik.

Maree, K. (Ed.) (2007b). *Shaping the story: A guide to facilitating narrative counseling*. Pretoria, South Africa; Van Schaik.

Maree, J. G., & Beck, G. (2004). Using various approaches in career counselling for traditionally disadvantaged (and other) learners: Some limitations of a new frontier. *South African Journal of Education, 24*(1), 80–7.

Maree, J. G., Bester, S. E., Lubbe, C., & Beck, G. (2001). Postmodern career counselling to a gifted Black youth: A case study. *Gifted Education International, 15*, 325–39.

Maree, K., & Molepo, M. (2006). The use of narratives in cross-cultural career counselling. In M. McMahon & W. Patton (Eds.), *Career counselling: Constructivist approaches* (pp. 69–81). London: Routledge.

Maree, K., & Molepo, M. (2007). Changing the approach to career counselling in a disadvantaged context: A case study. *Australian Journal of Career Development, 16*(3), 62–70.

McMahon, M., Arthur, N., & Collins, S. (2008a). Social justice and career development: Looking back, looking forward. *Australian Journal of Career Development, 17*(2), 21–9.

McMahon, M., Arthur, N., & Collins, S. (2008b). Social justice and career development: Views and experiences of Australian career development practitioners. *Australian Journal of Career Development, 17*(3), 15–25.

McMahon, M., Patton, W., & Watson, M. (2005a). *My system of career influences*. Camberwell, Australia: ACER.

McMahon, M., Patton, W., & Watson, M. (2005b). *My system of career influences (MSCI) facilitators' guide*. Camberwell, Australia: ACER.

McMahon, M., Watson, M., & Patton, W. (2010a). *My system of career influences adult version*. Unpublished manuscript.

McMahon, M., Watson, M., & Patton, W. (2010b). *My system of career influences (MSCI) adult version*. Facilitators' guide. Unpublished manuscript.

Mkhize, N. J. (2004). Dialogism and African conceptions of the self. In D. Hook, N. J. Mkhize, P. Kiguwa, & A. Collins, (Eds.). *Critical psychology* (pp. 53–83). Cape Town: UCT Press.

Mkhize, N. (2005). The context of career counselling: Lessons from social constructionism and hermeneutics. *Perspectives in Education, 23*(3), 93–105.

Mkhize, N., & Frizelle, K. (2000). Hermeneutic-dialogical approaches to career development: An exploration. *South African Journal of Psychology, 30*(3), 1–9.

Mnyaka, M., & Motlhabi, M. (2005). The African concept of Ubuntu and its socio-moral significance. *Black Theology, 3*, 215–37.

Mpofu, E. (2005). Selective interventions in counseling African-Americans with disabilities. In D. A. Harley & J. M. Dillard (Eds.), *Contemporary mental health issues among African Americans* (pp. 235–54). Alexandria, VA: American Counseling Association.

Mpofu, E., Crystal, R., & Feist-Price, S. (2000). Tokenism among rehabilitation clients: Implications for rehabilitation education. *Rehabilitation Education, 14*, 243–56.

Mpofu, E., Gudyanga, E., & Ngara, C. (2007). Constructions of giftedness among the Shona of Central-Southern Africa. In S. N. Phillipson & M. McCann (Eds.), *What does it mean to be gifted?: Sociocultural perspectives* (pp. 225–52). Mahwah, NJ: Lawrence Erlbaum.

Mpofu, E., & Harley, D. R. (2006). Racial and disability identity: Implications for the career counseling of African Americans with disabilities. *Rehabilitation Counseling Bulletin, 50*, 14–23.

Nelson, G., Prilleltensky, I., & MacGillivary, H. (2001). Building value-based partnerships: Toward solidarity with oppressed groups. *American Journal of Community Psychology, 29*(4), 649–77.

Nicholas, L., Naidoo, A. V., & Pretorius, T. B. (2006). A historical perspective of career psychology in South Africa. In G. B. Stead & M. B. Watson (Eds.), *Career psychology in the South African context* (2nd ed., pp. 1–10). Pretoria, South Africa: Van Schaik.

Patton, W., & McMahon, M. (2006). Constructivism: What does it mean for career counselling? In M. McMahon & W. Patton (Eds.), *Career counselling: Constructivist approaches* (pp. 3–15). London: Routledge.

Patton, M., McMahon, M., & Watson, M. (2006). Career development and systems theory: Enhancing our understanding of career. In G. B. Stead & M. B. Watson (Eds.), *Career psychology in the South African context* (2nd ed., pp. 65–78). Pretoria, South Africa: Van Schaik.

Pillay, Y. (2005). Racial identity as a predictor of the psychological health of African American students at a predominantly White university. *Journal of Black Psychology*, *31*, 46–66.

Ramose, M. B. (1999). *African philosophy through Ubuntu*. Harare, Zimbabwe: Mond Books.

Reid, H. L. (2006). Usefulness and truthfulness: Outlining the limitations and upholding the benefits of constructivist approaches for career counselling. In M. McMahon & W. Patton (Eds.), *Career counselling: Constructivist approaches* (pp. 30–42). Abingdon, OXON: Routledge.

Repetto, E., Malik, B., Ferrer-Sama, P., Manzano, N., & Hiebert, B. (2003). International competencies for educational and vocational guidance practitioners: Final report to the General Assembly of the International Association for Educational and Vocational Guidance. Bern, Switzerland. Retrieved February 21, 2007 from http://www.iaevg.org/IAEVG/.

Rogers, C. (1980). *A way of being*. New York: Mariner Books.

Sampson, A. (1999). *Mandela: The authorized biography*. New York: Knopf.

Schiele, J. H. (1996). Afrocentricity: An emerging paradigm in social work practice. *Social Work*, *41*(3), 284–94.

Speight, S. L., & Vera, E. M. (2004). Social justice, ready or not? *The Counseling Psychologist*, *32*, 109–18.

Stead, G. B. (1996). Career development of black South African adolescents: A developmental contextual perspective. *Journal of Counseling and Development*, *74*, 270–5.

Stead, G. B. (2004). Culture and career psychology: A social constructionist perspective. *Journal of Vocational Behavior*, *64*, 389–406.

Stead, G. B., & Watson, M. B. (1998). Career research in South Africa: Challenges for the future. *Journal of Vocational Behavior*, *52*, 289–99.

Stead, G. B., & Watson, M. B. (2006). Indigenisation of career psychology in South Africa. In G. B. Stead & M. B. Watson (Eds.), *Career psychology in the South African context* (2nd ed., pp. 181–90). Pretoria, South Africa: Van Schaik.

Sue, D. W., & Sue, D. (2003). *Counseling the culturally diverse: Theory and practice*. New York: John Wiley & Sons.

Tlhabano, K., & Schweitzer, R. (2007). A qualitative study of the career aspirations of resettled young Sudanese and Somali refugees. *Journal of Psychology in Africa*, *17*(1–2), 13–22.

Toporek, R. L., & Chope, R. C. (2006). Individual, programmatic, and entrepreneurial approaches to social justice: Counseling psychologists in vocation and career counseling. In R. L. Toporek, L. H. Gerstein, N. A. Fouad, G. Roysircar, & T. Israel, (Eds.), *Handbook for social justice in counseling psychology: Leadership, vision, and action* (pp. 276–93). Thousand Oaks, CA: SAGE Publications.

Toporek, R. L., Gerstein, L. H., Fouad, N. A., Roysircar, G., & Israel, T. (Eds.). (2006). *Handbook for social justice in counseling psychology: Leadership, vision, and action*. Thousand Oaks, CA: SAGE Publications.

Toporek, R. L., & Williams, R. A. (2006). Ethics and professional issues related to the practice of social justice in counseling psychology. In R. L. Toporek, L. H. Gerstein, N. A. Fouad, G. Roysircar, & T. Israel, (Eds.), *Handbook for social justice in counseling psychology: Leadership, vision, and action* (pp. 17–34). Thousand Oaks, CA: SAGE Publications.

Watson, M. B. (2006). Career counselling theory, culture and constructivism. In M. McMahon & W. Patton (Eds.), *Career counselling: Constructivist approaches* (pp. 45–56). Abingdon, OXON: Routledge.

Watson, M., & McMahon, M. (2005). Postmodern (narrative) career counselling and education. *Perspectives in Education*, *23*(2), vii–ix.

Watson, M. B., & Stead, G. B. (2002). Career psychology in South Africa: Moral perspectives on present and future directions. *South African Journal of Psychology*, *32*(1), 26–31.

Watson, M. B., Stead, G. B., & Schonegevel, C. (1998). Does Holland's hexagon travel well? *Australian Journal of Career Development*, *7*(2), 22–6.

Watts, A. G. (1996). The changing concept of career: Implications for career counseling. In R. Feller & G. Walz (Eds.), *Career transitions in turbulent times: Exploring work, learning and careers* (pp. 229–36). Greensboro, NC: ERIC/CASS.

Wolf, D. M., & Kolb, D. A. (1980). Career development. personal growth, and experimental learning. In J. W. Springer (Ed.), *Issues in career and human resource development* (pp. 1–11). Madison, WI: American Society for Training and Development.

SELF-CHECK EXERCISES

1. Give an outline of the evolving nature of career counseling with examples from the African cultural context.
2. Define career counseling from alternative cultural perspectives.
3. What is the utility of the construct of *Ubuntu* in understanding career development counseling in African cultural contexts?
4. Evaluate narrative theory as an approach to the career development counseling of people of African ancestry.

FIELD-BASED EXPERIENTIAL EXERCISES

1. Interview two or three people of African ancestry and discuss the relative role of *Ubuntu* in their lives. Compare and contrast their responses.
2. Interview a career counselor about the approaches he or she uses when counseling clients of African ancestry.
3. Observe a career counselor in practice and take note of how the career counselor utilizes career assessment techniques within the contexts of his or her clients.
4. Discuss with a career counselor his or her understanding and application of social justice in practice.

MULTIPLE-CHOICE QUESTIONS

1. A definition of career development would include which of the following aspects:
   a. Context
   b. Change over time
   c. Organizational promotion
   d. An individual's culture

2. The African cultural concept of *Ubuntu* is characterized by:
   a. Respecting the human dignity of others
   b. Caring and sensitivity to others' needs
   c. Human interdependence
   d. Connectedness to material symbols
3. The literature describes racial identity in terms of developmental statuses that include:
   a. Pre-encounter
   b. Internationalization
   c. Encounter
   d. Immersion–emersion
4. Career counselors could develop social justice competencies in which of the following areas?
   a. Knowing the potential impact of systemic forces such as oppression on clients
   b. Learning career counseling and career assessment competencies
   c. Developing a capacity for multiple roles and multiple levels in career development interventions
   d. Increasing access and availability of culturally appropriate career services and resources
5. Narrative approaches to career counseling encourage:
   a. Consideration of the contextual and cultural location of career issues
   b. Clients to actively engage in an interactive and dynamic process in which they construct their own reality within the environments in which they live
   c. A step-by-step process led by an expert career counselor
   d. The use of qualitative career assessment processes

Answers to the multiple-choice questions are provided at the back of the book

19 Counseling People with Disabilities

Elias Mpofu, Grace Ukasoanya, Anniah Mupawose, Debra A. Harley, John Charema, and Kayi Ntinda

OVERVIEW. The counseling needs of people with disabilities in African settings have received relatively little attention in the published literature, despite the fact that a majority of Africans, or their families, experience disability in their lifetimes. The disabilities arise mostly from avoidable causes such as inadequate health care systems, civil strife, marginal or failing national economies, and lack of enforcement of disability rights by national governments. This chapter addresses conceptions of disability from an African cultural heritage perspective and counseling interventions to address disability-related needs in those settings. Legal and professional issues that influence the availability of psychosocial services to people with disabilities in sub-Saharan Africa are considered. Counseling enhances health and quality of life in people of African descent with disabilities.

LEARNING OBJECTIVES

By the end of the chapter, the reader should be able to:

1. Define disability-related terms.
2. Explain the likely influence of culture on disability identity in an African cultural heritage setting.
3. Identify and describe the needs in people of African descent with disabilities that counseling services would meet.
4. Outline the typical counseling interventions that have been used in counseling people with disabilities in African settings and the rationale for their use.
5. Evaluate the role of community-based approaches in counseling people of African descent with disabilities.
6. Suggest and discuss ways in which counseling services for African cultural heritage people with disabilities could be enhanced.

INTRODUCTION

The prevalence of disabilities in sub-Saharan Africa would be expected to be among the highest in the world owing to underdeveloped health care systems, lower health literacy in the general population, and elevated levels of poverty and disease compared to the developed countries (Lopez, Magweva, & Mpofu, 2007; Mpofu, Peltzer, Shumba, Serpell, & Mogaji, 2005). Disability can significantly affect an individual's social role valuation in the African society (Devlieger, 1998a,b). Wolfensberger (1991, 1999) was of the view that people's well-being and social positioning were determined by the social roles they play. The experiences of individuals with disabilities are often characterized by multiple rejections, downgrading, deindividualization, and stigmatization (Lustig & Strauser; 2007; Wright, 1991). Disability may lead to significant sociocultural disadvantage from limited access to resources for community participation and from expenses related to medical and personal care and transportation. Without prompt rehabilitation interventions, as is usually the case, the psychosocial burdens associated with disability increase, and consequently the lives of individuals with disabilities are significantly altered for the worse.

This chapter discusses counseling services for people with disabilities in the sub-Saharan African context, which is the region populated mostly by people of an African cultural heritage. Sub-Saharan Africa is a vast geocultural region, and the evolution and maturity of psychosocial services for people with disabilities varies widely between countries. For instance, some of the countries have more advanced rehabilitation services (e.g., South Africa and Zimbabwe) in comparison to others (e.g., Botswana, Rwanda, Tanzania, and Zambia). A large number of countries in sub-Saharan Africa share a history of civil wars (e.g., Angola, Liberia, Mozambique, Somalia, Sudan, Rwanda, Uganda, Zimbabwe), and strong advocacy for disability rights movements (e.g., South Africa, Zimbabwe), which influenced the development of counseling services for people with disabilities in the individual countries, and also regionally. Thus, we examine counseling services for people with disabilities in sub-Saharan Africa fully conscious of the diversity in the development of psychosocial services in countries within the region, and considering best practices that we can discern from country and regional practices. We examine concepts and practices related to disability counseling, taking into account national, regional, and international policies. We consider gaps in the knowledge base in counseling practices with people with disabilities in the African context

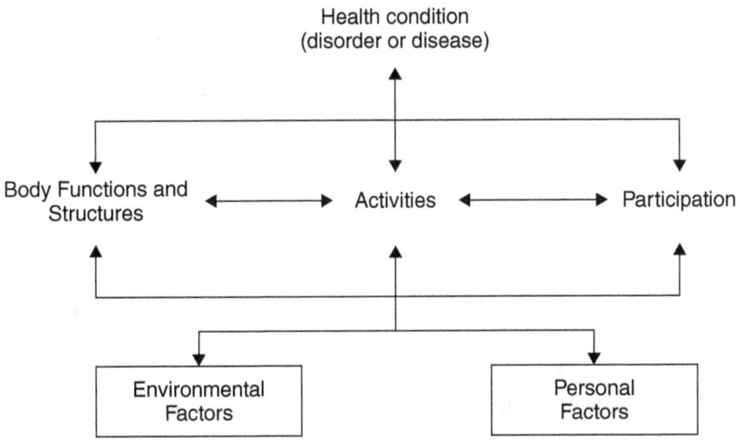

Figure 19.1. Interactions between the components of the ICF. (From *The International Classification of Functioning, Disability, and Health*, p. 18. World Health Organization, 2001, Geneva, Switzerland).

that could be addressed by research and other evidence-informed practices.

IMPORTANCE, DEFINITION, AND SCOPE OF KEY TERMS AND CONCEPTS

How disability is defined determines, in part, its perceived prevalence, impact on social systems, and appropriate interventions to enable those at risk from disadvantage because of a disability. The International Classification of Functioning, Disability, and Health (ICF: WHO, 2001) is the gold standard for defining disability and widely endorsed by countries in sub-Saharan Africa.

Disability

The ICF defines disability in reference to impairments, activity limitations, and participation restrictions from a physical or mental condition in the context of environmental factors. According to the ICF, impairments are physical manifestations of dysfunction in the body structures or functions. They may not necessarily translate into a disability and do not necessarily imply the presence of a disorder or disease. However, a disability impacts a person's ability to perform major life activities such as walking, breathing, eating, seeing, hearing, and communicating to a level beyond that experienced by the average person. A disability could result from impairment, particularly in the context of environmental barriers (i.e., physical or social) that hamper a person's participation. Thus, *disability* refers to "the outcome or result of a complex relationship between an individual's health condition and personal factors, and of the external factors that represent the circumstances in which the individual lives" (WHO, 2001, p. 17). *Disability* is about the individual, societal, and body-related aspects of impairments, activity limitations, and participation restrictions in the sociocultural environment. It is about activity and participation limitations due to significant health conditions and in normative or everyday environments.

Figure 19.1 illustrates the components and interactions that can be used to describe the relationship between disability and functioning (WHO, 2001, p. 18).

Use of impairment-oriented definitions of disabilities would impose greater functional limitations on people with disabilities in the African cultural heritage tradition than would definitions that are activity and participation oriented. For instance, misunderstanding of presenting disability related functional limitations by family and community could lead to social rejection or stigmatization (see Chapter 1, this volume). For instance, in the case of disability from brain injury, accompanying cognitive deficit may be perceived by others as laziness; emotional dysregulation associated with brain injury may be viewed as attention seeking behavior. People of African heritage, who prioritize solutions to practical problems of living, may prefer counseling for successful community living with others rather than focused mostly on perceived personal issues.

Activity- and participation-oriented definitions of disability are appropriate culturally in the largely subsistence economies of sub-Saharan Africa, where what one does to contribute to the good of the collective (e.g., extended family) earns a status of competence and respect. In the cultural societies of sub-Saharan Africa, impairment per se does not imply having a disability in the absence of task and social role performance.

Distinguishing between Disability and Illness

Persons with disabilities are not necessarily sick. Sickness or illness typically involves a subjective feeling of lack of well-being, such as pain or other physical or psychological strain (Finkelstein & French, 1997). For instance, an individual with a visual impairment is not sick. However, some illnesses, if untreated, can cause a disability (e.g., measles causing visual impairment). Some disabilities can cause illness (e.g., a person with spinal cord injury who may develop decubitus ulcers or pressure sores). Also, disability and illness may coexist (e.g., mental illness is both an illness and a disability).

Disabilities do not lead to activity or participation limitations across all situations. Persons with specified disabilities may function differently from others in some settings rather than others. They can function better in disability-friendly environments or with appropriate assistive aids.

Not all disabilities are visible. Some mental and physical disabilities may not have clear markers. Learning disabilities and personality disorders are types of invisible disabilities. Chronic fatigue syndrome is an example of a physical disability that is not visible. Chronic fatigue syndrome is

Discussion Box 19.1: Cultural Issues that Impact the Transportability of Disability and Rehabilitation Concepts from Western to African Settings

Perspectives on disability and rehabilitation have changed over the years from being predominantly medically based to socially based views. Yet, it should be noted that both these views on disability and rehabilitation are American and European originated. Therefore, when exporting these views to developing countries, caution should be taken, because the socioeconomic and political systems found in developed countries are different from African developing countries (Turmansani, Vreede, & Wirz, 2002). For example, most African countries lack resources for welfare systems and they are not as savoir-faire with the concepts of human rights and equality in the same way developed countries are. As a result, when Western technologies are imported to Africa via CBR programs, they do not always achieve the expected impact or outcomes on the community (Pollard & Sakellariou, 2008; Turmansani et al., 2002). This reduced impact is due in part by failure of international funding organizations to take into account the local values and traditions concerning the notion of disability and rehabilitation, and society's response to them (Myezwa & M'Kumbuzi, 2003, Ojwang & Hartley, 2001).

Questions

1. What could the government and international donors have done to encourage more participation from the relevant stakeholders?
2. What cultural issues and definitions should have been initially addressed by the international donors?
3. Where should the emphasis in terms of benefit be placed? Individual or family? And why?

Case Study 19.1: Effects of the Environment on Living with a Disability

Merjury is a nineteen-year-old Black woman from a poor family on one of Zimbabwe's commercial farms. She has a developmental disability that hampers use of her legs. She wobbles significantly when walking and often needs some support for sustained mobility. About five years ago, a nongovernmental organization donated a wheelchair to Merjury. However, currently wheelchair is not working because of a mechanical problem with one of the wheels. Even before it broke down, it was of limited use as a mobility aid to Merjury because of lack of pavement and ramps in Merjury's village and homestead. Most roads in Merjury's village are footpaths, some of which were paved by foraging livestock. In addition, the area has significant levels of soil erosion, which adds to Merjury's mobility problems.

Merjury's parents have been on the farm for the past ten years. Merjury is the third born in a family of eight children. She is the only child with a disability in the family. Only a few of the children completed seventh grade because of the lack of adequate schooling facilities on the farm and low parental education. None of the parents went to school.

Merjury, unlike her siblings, never attended school. Her father considered it a waste of resources to educate a female child who was likely to get him some wealth through marriage (i.e., via payment of lobola by a son-in-law). She had a very lonely childhood, as most family members spent more time on farm duties than at home. Things have not changed much for her, even at nineteen. She still spends a significant amount of time alone. However, currently, she is more involved with homekeeping and preparation of meals for the family and seems to take a great deal of pride in the role.

Merjury hopes to marry one day and to raise a family of her own. She says that she would prefer to stay on the farm because that is all the world she knows.

The case of Merjury shows that personal, disability, and environmental characteristics are often interwoven in their impact on the lives of people with disabilities and on their needs for counseling. A counselor working with Merjury would need to take into account the specific personal, disability, and environmental characteristics as well as the ways in which they may jointly influence Merjury's psychosocial adjustment.

a condition characterized by the experience of a persistent feeling of physical and mental exhaustion beyond that which is within the norm to most people and that cannot be explained by an identifiable organic cause. In most African context settings, visible disabilities tend to be more noticed and are more likely to be associated with stigma than invisible disabilities. As noted previously, the behavioral effects of invisible disabilities may lead to social ostracism from the misconception that the individual is deliberately failing in performing expected cultural roles.

Case Study 19.2: Cultural Influences on Using an Assistive Device

Nompumelelo was a ten-year-old girl with spastic quadriplegia. At the time of identification by the Department of Education, she had no previous schooling experience. She was from a poor working-class family. Her father worked for a meat packaging family in the local town. The family stayed in a makeshift home in an informal settlement in the town.

She needed a wheelchair for mobility. Subsequently, the Ministry of Health and Child Welfare provided a wheelchair gratis to Nompumelelo's family upon the recommendation of the Education Department. Reasons for granting a free wheelchair to Nompumelelo were to facilitate her school attendance as well as improve her quality of life as a person living with a disability.

Subsequently, it turned out that Nompumelelo's school attendance was erratic and with many unexplained absences. Investigation by the Department of Social Welfare revealed that her father had taken over the wheelchair for himself and was using it as his house chair. Apparently, the father, who ordinarily sat on a traditional three-legged wooden stool about thirty centimeters high, would not accept Nompumelelo sitting higher than he did. Culturally, the mother and children were all to sit at a height lower than that of the father. That seating order reinforced the father's authority over the family. The arrival of the wheelchair upset the seating order and symbolically threatened the father's authority. For that reason, Nompumelelo was dispossessed of her wheelchair and could not even use it to attend school.

Questions

1. Discuss how culture may have influenced perceptions of disability in the case of Nompumelelo.
2. How would you provide counseling in the context of the family's needs, including the cultural hierarchy?

Case Study 19.3: Disability and Care in a Tradition-Led Setting

Ngozi is a twenty-six-year-old woman with multiple sclerosis. Her husband is a forty-five-year-old trader who has been partnering with Ngozi in the sale of textile materials for five years. Ngozi's physical illness has continued to progress with associated physical debilitation. Ngozi and her husband live in the same compound as her father-in-law, mother-in-law, and other adult sibling in-laws. Neither Ngozi nor any member of the immediate or extended family understood the cause of her deteriorating health for the first two years of her disability. Three months ago, Ngozi was referred to the teaching hospital in the city by the new public health department in her village. They diagnosed her with multiple sclerosis and referred her back to the local public health agency with comprehensive information about her diagnosis, prognosis, and management regimen. At this point, Ngozi's in-laws began to blame her parents and her for this disability. It was interpreted as a rebound of a diabolical activity targeted against her husband by her parents. Although Ngozi's husband loved her, the presence of his parents made it difficult for him to provide extensive care to her.

Questions

1. Explain the experience of disability by Ngozi from a social role function perspective in an African setting. What other culturally grounded explanations are possible?
2. What are some barriers to Ngozi's in-laws in understanding her disability? How may these be overcome?

Prevalence of Disability

The types and extent of services perceived to be needed by individuals with disabilities are influenced by prevalence of disability in a particular setting. The World Health Organization (WHO) estimates that 10 percent of any population has disabilities. However, disability prevalence statistics from several sub-Saharan African countries suggest otherwise. For example, South Africa, with a population of approximately 46 million, has an estimated prevalence of disability of 5 percent of the total population (South Africa National Census, 2001). Zimbabwe had a population of approximately 11 million people (Central Statistical Office, 1998). Yet, in a survey of 100,000 people conducted in eight different rural districts of Zimbabwe as part of the community-based rehabilitation (CBR) program implementation, 3 percent of the population was estimated to have disabilities (Jelsma et al., 2002). In other CBR pilot study of areas in Zimbabwe the prevalence figures have varied from 1.5 to 4.5 percent (Chidyausiku & Nleya, 1998). A house-to-house

Discussion Box 19.2: Counseling for Social Support

In most countries in sub-Saharan Africa, such as Zambia, Botswana, and Malawai, unlike professional rehabilitation counselors, family members are easily accessible and available to clients with disabilities. These members remain a critical source of comfort and help particularly in communities where professional rehabilitation counselors are not available. One important role of such counselors in most countries in sub-Saharan Africa is to help strengthen family ties for adults with disabilities who may be socially neglected. In addition, counselors may seek to enhance the social network of adults with disabilities at risk for social isolation by linking them with the social groups such as religious organizations that offer social support. To be successful in helping clients establish and maintain social support systems, counselors need to address social, physical, cultural, and spiritual or religious aspects of well-being. This acknowledgment goes beyond the professional preparation that counselors routinely receive from their mostly Western counselor education programs.

Questions

1. What is the significance of social support in living with a disability in an African setting?
2. How could education and training better prepare counselors in African settings to best serve adult clients with significant disabilities?

survey in a low-socioeconomic status suburb of Harare (Zimbabwe) yielded a 5.6 percent prevalence rate of disability (Jelsma et al., 2002). Rwanda, a small land-locked country in the Great Lakes region of central Africa with a population slightly higher than 8.6 million, has an estimated disability prevalence rate of just less than 5 percent of the population (Thomas, 2005). However, about 800,000 Rwandese citizens died from genocide in the last decade that left millions with both physical and mental disabilities (Palmer, 2002), suggesting that the estimated low disability prevalence for that country is likely a gross underestimate. The ways in which national governments in sub-Saharan Africa collect disability prevalence data may leave many people with disabilities unidentified. Persons who could be regarded as having a disability, especially if it is not visible, may also not self-identify, as that would bring social stigma on them and family. Also, they would not self-identify as having a disability if they did not perceive themselves failing on culturally expected role functioning from a personal difference others regarded as a disability.

Conditions for Which Counseling May Be Sought

People with disabilities may seek counseling to address needs in four interdependent areas: social, physical, personal, and resource (Mpofu, 2002). Social needs may arise from negative societal attitudes, and are probably the most pervasive. They are reflected in negative expectations for success in persons with disabilities and in denying them equal opportunities.

Personal needs are attitudes toward one's own disability that may hamper adaptation or effective life participation. Disability consciousness is an important personal need for which counseling services would be helpful (Barnatt, 1996; Mpofu, 2002). Disability consciousness refers to one's awareness of sensitivity of the environment (e.g., community, workplaces) to disability-related differences. Environments that are supportive of disability-related differences (e.g., positive social attitudes, enabling structures and resources) may make disability-related differences less salient to persons with disabilities and typically developing others, which would enhance perceptions of similarities between persons with disabilities and others. Disability self-advocacy is important for addressing barriers in the environment that would lead to economic deprivation and limitations in choice of a preferred life style.

Personal needs could include a lack of disability management knowledge or skills that may add to difficulties beyond those that are objectively indicated by the type or severity of the disability. Personal counseling needs of people with disabilities at different ages are influenced by the interaction between their disability status and normative developmental needs. In this connection, it is important for counselors to keep in mind that current theories of human development may not accurately represent the developmental experiences of individuals with disabilities living in Africa.

Typically, physical needs are from physical–structural barriers such as disability-inaccessible buildings and transport and communication systems that deny persons with disabilities equal opportunities. Resource needs may arise from limitations in materials and support systems that could aid adaptation to disability. Limitations of resources such as medical, financial, and social support can be handicapping.

Social needs are the most intractable and often lead to personal, physical, and resource handicaps. Disadvantage from social needs is reversible through changes in social policies and with increasing knowledge of disability management. The social–cultural barriers that are faced by

Case Study 19.4: Communal Affiliation Effects on Living with a Disability

Tonya is a twenty-eight-year-old African American woman with a history of substance abuse and depression. She has gone through several treatment programs for substance abuse and has been hospitalized twice for depression. Her last hospitalization for depression was nine months ago. She lives in a rural area and had to leave for treatment each time. Given the size of her hometown, everyone is aware of her treatments and hospitalizations.

As the counselor, you also live in the same small town. While volunteering at a church yard sale, one of the church members remarked to you that she saw Tonya at the bar last night and she was drinking. She further commented that "someone like that needs to be on her knees praying all the time." Tonya is also a member of the same church.

Tonya still lives with her parents, who self-identify as born-again Christians. Both parents have made it clear that this is her last chance and if she messes up this time, she is "on her own." Tonya stated that she has been "free" of alcohol and any other drugs for the past three months. She is scheduled for an interview for a job as a school bus driver next week.

Questions

1. Discuss any cultural and community dynamics in this case.
2. How would you provide counseling in this case to address family issues and needs, including cultural hierarchy and religion?

persons with disabilities, and the unique socioeconomic experiences of people with disabilities, mark them as a minority. Minorities are often distinguished in being denied equal economic and social opportunities.

The Ordinariness of Disabilities

People with disabilities share many needs with typically developing others, for which they too would need counseling. However, people with disabilities may be counseled under the mistaken assumption that the needs they have are primarily caused by the disability. This may not be the case. For instance, if a person with a disability appears depressed, anxious, passive, and helpless, these symptoms are regarded by typically developing others as primarily caused by the disability. However, these very symptoms may be a normal reaction to negative discrimination, stigmatization, and denial of opportunities by typically developing others. For instance, society may exert pressure on the individual with a disability to act in a manner that is "expected" of persons with a disability. These undeclared expectations often translate to the person with a disability, that he or she must appear as if he or she is dependent, confused, or even sick. If the individual with a disability behaves in ways that minimize a disability-related difference, then he or she could be regarded as not having "come to terms" or accepted the disability. These negative societal expectations, which reflect minority status in persons with disabilities, are communicated to them with such persistence, intensity, and pervasiveness as to influence the way some persons with disabilities perceive, think, and feel. They may lead to counseling needs not necessarily arising from the objective fact of having a disability.

HISTORY OF RESEARCH AND PRACTICE IN COUNSELING PEOPLE WITH DISABILITIES

Research on disabilities in sub-Saharan Africa has focused on cultural perceptions important to the salience of disability in indigenous communities. The research has considered the types and perceived efficacy of counseling interventions in those communities, particularly of community-based programs and psychoeducational interventions.

Cultural Perceptions

Although persons with disabilities comprise a significant proportion of the population of sub-Saharan Africa (Murray & Lopez, 1996), ethnographic studies of East and Southern African cultures have reported the absence of a large number of Western terms for disabilities (Devlieger, 1995; Jackson & Mupedziswa, 1988). Also, anthropological studies suggest that among some East African tribes, children with disabilities are not any more socially stigmatized than children in general (Devlieger, 1995). This phenomenon may in part be explained by the fact that role function is culturally more important than personal attributes and also that in village settings, there is likely to be social support from the family to carry out expected social role functions successfully (Mpofu, 1999). On the one hand, some Africans with disabilities could enjoy wider social acceptance than their Western peers. For instance, certain forms of psychiatric and physical disabilities as defined in Western culture are considered spiritual gifts and worth of reverence rather than treatment (Devlieger, 1995; see also Chapter 1 this Volume,). On the other hand, native African cultures are less accepting of some common forms of physical and mental disabilities

Research Box 19.1: Social Acceptance with a Disability

Mpofu, E. (1999). *Social acceptance of early adolescents with physical disabilities*. Ann Arbor, MI: UMI Dissertation Services.

Objective: The goal of the study was to compare social acceptance of African students with a visible physical disability and typically developing others.

Method: Social acceptance data were collected from 235 adolescents with physical disabilities and 231 typically developing adolescents from the same schools. The social acceptance data were from 8,009 classmates and the students with physical disabilities themselves.

Results: Students with physical disabilities had social acceptance ratings similar to those of typically developing others. However, students with disabilities were twice as likely to be nominated for negative behaviors (e.g., unreliable, lazy, aggressive) compared to their typically developing peers.

Conclusion: Students with physical disabilities were as socially accepted as peers without a physical disability. Having a visible disability made it more likely that a negative behavioral trait would be ascribed. The sources of the negative attributions were unclear.

Questions

1. Explain the fact that social acceptance statuses in students with physical disabilities and typically developing others would be similar in this African school context.
2. How may the perceived negative behavioral perceptions by peers be explained?
3. What counseling needs are implied by the findings of the study? How would you go about addressing them?

(e.g., epilepsy; cerebral palsy), as persons with these conditions are seen as victims of misfortune cast by avenging spirits or demons due to previous misdeeds by their parents or ancestors (Devlieger, 1995; Mpofu & Harley, 2002). In some African cultures, having a disability is considered a punishment for a social transgression by the individual or family of origin. For instance, the Shona of Mozambique and Zimbabwe may say "Mwari akamuseka" (God laughed at him or her) with reference to a person with a disability. The Ndebele of South Africa and Zimbabwe say "Umlimo wamuhleka" to mean the same. Thus, a disability may be considered personal in both its origins and consequences.

In most African cultures, people with developmental disabilities are socially stigmatized. Immediate and extended family may also be socially ostracized for presumed complicity in the primary violation of social norms that caused the disability (Jackson & Mupedziswa, 1988; Whyte, 1991). Also, being female is associated with lower social status in African cultures (Bourdillon, 1987). Anecdotal evidence suggests that African males with disabilities are likely to have higher levels of social participation than females with disabilities.

Social acceptance with a disability is mediated by perceived adequacy of role function and social support to succeed in expected social roles. Family or the village community rather than professional counselors tend to provide counseling to people with disabilities for effective community participation.

A question of interest is how counseling needs are communicated and perceived by the participants in the family or village setting. Quite clearly, family and village mentors appear to have an intuitive understanding of the needs of their members with a disability. The fact that counseling needs related to a disability are often directly connected to normative functional roles for community members makes it easier for others to provide appropriate and timely help. Family social support and village mentors would not be available to those with disabilities in urban areas, and professional counselors are more involved in working with clients with disabilities in those settings (Mpofu, 1999). Clients may perceive to be receiving counseling that does not necessarily address their needs.

Community-based Rehabilitation Services

The involvement of people with disabilities, family members, and community members working with local resources and through local organizations is the key element of community-based rehabilitation (CBR). CBR attempts to maximize the full potential and functions of persons with disabilities in their natural environment within the family and the community (Ndawi, 2000). It seeks to enhance the quality of life for people with disabilities and their families, meeting basic needs and supporting their inclusion and participation. CBR encompasses several life space domains: health, education, livelihood, and social empowerment.

The typical CBR model includes a three-tier system (Judd, 2003). In the first tier are volunteer lay members of the community (local supervisors), and they are trained in basic rehabilitation techniques for common disabilities.

Discussion Box 19.3: Marketing Disability

Consider the following excerpt from an interview with an African American with a disability:

"In one position I was hired to be the future accountant but was used to raise funds for the program. I was the only ... person with a disability on the staff. The position required that we go to the capital city, and meet with someone about seeking funds to finance the program. We succeeded in obtaining the funds necessary to keep the program going for quite sometime.

On another occasion I worked as a counselor, and was the only disabled ...working on the floor. I feel I was used to inspire patients to do their best to get better as quickly as possible. I obtained those jobs and was willing to work in the positions ... it didn't really bother me a great deal. I was glad to be able to help others that were not as fortunate as I."

Questions

1. What is your reaction to the needs that employer-counselors sought to meet with this individual with a disability?
2. How would you have counseled this individual about his work role experiences?

They provide direct services to people with disabilities in their homes, community centers, and community clinics (Judd, 2003). The second tier consists of district rehabilitation professionals who train and supervise the local supervisor. These professionals include medical and allied health professionals (Judd, 2003). The third tier is the national coordination, typically the government, in corroboration with a nongovernmental organization. Participation is crucial at all these levels, especially the community, for the sustainability of CBR (Hartley, Ojwang, Baguwemu, Ddamulira, & Chavuta, 2005;). Most CBR programs in Africa are funded by international donor agencies without which these programs would lack the necessary resources and would also not be sustainable. We consider a few illustrative cases from across sub-Saharan Africa.

CBR programs in Ethiopia have provided a wide range of training activities to people with disabilities and their communities. For instance, many Ethiopians with disabilities have trained in agricultural production and the maintenance of orthopedic appliances and workshops. CBR programs in Kenya have been aimed at increasing the participation of persons with disabilities in normative community activities such as vocational training and education for jobs in the local market. In Uganda, CBR training programs are offered to teachers, school administrators, community leaders, and parents on various topics including prevention of disabilities, early identification, inclusion in mainstream schools, and effective coordination of services (Ojwang & Hartley, 2001).

CURRENT PRACTICES

The vast majority of the indigenous Africans use both traditional (nonformal) and modern rehabilitation services (Mpofu, 2000; Mpofu & Harley, 2002; see also Chapter 1, this volume). In all African countries, not-for-profit (i.e., nongovernmental organizations [NGOs]) have played a key role in the development of rehabilitation services, often influencing national policies, personnel education, and training. We address these within the context of specific approaches that we discuss below. Psychoeducational interventions in the postmodern paradigm have great potential in counseling people with disabilities in African settings. Community-based approaches remain an effective intervention in these settings.

Postmodern Psychoeducational Approaches

Choice of technique or strategy is a key consideration in counseling people of African descent with disabilities. Postmodern approaches to counseling are those that value lived experiences and local perspectives. These approaches are different from classical or modern psychoeducational approaches in that have a bias toward counselor rather than client perspectives. Often, understanding lived experiences in local contexts results in more responsive counseling interventions than would be the case with interventions based on assumed transferability of counseling approaches across settings.

Postmodern approaches that work in counseling people of African descent with disabilities include memory healing (Nwoye, 2005) and narrative therapy (Farber, 2002; see also Chapter 2, this volume). People of African descent use these as primary communication tools, especially in life-changing circumstances such as chronic illness or disability.

Memory Healing

Memory healing has been used to counsel individuals with HIV and AIDS in Africa (Nwoye, 2008; William, 1996). The four-part memory paradigm comprises the following components: fact, behavioral, event, and prospective memories which become scaffolds for developing coping strategies in living with a disability. First, with an acquired disability, the *fact memory* helps the client understand the what, how, when, where, and wherefore associated with the disability. The client needs an understanding of the disability and the implications of the disability to his or her life. Second, the *behavioral memory* helps the client to comprehend perceptions of significant others about the disability and how that will impact their attitudes toward him or her. It involves the search for historical and cultural background resources regarding how to respond to the disability. Third, *event memory* is intended to address the client's preoccupations with the magnitude or severity of the disability. The client may seek answers and reassurance from multiple sources: healer, counselor, family, friends and acquaintances, and medical practitioners. The client may explore multiple descriptions of the crisis and how its challenges can be transcended (Nwoye, 2008). Fourth, the *prospective memory* is a concept relevant to helping clients to focus on life goals, including personal-familial goals.

Memory healing provides an organizing framework around which the counselor listens to the client's narratives and works with the client to identify concerns, and personal-familial resources for responding to the needs influenced by having a disability. The client needs assistance with putting the prospective memory into proper perspective and fully addressing them.

Ritual Theory

Turner (1980) developed the ritual theory based on the life experiences of Central African people. Turner proposes that social drama occur out of traumatic life events. This drama starts with a perception of breach of normalcy and results in crisis of disorientation and destabilization and a search for stabilization again. For instance, the onset of congenital or acquired disability represents a breach to normal order of life. The result is often disorientation, confusion, and loss of sense of coherence. This loss of coherence is particularly acute with the onset of severe mental illness. Severe mental illness is not well understood in the many indigenous communities of Africa and often ascribed to possession avenging spirits or demons. Loss of coherence calls for efforts by the individual with a disability, and his or her family and community, to seek to "redress" the situation or to mitigate the disorientation and confusion from the experience of a disability to the best extent possible (Geertz, 1983; Nwoye, 2008).

The goals of redressive actions in counseling people with disabilities is to broaden their self-awareness in living with a disability, improve access to resources, and offer relief to an individual with disability and his or her family (Nwoye, 2008, p. 23). In the African context, redressive actions in counseling comprise various parts. First, hidden inaccuracies and faulty generalizations are challenged using humor and metaphors. Metaphors and analogies that depict cultural values are used to present a balanced perspective of the disability and to prompt the client to appreciate the personal responsibilities that would be necessary in the process of adjustment to disability. Second, the counselor discloses an example story of someone in the community successfully living with a disability. The lessons from the storytelling create room for the client to reconstruct options for successful living with a disability. Third, the counselor assists in reframing the client's perspectives that are associated with emotional issues such as anger, guilt, and fear in living with a disability. The client may view living with a disability differently and thereby limit the spread of negative emotions.

Narrative Theory

Traumatized people make sense of their experiences by constructing and presenting subjective narratives (see also Chapters 2 and 15, this volume). Narratives serve positive self empowering as well as negative self-mortifying purposes (Besley, 2002; Speedy, 2000; Windsale & Monk, 1999). These narratives are often emotionally charged. In the African setting, the individual with disability values his or her personal story and the subjective mapping of his or her experiences. Storying about "how I got here" is a self-empowering first step in making coping choices among African cultural heritage people. A valuable component of counseling is creating a space for listening to these narratives with respect, acknowledging the stories of the client while helping him or her to reconstruct the stories by incorporating more objective and relevant empowering information into the story (Farber 2002; Geertz, 1983).

Following Faber's (2002) narrative therapy approach, the counselor may start with creating a warm-accepting space for the individual to explore his or her story, and to invest emotional and culture-laden perspectives in the story. The counselor listens carefully in preparation for assisting the client to enlarge his or her views and incorporate more helpful values for reorganization, reorientation, and reengagement with life. For example, the counselor may assume an orientation of not knowing the experiences of the client and willingness to learn from the client. He or she listens for orientation and teaching from the client. Drawing from deep cultural understanding, the counselor asks questions to assist the client in re-listening to his or her own narrative and the gaps in his or her narrative. The client's initial narrative may be focused more on the losses, woes, and generalized sense of catastrophe as a way of reaching out to the community for understanding and empathy. In that case, the counselor assists the client in reconstructing his or her narrative to include awareness of how the disability is only a part of who the client is as a person, in the family and community.

Psychosocial Support Services

Psychosocial support services (PSS) for individuals with disabilities have increased substantially in recent years in Africa (Mpofu, et al., 2007). This increase is accounted for by the AIDS pandemic as well as the upsurge of wars and political turmoil in many parts of Africa (see also Chapters 14, 15, and 16, this volume). PSS for individuals with disabilities include disabilities education and disability advocacy to increase access to resources and participation by people with disabilities (Rule, Lorenzo, & Wolmarans, 2005). Individuals and their significant others are supported by PSS facilitators ranging from trained nurses, social workers to volunteer peer and elder counselors to explore the life meanings that are associated with disability. Support services simultaneously target the individual who is experiencing disability and the family that is experiencing disruptions. Support service providers often live in the immediate communities and are expected to respond rapidly to crisis calls.

The major service provision model is integrative helping. Many resources are simultaneously accessed for each case. For example, PSS for an individual with epilepsy will include services from the health center, health and safety education department, and counseling services where available. The support services for the individual with serious mental illness will include the administration of clinical drugs, psychosocial counseling for significant family members, and mental health education as well as traditional and religious healing (Baron, 2002). In line with this integrative model, the components of PSS facilitators training involve an integration of basic physiotherapy, social work, community development, advocacy, and counseling contents. The efficacy of this PSS model has been demonstrated among refugee populations in Uganda, Liberia, and Rwanda (Baron, 2002; Lopez, 2007).

Legal and Professional Issues

In sub-Saharan Africa, rehabilitation is perceived primarily as enhancing national development through enabling the economic participation of all citizens. The vast majority of Africans with disabilities are excluded from schools and opportunities to work. Their rehabilitation adds to the human resource base for community and national development. Rehabilitation counseling is an important pillar of these efforts and aimed mostly at citizenship rights education and the use of opportunity equalization policies and programs.

Rehabilitation and disability-related policies adopted by national governments in the six sub-Saharan African nations are mostly modeled after United Nations Conventions. For example, most African countries adopted rehabilitation and disability-related international charters, conventions, and cooperation agreements such as the UN Convention on the Rights of the Child (1989), The United Nations Convention on the Rights of Persons with Disabilities (2006), the Standard Rules on the Equalization of Opportunities for Persons with Disabilities (1993), the Salamanca Statement and Framework for Action on Special Needs Education (1994), Millennium Development Goals focusing on Poverty Reduction and Development (2000), and EFA Flagship on Education and Disability (2001).

Following the adoption of the United Nations Standard Rules on equal opportunities for people with disabilities, the Tanzanian government established a National Council for the Disabled (NCD) to address the socioeconomic of citizens with disabilities (Policy & Legislation, 2006). The NCD is made up of the following government departments: Education and Culture, Health, Labour, and Youth Development. The Tanzanian government adopted a quota employment system by which 2 percent of positions by employers in both the public and private system are reserved for people with disabilities. The government of Botswana's national vision states that by 2016 Botswana should be a "compassionate and caring nation" as evidenced by adoption of policies and programs that addresses the needs of vulnerable groups, including people with disabilities. To that effect, the Botswana government's Revised National Policy on Education (RNPE, 1994) commits it to providing education for all children in the next twenty-five years. In addition, the government of Botswana has a National Policy on the Care for People with Disabilities and for the provision of assistive devices to people with disabilities to enhance their community inclusion.

In post-apartheid South Africa, rehabilitation and disability-related policies are considered human rights issues. Consequently, at independence from apartheid rule in 1994, a Disability Directorate was established within the Office of the Vice-President, indicative of how important disability and human rights were held to be. In 1997, the South African government produced the White Paper on the Integrated National Disability Strategy (Office of the Deputy President, 1997), which outlined policies and strategies for equalizing opportunities, such as the creation of work opportunities for people with disabilities through the development and maintenance of state-supported small to medium business enterprises.

Rwanda's national constitution promotes the rights and dignity of persons with disabilities, and the Rwandese Government's 10-Year National Development Plan includes a specific paragraph on disability (Thomas, 2005). Other relevant governmental rehabilitation and disability-related initiatives include the National Policy for the Protection of the Handicapped for the equalization of opportunities among citizens regardless of disability. A Rwandan government supported national disability organization, the Federation of Associations and Centres of the Handicapped in Rwanda (FACHR), provides office space and limited financial support for small business enterprises by citizens with disabilities. Several other agencies offer organizational and public awareness supports; these include National Assistance Fund for Needy Survivors of Genocide and Massacres in Rwanda (NFGMR), General Association of Disabled People in Rwanda (AGHR), Rwandan Union of the Blind (RUB), Rwandan Association of the Deaf (RNAD), and Federation Rwandaise Handi Sport (FERHANDIS). The Handicap International provides material and technical support to governmental rehabilitation centers. The Christian Blind Mission (CBM) operates a center in the capital city of

Kigali, and groups such as One Love and Gatagara provide prosthetics, orthotics, and technical assistance.

The Zambian government, through its Ministry of Community Development and Social Services (MCDSS), addresses the human rights of people with disabilities, including their rights to education, employment, and health (Ngoma, 2007). Other government departments involved in creating, promoting, and supporting conditions that equalize opportunities for people with disabilities are the Ministries of Health, Education, and Youth, Sport, and Child Welfare. For example, during 2006, the Zambian Ministry of Health coordinated efforts with the Ministries of Education, Youth Sport, and Child Welfare, and an NGO (i.e., the Zambia Association for the Physically Disabled [ZAPD]) to develop a CBR policy to increase access to rehabilitation services. The Zambian CBR policy advocates for a proactive approach for the prevention, treatment, and rehabilitation of all forms of disability. A proactive preventive approach (e.g., treat the hypertension rather than rehabilitate the stroke) is a priority in the Zambian CBR national program.

To our knowledge, only four African countries (i.e., Cameroon, South Africa, Uganda, and Zimbabwe) have disability legislation. For example, the Zimbabwe government passed disability legislation (i.e., Disabled Persons Act, 1994). The Zimbabwe Disabled Persons Act makes a provision for equal opportunity and access for people with disabilities. However, the practical effect is limited by the fact that the Act absolves the Zimbabwe government from litigation for lack of nonadherence with its own disability law. Cameroon's Law No. 83/13 of July 21, 1983, as operationalized by presidential decree (i.e., Decree No. 90/1516 of 26 November 1990), provides the guidelines for the rehabilitation and education of person with disabilities in the country. The law provides for health care for people with disabilities and their education in inclusive settings. The intent of the law is still to be achieved for the majority of Cameroonians with disabilities who mostly are unaware of or have no access to state-mandated rehabilitation services. Rehabilitation-related policies are still to translate into legislation in four of the six countries under review.

In general, rehabilitation and disability-related policies within national states lack adequate interagency coordination, with the result that implementation of stated policies is not effective. National governments tend to underfund rehabilitation and disability-related agencies, with the result that intended policy outcomes are not achieved.

The vast majority of citizens of sub-Saharan Africa with mental health needs receive rehabilitation services from family, traditional healers, and faith-based organizations (Lopez et al., 2007; Mpofu, 2000, 2006). None of the national governments of the six countries under review have formal policies for family-supported rehabilitation or those provided by traditional healers and faith-based organizations (Mpofu & Harley, 2002; Serpell, Mariga, & Harvey, 1993). The Zimbabwe government has a Traditional Healers Act (THA) that recognizes health care services by traditional healers. However, the THA does not specifically address rehabilitation counseling for disability-related issues.

ISSUES FOR RESEARCH AND OTHER FORMS OF SCHOLARSHIP

To be effective, psychosocial services must be based on a reliable census of those to be served, the specific needs they have, and the types of resources relevant to the needs identified. We noted in a previous section that national governments in sub-Saharan Africa appeared not to have reliable enrollment data on those with disabilities. Other issues that influence the quality of rehabilitation counseling services in sub-Saharan Africa include the lack of appropriately trained counselors, the underdevelopment of the research base on theories to guide counseling interventions in Africa context settings, and lack of evidence-informed CBR programs.

Inaccurate Prevalence Figures

We conclude from the negative discrepancy between the national disability prevalence estimates and WHO disability population estimates that none of the countries under review has reliable data on the prevalence of disabilities in their populations. This information gap may, in part, be from lack of personnel with training and education in the identification of disabilities (Mpofu et al., 2007). Inconsistencies in disability prevalence statistics within country are explained by the fact that different studies use different inclusion criteria (Jelsma et al., 2002).

Underreporting of disabilities by African national governments and international agencies disenfranchises millions of African citizens of their rights to health, education, and political redress. For example, national governments would have more resources allocated to their rehabilitation and disability-related policy implementation with larger and more realistic disability prevalence figures, portending a larger political constituency whose unique needs would not be easily ignored. The African Union (AU) declared 1999–2009 to be the African Decade of Disabled Persons. The extent to which this resolution will influence rehabilitation and disability-related policies and service personnel education and training in African Union member nations remains to be seen.

Counselor Training and Education

To successfully counsel individuals of African descent with disabilities, counselors must understand that clients evaluate the counseling process through cultural filters. For instance, studies on Americans of African descent in mental health counseling reported that the clients formed their opinions about the counselor very early in

Research Box 19.2: Counseling and Psychological Services

Kearney, L. K., Draper, M., & Baron, A. (2003). Counseling utilization by ethnic minority students. Counseling & Mental Health Center, The University of Texas at Austin. Retrieved from http//:www.utexas.edu/student/cmhc/research/rescon.html

Objective: The goal of the study was to examine counseling utilization and outcomes for ethnic minorities on university campuses.

Method: A sample of 1,166 African American, Asian American, Caucasian, and Hispanic help-seeking university students from more than forty universities nationwide filled out the Outcome Questionnaire at the first and last therapy sessions.

Results: Caucasian students attended significantly more sessions than all other groups. Further, the greatest distress was found at intake in Asian American clients, followed by Hispanic, African American, and Caucasian students. All groups appeared to benefit from therapy, as noted by a decrease in symptoms, but none of the groups met criteria for clinically significant change.

Conclusion: These findings offer some hope that university counseling centers, with their greater emphasis on multicultural awareness, may be providing better treatment for ethnic minority students than would be received in community health centers, where such training for therapists is not emphasized. Unfortunately, because the study did not include information about the multicultural training therapists had received, conclusive evidence that this is the case cannot be found in this particular study.

Questions

1. Explain why Caucasian students attended more counseling sessions than all other groups combined.
2. How many barriers to attendance can you identify for African American students?
3. What counseling needs are implied by the findings of the study? How would you go about addressing them?

the process and that assessment affected their engagement in the counseling process (Fabian & Edwards, 2005; Harley, 2005). Clients of African descent prefer to work with counselors with whom they have a sense of comfort, and who share similar life ideologies with them. It is noteworthy that these clients were willing to engage actively in counseling with counselors who understood their world and accepted their meaning without having prejudgmental attitudes. This expectation for cultural concordance is applicable to Africa given that most professional counselors are Western styled or trained. The Western styled or trained counselor and the indigenous African with a disability may not share similar cultural perspectives implicitly and explicitly. Effectiveness of counseling by individuals of African descent for individuals of African descent with disabilities will be predicated on cultural sensitivity by the counselors.

Multicultural Education

The trend that social programs and public policy for persons with disabilities in non-Western countries are generally adopted from Western countries (Whyte & Ingstad, 1995) make it more than likely that Western social constructs for disabilities will be (mis)applied to non-Western countries without prior study. For instance, psychoeducational counseling intervention, based on Western theories and models, may be misapplied or applied in ways that may not be culturally sensitive. Multicultural models of counseling (Lewis, 2006) could serve as frameworks for integrating the arts and science of theory-driven Western counseling models with dynamic African culture, in order to best serve the client.

Counseling Outcomes

Counselors of Africans with disabilities may be involved in counseling for independent living and socioeconomic productivity. In that regard, it is important to keep in mind both the cultural appropriateness of independent living and socioeconomic productivity for particular clients. Consideration needs to be given to the changing self-perceptions of Africans toward Western, individualist self-perceptions and conceptions of productivity. Counselors need to determine and act on the client's preferred living arrangements and productivity status. It would be inappropriate, for example, to counsel a client whose desired living arrangements and sense of socioeconomic productivity are with extended family toward Western type, individualistic independence. At the same time, counselors working with Africans with disabilities should guard against perceiving clients in stereotypical ways that could lead them to the equally mistaken view that their clients must, of necessity, prefer collectivistic-oriented living arrangements and productivity because they are Africans. The ideal condition is to counsel the clients to make choices of living arrangements and productivity that are consistent with their needs and least likely to harm their well-being and that of others.

Community-focused Approaches Are Important

Rehabilitation counseling and other social service delivery systems often overlook available counseling and health supportive resources in African context neighborhoods (e.g., churches, community organizations, kinship networks) (Lawson & Kim, 2005). People of African descent tend to prize sense of community. Service models likely to work for them are those in which they are recognized and included in societal, organizational, and service delivery resources.

Community-based rehabilitation services, in the United States for African Americans, should include models based on the holistic approach, including all parts of the culture within the larger context (Wilson, Edwards, Alston, Harley, & Doughty, 2001). According to Barrio (2000), "research shows that some rehabilitation approaches based on Western models may produce adverse effects when used with patients from ethnic minority groups" (p. 879).

Evidence Informed CBR Programs Are Needed

CBR programs provide the most cost-effective and integrative modes of interventions for people with chronic and common health problems in African settings. However, the process and effectiveness of these interventions still needs to be adequately addressed (FinkenflÜgel, Cornielje, & Velema, 2008). FinkenflÜgel et al. (2008) have asserted that robust and easy to use indicators of CBR programs need to be developed to determine if stated program interventions are effective. These indicators need to be standardized so that they can be used across similar aspects of different programs so as to generate synchronicity of evidence-based practice across Africa.

SUMMARY AND CONCLUSION

Disability carries significant opportunity cost from social stigma by typically developing others. Counseling needs may arise from the need to live positively with a disability and to counteract barriers to full community participation. In African cultural heritage settings, families provide much of the rehabilitation counseling of a member with a disability, more than do professional counselors. CBR programs are used to equate opportunity for individuals with disabilities through psychoeducational and vocational training. A variety of psychoeducational interventions rooted in Africanist world views appear to hold promise for counseling individuals with disabilities.

REFERENCES

Barnatt, S. N. (1996). Disability culture or disability consciousness? *Journal of Disability Policy Studies*, 7(2), 1–19.

Baron, N. (2002). Community based psychosocial and mental health services for southern Sudanese refugees in long term exile in Uganda. In J. de Jong (Ed.), *Trauma, war, and violence: Public mental health in socio-cultural context* (pp. 157–204). New York: Kluwer Academic/Plenum Press.

Barrio, C. (2000). The cultural relevance of community support programs. *Psychiatric Services*, *51*, 879–84.

Besley, T. (2001). Foucauldian influences in narrative therapy: An approach for schools. *Journal of Educational Enquiry*, *2*(2), 72–93.

Besley, T. (2002). *Counseling youth Foucault, power, and the ethics of subjectivity*. Abingdon, UK: Praeger.

Chidyausiku, S., & Nleya, C. (1998). Country Report – Zimbabwe. In H. Cornielje, J. Jelsma, & A. Moyo (Eds.), *Research informed rehabilitation planning in Southern Africa* (pp. 112–13). Harare, Zimbabwe: SAFOD.

Chimedza, R. M., & Peters, S. (1999). Disabled people's quest for social justice in Zimbabwe. In F. Armstrong & L. Barton (Eds.), *Disability, human rights and education* (pp. 7–23). Buckingham, UK: Open University Press.

Dell Orto, A. E. (2003). Coping with the enormity of illness and disability. In R. P. Marinelli & A.E. Dell Orto (Eds.), *The psychological and social impact of disability* (3rd ed., pp. 333–5). New York: Springer.

Devlieger, P. J. (1995). Why disabled? The cultural understanding of physical disability in an African society. In B. Ingstad & S. R. Whyte (Eds.), *Disability and culture* (p. 3–32). Berkeley: University of California Press.

Devlieger, P. J. (1998a). Vocational rehabilitation in Zimbabwe: A socio-historical analysis. *Journal of Vocational Rehabilitation*, *11*, 21–31

Devlieger, P. J. (1998b). Physical "disability" in Bantu languages: Understanding the relativity of classification and meaning. *International Journal of Rehabilitation Research*, *21*, 63–70.

Disabled Persons Act. (1992). Harare, Zimbabwe: Government Printers.

Fabian, E. S., & Edwards, Y. V. (2005). Community mental health and African Americans. In D. A. Harley & J. M. Dillard (Eds.), *Contemporary mental health issues among African Americans* (pp. 225–35). Alexandria, VA: American Counseling Association.

Farber, E. W. (2002). Existential treatment with HIV/AIDS clients. In R. F. Massey & S. W. Massey (Eds.), *Comprehensive handbook of psychotherapy* (Vol. 3, pp. 303–31). New York: John Wiley & Sons.

Finkelstein, V., & French, S. (1997). Towards a psychology of disability. In J. Swain, V. Finkelstein, S. French, & M. Oliver (Eds.), *Disabling barriers-enabling environments* (pp. 27–33). Thousand Oaks, CA: SAGE Publications.

FinkenflÜgel, H. Cornielje, H., & Velema (2008) The use of models of evaluation of CBR programmes. *Disability and Rehabilitation*, *30*(5), 348–54.

Geertz, C. (1983). *The interpretation of cultures*. New York: Basic Books.

Harley, D. A. (2005). The Black church: A strength-based approach in mental health. In D. A. Harley & J. M. Dillard (Eds.), *Contemporary mental health issues among African Americans* (pp. 191–202). Alexandria, VA: American Counseling Association.

Hartley, S., Ojwang, P., Baguwemu, A., Ddamulira, M., & Chavuta, A. (2005). How do carers of disabled children cope? The Ugandan perspective. *Child: Care, Health & Development*, *31*(2), 167–80.

Jackson, H., & Mupedziswa, R. (1988). Disability and rehabilitation. *Journal of Social Development in Africa*, *3*, 21–30.

Jelsma, J., Mielke, J., Powell, G., Fox, B., Weerdt, W. D., & Cock, P. D. (2002). Disability in an urban black community in Zimbabwe. *Disability and Rehabilitation*, *24*, 851–9.

Judd, T. (2003). Rehabilitation of emotional problems of brain disorders in developing countries. *Neuropsychological rehabilitation*, *13* (1/2) 307–25.

Lawson, E. J., & Kim, Y. J. (2005). Collaborators: Mental health and public health in the African American community. In D. A. Harley & J. M Dillard (Eds.), *Contemporary mental health issues among African Americans* (pp. 205–22). Alexandria, VA: American Counseling Association.

Lewis, S. (2006). Three-factor model of multicultural counselling for consumers with disabilities. *Journal of Vocational Rehabilitation*, *24*(3), 151–9.

Lustig, D., & Strauser, D. (2007). The causal relationship between chronic poverty and disability. *Rehabilitation Counseling Bulletin*, *50*, 194–202.

Mpofu, E. (1999). *Social acceptance of Zimbabwean adolescents with physical disabilities*. Ann Arbor, MI: UMI Dissertation Services.

Mpofu, E. (2002). Disability and rehabilitation in Zimbabwe: Lessons and implications for rehabilitation practice in the U.S. *Journal of Rehabilitation*, *68*(4), 20–5.

Mpofu, E. (2006). Majority world health care traditions intersect indigenous and complementary and alternative medicine (Editorial for Special Issue on Indigenous Healing Practices). *International Journal of Disability, Development and Education*, *53*, 375–9.

Mpofu, E., & Harley, D. A. (2002). Disability and rehabilitation in Zimbabwe: Lessons and implications for rehabilitation practice in the U.S – Disability and rehabilitation in Zimbabwe. *Journal of Rehabilitation*, *68*(4), 26–33.

Mpofu, E., Peltzer, K., Shumba, A., Serpell, R., & Mogaji, A. (2005). School psychology in sub-Saharan Africa: Results and implications of a six country survey. In C. Frisby & C. R. Reynolds (Eds.), *Comprehensive handbook of multicultural school psychology*. New York: John Wiley & Sons.

Mpofu, E., Zindi, F., Oakland, T., & Peresuh, M. H. (1997). School psychology practices in East and Southern Africa: Special educators' perspective. *Journal of Special Education*, *31*, 387–402.

Mpofu, E., Jelsma, J., Maart, S., Levers, L. L., Montsi, M. R., Thlabiwe, P., et al. (2007). Rehabilitation in seven sub-Saharan African countries: Policies, personnel training and education. *Rehabilitation Education*, 21, 223–230.

Murray, C. J. L., & Lopez, A. D. (1996). *The global burden of disease series*. Boston, MA: Harvard School of Public Health.

Myezwa, H., & M'kumbuzi, V. R. P. (2003). Participation in community based rehabilitation programmes in Zimbabwe: Where are we? *Asia Pacific Disability Rehabilitation Journal*, *14*(1), 18–28.

Ndawi, O. P. (2001).The role of legislation in facilitating CBR in Zimbabwe. In S. Hartley (Ed.), *CBR: A participatory strategy in Africa*. London: University College London

Ngoma, M. S. (2007). *An overview of rehabilitation services in Zambia*. Unpublished manuscript.

Nwoye, A. (2005). Memory healing processes and community intervention in grief work in Africa. *ANZJFT*, *26*(3), 147–54.

Nwoye, A. (2008). Memory and narrative healing processes in HIV counseling: A view from Africa. *Contemporary Family Therapy*, *30*, 15–30.

Office of the Deputy President. (1997). Integrated national disability strategy. Retrieved December 14, 2005 from http://www.polity.org.za/govdocs/white_papers/disability1.html

Ojwang, V. P., & Hartley, S. (2001). Community based rehabilitation training in Uganda: An overview. In S. Hartley (Ed.), *CBR: A participatory strategy in Africa*. London: University College London

Palmer, I. (2002). Psychosocial costs of war in Rwanda. *Advances in Psychiatric Treatment*, *8*, 17–25. Retrieved December 16, 2006 from http://apt.rcpsych.org/cgi/content/full/8/1/17

Republic of Rwanda. (2003). *Constitution of the Republic of Rwanda*. Kigali, Rwanda: Official Gazette of the Republic of Rwanda.

Rule, S., Lorenzo, T., & Wolmarans, M. (2006). Community-based rehabilitation: New challenges. In B. Watermeyer, L. Swartz, T. Lorenzo, M. Schneider, & M. Priestley. M. (Eds.), *Disability and social change: A South African agenda* (pp. 273–90). Cape Town: HSRC Press.

Serpell, R., Mariga, L., & Harvey, K. (1993). Mental retardation in African countries: Conceptualization, services and research. *International Review of Research in Mental Retardation*, *19*, 1–34.

South African Government Communication and Information System. (2005). *Pocket guide to social development*. Retrieved June 30, 2006 from http://www.gcis.gov.za/docs/publications/pocketguide/social05.pdf

Speedy, J. (2000). The 'storied' helper. *European Journal of Psychotherapy Counselling and Health*, *3*(3), 361–74.

Thomas, P. (2005). Mainstreaming disability in development: Country-level research:Rwanda country report. Report for the DFID (UK's Department for International Development) Disability Knowledge and Research (KaR) Programme. Retrieved December 13, 2006 from http://www.disabilitykar.net/pdfs/rwanda.pdf

Turner, V. (1980). Social dramas and stories about them. *Critical Inquiry*, *7*(4), 141–68.

UNESCO. (1994). *The Salamanca Statement and Framework for Action on Special Needs Education*. Paris: Author.

United Nations. (2006). Convention on the rights of persons with disabilities. Retrieved February 9, 2008 from http://www.un.org/esa/socdev/enable/plenaryofga06.htm

Whyte, W. F. (Ed.) (1991). *Participatory action research*. London: SAGE Publications.

Whyte, S. R., & Ingstad, B. (1995). Disability and culture: An overview. In B. Ingstad & S. R. Whyte (Eds.), *Disability and culture* (pp. 3–32). Berkeley: University of California Press.

Wilson, K. B., Edwards, D. W., Alston, R. J., Harley, D.A., & Doughty, J. D. (2001). Vocational rehabilitation and the dilemma of race in rural communities: Sociopolitical realities and myths from the past. *Journal of Rural Community Psychology*, *E-4*(1), 55–81.

Winslade, J., & Monk, G. (1999). *Narrative counseling in schools: Powerful and brief*. Thousand Oaks, CA: Corwin Press.

Wolfensberger, W. (1991). *A brief introduction to Social Role Valorization as a high-order concept for structuring human services*. Syracuse, NY: Training Institute for Human Service Planning, Leadership and Change Agency: Syracuse University

Wolfensberger, W. (1999). Concluding reflections and a look ahead into the future for Normalization and Social Role Valorization. In R. J. Flynn & R. Lemay (Eds.), *A quarter-century of Normalization and Social Role Valorization: Evolution and impact* (pp. 489–504). Ottawa: University of Ottawa Press.

World Health Organization (WHO). (1980). International classification of impairments, disabilities and handicaps: A manual of classification relating to the consequences of disease. Geneva: Author.

World Health Organization (WHO). (2001). *International Classification of Functioning, Disability and Health*. Geneva: Author.

Wright, B. A. (1991). Labelling: The need for person-environment individuation. In C. R. Snyder & D. R. Forsyth (Eds.). *Handbook of social and clinical psychology: The health perspective* (pp. 469–87). Elmsford, NY: Pergamon.

SELF-CHECK EXERCISES

1. Distinguish among impairment, disability, and participation. How are they related?
2. How is knowledge of the difference between impairment and disability and participation useful to counselors of people with disabilities?
3. Explain the likely higher prevalence of disability in developing African countries.
4. What, if any, is the relationship between disability and illness?
5. Identify four types of disability-related needs for which counseling may be necessary. What are the roles of (a) personal, (b) disability-related, and (c) environmental factors in the experience of disability? Discuss with reference to selected characteristics.
6. Show how personal, disability, and environmental characteristics may interact in their impact on the experience of disability. Discuss with reference to a case example you created.
7. What counseling goals would you have for Merjury? How would you go about meeting them? What resources (e.g., material, human, other) would be useful in counseling Merjury? How are the needs related to each other?

FIELD-BASED EXPERIENTIAL EXERCISES

1. Interview several people in your community on how they identify a person to have a disability. How do the identification criteria used by people in your community compare with those used by the WHO?
2. Interview a person with a disability and determine (a) the experiences that place him or her in minority status, (b) the person's awareness of being a minority, and (c) the personal minority statuses he or she recognizes. Explain your findings.
3. Interview a person with a disability to determine the needs they perceive to require counseling. On the basis of your interview, determine the extent to which the person has disability consciousness. To what extent would the construct of disability consciousness apply to your community?
4. Interview an individual with a disability on his or her experience with disability-related societal discrimination. Evaluate the extent to which the individual's reaction was rational or appropriate to the circumstances. What would be your counseling goals with the individual?

MULTIPLE-CHOICE QUESTIONS

1. According to the ICF, disability refers to:
   a. Impairments and participation restrictions from a physical or mental condition in context of environmental factors
   b. Mental condition in the context of environmental factors
   c. Impairments, activity limitations, and participation restrictions from a physical or mental condition in the context of environmental factors
   d. Activity limitations
   e. None of the above
2. Disability is about:
   a. The individual, societal, and body-related aspects of impairments, activity limitations, and body-related aspects of impairment, activity limitations, and participation restrictions in the sociocultural environment
   b. Activity limitations
   c. Participation restrictions in the sociocultural environment
   d. Stigma and ostracism
   e. All of the above
3. People with disabilities may seek counseling to address needs in the following interdependent areas:
   a. Social
   b. Physical
   c. Personal
   d. Resource
   e. All of the above
4. Which of the following is true of disability prevalence data in sub-Saharan Africa?
   a. There is low disability prevalence in many countries in sub-Saharan Africa.
   b. The ways in which national governments in sub-Saharan Africa collect disability prevalence data may leave many people with disabilities unidentified.
   c. Persons with disability always self-identify, hence increased prevalence data.
   d. Persons with disability are known in many sub-Saharan Africa areas.
   e. None of the above.
5. Which of the following is true about having a disability in some African cultures?
   a. Disability is considered a punishment for a social transgression by the individual or family of origin.
   b. Disability is a culturally accepted condition.
   c. Disability is not inability.
   d. Disability is not stigmatized.
   e. All of the above.
6. Fill in the blanks. For the sustainability of a CBR program in Africa ___________ and ___________ are crucial
   a. community involvement and funding
   b. government and nongovernmental organizations

c. community involvement and health care clinic
d. community and psychoeducational programs
e. community training and education

7. Culturally speaking, certain disabilities are socially stigmatized more than others. Which of these disabilities would be the least stigmatized?
a. Female with a disability
b. Male with a disability
c. Person with a disability
d. Family members (immediate and extended) of a person with a disability
e. Person who presents with chronic fatigue syndrome

8. Which of the following components does not belong to the ICF classification?
a. Body function and structure
b. Resources
c. Participation
d. Environmental factors
e. Activities

9. People with disabilities may seek counseling to address:
a. Social, physical, personal, and resource needs
b. Physical and personal needs
c. Social, physical, personal, and family needs
d. Social, physical, psychological, and mental needs

Answers to the multiple-choice questions are provided at the back of the book

PART 4
THE FUTURE OF COUNSELING IN AFRICAN HERITAGE SETTINGS

20 Counseling in African Cultural Heritage Settings: The Challenges and Opportunities

Elias Mpofu, Terri Bakker, and Lisa Lopez Levers

OVERVIEW. This chapter integrates and synthesizes many elements of the interdisciplinary discourse, regarding counseling people of African ancestry, that have been offered in the previous chapters. In considering the challenges and opportunities inherent in counseling people of African ancestry, the authors discuss how world view can influence help-seeking predispositions; they detail the necessity of ecoculturally relevant psychological assessments; they emphasize how historical legacies can influence health and well-being; they point to the influences of Western psychology and postcolonial oppression; and, finally, they propose the relevance of community-level counseling interventions with people of African ancestry. The chapter concludes by endorsing the importance of culturally diverse and culturally relevant counseling interventions when working with people of African ancestry.

LEARNING OBJECTIVES

By the end of the chapter, the reader should be able to:

1. Critically discuss the notion of people of African ancestry in terms of identity and diversity.
2. Discuss the impact of world view on African health and help-seeking behavior.
3. Discuss the role of ecoculturally relevant assessment and research in improving counseling in African settings.
4. Explain how historical legacies have an impact on mental health and service utilization in African communities.
5. Critically discuss the tension between Western versus Africentric psychology and ways of resolving this tension in counseling practices.
6. Explain the concept of postcolonial oppression and show how this has an impact on health and well-being in African communities.
7. Explain the relevance of community-based interventions and empowerment to health and well-being in African settings.

INTRODUCTION

The notion of people of African ancestry raises questions in others about the identities of those subsumed under this rubric, owing to the diversity in the cultural heritages of those who claim such an identity (Mpofu, 2005). Claims to a Western culture or Asian culture are similarly based on the presumption of the existence of generic values that mark those heritages to be different from others, even though they may have considerable diversity within those cultures. Within African cultural heritage settings, there is considerable diversity in cultural aspects salient to subgroups within the same generic cultural mix for which creative or innovative approaches to counseling service provision would be necessary. However, it is the opinion of the authors that there are identifiable political, social, and psychological factors that differentiate communities of African ancestry from other communities and that require the use of culturally responsive therapeutic modalities.

Discussions that seek to address needs in such broadly constructed groupings are constrained in their generalization to sociocultural strata within the generic groupings. Nonetheless, the diversity of self-identities also speaks to the richness of cultural resources that could be applied to address the needs of those who subscribe to specific identities. Like in many other cultural settings in which there are needs that counseling services would meet, such needs span the full range of the life space: physical health, mental health, emotional concerns, lifestyle, community living, and spiritual dimensions. The chapters in this book attest to a dire necessity for appropriate services to address these needs, as well as to the richness of cultural and other resources available to those sensitive to the specific African contexts involved.

WORLD VIEW INFLUENCES HELP-SEEKING PREDISPOSITIONS

Aspects of African cosmology are important to understanding health and well-being in African heritage culture communities. For instance, African traditional healers are believed by many to be credible helpers in their multiple ontological personhoods: doctor, healer, counselor, advisor, cultural broker, and conduit to the ancestors and the spiritual realm. Cosmology is the branch of metaphysics that studies the nature and origin of the universe. Ontology is the branch of metaphysics that studies the nature of being and existence. About 80 percent of

Africans seek health care services – and by extension, mental health care services – from traditional healers.

A major premise of this book is that cultural relevance may determine (1) the utilization of counseling services, (2) their perceived service accessibility, and (3) outcome efficacy. The world view that traditional healers share with their clients is important for professional counselors to understand. Professional counselors interact with clients who elect to receive treatment from traditional healers, either sequentially or concurrently with modern counseling services. An understanding by professional counselors of the role that traditional healers play in mediating health services for the majority of clients can increase their perceived credibility and effectiveness with clients (Mpofu, 2003). The setting up of transparent referral systems to network traditional healing services that clients elect to use would benefit many clients who often use both modern and traditional health services with little professional oversight. The lack of professional oversight potentially could harm the clients who may receive contradictory treatment regimens from well-meaning health care providers in the nonformal and formal health care service sectors (Mpofu, 2006).

ECOCULTURALY RELEVANT ASSESSMENTS AND RESEARCH ARE NECESSARY

Effective counseling interventions are based on evidence from appropriate assessment. A majority of assessment instruments and procedures used in African cultural heritage settings have been developed predominantly within a Western-based environment, largely reflecting Euro-American values and notions of health and well-being. It would be important for providers of counseling services in Africanist settings to consider the crosscultural applicability of assessment instruments and procedures they use in intervention planning. Instruments designed for use with predominantly Western Caucasian populations may be inappropriate for use with people of African ancestry. However, the relevance of specific assessment methods is a complex issue. Some Western instruments may be readily adapted for use, while others may remain inappropriate. This complexity reflects the tension between Western and Africentric approaches to psychology, as discussed later in this chapter.

The research that informs counseling interventions with people of African ancestry is another important area for consideration in the design and use of counseling interventions with people of African ancestry. Specifically, an Africanist world view and indigenous knowledge are essential to (1) asking culturally relevant research questions that lead to the answers that can inform best counseling practices in Africanist settings, and (2) understanding the patterns of client demographics and counseling service utilization that are important for the appropriate targeting of such services. In this volume, the contributing authors document the relevance of indigenous culture to contemporary counseling practices, identifying the major strategies used in African settings, the research associated with each, and the gaps in the research literature. The authors also discuss the need for culturally relevant research endeavors that can lead to more Africentric approaches to counseling interventions.

HISTORICAL LEGACIES INFLUENCE HEALTH AND WELL-BEING

Culture cannot be divorced from history and socioeconomic issues. In African contexts, cultural practices are interwoven with historical, political, and socioeconomic realities. Many of the issues faced by people of African descent are those that are faced by disadvantaged people all over the world and that may be similar to issues faced in many developing countries. For example, many people may consult traditional or religious healers, not only because of cultural beliefs, but simply because these may be the only service providers to whom they have easy access. Access to health care services may be limited for people who live in undeveloped parts of a country, as well as for those subjected to political oppression, a lack of educational opportunities, and so forth. These all play into their use and knowledge of counseling and healing practices. In addition, African communities are increasingly and unevenly transformed through processes of globalization. Traditional family and community values may remain strong among some people, while others may reject traditional values in favor of new forms of relationship, family structures, and ways of defining personal identities. This occurrence may be especially the case for those who may view themselves as disadvantaged within traditional values systems, such as women and gays. Again, current liberatory values may enter into and confound historical influences, depending on the specific circumstances of a person or community.

INFLUENCES OF WESTERN PSYCHOLOGY

The hegemonic influences of Western psychological theories and methods may have adversely influenced counseling theory and practice in African settings, and research informing transformations that better account for culture in service provision is needed (see also Chapter 6, this volume). Hegemony refers to the leadership or dominance of one nation or social group over another. Nonetheless, pursuing a purely indigenous psychology, through the uncritical exclusion of Western psychology, could result in an unwanted shift to insularity and cultural specificity (Mpofu, 2002, 2006). Africentric cultural heritages are part of the global network of cultures, and they exchange cultural elements with other cultures. However, these cultural exchanges may be one-sided and unequal for some sectors of African cultural heritage communities, especially for those with a history of political and economic exploitation by competing cultures. For example, Western (neo)colonial influences may lead to the undervaluing of enabling values in Africanist communities. The scars of racism and colonization on the mental health of people of African ancestry may have intergenerational influences. Counseling practices based on liberation psychology could be useful when addressing the effects of oppression in a restorative manner. For instance, professional counselors would be more effective in their interventions if they were to integrate culture-specific theories and interventions into contemporary Western approaches; reconfigure traditional models; and implement novel, culturally sensitive strategies in assisting clients.

POSTCOLONIAL OPPRESSION

Many African communities have had to contend with ongoing oppression by postcolonial ruling oligarchies that have no regard for human rights and the rule of law. *Oppression* refers to various forms of discriminatory practices that entail some form of abuse of power and internalization of a sense of powerlessness (see also Chapters 5 and 6, this volume). An oligarchy is a political system or form of government in which only a few have power. Significant compromises to the health and well-being of the citizens of many postcolonial African nations have resulted from political oppression and abuse of the citizenry by self-serving leader-dictators; this has transpired in ways that rival and surpass the evils of colonialism. Counselors, in some postcolonial communities ruled by dictatorial regimes, could be involved in trauma counseling, perhaps even more than other counseling services.

Some conflicts on the African continent emanated from ethnolinguistic divisions that were associated with the colonial period and subsequently fanned by ruling tribal cabals. Consequently, diversity training and management becomes a central aspect of citizenship counseling. There also may be a need for citizenship counseling, as citizens under despotic postcolonial regimes may not be aware of their rights under international human rights conventions or national constitutions and laws. Citizenship counseling could play a central role in creating tolerance in diverse societies, as well as in embracing other democratic values necessary to sustainable health and well-being.

COMMUNITY-LEVEL INTERVENTIONS ARE RELEVANT

Community-level interventions are likely to reach more persons with counseling needs in African context settings, especially given the cultural importance of community action in many Africanist settings. Community counseling is dedicated to critically analyzing the situation of oppression and developing strategies that contribute to liberation from constraints on thought, action, and space. Many communities of interest exist in African cultural heritage settings, and the alignment of services needs to be tailored to the specific needs of these communities; this is particularly important for their health and well-being. For example, Africa now hosts many refugee communities, perhaps more than any other continent in the world (see also Chapter 11, this volume). It also hosts the largest number of children who have been orphaned by the HIV and AIDS pandemic and perennial civil wars. Emergent communities from these sociopolitical upheavals have unique needs that are best served with well targeted counseling interventions.

Empowerment is a central goal in community counseling and refers to one's development of a sense of collective efficacy or control over the institutions that affect one's life (Rappaport & Seidman, 2000). Citizenship counseling, as previously discussed, allows for self-determination and collective well-being through social participation (Wandersman & Florin, 2000).

SUMMARY AND CONCLUSION

This book demonstrates that people of African descent exist in spaces of cultural fluidity and heterogeneity where culture interfaces with class, economic factors, political realities, and global issues. This aspect carries over into the counseling situation where there is a tension among African cosmologies, Western counseling practices, and the challenges posed by contemporary realities that people face in complex, real-life situations. The task of counselors and mental health workers in the African context appears to be to implement novel, culturally sensitive strategies in assisting people. Counselors working in this context must learn to draw innovatively from a diversity of approaches and world views to forge a new kind of holistic, systemic counseling that would be appropriate to their clients.

The authors contributing to this volume are from diverse geographical and discursive landscapes. However, they have in common personal experience, knowledge, and a familiarity with local African contexts that they bring to their respective chapters. There is a sense of discovery, dedication, and newness embedded in the chapters comprising this volume. It is hoped that such a sense of discovery, dedication, and openness to innovation will be taken further into the future by readers of this book.

REFERENCES

Mpofu, E. (2002). Psychology in Africa: Challenges and prospects. *International Journal of Psychology*, *37*, 179–86.

Mpofu, E. (2003). Conduct disorder: Presentation, treatment options and cultural efficacy in an African setting. *International Journal of Disability, Community and Rehabilitation*, *2*(1), http://www.ijdcr.ca/VOL02_01_CAN/articles/mpofu.shtml.

Mpofu, E. (2005). Selective interventions in counseling African-Americans with disabilities. In D. A. Harley & J. M. Dillard (Eds.), *Contemporary mental health issues among African Americans* (pp. 235–54). Alexandria, VA: American Counseling Association.

Mpofu, E. (2006). Majority world health care traditions intersect indigenous and complementary and alternative medicine

(Editorial for Special Issue on Indigenous Healing Practices). *International Journal of Disability, Development and Education, 53*, 375–9.

Rappaport, J., & Seidman, E. (2000). *Handbook of community psychology*. New York: Kluwer Academic/Plenum Press.

Wandersman, A., & Florin, P. (2000). Citizen participation and community organizations. In J. Rappaport & E. Seidman (Eds.), *Handbook of community psychology* (pp. 43–64). New York: Kluwer Academic/Plenum Press.

SELF-CHECK EXERCISES

1. Discuss the notion of people of African ancestry in terms of identity and diversity.
2. How may world view influence help-seeking behavior in people of an African cultural heritage?
3. Explain the role of ecoculturally relevant assessment and research in improving counseling in African settings.
4. Describe some historical legacies that have an impact on mental health and service utilization in African communities.
5. Explain the concept of postcolonial oppression and show how this has an impact on health and well-being in African communities.
6. What is the relevance of community-based interventions and empowerment to health and well-being in African settings?
7. Write your own summary of what you have learned from this book. Formulate a brief outline of what you would consider an appropriate approach to counseling people of African descent.
8. Make two lists, one of the challenges and the other of the opportunities associated with providing counseling services to people of African ancestry. Identify ways that a counselor, working with a systemic mind set, might advocate for changing some of the challenges into opportunities. Identify ways that some of the opportunities can be informed by greater cultural awareness.

FIELD-BASED EXPERIENTIAL EXERCISES

1. Collect articles from local newspapers that illustrate inequities in health care and social service provision to people of African ancestry. Try to trace the origin of each particular inequity to some of the contextual issues identified in this and other chapters in this book.
2. Interview a willing elder from a traditional community of African ancestry, asking about health care experiences in his or her life. Record the interview, if the person is willing, or take detailed notes. Later, transcribe the interview or reconstruct it from your notes. Try to identify historical and contextual issues that have had an impact on the ability of this person to access health care.

MULTIPLE-CHOICE QUESTIONS

1. The presumption of generic values applies to:
   a. Cosmology
   b. Ontology
   c. Philology
   d. Linguistics
   e. Culture
2. People of African ancestry use:
   a. Biomedical services exclusively
   b. Traditional health services exclusively
   c. Both modern and traditional health services
   d. Modern mental health services exclusively
   e. Pharmacies exclusively
3. A majority of assessment instruments and procedures used in African cultural heritage settings have been developed predominantly:
   a. By psychologists
   b. By psychometritians
   c. By psychiatrists
   d. Within a Western-based environment, largely reflecting Euro-American values and notions of health and well-being
   e. All of the above
4. In terms of relevant community-level interventions, one central goal in community counseling is:
   a. Empathy in the individual counseling relationship
   b. Ethnography
   c. Empowerment
   d. Hegemony
   e. None of the above
5. Among the persistent challenges for many postcolonial African societies that result in significant lack of well-being in the general population include:
   a. Poverty
   b. Cultural awareness
   c. Civil strife
   d. Human rights abuses
   e. a, c, and d

Answers to the multiple-choice questions are provided at the back of the book

Counseling People of African Ancestry Multiple Choice Answers

Chapter 1. Indigenous Healing Practices in sub-Saharan Africa

1. c
2. e
3. a
4. d
5. c
6. d

Chapter 2. The Role of the Oral Tradition in Counseling People of African Ancestry

1. a
2. d
3. b
4. d
5. c

Chapter 3. Assessment for Counseling Intervention

1. a
2. c
3. b
4. b
5. b

Chapter 4. Research on Counseling in African Settings

1. a
2. a
3. a
4. a
5. d
6. c
7. b
8. d
9. a
10. b

Chapter 5. Deconstructing Counseling Psychology for the African Context

1. e
2. c
3. d
4. d
5. e
6. d
7. e
8. a
9. a
10. c

Chapter 6. Racial Oppression, Colonization and Identity: Toward an Empowerment Model for People of African Heritage

1. b
2. a
3. b
4. e
5. d
6. a
7. b
8. e
9. e

Chapter 7. School Counseling

1. b
2. b
3. c
4. c
5. e
6. a
7. b
8. c

Chapter 8. Counseling Students at Tertiary Institutions

1. a
2. e
3. c
4. c
5. e
6. b
7. c
8. d
9. c
10. c

Chapter 9. Family Therapy within the African Context
1. b
2. c
3. c
4. a
5. c
6. a
7. a

Chapter 10. Pastoral Care and Counseling
1. d
2. c
3. d
4. a
5. c
6. d
7. d
8. e
9. d
10. d

Chapter 11. African Refugees: Challenges and Prospects of Resettlement Programs
1. c
2. d
3. b
4. d
5. a

Chapter 12. Counseling Orphans and Vulnerable Children in Africa
1. a
2. b
3. d
4. d
5. d
6. c
7. d
8. a
9. d
10. a
11. d

Chapter 13. Diversity Counseling with African Americans
1. b
2. c
3. c
4. a
5. d

Chapter 14. Resolving Conflict in Africa: In Search of Sustainable Peace
1. c
2. a
3. c
4. c
5. d
6. b
7. b

Chapter 15. Counseling for Trauma
1. b
2. c
3. a
4. b
5. a
6. b
7. c
8. a
9. d
10. a

Chapter 16. HIV and AIDS Counseling
1. d
2. c
3. a
4. b
5. a

Chapter 17. Substance Use Disorder Counseling
1. d
2. e
3. d
4. b
5. b
6. c
7. e
8. b
9. c
10. d

Chapter 18. Career Counseling People of African Ancestry
1. b
2. c
3. b
4. d
5. b

Chapter 19. Counseling People with Disabilities
1. c
2. a
3. e
4. b
5. a
6. a
7. e
8. b
9. a

Chapter 20. Counseling in African Cultural Heritage Settings. The Challenges and Opportunities
1. e
2. c
3. d
4. c
5. e

Index

Note: Italicized letters after page numbers are used in this index to indicate the following: *ce* = case example; *cs* = case study; *db* = discussion box; *f* = figure; *ib* = information box; *rb* = research box; and *t* = table.

AACHRD (African Advisory Committee for Health Research and Development), 7
Abdi, Y. O., 28–29
Abduli-Adil, J., 100
Abong, J. T., 65
abortion, 185*db*
ACA (American Counseling Association), 52*db*
academic pressure, 131
ACE (Adverse Childhood Experiences) study, 234
Ackerman, Nathan, 142, 147
Ackermann, E., 160
"acts of God," 22
Acute Stress Reaction (ASR), 229. *See also* trauma; trauma counseling
Adair, J. G., 86, 88
Adams, G. A., 233–234
addiction recovery, 275. *See also* substance use disorder counseling
Adverse Childhood Experiences (ACE) study, 234
adversity/suffering, 22
AfCA (African Counseling Association), 205
African Advisory Committee for Health Research and Development (AACHRD), 7
African Americans. *See also* diversity counseling
  career counseling of, 286–288
  cultural phenomena and, 201
  demographic shifts, 201–203
  errors in research studies on, 196
  ethnic identity of, 105*rb*
  health and wellbeing of, 193–194
African counseling community, 204*t*
African cultural heritage settings
  ancestry/identity, 313
  assessment/research methods, 314
  community-level interventions, 315
  empowerment, 315
  help-seeking predispositions, 313–314
  historical legacies and, 314
  post-colonial oppression and, 315
  Western psychology, influences of, 314–315
Africanist churches, 150. *See also* Black church
African migration, historical aspects of, 94–95
"African personality," 76, 78*f*
African psychology, 42–43. *See also* assessment procedures
African refugees
  career aspirations of, 287*rb*
  cultural/diversity issues, 173–176
  definitions of, 166
  economic participation of, 171
  history of, 167
  hosting agencies, 170
  hosting/exporting countries, 167–168
  hosting policies/practices, 170–171
  initiatives on, 167–169
  legal issues, 175–176
  local attitudes toward, 171
  push/pull migration factors, 169
  refugee camp locations, 170
  research, issues for, 176
  status phasing, 172*db*
  UNHCR, role of, 170, 177
  women and children, 171, 176*rb*
African spirituality, 156*db*, 160
African worldview, 155
age, vulnerability and, 234–235. *See also* trauma; trauma counseling
Aggleton, P., 253
Aguilar-Kitibuti, A., 52
AIDS. *See* HIV/AIDS
AIDS and Society Research Unit (ASRU), 65–66
AIDS stigma reduction, 257*rb*
Akeroyd, A. V., 253
Alarcon, R. D, 145
alcohol. *See* Global Alcohol Database (GAD)
alcoholism, 101–102. *See also* substance use disorders
Allen, K., 215*db*
Allwood, C. M., 75, 79
alternative/complementary approaches, 83
Alternative Models of Care program, 184
amabali, 27
American Association for Marriage and Family Therapy, 150
American Counseling Association (ACA), 52*db*
American Psychological Association (APA), 52*db*
American School Counselor Association (ASCA), 52*db*
Ames, D., 79
ancestors, role of, 160
ancestral spirits, counter claims of, 6*cs*
Ancis, J. R., 143, 145

Anderson, Harlene, 148
Andiman, W., 258
anecdotes, use of, 30
anger issues, 202*db*
Ani, C., 183
animal sacrifice. *See* sacrificial rites
Ankrah, E. M., 255
ANPP (Association of Niger Psychologists and Psychiatrists), 53
Anstey, M., 210
antiretroviral therapy (ART), 256*rb*. *See also* HIV/AIDS counseling research
APA (American Psychological Association), 52*db*
archetypes/archetypal motifs, 23, 33–34
aroma therapy, 12
Arthur, N., 289
ASCA (American School Counselor Association), 52*db*
ASR (Acute Stress Reaction), 229. *See also* trauma; trauma counseling
ASRU (AIDS and Society Research Unit), 65–66
assessment procedures/criteria. *See also* consultation practices; indigenous counseling practices
  anecdotes, use of, 30
  assessor competency, 51–52
  Black psychology, influence of, 42–43
  conceptualization/classification of illness, 45–46
  content, appropriateness of, 46–47
  cross-cultural dilemma, 43*db*
  culturally specific tests/techniques, 42, 50–51
  deviant behavior, 45
  ethical considerations, 53
  history of, 41–42
  legislative implications, 52–53
  linguistic equivalence, 46
  measurement, types of, 47
  multicultural approaches/trends, 43, 44
  recent developments in, 42
  RESPECTFUL model, 47
  self-knowledge and, 44–45
  symptoms, meaning of, 45
  test design/development, 46*rb*, 47, 53–54
  in Traditional Healing paradigm, 47–48
  western/indigenous approach interface, 48, 53
assessor competency, 51–52
assistive devices, 297*ce*
Association for the Promotion of Traditional Medicine (Senegal), 7–8
Association of Niger Psychologists and Psychiatrists (ANPP), 53
asylum countries, 167–168. *See also* African refugees
asylum seekers, 36*rb*. *See also* African refugees
Atkinson, D. R., 32
attire, use of, 9
Atwine, B., 183
Augsburger, D. W., 161
autobiographical memory, 241
AVERT, 253
avoidance symptoms, 230–231. *See also* trauma; trauma counseling

Baaz, M., 211
Babbie, E., 79
Baeten, J. M., 254–255
Bajunirwe, F., 183
balance, notion of, 162
Barnhardt, R., 59*db*
Bate, S. C., 160
Bateson, Gregory, 142, 147
Baumann, L. J., 188
Becvar, D. S., 150
Becvar, R. J., 150
behavioral therapy, 147. *See also* family therapy
behavior problems, approaches to, 29*db*
Bekker, S., 44
Bell, E., 126–127
Bellagamba, A., 160
Ben-Amos, D., 27
bereavement counseling, 188*cs*
Berry, J. W., 75, 79
Bettelheim, B., 24
Bhusumane, D-B., 62–63, 65
Biblical counseling, 157. *See also* pastoral care
bicultural competencies, 202*rb*
Biddlecom, A. E., 253
Biesheuvel, S., 29
Biko, Steve, 93
biological variation, 201
Bishop, B. J., 85
Black church, 200. *See also* Africanist churches
Black family pathology, myth of, 95*db*
Blackness. *See* "neurosis of Blackness"
Black psychology, 42–43. *See also* assessment procedures
Black Skin/White Masks (Fanon), 99
Bleek, Wilhelm, 26
Bloomfield, D., 214
Bodibe, R. C., 32
bodily movement therapies, 9
body language, 200–201
Bokhorst, F., 126–127
Bor, R., 255
Bosch, D. J., 160
Boscolo, Luigi, 147
boswagadi, 66
Botswana
  disability policies in, 303
  psycho-educational intervention in, 66*rb*
  school counseling in, 114
Bowen, M., 142
Bowman, B., 81–82
Boyd-Franklin, N., 143
Brockerhoff, M., 253
Buhrmann, M. W., 29
Bujo, B., 160–161
Bulhan, H. A., 76, 148–149
Burkard, A. W., 203
Burr, V., 76
Burton, John, 222
Burton, L. M., 145–146
Burton's Human Needs Theory, 211–213. *See also* conflict/conflicts
Burundian conflict, 215–217. *See also* conflict/conflicts

CACREP (Council for Accreditation of Counseling Related Educational Programs), 52*db*
Cameroon, disability legislation in, 304
Campbell, C., 253, 254, 255*db*
Canadian Council for Refugees, 169*db*. *See also* African refugees
Cantor-Graae, E., 183
Care Counsellors of Malawi, 149
career choices, 113*db*, 136. *See also* school counseling
career counseling
  of African Americans, 286–288
  of African refugees, 286–287
  and career choice, 136
  contextual influences/approaches, 84*rb*, 282
  current issues in, 288–289
  Holland's Hexagon Model, 286*rb*
  importance of, 82

interest inventories, 288*db*
narrative approaches, 290
revising/redefining process of, 281–282
social justice perspective, 289–290
ubuntu in, 283–285, 290
Carney, C. G., 27–28
CATT (Children's Accelerated Trauma Treatment), 242
CBR (community-based rehabilitation services), 296*db*, 300–301, 306. *See also* disability counseling research/research needs
Cecchin, Gianfranco, 147
Celum, C., 254–255
Center for Disease Control, 251*ib*
Chaava, T., 81
Chagonda, T., 135
Chatelain, Clara de, 26
Chavunduka, G. L., 5
Cheatham, H. E., 204
Chen, C. P., 30–31, 33
Chigunta, F., 77
child, definition of, 180–181
child abuse counseling intervention, 124*cs*
Child Line, 64
child molestation, 174*cs*
child-rearing patterns, 96
children. *See also* African refugees; orphans; other vulnerable children (OVC)
HIV/AIDS and, 251
rights and protections needs of, 174*rb*
Children living in a world with AIDS, 182
Children on the Brink Report, 180, 181, 182
Children's Accelerated Trauma Treatment (CATT), 242
child soldiers, 183, 215*db*
Chinweizu, 99
Chipandambira, K. S., 133*rb*
Choudree, R., 218
Christian missionaries, 113–114
Christian traditions, 156. *See also* pastoral care
Christie, G., 32
church. *See* Africanist churches; Black church
Church, A. T., 85
citizenship counseling, 315
civil wars. *See* conflict/conflicts
Clacherty & Associates, 256
Clark, M., 210
cleansing measures, 12
Clinebell, H. J., 157
Cluver, L., 183
Coates, T. J., 254–255, 256
Code of Ethics (American Association for Marriage and Family Therapy), 150
Coercive Theory, 169–170. *See also* African refugees
Coetzee, M., 64
cognitive therapy, 147. *See also* family therapy
coherence. *See* sense of coherence (SOC)
Coleman, R., 84, 195, 197
collaborative language systems approach, 148
collective grief, 101
collectivism/collectivist cultures, 96–97, 199
colonization/colonialism
decolonization of the mind, 100–101
family structures and, 96
higher education in, 127
historical aspects of, 94–95
mental colonization, 99–100
psychological imperialism, 98
racial oppression and, 96–97
racist thinking in, 97
school counseling under, 113–114
Commission for Research Partnerships with Developing Countries (KFPE), 67*db*
communality, wellbeing and, 162
communication styles, 200–201
communication theories, 147. *See also* family therapy
community, role of, 160
community-based interventions, 258
community-based rehabilitation (CBR) services, 296*db*, 300–301, 306. *See also* disability counseling research/research needs
conceptual incarceration, 99
condom use, 255*db*
conflict/conflicts
Burundian conflict, 215–217
cost of, 209
in Darfur, 222
epistemological aspects, 212–213
identity politics in, 214–215
life cycle of, 210
as "new wars," 214
number of, 209
perceptions of, 209–210
political leadership, 217
psychology of, 213–214
in Rwanda, 216*db*
theoretical issues in genesis of, 213*t*
theories/approaches to understanding, 210–213
typologies of, 210
unique nature of, 209
conflict resolution
African vs. Western approaches to, 218–219
considerations/predictions in, 211–212
legal issues, 222
peace agreements, 214
positive/negative peace, 217–218
psychological factors in, 221–223
religion and, 220*rb*
research, issues for, 222
restorative justice, 218
in schools, 119*rb*
socio-psychological approaches, 219–220, 221
conflict theorists, 211
Congo. *See* Democratic Republic of the Congo (DRC)
CONNECT, 143
construct bias, 45*ib*
consultation, reasons for, 4–5
consultation practices. *See also* assessment procedures/criteria
continuous out-patient consultation, 14–15
episodic out-patient setting, 14
family/community consensus, 13
healer-patient dynamics, 13
in-patient setting, 15
overview of, 16
Contemporized-Themes Concerning Blacks Test (C-TCB), 50–51
content, appropriateness of, 46–47
contextualist model/theory, 42, 79–80
Convention on the Rights of the Child (CRC), 182
Coser, L., 210
Council for Accreditation of Counseling Related Educational Programs (CACREP), 52*db*
counseling
defined, 58
group work, 31–32
indigenous models for, 63*rb*
language/cultural differences in, 32–33
racial/ethnic differences in, 203*rb*
reasons for, 60
world view, consideration of, 32

counseling psychology. *See also* indigenous counseling practices
  in African contexts, 75–76
  "African personality," 76
  career counseling, 82, 84*rb*
  contextualist perspective, 79–80
  culture, notion of, 76
  emic vs. etic research strategies, 79
  "Family," notion of, 77
  historical context, 80
  HIV/AIDS challenge, 81
  modernization, effects of, 81
  participator methods, 84
  poverty/under-development, 82
  racism and, 81–82
  research methods/approaches, 79–80, 86–88
  role of, 88
  self, conceptualization of, 76
  universalism vs. particularism, 77–79
  "youth," conceptions of, 77
counseling-related research
  African indigenous healing, 58–59
  counseling services, role of, 60
  current trends in, 65–66
  disaster mental health responses, 60–61
  funding bodies and, 59–60
  health counseling, 62
  HIV/AIDS counseling, 61–62
  key concepts, 57–58, 69–70
  mental health outcomes, 61
  on orphans/OVCs, 64
  psycho-educational practices, 65–66
  reasons for counseling, 60
  rehabilitation counseling, 64–65
  trauma counseling, 62–64
  Western approaches, transportability of, 59
counseling strategies/techniques, in diverse settings, 33
counselor education programs, 52*db*
counselor training, 137–138
Coury, D., 181
crisis-intervention hot line, 64
cross-cultural counseling, 32–33, 43*db*, 45*ib*
Crossley, M., 67
C-TCB (Contemporized-Themes Concerning Blacks Test), 50–51
cultural diversity, definition of, 194–195
cultural factors
  for African refugees, 173
  in family therapy, 145–146
cultural integration/differences, 173–174, 175. *See also* African refugees
culturally intentional counselor, 42*ib*
culturally relevant assessments, 51*rb*
culturally specific tests, 50–51
cultural mistrust, 193, 195
culture, notion of, 76
culture-specific treatments, 199–204
Cunha, M., 253
cybernetics, 146–147

Dana, R. H., 52
dancing, 31
Dandala, H. M., 282
D'Andrea, M., 47
Daniels, J., 47
Darfur conflict, 222. *See also* conflict/conflicts
Darling, C. A., 144
Dasen, P. R., 26
Davies, P., 253
Deacon, H., 186
De Beer, J. P., 126–127
debriefing, 239
debt, third-world, 94
decolonization, of the mind, 100–101
De la Rey, C., 88
deliverance, 162
Democratic Republic of the Congo (DRC), 215*db*
democratization, emergence of, 171
Denby, R. W., 199
dependence, psychological, 268. *See also* substance use disorders
depression, 182–183, 231*cs*
developmental approach, to counseling, 131, 187–188
deviant behavior, location of, 45
Dhlomo, R. M., 282–283
diagnostic process, divination in, 5–7
Diaz-Vivar, N., 52
Diemer, M. A., 202
disability
  assistive devices, 297*ce*
  care in traditionalist settings, 297*ce*
  communal affiliation effects and, 299
  counseling services sought for, 298–299
  definition of, 295
  environmental characteristics and, 296*ce*
  functioning and, 295
  vs. illness, 295–296
  marketing of, 301*db*
  ordinariness of, 299
  prevalence of, 297–298
  psychosocial support services (PSS), 302–303
  social role valuation, 294
  social support for, 298*db*
  visibility/invisibility of, 295–296
disability counseling practices
  legal/professional issues, 303–304
  memory healing, 301–302
  narrative theory, 302
  post-modern psychoeducational approaches, 301
  ritual theory, 302
disability counseling research/research needs
  community-based rehabilitation (CBR) services, 300–301, 306
  counseling outcomes, 305–306
  counseling utilization, 305*rb*
  cultural perceptions, 299–300
  multicultural models, 305
  prevalence figure inaccuracy, 304
  social acceptance, 300*rb*
disasters, mental health responses, 60–61
discrimination. *See* perceived discrimination
dissociation, 231. *See also* trauma; trauma counseling
diverse settings, counseling strategies in, 33
diversity counseling
  Afrocentric worldview in, 204–205
  aims of, 194–195
  culture specific treatment, 197–198
  demographic shifts and, 201–203
  evidence-based practices (EBPs), 195–196, 197
  family therapy, 199
  gender sensitivity, 200
  identity counseling, 198–199
  interdisciplinary nature of, 204
  mental health services, 199
  minister's intervention, 200*db*
  multicultural competencies, 196*db*
  multicultural context of, 194–195, 205
  non-verbal language, 200–201
  professional issues, 203–204
  psychological interventions, 198*t*

relationship factors, 201
research, issues for, 201–203, 205
spirituality/religiosity, 200
terminology of, 194
divination
art of, 7*db*
in diagnosis, 5–7
forms of, 83
divinity, role of, 160–161. *See also* pastoral care
Doherty, W. J., 146
donor agencies, 59–60
dop-system (tot system), 101–102
"double consciousness," 99
Draguns, J. G., 42, 46
Draman, R., 213
dramatic flair, use of, 9
DRC (Democratic Republic of the Congo), 215*db*
dream interpretation, 10–11
drugs. *See* substance use disorders
DSM-IV
PTSD diagnostic classifications, 231
substance use disorders, 267
Dubois, W. E. B., 99
Duncan, N., 81–82
Durham, D., 77

Eastern and Southern African Regional Initiative on Traditional Medicine and AIDS, 7–8
Ebersöhn, L., 76
EBPs (evidence-based practices), 195–196, 197
educational counseling, 112. *See also* school counseling
educational psychologist, training adequacy, 120*t*
education programs, for counselors, 52*db*
Edwards, D. J. A., 239–240, 242
Edwards, S. D., 282–283
efficacy, evidence of, 67
Egan, G., 158
Elbert, T., 63–64
emergent self (*umuntu*), 283–284
emic perspective, 67–68, 79, 195*db*
emotional intelligence, 112–113. *See also* school counseling
emotional stability, 233
empowerment, 315. *See also* Jamestown Community Project (JCP)
enactment, use of, 9–10
engagement/meaningfulness, 233. *See also* trauma counseling
environmental control, 201
epistemological changes, in counseling, 28–29
epistemological pluralism, 29*db*
epistemology, meaning of, 156–157
Epston, David, 148
Erasmus, Elrika, 149*rb*
Erikson, E. H., 188
Eth, S., 186
ethical considerations, 53, 68–69, 124
ethical practices
among traditional healers, 16
characteristics of, 53*ib*
in family therapy, 150
ethnic conflicts, 209–210, 216*db*. *See also* conflict/conflicts
ethnic differences
in counseling utilization, 305*rb*
in substance use disorders, 270
ethnic identity, in African-Americans, 105*rb*
ethnocultural counseling model, 63*rb*
ethnographic research, 68*cs*
ethnopsychology, establishment of, 29
etic perspective, 67–68, 79, 195*db*
Eurocentric concepts, of self, 76
European fairytales, 26
Everly, G. S., 239
evidence-based practices (EBPs), 195–196, 197
evil spirits, 87*db*
existential healing, 159*t*
exorcism, 162
expectation, use of, 9
experiential approach, 147. *See also* family therapy
extended family
career choice influence, 285
idea of, 181
as source of support, 182*db*
external control (EC), 201
externalizing, notion of, 162–163
externalizing behaviors, 183. *See also* other vulnerable children (OVC)

fables, 27. *See also* folktales
Fairbank, J. A., 233–234
fairytales (European), 26–27, 144–145
faith healers, 58–59
family, idea of, 77, 144–145, 181
family pathology. *See* Black family pathology, myth of
Family Process (research journal), 143
family structures, 96
family support, 131
family therapy
in African context, 142–143
approaches to, 146–147
bias, sources of, 146*db*
cultural factors, 145–146
cultural sensitivity in, 151*rb*
definitions of family, 144–145
in diversity counseling, 199
ethical issues, 150
family functions, 144
gender roles, 146
history of, 143
modalities of, 147–148
multigenerational family dynamics, 148*cs*
narrative approaches, 148
poverty/economic marginalization, 146
practices, comparisons of, 150–151
professional issues, 149–150
research issues, 143, 151
role of, 142, 152
scope of need, 143–144
social constructionist approaches, 148
in substance use disorders, 273–274
Fanon, F., 99, 100, 101
Farber, E. W., 302
Farm Orphan Support Trust (FOST), 185–186
Farooqi, Y. N., 150–151
Fasser, R., 150
feminism, 146. *See also* gender roles
fetal alcohol syndrome, 101–102
financial assistance, 135–136
Finkenflügel, H., 306
Firelight Foundation, 184, 185
first-order cybernetic position, 146–147
Fisher, R., 210, 212–213
flashbacks, 230. *See also* trauma; trauma counseling
Fleming, A., 195
Flisher, A. J., 126–127
Florsheim, P., 44
folklore, 27
folklorist, role of, 23

folk-oriented research, 69
folktales
  classification of, 27–28
  fables, 27
  folklore, 27
  interventive use of, 33
  legends, 27
  Litokotoko, 33, 34–36
  The Meat of Tongues, 35
  myths, 27
  perspectives on, 25–26
  problems addressed by, 28
  rationale for studying, 24–25
  Two Brothers, 25*db*
  Two-Headed Snake (folk tale), 69*db*
Fonchingong, C. C., 65
FOST (Farm Orphan Support Trust), 185–186
Foster, D., 98–99
Foster, G., 181
Fouche, P., 28, 81, 88
Foulks, E. F., 145
Foxcroft, C. D., 47
Framework for the Protection, Care, and Support of Orphans and Vulnerable Children Living in a World with HIV and AIDS, 182, 184, 258
Frank, M. E., 160–161
Freeman, M., 196
Frykholm, B., 275
fumigation, 12
functionalist school, 211
funding bodies, 59–60

Gacaca Tribunals, 219
GAD (Global Alcohol Database), 269–270
Gaidzanwa, R. B., 127, 135–136
Gale, J., 146
Galton, Francis, 41
Galtung, F., 210
Gardner, F., 183, 186
garments, use of, 9
"Gate of Return," 97*db*
Gauri, V., 256
Geballe, S., 258
Gehman, R. J., 160–161
gender, trauma and, 234, 236
gender accessibility, use of, 9
gender roles
  in family therapy, 146
  in pastoral care, 163
  tertiary students and, 130–131
gender sensitivity, 200
General Systems Theory, 146. *See also* Teddy Bear Therapy (TBT)
genocide, 216*db*
genograms, 199
Germann, S., 188
Ghai, Y., 214
Ghana, 48
Ghana Psychological Association (GPA), 53
Gielen, U. P., 144
Gist, R., 232
Gladding, S. T., 150
Global Alcohol Database (GAD), 269–270
Global Initiative for Traditional Systems of Health, 7–8
God, disregard for, 22
God-images, 158, 160–161. *See also* pastoral care
Goldenberg, H., 150*db*
Goldenberg, I., 150*db*
Goldgeier, J., 222–223
Goldman, E., 255
Goolishian, Harry, 148
Gordon, E. W., 197*db*
Gould, W., 84
government policies, for OVCs, 185
GPA (Ghana Psychological Association), 53
grandparents, as caregivers, 144–145. *See also* family therapy
Grantham-McGregor, S., 183
Great Snake legend, 22, 26. *See also* folktales
grief, collective, 101
group activities, in treatment efforts, 9
group work, 31–32, 36*rb*
Gruendel, J., 258
guidance, 113, 121*db*. *See also* school counseling
guilt experiences, 161*db*

Hagg, G., 218
Hagmann, T., 218
Haines, D. W., 173
Haley, Jay, 142, 147
hardiness, 233–234. *See also* trauma counseling
Harley, D. A., 200, 204
Harriet Shezi Clinic, 185
Harris, T., 146
Hayes, N., 76, 88
health, notions of, 161–162
health counseling, 62
hegemonic influences, 314–315
Hellenism, 155
help-seeking preferences, 3
hermeneutics, 155
heroin, 267, 274*rb*. *See also* substance use disorders
heterosexual orientation, 131
Hickson, J., 29, 32
higher education, institutions of. *See* tertiary institutions, counseling in
Hiltner, S., 159
Hirschowitz, R., 236–237
historical legacies, implications of, 95–97
HIV/AIDS
  bio-physiological aspects of, 250
  children and, 251
  coping with, 252
  counseling psychology and, 81
  deaths from, 249
  global impact, 249
  herbal remedy research, 7–8, 12–13
  infection rates, 93
  infection/symptom description, 250
  intravenous drug use (IDU), 266
  people living with/affected by, 249, 250
  psychosocial impacts of, 260
  socio-economic vulnerability, 249
  transmission of, 251*ib*
  vulnerabilities, experience of, 250
HIV/AIDS counseling
  community interventions/support, 252, 258, 259
  culture, influence of, 259
  global/regional responses, 257–258
  history of research/practice in, 252–253
  lay counselors, 252
  memory box counseling technique, 186
  need for, 250
  of orphans and OVCs, 258–259
  pandemic responses, 61–62
  pastoral care case study, 157*cs*
  photovoice technique, 80*rb*
  play, as therapeutic tool, 149*rb*

RAMs for, 66*rb*
research, issues for, 259–260
at tertiary educations institutions, 133–134
HIV/AIDS counseling research
family system impact, 255
gender issues, 254
health communication, 255
male circumcision, 254–255
migration, influence of, 253
orphan children, 255
policy/political dimensions, 256
prevention programming, 255
risk behaviors, 253
serodiscordant couples, 254*cs*
transactional sex, influence of, 253–254
voluntary counseling and testing (VCT), 255–257
youth, sexual decision making of, 254–255
Holdstock, T. L.
cultural beliefs, 76, 77
indigenization of psychology, 85
psyche, role of the, 76
universalism vs. particularism, 77–79
Holford, L., 237*db*
holistic treatment, emphasis on, 8–9
Holland's Hexagon Model, 286*rb*
Hollis, A. R., 24
Holmes, K., 67
home visits, 14
homosexual orientation, 131, 175*cs*
Hook, D., 99, 100
hot lines, for crisis intervention, 64
Howitt, D., 76, 94, 97
Huber, C. H., 150
Huber, U., 84
human person, African concept of, 163
Human Sciences Research Council Guidance Working Committee, 114
Hutus, 216*db*
Huysamen, G. K., 41
Hwang, K., 42
Hyder, A. A., 256
hyper-arousal symptoms, 231. *See also* trauma
hypothetico-deductive model, 41

IANSA (International Action Network on Small Arms), 209
ICC (International Criminal Court), 222
ICF (International Classification of Functioning, Disability and Health), 295
identity counseling, 198–199. *See also* diversity counseling
identity politics, 214–215. *See also* conflict/conflicts
IDU (intravenous drug use), 266–267. *See also* substance use disorders
iintsomi, 27
illness, conceptualizations/classifications of, 45–46, 161–162
imideni, 181
imilando, 27
immanency, role of, 161. *See also* pastoral care
imperialism. *See* psychological imperialism
incarceration. *See* conceptual incarceration
indigenizing psychology, 85, 88
indigenous counseling practices
alternative/complementary approaches, 83
examination of, 82–83
indigenous health care
counseling-related research, 58–59
definition of, 3, 15
help-seeking preferences, 3
intervention strategies, 3–4
legal/professional issues, 15–16
local culture, 3
national/international influences, 7–8
research, issues for, 16
scope of practice, 4
in substance use disorders, 271–272
value of, 3, 16
indigenous health care, current practices
cleansing measures, 12
dream interpretation, 10–11
etiology of health conditions, 8
expectation, use of, 9
group activities, 9
healer-patient dynamics, 13
HIV/AIDS treatment, 12–13
holistic emphasis, 8–9
naming process, 10
patient adherence, 13–14
physical activity, 9
sacrificial rites, 12
scarification, 12
symbolism/enactment, 9–10
treatments, 9, 16
indigenous health care, research in
divination process, 5–7
HIV/AIDS management, 7–8
orally transmitted knowledge, 4
psychosis management, 6*db*
reasons for consultation, 4–5
wellbeing/disease concepts, 5
indigenous knowledge, 58
indirective counseling, 163
injection drug use, 266*t*. *See also* substance use disorders
in-patient treatment centers, 15
integrationist approach, 42
intelligence, construction of, 96–97
interest inventories, 288*db*. *See also* career counseling
internal control (IC), 201
internalized racism, 99. *See also* racism
internalizing behaviors, 182–183. *See also* other vulnerable children (OVC)
International Action Network on Small Arms (IANSA), 209
International Child Rights Declaration, 64
International Classification of Functioning, Disability and Health (ICF), 295
International Criminal Court (ICC), 222
international students, 129–130. *See also* tertiary institutions, counseling in
International Test Commission (ITC), 53
interpretation of dreams, 10–11
interviews, conducting, 68*cs*
intoxication, 267–268. *See also* substance use disorders
intrastate conflict, 209–210. *See also* conflict/conflicts
intravenous drug use (IDU), 266–267. *See also* substance use disorders
Ipser, J., 88
Islamic traditional healers, 150–151
ITC (International Test Commission), 53
item bias, 45*ib*

Jackson, D. D., 147
Jackson, K.A., 158
Jackson, R., 217
Jamestown Community Project (JCP)
genesis of, 102
implementation of, 102–103
as prevention approach, 103
response to, 103–104

Jayasuriya, D. C., 7, 15
Jayasuriya, S., 7, 15
Jelsma, J., 64
job-finding skills, 136–137. *See also* career counseling
Jobson, L., 238*rb*
Joint Learning Initiative on Children and HIV/AIDS, 182
Jones, James, 101
Juhnke, G. A., 43
Jung, C. G., 23, 33–34
justice, restorative, 218

Kagwanja, P., 218
Kaldor, Mary, 214
Kamanzi, D., 62–63
Kampmeyer, K. L., 146
Kanabus, A., 188
Kardiner, A., 98
Karunakara, U., 63–64
Kasayira, J. M., 133*rb*
Katigbak, M. S., 85
Kawagley, A. O., 59*db*
Keane, T. M., 233–234
Kelly, M. J., 134*db*
Kelman, Herbert, 222
Kenyon, B., 188
KFPE (Commission for Research Partnerships with Developing Countries), 67*db*
Kim, U., 42, 79
King, D. W., 233–234
King, L.A., 233–234
King, R. U., 238*db*
kin network, 77
Kinoti, H. W., 155
Kiriswa, B., 162, 163
Kirkpatrick, J., 44
Kirmayer, L. J., 44, 47
Klaschik, C., 63–64
Knappert, J., 33
Knight, D., 213
Kolb, D. A., 281–282
Korman, M., 53
Kriel, A., 160–161
"kufemba," 14
Kunz, E. G., 169
Kwok Leung K., 79

Lamprecht, J. C., 136
language
  cultural differences, 32–33
  use of, 162
Lartey, E. Y., 80, 81, 156
Lassiter, J. E., 76–77
latent conflict, 210. *See also* conflict/conflicts
law, on refugees, 175–176. *See also* African refugees
laying on of hands, 162
Lee, C. C., 199
Lee, W. M. L, 202–203
legacies, implications of historical, 95–97
legends, 27. *See also* folktales
legislation, implications of, 52–53
Lehobye, K., 64
Leilde, A., 44
Lesolang-Pitje, N., 15
Letamo, G., 259
Lett, J., 79
Levers, L. L.
  client empowerment, 58
  district health systems, 62
  ethnographic research, 68*cs*
  existential counseling, 59
  orphans, teachers' knowledge of, 64
  psychological pluralism, 28–29
  rehabilitation counseling, 64
  trauma counseling, 62–63
  violence, educational effects of, 64
Lewis, S., 188
liberation psychology, 98–99, 100. *See also* Jamestown Community Project (JCP)
Lickel, B., 79
Lieberman, E., 256
Life Line International, 62
lifeskills curriculum, 117. *See also* school counseling
linguistic/cultural diversity, 129
linguistic equivalence, 46
linguistics/sociolinguistics, 200–201
Litokotoko (folktale), 33, 34–36
Littlewood, R, 45
Lobo, E., 95*db*
Logan, S. M. L., 196
Long, M. W., 162
Louw, D. J., 158
Lucas, S., 258
Lumumba, H., 83
Lynch-Brown, C., 27

Maafa, concept of, 100, 101
Maart, S., 64
Maat, concept of, 101
Macleod, C., 76, 88
MacPhail, C. L., 254, 255*db*, 256
Madanes, Cloe, 147
Magweva, I., 62
Makame, V., 183
Makanjuola, R. O. A., 9–10
Maki, D. R., 59, 68*cs*
Makunga, N. V., 282–283
Malawi
  school counseling in, 114
  teacher/counselor training, 116
Malema, N., 64, 65
Mallmann, S., 258
Malott, K. M., 28–29
Mandela, Nelson, 222, 282
manifest conflict, 210. *See also* conflict/conflicts
Mannoni, O., 98
Mapfumo, J., 128*rb*
Maree, K.
  career choices/counseling, 82, 113*db*, 286, 288
  cultural systems, 76, 85
  school counseling/psychologists, 115*cs*, 117
marketing, of traditional medicines, 15–16
marriage therapy, 86*db*
Martin-Baro, I., 98–99
masekitlana, 118*rb*
Mashego, T-A. B., 254
Matsuo, H., 235
"maturing out" hypotheis, 274
Mbeki, Thabo, 217, 222
Mbuagbo, T. O., 65
McCulloch, J., 98
McGoldrick, M., 145
McIntyre, K. P., 235
Mdleleni-Bookholane, T. N., 188
meaningfulness/engagement, 233. *See also* trauma counseling
measurement, types of, 47
The Meat of Tongues, 35. *See also* folktales

memorate, 24, 30. *See also* folktales
memory, autobiographical, 241
memory box technique, 186. *See also* other vulnerable children (OVC), counseling strategies for
memory healing, 301–302. *See also* disability counseling practices
mental disorders, treatment sought for, 4–5
mental health outcomes, 61
mental health services, racism in, 197*db*
Mental Research Institute, 147
metaphors, use of, 162
methamphetamine, 270–271. *See also* substance use disorders
method bias, 45*ib*
Meya, A. F., 249
Mhlope, Gcina, 23
migration, African. *See also* African refugees
  Coercive Theory, 169–170
  historical aspects of, 94–95
  "Push and Pull" Theory, 169
Milan group, 142
Milan systemic approach, 147. *See also* family therapy
Millennium Summit, 182
Miller, R., 255
Miller, W. R., 158
Minuchin, Salvador, 142, 147
Mitchell, C., 213
Mitchell, J. T., 239
Mkhize, N., 75
Mnyaka, M., 282
mobility devices, 297*ce*
modernization, effects of, 81
Moergeli, H., 233
Molepo, M., 76, 286, 288
molestation, child, 174*cs*
Monk, G., 202, 204–205
Montsi, M. M. R., 64
Moret, L. B., 146
Morris, E. K., 79
Morrison, N., 235
Morten, G., 32
Mortland, C. A., 173
Motlhabi, M., 282
Moynihan Report, 95*db*
Moyo, H. J., 128
Mpofu, E., 62, 64, 117
Msimanga-Ramatebele, S. H., 65
Mtetwa, S., 160
Mudenda, Choolwe, 170, 171
Mugabe, Robert, 217
Mukamana, D., 62–63
multicultural competencies, 137*db*, 196*db*
multiculturalism. *See also* diversity counseling
  assessment procedures and, 43, 44
  definition of, 44
  factors in diagnosis, 44
  terminology of, 194
multi-lingualism, use of, 9
Murithi, T., 217, 218
Musingarabwi, S., 133*rb*
Musisi, S., 183, 235
Mutepfa-Mhaka, M., 184
Mutual Story Telling Technique, 186
myths, 27. *See also* folktales
Mzimkulu, K. G., 12

Nagel, B., 235
Naidoo, A. V., 103
naming process
  diagnosis in, 5–7, 10
  healer practices, 11*db*
  as therapeutic technique, 10–11
narrative counseling. *See also* oral traditions
  assessment process in, 48–49
  for careers, 290
  in family therapy, 148
  focus of, 49
  in pastoral care, 157*db*, 163
  power-sharing dialogue, 48–49
  research, issues for, 49*ib*
  in tertiary institutions, 132
  value of, 30–31
  as worldview strategy, 48
narrative exposure therapy (NET), 63–64
narrative questions, 30*cs*
National Council for the Disabled (NCD), 303
National Guidance and Counseling Association (NGCA), 53
natural disasters, mental health responses, 60–61
nature, forces of, 22
NCD (National Council for the Disabled), 303
Ndlovu, S., 135
negative peace, 217–218
Nell, V., 32
Nelson Mandela Children's Trust Fund (NMCF), 184
neo-colonialism, description of, 94
NET (narrative exposure therapy), 63–64
Neuner, F., 63–64
"neurosis of Blackness," 99
New Africa Foundation, 184
"new wars," 214. *See also* conflict/conflicts
New York Protocol (1967), 175–176. *See also* African refugees
NGCA (National Guidance and Counseling Association), 53
Ngcobo, H. S. B., 282–283
Ngoma, Mary, 170, 171
NGOs, influences/priorities of, 59–60
Nkrumah, K., 217
Nobles, Wade, 43, 99
non-verbal language, 200–201
Norcross, J. C., 197
Nsamenang, A. B., 75, 79–80, 85
Nwoye, A., 143, 145, 149, 150
Nyanhongo, S., 133*rb*
Nyblade, L., 256
Nyirongo, L., 163

Oakland, T., 117
OAU (Organization of African Unity), 7
Obama, Barack, 100*db*
Obot, I., 269–270
Oden, T. C., 159
Oedipus, 24*db*
O'Kearney, R. T., 238*rb*
Olley, B. O., 65, 183
Operario, D., 183
optimism, 233. *See also* trauma counseling
oral traditions. *See also* folktales
  "acts of God" and, 22
  background on, 23–24
  counseling questions and, 23
  as education aid, 24–25
  Great Snake legend, 22, 26
  moral messages, 25
  singing and dancing, 31
  storytelling in, 22, 31
  uses of, 24, 36–37
O'Reilly, K., 253
Organization of African Unity (OAU), 7

Orisa cults, 14
Orkin, M., 236–237
orphans. *See also* other vulnerable children (OVC)
  counseling of, 258–259
  counseling-related research on, 64
  definition of, 181
  HIV/AIDS counseling research on, 255
Osman, A., 219
Ost, L. G., 63
"other," definition of, 97
other vulnerable children (OVC)
  community-based responses, 184
  coping capacity of families, 184
  counseling of, 64, 258–259
  depression/internalizing behaviors, 182–183
  essential services, access to, 184–185
  externalizing behaviors, 183
  gaps in support for, 183–184
  key terms/concepts, 180–182, 189
  legal protections, 185
  legislative contradictions, 185*db*
  raising awareness/support for, 185–186
  research, issues for, 188
  statistics on, 180
  street children, 183*rb*
  UN strategies and goals, 181–182
other vulnerable children (OVC), counseling strategies for
  bereavement counseling, 188*cs*
  developmental approach, 187–188
  memory box technique, 186
  support groups, 187
  Teddy Bear Therapy (TBT), 186–187
  three stage approach, 186
Outcome Framework for 2009–2011, 182
out-patient consultation, 14
OVC. *See* other vulnerable children (OVC)
Ovesy, L., 98
Owusu-Bempah, J., 76, 94, 96, 97
Oxfam International, 209

Pack-Brown,S., 195
Painter, T. M., 256
participator methods, 84
pastoral care
  African traditions, 156–157
  ancestors, role of, 160
  Christian traditions, 156
  community, role of, 160
  counseling strategies/techniques, 162–163
  existential healing, 159*t*
  God-images, role of, 160–161
  health/illness, notions of, 161–162
  history of research/practice in, 158–160
  HIV patient, case study of, 157*cs*
  immanency, role of, 161
  key concepts, 155–156
  psychological perspective in, 157–158
  research, issues for, 163
  stages in, 158–159
  systemic framework of, 163–164
  theological assessment in, 158
patient adherence, 13–14
Patra, J., 269–270
Patterson, Gerald, 147
Patterson, L. E., 58
Paunovi, N., 63
peace, notion of, 162
peace making, 218
pedagogical method, 163
Pederson, P. B., 137
Pells, K., 62–63
Peltzer, K., 14, 68, 254
Pengpid, S., 254
perceived discrimination, 98–99
Perry, J. C., 121*db*
Pershing, L., 24
personal development counseling, 112–113. *See also* school counseling
personal reflections, 144*db*
Pettifor, A., 256
pharmaceuticals, regulation of, 15–16
photovoice research technique, 80*rb*
physical activity, in treatment efforts, 9
Pike, K. L., 79
play, as therapeutic tool, 118*rb*, 149*rb*. *See also* school counseling
poets, role of, 23
political conflicts, 171. *See also* African refugees; conflict/conflicts
political leadership, 217
Porter, R. E., 173–174
positionalities, 200, 205
positive peace, 218
positivism, 88
possession, divination in, 5–7
possession cults, 14
postcolonial period
  higher education in, 127–128
  school counseling in, 114
postmodern counselors, 147
post-traumatic stress disorder (PTSD)
  assessment and treatment, 239–241
  CATT, 242
  counseling for, 62–64
  in dependent/interdependent cultures, 238*rb*
  diagnosis in, 231
  individual responses to, 233*cs*
  lasting effects of trauma, 231–232
  play, as therapeutic tool, 118*rb*
  rape and, 235*cs*
  symptom identification, 230
  Western psychiatry and, 232*db*
post-traumatic stress management (PTSM), 239
Potgieter, E., 64
poverty, 82, 146
predatory state, 217. *See also* conflict/conflicts
presidents-for-life phenomenon, 217. *See also* conflict/conflicts
Prince, R., 83
prison population statistics, 93
"protectors," 28
PSS (psychosocial support services), 302–303. *See also* disability counseling practices
psychoactive substances. *See* substance use
psychodynamic approach, 147. *See also* family therapy
psychodynamic psychotherapy, 272
psychoeducation, 239, 240*cs*
psycho-educational practices, 65–66. *See also* counseling-related research
psychological approach, to conflict, 210–211. *See also* conflict/conflicts
psychological decolonization, 100–101
psychological dependence, 268. *See also* substance use disorders
psychological imperialism, 98
psychological interventions, with diverse groups, 198*t*
psychologists, multicultural competence of, 137*db*
psychology. *See* counseling psychology

Psychology of Colonization (Mannoni), 98
psychosis management, 5
psychosocial support services (PSS), 302–303. *See also* disability counseling practices
psychosomatic illness/disorders, 4–5
psychotherapy, play in, 149*rb*
PTSD (post-traumatic stress disorder)
  assessment and treatment, 239–241
  CATT, 242
  counseling for, 62–64
  in dependent/interdependent cultures, 238*rb*
  diagnosis in, 231
  individual responses to, 233*cs*
  lasting effects of trauma, 231–232
  play, as therapeutic tool, 118*rb*
  rape and, 235*cs*
  Western psychiatry and, 232*db*
PTSM (post-traumatic stress management), 239
public health codes, 15
"Push and Pull" theory, 169. *See also* African refugees
Pynoos, R., 186

"Rab" healer group, 14
race, in counseling, 82*db*
race relations, 93
racial/ethnic differences, in counseling, 203*rb*
racial justice perceptions, 46*rb*
racial oppression. *See also* Jamestown Community Project (JCP)
  actions of colonialist, 96–97
  collectivist cultures and, 96–97
  community intervention, 101–102
  decolonization of the mind, 100–101
  family structures and, 96
  historical aspects of, 93–95, 105
  liberation psychology, 98–99
  mental colonization, 99–100
  psychological functioning and, 93–94
  psychological imperialism, 98
  psychological manifestations of, 98–99
  racist thinking, 97
  research considerations, 103–105
  slavery/slave trade and, 96
racism
  counseling, affects on, 193
  counseling psychology and, 81–82
  internalized, 99
  in mental health services delivery, 197*db*
Ramokgopa, I. M., 188
Ramose, M. B., 282
Ramphele, Mamphela, 234
rape, counseling for, 235*cs*, 237*db*
Raphael, B., 61
Rapid Appraisal Methods (RAMs), 66*rb*
Reber, A. S., 265
recognition, need for, 210. *See also* conflict/conflicts
Rees, H., 256
reflexive practice/methodology, 84–85
refugees. *See* African refugees
regalia, use of, 9
rehabilitation counseling, 64–65
Rehm, J., 269–270
Reilly, G., 214
relapse, 268. *See also* substance use disorders
religion/religiosity, 130, 200, 220*rb*
remittances, 96
Remley, T. P., 150
research, facilitation of, 68*cs*
research, issues for. *See also* counseling-related research
  on African refugees, 176, 177
  assessor competency, 51–52
  in conflict resolution, 222
  counselor training, 137–138
  in disability counseling, 304–306
  in diversity counseling, 201–203, 205
  emic vs. etic perspectives, 67–68
  ethical considerations, 53, 68–69
  evidence of efficacy, 67
  in family therapy, 151
  folk-oriented research, 69
  in HIV/AIDs counseling, 259–260
  indigenizing psychology, 85, 88
  indigenous approaches, 16, 85–86
  interdisciplinary approaches, 67–68
  legislative implications, 52–53
  marriage therapy, 86*db*
  in narrative counseling, 49*ib*
  for OVCs, 188
  racial oppression, 103–105
  reflexive practice/methodology, 84–85
  resource scarcity, 138
  in school counseling, 119–122
  in substance use disorder counseling, 276–277
  in trauma counseling, 243–244
research, participatory approaches, 80*rb*
research partnership, principles for, 67*db*
resettlement problems, 174–175. *See also* African refugees
resilient individuals, 232–233
resource needs, 131
RESPECTFUL model, 47
restorative justice, 218
Reviere, R., 59
Rider, E. A., 131
ritual enactment, use of, 9–10
ritual theory, 302. *See also* disability counseling practices
Roberts, H., 85–86
Robertson, B. A., 271
Robins, L., 275
Roerecke, M., 269–270
Rogerian technique, 157*db*
Rollock, D., 197*db*
Roopnarine, J. L., 144
Roos, V., 64
Roscoe, A. A., 69*db*
Roth, W. T., 63
Rotter, J., 201
Ruane, I., 130, 137
Rudnick, H., 15
Rwanda, 303–304
Rwandan conflict/genocide, 216*db*, 219, 238*db*, 242

SAAMFT (South African Institute of Family Therapy), 143
sacrificial rites, 12, 14–15
Saferworld, 209
Sammons, P., 295
Samovar, L. A., 173–174
Sanchez, G., 27
sangomas/shamans, 83
SAP (World Bank/IMF Structural Adjustment program), 171
Satir, Virginia, 147
Savickas, M. L., 23, 30*cs*
Sayson, R., 249
scarification, 12
Schauer, E., 63–64
Scheub, H., 27
Schipani, D. S., 157
Schnyder, U., 233

Schoffeleers, J. M., 69*db*
Schonegevel, C., 286
school counseling. *See also* tertiary institutions, counseling in
  allied services, 117
  career choices, 113*db*
  child abuse intervention, 124*cs*
  educational, 112
  guidance, 113
  history of, 113–115
  organizational structure/service provision, 116
  personal development, 112–113
  play, as therapeutic tool, 118
  professional/ethical issues, 118
  psychologists, training adequacy of, 120*t*
  purposes of, 111–112, 122
  research, issues for, 119–122
  school psychologists, 117
  services offered, 117
  social development, 112
  teacher qualifications, 116–117
  violence prevention, 119*rb*
  vocational, 112
Scientific and Technical Research Commission (STRC), 7
second-order cybernetic position, 147
Seidel, J., 84
self, conceptualization of, 76
self, emergent view of (*umuntu*), 283–284
self-knowledge, 44–45
self-perceptions/self-worth, 112
senile dementia, 8*db*
sense of coherence (SOC), 233–234. *See also* trauma counseling
seriti, 160
Setiloane, G. M., 160–161
sexual orientation, 131
sex work, HIV/AIDS and, 254*cs*
shamans/sangomas, 83
shame culture, 161*db*
Shmukler, D., 32
Sigelman, C. K., 131
Silverman, P. R., 188
Simbayi, L. C., 253
singing, 31
Sinha, D., 85
Skhakhane, Jerome, 160
Skinner, D., 181
Skinner, J., 60
slavery/slave trade, 94–95, 96, 97*db*
Slutkin, G., 253
Smart, R., 181
Smith, C., 237*db*
Smith, L. T., 67, 87
Smith, T. B., 199
Snyman, S., 150
SOC (sense of coherence), 233–234. *See also* trauma counseling
social constructionist approaches, 148. *See also* family therapy
social development counseling, 112. *See also* school counseling
social justice, 289–290
social organization, 201
social-psychological approaches, to conflict, 219–220, 221
social support, 232–233. *See also* trauma counseling
Société Générale de Belgique, 94
Society for Student Counseling in Southern Africa (SSCSA), 137
socio-emotional skills, use of, 9
sociological approaches, to conflict, 211. *See also* conflict/conflicts
Sodi, T., 133*rb*
Somerai, P., 130–131, 135
Sonn, C. C., 85
soul, 155. *See also* pastoral care
South Africa
  disability policies in, 303
  drug scene in, 270*db*
  multiculturalism in, 44
  oral tradition in counseling, 37
  psychological assessment tools in, 41
South African Institute of Family Therapy (SAAMFT), 143
Sow, I., 78*db*
spatial needs, 201
Speight, S. L., 105
Sphinx, riddle of the, 24*db*
spirit meditation cults, 14–15
spirit mediumship, 83
spirit possession, 5–7, 87*db*, 162
spirits, role in health conditions, 8
spirituality, 130, 155, 200. *See also* pastoral care
SSCSA (Society for Student Counseling in Southern Africa), 137
SSI (Strong Interest Inventory), 288*db*. *See also* career counseling
Standards for Multicultural Assessment (AAC), 52
Stead, G. B., 81, 285–286, 288
Stellenbosch, community intervention, 101–102
Stephney, I., 186
Stevens, G., 81–82
stigma. *See* AIDS stigma reduction
storytellers/storytelling
  importance of, 31
  in pastoral care, 163
  in psychotherapeutic group work, 36*rb*
  role of, 23
Straker, G., 28–29, 182–183
STRC (Scientific and Technical Research Commission), 7
street children, 183*rb*. *See also* other vulnerable children (OVC)
Strong Interest Inventory (SSI), 288*db*. *See also* career counseling
structural approach, 147. *See also* family therapy
student clubs/associations, 135
Subbarao, K., 181
substance abuse, 132–133
substance use
  ethnic differences in, 270
  history of, 265, 268
  in modern period, 269–271
  in pre-colonial period, 268–269
  for recreational purposes, 265
substance use disorder counseling
  access to treatment, 275–276
  collaborative efforts, 271–272
  contextual factors, 275
  family therapy, 273–274
  heroin dependence recovery, 274*rb*
  "maturing out" approaches, 274
  multidisciplinary approach, need for, 277
  phases of recovery, 275
  professional skills development, 276
  psychodynamic psychotherapy, 272
  regulation of, 275
  research, issues for, 276–277
  residential treatment, 273*cs*
  transpersonal psychology, 272
substance use disorders
  co-morbid mental health disorders, 268, 269*cs*
  as defined in DSM-IV-TR, 267
  dependence, features of, 267
  as disease, 267*db*
  intravenous drug use (IDU), 266–267
  psychological dependence, 268

relapse, 268
social-cultural influences, 266
social impact, 266
substance intoxication, 267–268
substance withdrawal, 268
Sue, D., 202
Sue, D. W., 32, 195–196, 201, 202
suffering/adversity, 22
Summerfield, D., 232*db*
support groups, for OVCs, 187
survivors of violence, counseling models for, 63*rb*
Svensson, Isak, 220*rb*
symbols/symbolism, use of, 9–10, 162
symptoms, meaning of, 45
systems approach, to counseling, 131

Tanzania, disability policies in, 303
TAT (Thematic Apperception Test), 50
Taylor, C. W., 158
TBT (Teddy Bear Therapy), 186–187
TCB (Themes Concerning Blacks Test), 50
teachers/guidance counselors, 116–117. *See also* school counseling
Teddy Bear Therapy (TBT), 186–187
Tempels, P., 160–161
Terrell, F., 194
tertiary institutions, counseling in. *See also* university students, issues faced by
academic pressure, 131
career choice, 136
case studies, 130–136
counseling settings, 132
counselor training, 137–138
developmental approach, 131
family support, 131
financial assistance, 135–136
gender roles, 130–131
vs. high-school counseling, 128*rb*
history of, 127–128
international students, 129–130
job-finding skills, 136–137
key concepts, 127
linguistic/cultural diversity, 129
narrative approach, 132
religiosity and, 130
resource needs, 131
student clubs/associations, 135
student diversity, 126–127, 138
systems approach, 131
test design/development, 46*rb*, 47
Tetlock, P.E., 222–223
THA (Traditional Healers Act), 304
Theis, M., 58
Thematic Apperception Test (TAT), 50
Themes Concerning Blacks Test (TCB), 50
theology/theological assessment, 155, 158. *See also* pastoral care
third-world debt, 94
Thlabiwe, P., 64
thokolosi, 66
"tik." *See* methamphetamine
time orientation, 201
Tomlinson, C., 27
tot system (dop-system), 101–102
touch, 162
Traditional and Modern Health Practitioners Together Against AIDS (Uganda), 7–8
traditional healers
counseling-related research, 58–59
Islamic views, 150–151
pastoral care and, 156
Traditional Healers Act (THA), 304
Traditional Healing paradigm, 47–48
training, of traditional health workers, 15
transpersonal psychology, 272
trauma
age and, 234–235
avoidance symptoms, 230–231
childhood experiences, 234, 236
children refugees and, 173*cs*
diagnostic classifications, 231
gender and, 234, 236
hyper-arousal symptoms, 231
lasting effects of, 231–232
prolonged exposure to, 234, 236
re-experiencing symptoms, 230
responses to, 229–230, 233*cs*, 234, 244
traumatizing events, 229
trauma counseling
assessment and treatment, 239–241
autobiographical memory, 241
emotional stability, 233
engagement/meaningfulness, 233
immediate support, 239
individualized treatment, 241–242
integrative model for, 242
intervention models, 238–239
PTSD, 230
resilience/resilient individuals, 232–234
social support, 232–233
symptom identification, 230*cs*
trust development/support systems, 241
trauma counseling, research on
childhood experiences, 236
community impacts, 236–238
cultural context, 235, 238*rb*
"culture of violence," 238
gender issues, 236
issues for, 243–244
prolonged trauma exposure, 236
PTSD, 62–64
tribal lore, 23
tribe, use of term, 97
Trickster, 25
TRIOS cultural orientation, 101
Truth and Reconciliation Commission (TRC), 31, 219
Tuckwell, G., 137*db*
Turner, V., 302
Turton, R. W., 29
Tutsis, 216*db*
Tutu, Desmond, 22, 31, 37
Two Brothers (folktale), 25*db*
Two-Headed Snake (folktale), 69*db*

ubuntu
in African diaspora, 22–23
in career counseling, 283–285, 290
counseling promotion and, 30
cultural concept of, 31, 160, 218, 282–283
umndeni, 181
umona, 162
umuntu, 283–284
UNAIDS reports, 249
UN Convention Relating to the Status of Refugees, 175–176. *See also* African refugees
under-development/poverty, 82
UNESCO, 218

UNHCR (United Nations High Commissioner on Refugees), 170, 174*rb*
United Nations Conventions, on disability policy, 303
United Nations High Commissioner on Refugees (UNHCR), 170, 174*rb*
University of Kwazulu, 15
university students, issues faced by. *See also* tertiary institutions, counseling in
  adjustment to environment, 132
  common issues/needs, 132, 133*rb*
  emotional difficulties, 134
  faculty/academic challenges, 135
  health-related issues, 132
  residence/accommodation, 134–135
  sexual health, 133–134
  substance abuse, 132–133
Usiko Program, 104*cs*

van der Westhuizen, Carol N., 115*cs*
Van Dyk, A. C., 258
Van Dyk, P., 188
Van Wyk, S. B., 103
VCT (voluntary counseling and testing), 61–62, 255–257
verbal communication, 200–201
Vetter, H., 52
village cleansing ceremony, 14
"Vimbuza" healer group, 14
violence
  counseling models for survivors of, 63*rb*
  educational effects of, 64
  prevention in schools, 119*rb*
violent crime, 236–237
vocational counseling, 112. *See also* school counseling
voluntary counseling and testing (VCT), 61–62, 255–257
Von Franz, M-L., 33
Vontress, C. E., 195*db*
Vorster, Carl, 186–187
vulnerability, age and, 234–235. *See also* trauma; trauma counseling
vulnerable child, defined, 181. *See also* other vulnerable children (OVC)

Waldorf, D., 274
Wallace, Barbara, 101, 105
Wampold, B. E., 195, 197
war, impacts on children, 183
Waruti, D. H., 155
Watkins, C. E., 194
Watson, M. B.
  career counseling/research, 285–286, 288
  contextual sensitivity, 286
  counseling theories, 28
  HIV/AIDS counseling, 81
  indigenizing theory, 88
  modernization, effects of, 81
Watts, R., 100, 105
Watzlawick, P., 147
Webb, N. B., 188
Welfel, E. R., 58
wellbeing, 162, 233
Western approaches
  assessment methods, 48, 53
  combining indigenous practice with, 85–86
  psychological imperialism in, 98
  self concept and, 76
  transportability of, 59
Western knowledge systems, 59*db*
Whaley, A. L., 193
wheelchairs, 297*ce*
Whitaker, Carl, 147
White, J., 44
White, Joseph, 42–43
White, Michael, 49, 148
Williams, Robert, 50
Windling, T., 28
Winick, C., 274
wisdom counseling, 156–157
witchcraft, 17–16
witch doctors, 83
witch-hunting ceremony, 14
withdrawal, 268. *See also* substance use disorders
Wolf, D. M., 281–282
Wolfensberger, W., 294
women. *See* gender roles
Wood, B., 166
Woodall, S. J., 232
word usage, 201
World Bank/IMF Structural Adjustment program (SAP), 171
World Conference on Racism, Racial Discrimination, Xenophobia, and Related Intolerance, 82
World Fit for Children Declaration, 182
World Health Organization (WHO)
  disability prevalence estimates, 297–298
  Global Alcohol Database (GAD), 269–270
  traditional healing definition, 3
  training seminars/workshops, 15
world view
  consideration of, 32
  as key concept, 57
Wretched of the Earth (Fanon), 100

Xhosa tradition
  cleansing treatment, 12
  psychosis management, 6db
  umona, 162

Yang, K., 42
Young, M. J., 24
"youth," conceptions of, 77

Zambia
  disability policies in, 304
  teacher/counselor training, 116
Zane, N., 195–196
zar healing, 14, 83
Zartman, I., 217–218
Zhang, N., 203
Ziemba, S. J., 146
Zimbabwe
  disability legislation in, 304
  school counseling in, 114
Zimbabwe Institute of Systems Therapy, 143
Zimbabwe National Traditional Health Practitioner Association, 7–8
Zulu traditions
  family, idea of, 181
  Great Snake legend, 22
  healers in, 83

For EU product safety concerns, contact us at Calle de José Abascal, 56–1°, 28003 Madrid, Spain or eugpsr@cambridge.org.

www.ingramcontent.com/pod-product-compliance
Lightning Source LLC
LaVergne TN
LVHW080058220926
848484LV00007BA/1856